Thieme

Diagnostic Imaging of the Foot and Ankle

Ulrike Szeimies, MD
Head of Department
München-Harlaching Imaging Center
Munich, Germany

Axel Staebler, MD
Professor of Radiology
München-Harlaching Imaging Center
Munich, Germany

Markus Walther, MD
Professor of Orthopedic Surgery
Medical Director
Head of the Department of Foot and Ankle Surgery
Schön Klinik München-Harlaching
FIFA Medical Center Munich
Munich, Germany

532 illustrations

Thieme
Stuttgart • New York • Delhi • Rio

Library of Congress Cataloging-in-Publication Data
Szeimies, Ulrike, author.
[Bildgebende Diagnostik des Fusses. English]
Diagnostic imaging of the foot and ankle / Ulrike Szeimies, Axel Staebler, Markus Walther.
Translation of: Bildgebende Diagnostik des Fusses / Ulrike Szeimies, Axel Staebler, Markus Walther. Stuttgart: Thieme, 2012.
Includes bibliographical references and index.
ISBN 978-3-13-176461-4 (alk. paper) – ISBN 978-3-13-176471-3 (e-ISBN)
I. Staebler, Axel, author. II. Walther, Markus, 1967-, author. III. Title.
[DNLM: 1. Foot Diseases–diagnosis. 2. Magnetic Resonance Imaging–methods. 3. Tomography, Spiral Computed–methods. WE 880]
RD563
617.5'8507543–dc23
2014023829

This book is an authorized translation of the German edition published and copyrighted 2012 by Georg Thieme Verlag, Stuttgart. Title of the German edition: Bildgebende Diagnostik des Fußes

Translator: Terry C. Telger, Fort Worth, TX, USA

Illustrator: Roland Geyer, Weilerswist, Germany

Thieme Publishers Stuttgart
Rüdigerstrasse 14, 70469 Stuttgart, Germany
+49 [0]711 8931 421, customerservice@thieme.de

Thieme Publishers New York
333 Seventh Avenue, New York, NY 10001 USA
+1 800 782 3488, customerservice@thieme.com

Thieme Publishers Delhi
A-12, Second Floor, Sector-2, Noida-201301
Uttar Pradesh, India
+91 120 45 566 00, customerservice@thieme.in

Thieme Publishers Rio, Thieme Publicações Ltda.
Argentina Building 16th floor, Ala A, 228 Praia do Botafogo
Rio de Janeiro 22250-040 Brazil
+55 21 3736-3631

Cover design: Ulrike Szeimies, MD & Thieme Publishing Group
Typesetting by DiTech Process Solutions Pvt. Ltd., India

Printed in India by Replika Press Pvt. Ltd.

ISBN 9783131764614

Also available as e-book:
eISBN 9783131764713

To my beloved daughter Emilia
Ulrike Szeimies

To my beloved wife Susann
Axel Staebler

To all those dedicated to treating patients with foot and ankle disorders
Markus Walther

Contents

Preface

"Help, a difficult foot in MRI!" – Surely this is a common thought, especially if the referring foot surgeon is known for requesting very specific information. In creating this book, the editors (two radiologists and one foot surgeon) agreed that only clinical–radiologic correlation combined with expertise in the treatment of foot disorders could lead to an improved interpretation of pathologic findings. As in many areas of medicine, in radiology we are experiencing a trend toward subspecialization, as we move from method-centered to organ-centered diagnosis. The exchange of specialized knowledge with a clinical colleague is crucial in understanding such a biomechanically complex joint system as the foot. This book is intended to provide a concise, practical, fully illustrated guide to image interpretation from a clinical perspective, and always with reference to therapeutic options. Recommendations on protocols and diagnostic routines are based mainly on considerations of patient care, giving due attention to theoretical background while keeping an eye on the economic pressures that bear on a radiology practice.

The editors and authors hope that this guide to foot imaging will be of significant practical help in the everyday practice of image interpretation and will awaken in some readers a passion for the diagnosis of foot disorders.

Ulrike Szeimies, MD
Axel Staebler, MD
Markus Walther, MD

Contributors

Ruediger Degwert, MD
Department of Individual Back Therapy
Ambulatory Sports Trauma Center
Munich, Germany

Hartmut Gaulrapp, MD
Specialty Practice for Orthopedics and Pediatric Orthopedics
Munich, Germany

Sigurd Kessler, MD
Professor of Surgery
Center for Foot and Ankle Surgery
Schön-Klinik Hospital at München-Harlaching
Munich, Germany

Anke Roeser, MD
Center for Foot and Ankle Surgery
Schön-Klinik Hospital at München-Harlaching
Munich, Germany

Axel Staebler, MD
Professor of Radiology
München-Harlaching Imaging Center
Munich, Germany

Ulrike Szeimies, MD
Head of Department
München-Harlaching Imaging Center
Munich, Germany

Markus Walther, MD
Professor of Orthopedic Surgery
Medical Director
Head of the Department of Foot and Ankle Surgery
Schön Klinik München-Harlaching
FIFA Medical Center Munich
Munich, Germany

Abbreviations

ACR	American College of Rheumatology
AO	Arbeitsgemeinschaft für Osteosynthese
AOFAS	American Orthopedic Foot and Ankle Society
AP	Anteroposterior
ASIF	Association for the Study of Internal Fixation
AVN	Avascular necrosis
CRPS	complex regional pain syndrome
CT	computed tomography
3D	three dimensional
DMARD	disease-modifying antirheumatic drug
DNOAP	diabetic neuropathic osteoarthropathy
DP	dorsoplantar
fat-sat	fat saturated
HLA	human leukocyte antigen
ICI	Integral Classification of Injuries
IV	intravenous
MPR	multiplanar reformatting
MRI	magnetic resonance imaging
NOAP	neuropathic osteoarthropathy
NSAID	nonsteroidal anti-inflammatory drug
OTA	Orthopaedic Trauma Association
PA	posteroanterior
PD	proton density
PVNS	pigmented villonodular synovitis
STIR	short-tau inversion recovery
TNF	tumor necrosis factor
VR	volume rendering
WHO	World Health Organization

Chapter 1

Imaging Techniques

1 Imaging Techniques

1.1 Magnetic Resonance Imaging (MRI)

U. Szeimies

1.1.1 Imaging Strategy

MRI of the Foot: General Aspects

MRI System

It is still basically true that higher field intensity in MRI means higher resolution, and thus better image quality. The advantages of a 3-tesla (3-T) system are obvious, and its ability to depict fine details still has the power to fascinate the observer. The direct visualization of neural structures, tiny fascicles in the ligaments, and especially the hyaline articular cartilage, provides a high confidence level in the detection of pathology. On the other hand, a 3-T system is more susceptible to artifacts than a 1.5-T system in patients with internal fixation materials, and this may be a significant problem at large foot and ankle centers, for example. It should be added that modern 1.5-T MRI systems with multi-channel coil technology can achieve a resolution comparable to that of a 3-T system. The 1.5-T field does involve a more time-consuming protocol, however.

Coil, Positioning

A high-resolution multi-channel coil for the detailed evaluation of fine structures in a high-field system (1.5 T or higher) delivers high anatomical precision. Whenever possible, the patient is positioned prone with the foot in plantar flexion and optimally padded within the coil. That position is comfortable for the patient and should cause fewer motion artifacts than imaging in the supine position. It can also prevent artifacts that appear when the tendon is at a 54.7° angle to the B_0 magnetic field ("magic angle" phenomenon), causing increased intratendinous signal intensity that can mimic pathologic changes.

Sequences

Standard MR sequences are available for foot imaging and are especially useful for investigating generalized foot pain and evaluating the bone marrow and soft tissues. Special sequences are also available in which the sequence parameters and slice selection are individually tailored for a specific investigation. See examples under Special Sequences for Specific Investigation (p.2).

The standard MR sequences are as follows:

- Coronal > T1-weighted
- Sagittal and coronal PD (proton-density) weighted fat-sat (with fat saturation)
- > Axial T2-weighted
- Axial and sagittal T1-weighted fat-sat after intravenous (IV) contrast administration

A high-resolution square matrix (384 × 384, 448 × 448, or 512 × 512) is generally recommended for high-resolution imaging of the foot and ankle. Thin imaging sections are also advised, using a maximum slice thickness of 2 to 2.5 mm.

Contrast Medium

Except in acute trauma cases, MR images should be acquired with IV contrast medium, because conditions such as chronic overuse syndromes (affecting joints, tendons, capsuloligamentous structures, or fibro-osseous junctions) can be appreciated only on contrast-enhanced images showing increased uptake in the fibrovascular tissue. Recently, it has been stressed that contrast-enhanced MRI should include an assessment of renal function (creatinine clearance). If current blood work is not available, the clearance value can be quickly determined with a test kit by taking a small blood sample from the finger tip or earlobe.

Special Sequences for Specific Investigations

- *Anterior syndesmosis* (oblique sagittal/axial PD-weighted fat-sat sequence; ▶ Fig. 1.1 a): This oblique sagittal/axial angulation can display the full course of the anterior syndesmosis, which descends obliquely from the distal tibia to the fibula. This sequence will clearly show any fiber discontinuity or hemorrhagic areas in the tibiofibular syndesmosis.
- *Tendon pathology in the hindfoot and midfoot* (axial oblique T1-weighted fat-sat after contrast administration; ▶ Fig. 1.1 b): The tendons in the hindfoot (flexor and extensor tendons, and peroneal tendons) run at a 45° angle to the ankle joint. The axial oblique T1-weighted fat-sat sequence after contrast administration is prescribed at a 90° angle to the course of the tendons to give an optimum cross-sectional view of the tendons and their sheaths. This sequence and orientation will clearly show increased contrast uptake in the tendon sheaths or abnormal enhancement within those tendons that would indicate increased vascularity due to advanced intratendinous degeneration.
- *Morton neuroma* (axial and coronal T1-weighted sequences without contrast administration): These are the most important sequences for the evaluation of Morton neuroma. Due to its high cellularity, this mass appears hypointense within the hyperintense fat on unenhanced T1-weighted images and is often conspicuous by its bulbous or fusiform shape in the interdigital space. Often contrast administration adds little information, because Morton neuromas may show a variable degree of vascularity. The key identifying feature is the interdigital location of the mass (between the second and third or third and fourth metatarsal heads on the plantar side) and its shape (usually bulbous in the axial T1-weighted sequence and fusiform in the coronal sequence, extending into the plantar soft tissue).

In summary, an optimum MRI examination of the foot can be performed easily and routinely. Compromised image quality is often a result of economic constraints. High image quality requires a considerable investment of time, which is not always justifiable on purely economic grounds.

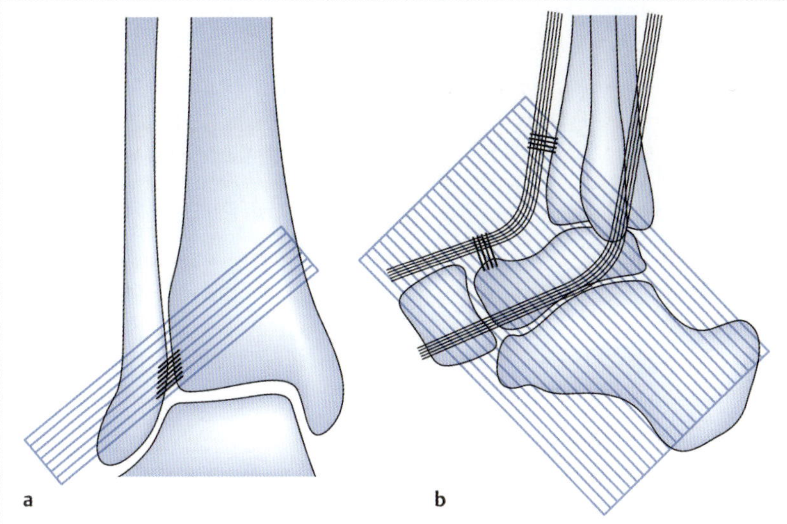

Fig. 1.1 a, b Special sequences for MRI of the foot.
a The anterior syndesmosis is evaluated with an oblique sagittal scan.
b Tendon pathology is evaluated with an oblique axial scan.

1.1.2 Post-Exercise MRI

A common problem in patients with foot pain is the intermittent nature of the complaints in response to weight bearing and exercise. Patients are often advised to rest the affected foot on their initial visit to a foot specialist, and a subsequent MRI examination is usually performed during a stress-free interval. Consequently, most patients are scanned at a time when they are not experiencing symptoms. They give a history of complaints that occur during or after physical exertion or athletic activity. In some cases MRI performed during an asymptomatic interval may fail to detect the pathology (e.g., deeply situated ganglia in the tarsal tunnel that exert a mass effect only during exercise, or instability of the peroneal tendons).

For a post-exercise MRI study, the patient is told to perform the exercise that typically causes the painful symptoms. If necessary the study is preceded by one or more units of running or training exercises that are likely to reproduce the pain. MRI scans are initiated only after the complaints have been elicited, and IV contrast administration should be used.

Post-exercise MRI has not yet been fully evaluated in studies, and its capabilities relative to "standard MRI" have not yet been definitively assessed. Also, studies should be done only by an experienced foot radiologist who will not misinterpret possible epiphenomena such as physiologic joint effusions or venous dilatation. Nevertheless, post-exercise MRI may be a helpful study, especially in athletes, in cases where prior images acquired elsewhere were negative and there is a new indication for MRI.

1.2 Multidetector-Row Spiral Computed Tomography (CT)

U. Szeimies

1.2.1 Positioning

- Comfortable supine position
- Avoid motion artifacts
- Scan only the affected foot in the supine position or with the foot resting on the cassette

1.2.2 Protocol

Isotropic voxels are necessary for optimum multiplanar reformatting (MPR) of the acquired data sets. Sample protocol:

- Slice thickness 0.5 mm
- Reconstruction increment 0.25 mm
- Pitch 0.875
- 120 kV
- 80 to 150 mA (use a reduced dose and strict selection criteria in children)

Images are reconstructed in three standard planes (axial, coronal and sagittal), while areas of special concern are evaluated in selected magnified views.

1.2.3 Indications

- *Initial work-up*:
  - Fractures (to assess axial malalignment in ankle fractures while clearly defining the fragments and looking for step-offs), especially metatarsal fractures
  - Severe sprains with equivocal radiographic features
  - Neuroarthropathy
  - Osteoarthritis (evaluating the extent of degenerative changes)
  - CT as an adjunct to MRI (ganglion cyst, unexplained bone marrow edema, further differentiation of tumors)
  - Coalition
  - As an aid to preoperative planning (e.g., calculation of the tibial torsion angle)
- *Postoperative imaging* (axial alignment, step-off in an articular surface, internal fixation materials)
- *Follow-up:*
  - Bony consolidation of fractures and nonunions
  - Localization and evaluation of internal fixation material (screw in the joint space, loosening; ▶ Fig. 1.2)

1.2.4 Special Techniques

- *3D imaging*; indications:
  - Complex fractures
  - Calcaneal fracture, evaluation of the subtalar joint surface

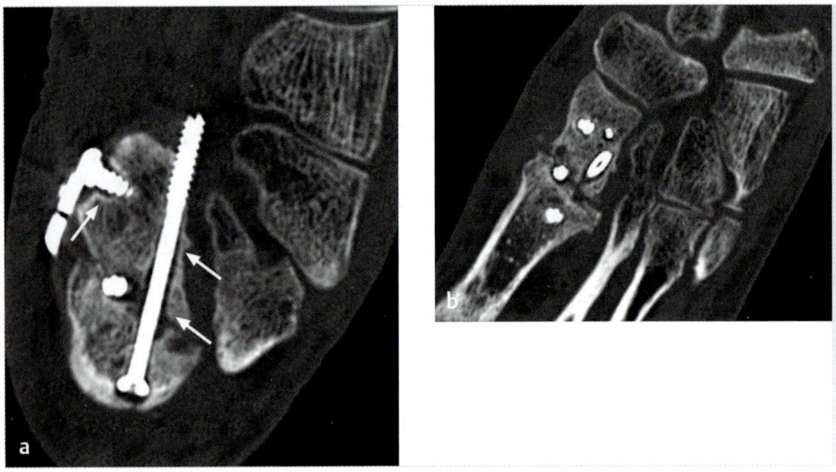

Fig. 1.2 a, b Persistent pain after fusion of the first tarsometatarsal joint in a 72-year-old woman.
a Oblique coronal multiplanar reformatting (MPR) image reconstructed along the screw through the first tarsometatarsal joint shows a fine zone of bone resorption around the arthrodesis screws (arrows). Bony consolidation around internal fixation material and the bony attachment of the material can be assessed accurately and with relatively few artifacts, even in small joints.
b Coronal MPR of the midfoot demonstrates nonunion of the first tarsometatarsal joint.

    - Tarsometatarsal (Lisfranc) and midtarsal (Chopart) joint lines
    - Interrelationship of the fragments
    - Axial malalignment
- *Side-to-side comparison:* Considered obsolete due to excessive radiation exposure
- *CT examinations in children:* Whenever possible, CT should be replaced by MRI due to radiation concerns (e.g., for investigating epiphyseal plate injuries, bone fractures involving the epiphyseal plate, or coalition). CT should be used only if MRI findings are equivocal.

1.3 Radiography

M. Walther

1.3.1 Forefoot

Weight-Bearing Radiographs of the Foot in Three Planes (▶ Fig. 1.3)

Indications

Standard radiographic series for the foot. Non–weight-bearing views of the foot are obtained only after trauma or surgery.

Positioning

- *DP (dorsoplantar) projection*:
    - Film flat on the floor
    - Patient standing on the cassette
    - Beam centered on the second tarsometatarsal joint
    - Tube 0° vertical
- *Lateral view*:
    - Film perpendicular to the floor, touching the medial side of the foot
    - Patient standing on the floor
    - Beam directed lateromedially, centered on the calcaneocuboid joint
    - Tube 0° horizontal

The determination of axial relationships on radiographs is subject to considerable variability. Couglin et al (2002) published a technique for determining bone axes based on designated reference points in the diaphysis. This technique was adopted by the AOFAS (American Orthopedic Foot and Ankle Society) as its standard for surgery of the forefoot.

Non–Weight-Bearing Radiographs of the Foot, Stress Radiographs

Indications

Non–weight-bearing radiographs of the foot are obtained in patients with suspected fractures and for postoperative evaluations and stress views.

Positioning

The patient lies on the X-ray table in a supine or lateral decubitus position (non–weight-bearing views are obtained only after trauma or surgery):

- *DP projection:*
    - Film horizontal on the X-ray table
    - Foot position: patient lies supine with the foot flat on the cassette
    - Beam centered on the second tarsometatarsal joint
    - Tube 0° vertical
    - If necessary, a forefoot adduction stress can be applied manually or with a mechanical apparatus (e.g., Telos device or Scheuba device).
- *Lateral view* (▶ Fig. 1.4 a):
    - Film horizontal on the X-ray table
    - Foot position: patient lies in lateral decubitus on the X-ray table with the affected foot down and resting on the cassette
    - Central ray focused on the calcaneocuboid joint
    - Tube 0° vertical
- *45° oblique views from the lateral side* (▶ Fig. 1.4 b):
    - Film horizontal on the X-ray table
    - Foot position: foot standing on the cassette and tilted 45° medially
    - Beam centered on the second tarsometatarsal joint
    - Tube 0° vertical
- *45° oblique view from the medial side* (e.g., an extra 45° inversion view is taken to evaluate the first tarsometatarsal joint after surgical fusion):
    - Film horizontal on the X-ray table

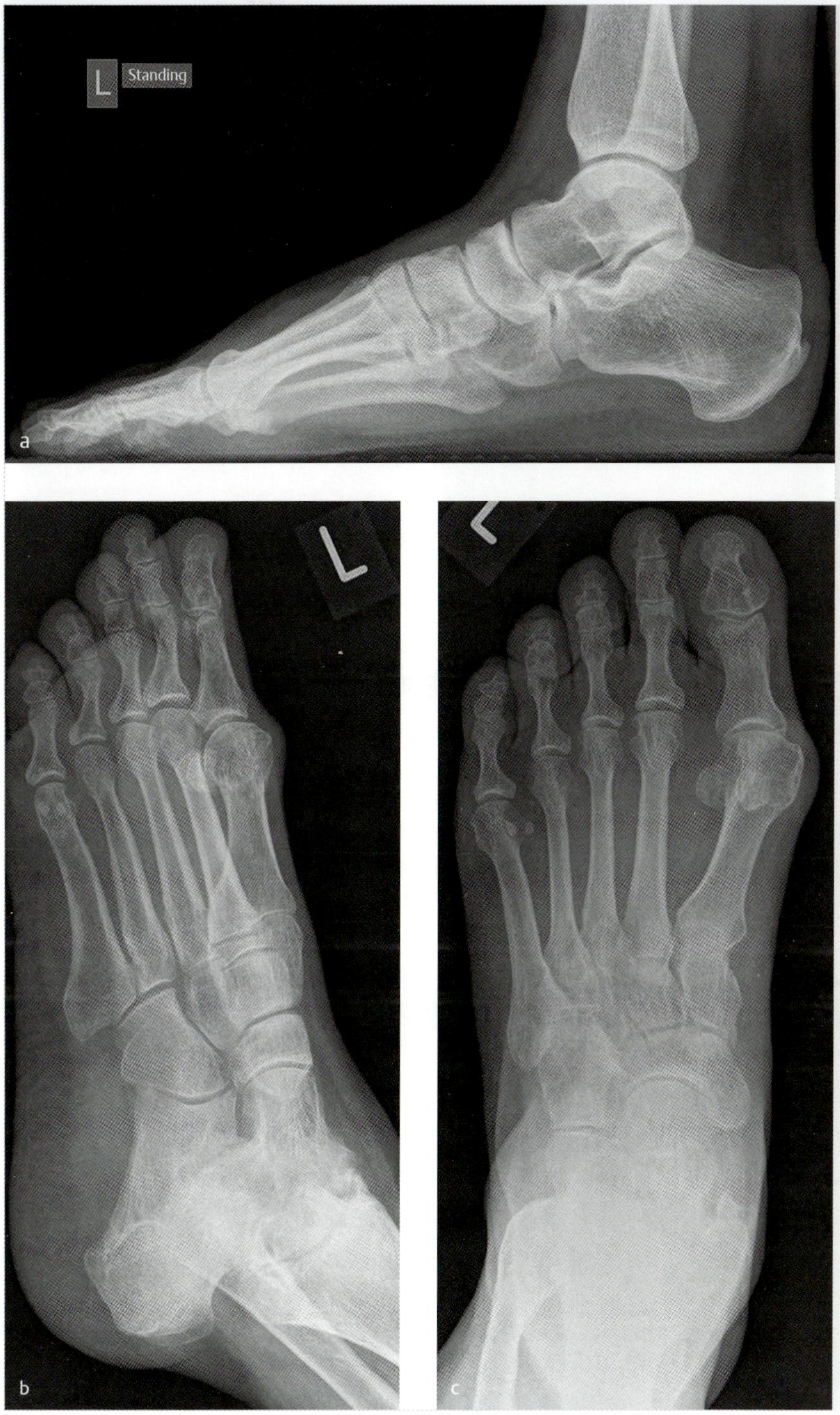

Fig. 1.3 a–c Weight-bearing radiographs of the foot in three planes. Standard series for evaluating deformities and degenerative diseases. These radiographs are the basis for most reconstructive surgical procedures on the foot. Angle determinations are all performed on weight-bearing radiographs. This series illustrates a hallux valgus deformity with degenerative changes in the subsesamoid joint space.
a Lateral view.
b Oblique view.
c DP view.

  - Foot position: foot standing on the cassette and tilted 45° laterally
  - Beam centered on the first tarsometatarsal joint
  - Tube 0° vertical

! Note

The stability of the calcaneocuboid joint can be evaluated on a non–weight-bearing DP radiograph while a forefoot adduction stress is applied. More than 10° of joint space opening is considered abnormal.

Toe Radiographs

Indications

Toe radiographs are obtained to evaluate toe injuries and other pathology.

Positioning

- DP projection
- Lateral oblique projection
- True lateral projection (rarely taken because the toes overlap in that projection)

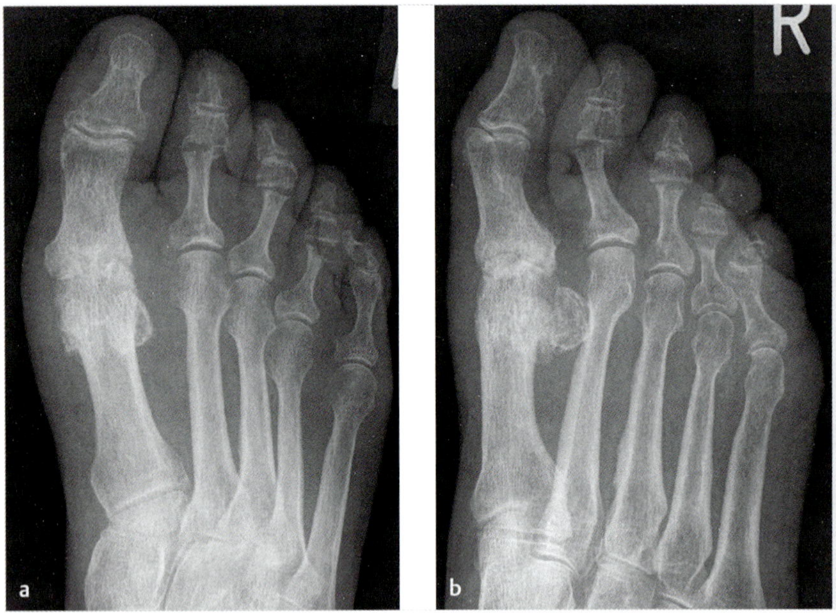

Fig. 1.4 a, b Non-weight-bearing radiographs of the forefoot in two planes. A weight-bearing radiograph could not be obtained in this patient due to severe arthritis of the first metatarsophalangeal joint.
a DP view.
b Oblique view.

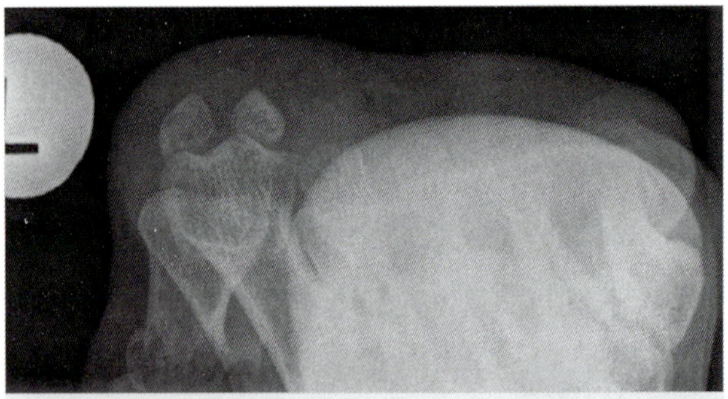

Fig. 1.5 Radiographic view of the sesamoids in their sulci, usually combined with radiographs of the foot in three planes. This view can demonstrate degenerative changes in the subsesamoid joint space, fragmentation due to sesamoid necrosis, subluxation of the sesamoids due to hallux valgus, or sesamoid irritation by metal following hallux surgery. The present image shows no abnormalities.

Toe projections are analogous to projections of the foot, except that the beam is centered on the second toe or on the toe with the presumed pathology.

Sesamoid Radiographs

Indications

Radiographs of the foot in three planes should be obtained in all patients with presumed sesamoid pathology.

Positioning

- *AP (anteroposterior) axial view of the sesamoids:*
  - Horizontal film position
  - Foot position: patient lies supine with the heel on the film plate, the ankle joint in 105° of plantar flexion, and traction applied with a strap to produce maximum dorsiflexion of the toes
  - Beam centered on the first metatarsophalangeal joint
  - X-ray tube 0° vertical
- *PA (posteroanterior) axial view of the sesamoids* (▶ Fig. 1.5):
  - Horizontal film position
  - Foot position: patient lies prone with the knee supported on a foam pad and the toes in maximum dorsiflexion
  - Beam centered on the first metatarsophalangeal joint
  - X-ray tube 0° vertical

! Note

Visualization of the sesamoids in their sulci is particularly helpful for evaluating degenerative changes in the subsesamoid joint space, unexplained complaints after hallux surgery, and sesamoid osteonecrosis. The sesamoid views are supplemented by radiographs of the big toe in three planes.

1.3.2 Hindfoot

Radiographs of the Ankle Joint in Two Planes

Indications

These are the standard projections for evaluating pathology in the talocrural joint.

Positioning

- *AP weight-bearing radiograph* (▶ Fig. 1.6):
  - Film is vertical and behind the ankle joint
  - Foot position: patient stands with the heel against the cassette and the axis of the foot parallel to the central ray
  - Beam centered on the ankle joint
  - X-ray tube 0° horizontal
- *Weight-bearing mortise view:*
  - Film is vertical and behind the ankle joint

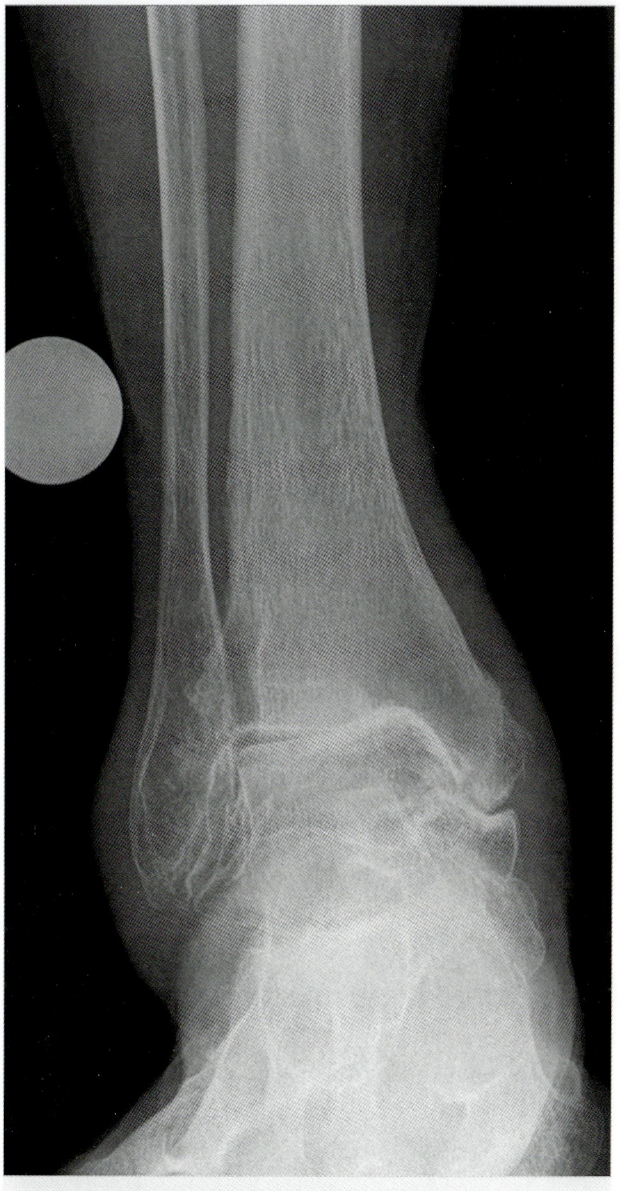

Fig. 1.6 AP weight-bearing radiograph of the ankle joint reveals degenerative joint changes with varus deformity.

- Foot position: patient stands with the heel against the cassette and the foot rotated internally until the axis of the ankle joint is parallel to the cassette
- Beam centered on the ankle joint
- X-ray tube 0° horizontal

- *Lateral ankle view:*
  - Film is vertical and medial to the ankle joint
  - Foot position: patient stands with the medial side against the cassette
  - Beam centered on the ankle joint
  - X-ray tube 0° horizontal

! Note

Oblique views in 45° of internal and external rotation supply additional information on the ankle mortise and talus. The internal rotation view is good for evaluating the distal fibula and subfibular region. The external rotation view clearly displays the posteromedial talus.

Non–Weight-Bearing Radiographs of the Ankle joint, Stress Radiographs

Indications

- Suspected fracture after trauma
- Stress views for evaluating (chronic) capsuloligamentous instabilities about the ankle joint

Positioning (▶ Fig. 1.7 and ▶ Fig. 1.8)

- *Non–weight-bearing AP projection:*
  - Film horizontal on the X-ray table
  - Foot position: patient lies supine on the table with the heel resting on the cassette (axis of the foot is parallel to the central ray)
  - Beam centered on the ankle joint
  - X-ray tube 0° vertical
  - If desired, a varus or valgus stress can be applied to the ankle manually or with a mechanical apparatus (e.g., Telos device or Scheuba device).
- *Non–weight-bearing mortise view:*
  - Film horizontal on the X-ray table
  - Foot position: patient lies supine on the table with the heel resting on the cassette (axis of the ankle joint is parallel to the cassette)
  - Beam centered on the ankle joint
  - X-ray tube 0° vertical
  - If desired, a varus or valgus stress can be applied manually or with a mechanical apparatus (e.g., Telos or Scheuba device).
- *Non–weight-bearing ankle lateral view:*
  - Film horizontal on the X-ray table
  - Foot position: patient is in lateral decubitus on the X-ray table with the affected foot down and resting on the cassette (axis of the foot is parallel to the central ray)
  - Beam centered on the ankle joint
  - X-ray tube 0° vertical
  - If desired, a drawer test can be performed by applying pressure to the front of the distal tibia while manually or mechanically stabilizing the calcaneal tuberosity.

Stress radiographs can be obtained by applying the stress manually or with a mechanical device. The standard pressure is 15 kPa. In an acute injury, stress radiographs are rewarding only when analgesia is administered (e.g., local anesthesia of the

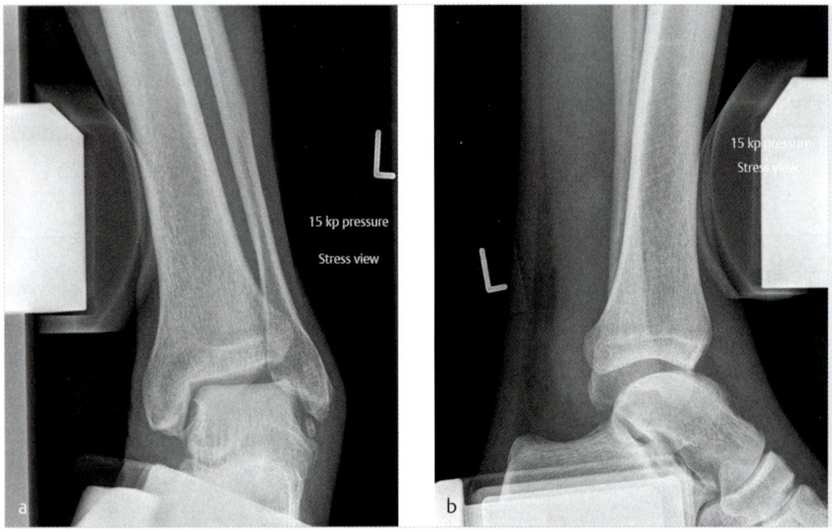

Fig. 1.7 a, b Stress radiograph of the ankle joint. Stress views are feasible only in patients without ankle pain. Increased joint space opening is diagnostic of capsuloligamentous laxity or a ligament tear. False-negative results are a possibility. Stress radiographs have become largely obsolete in the acute diagnosis of ligament tears.
a DP view.
b Lateral view.

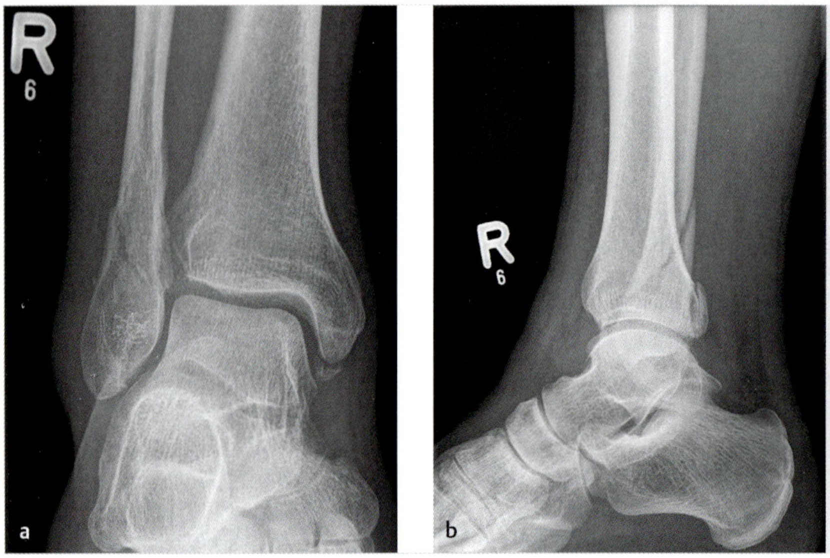

Fig. 1.8 a, b Non–weight-bearing radiographs of the ankle joint in two planes. These are the standard views for acute injuries, especially for suspected fractures. These radiographs show a fracture of the fibula and a chip fracture of the posterior tibial margin.
a DP view.
b Lateral view.

capsule and ligaments). Today, stress radiographs are of minor importance in the treatment algorithm for a lateral ankle sprain. Equivocal findings may be resolved by a side-to-side comparison, but this requires a higher radiation dose and should never be carried out to compensate for a lack of knowledge in radiographic anatomy or morphology.

! Note

The following signs on stress radiographs are considered abnormal:

- Anterior displacement of the talus > 2 mm in a side-to-side comparison
- Absolute talar displacement > 4 mm
- Lateral joint space opening > 10° in a side-to-side comparison
- Difference in the distance from the lateral distal talar margin to the fibular articular surface > 3 mm

Lateral radiographs are obtained in maximum dorsiflexion or plantar flexion with anterior or posterior impingement. AP radiographs are taken with eversion and dorsiflexion in patients with a suspected syndesmotic injury.

Broden View (▶ Fig. 1.9)

Indications

The Broden view is used to display the posterior facet of the subtalar joint.

Positioning

- *Medial oblique view:*
  - Film position horizontal on the X-ray table
  - Foot position: patient lies supine with the foot in internal rotation (45°) and the ankle joint at a 90° angle supported on a foam wedge

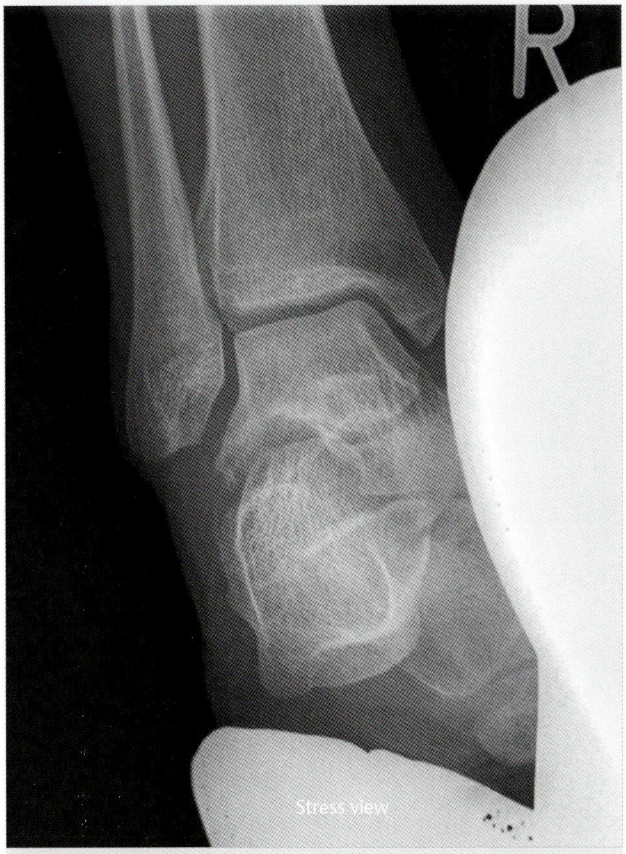

Fig. 1.9 Broden stress view. The Broden view is used to evaluate the stability of the subtalar joint in response to an inversion stress. This image shows slight joint space opening with rounded bone fragments on the lateral process of the talus following a sprain injury.

- Central ray is focused between the fibular apex and base of the fifth metatarsal
- X-ray tube: views are taken at 10°, 20°, 30°, and 40° angles from the vertical with the central ray angled cephalad

- *Lateral oblique view:*
  - Film position horizontal on the X-ray table
  - Foot position: patient lies supine with the foot in external rotation (45°) and the ankle joint at a 90° angle supported on a foam wedge
  - Central ray is focused between the medial malleolus and the tuberosity of the navicular bone
  - X-ray tube: views are taken at a 15° and 18° angle from the vertical with the central ray angled cephalad

! Note

The Broden view is a helpful intraoperative view during the open reduction and internal fixation of calcaneal fractures. CT has largely replaced the Broden view as a preoperative study. The medial oblique view can be obtained with a varus stress to evaluate subtalar joint stability.

Radiographs of the Calcaneus in Two Planes

Indications

Radiographs of the calcaneus in two planes are performed in patients with calcaneal fractures, after bony corrections, and in the diagnosis of Haglund exostosis and traction spurs.

Positioning

- *DP calcaneus axial projection:*
  - Film position horizontal on the X-ray table
  - Foot position: patient stands on the film with the tube behind the leg
  - Central ray is focused between the Achilles tendon insertion and the ankle joint
  - X-ray tube is angled anteriorly at a 25° angle from the vertical
- *Calcaneus lateral view:*
  - Film is perpendicular to the floor, placed against the medial aspect of the foot
  - Foot position: patient stands on the floor
  - Central ray from lateral to medial, centered on the calcaneus
  - X-ray tube: 90° from the perpendicular

! Note

Lateral views taken with 30° of internal and external rotation can detect calcifications on the calcaneal margins. Alternatively, CT or MRI can be used in clinically suspicious cases with negative radiographs.

Hindfoot Alignment View (Saltzman View, ▶ Fig. 1.10)

Indications

The Saltzman view is for evaluating the axial alignment of the hindfoot.

Positioning

- Film position: angled 20° from the vertical and 90° to the central ray
- Foot position: patient stands on a platform with the tube behind the leg and the cassette anterior to the foot
- Beam is centered on the ankle joint
- X-ray tube is angled 20° from the horizontal in a plantar direction

! Note

Hindfoot alignment views are an important aid in the work-up of calcaneal varus or valgus deformity and in the planning of hindfoot corrections.

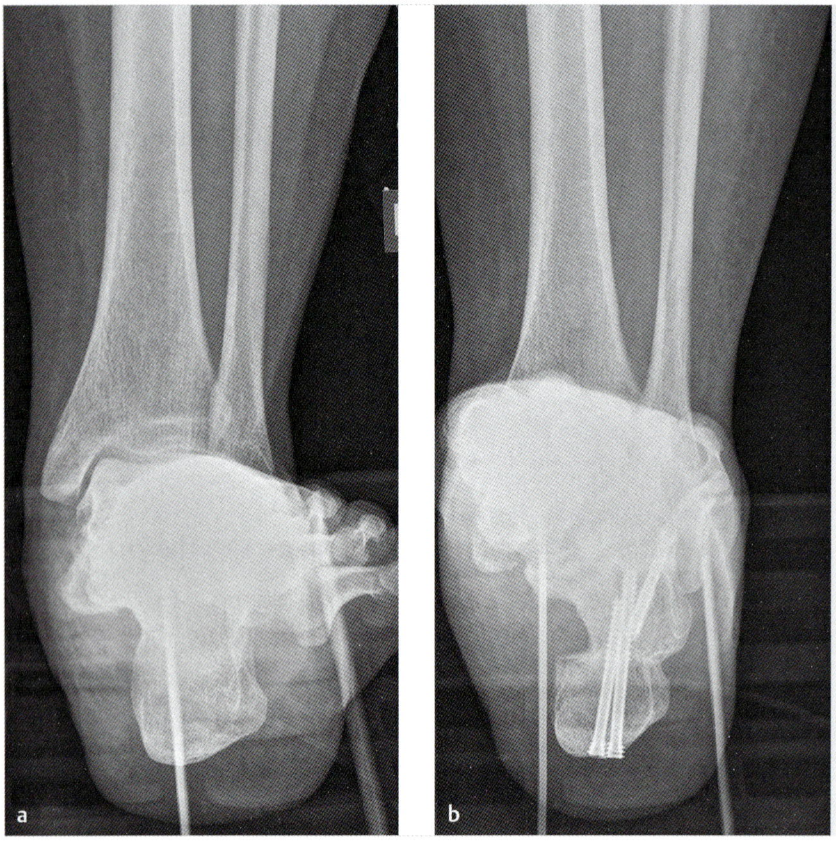

Fig. 1.10 a, b Saltzman view. The Saltzman view is used to evaluate calcaneal alignment. It has become increasingly important in recent years in the treatment of hindfoot deformities and is performed with weight bearing along with radiographs of the ankle joint in two planes.
a Patient with hindfoot valgus and forefoot abduction.
b Appearance following surgical correction by a calcaneal sliding osteotomy and calcaneal lengthening.

1.4 Ultrasound

H. Gaulrapp

Even in the foot and ankle, diagnostic ultrasound provides an "extended clinical finger," which should be performed personally by the clinical examiner in order to gain maximum information.

The patient is placed in a supine or prone position, supported if necessary with a padded roll. The affected structure is always scanned in two planes—longitudinal and transverse—using a 7.5- to 15-MHz linear transducer. A stand-off may be used on irregular surfaces and will improve resolution in the unfavorable near-field region, though it may sometimes cause troublesome reverberations. The use of a fluid-filled glove is not recommended owing to the presence of small air bubbles. The field of view and focus should be optimized for the region of interest (size, depth).

Besides the few standard sections recommended for the ankle joint by the DEGUM (German Society for Ultrasound in Medicine), additional planes have proven useful for scanning specific joint areas, tendons, and especially ligamentous structures.

Strengths of ultrasound:
- It can demonstrate fluids, soft tissues, joints, and bony surfaces.
- The power Doppler mode provides information on vascularity (e.g., angiogenesis in synovitis).
- Real-time imaging permits a unique dynamic–functional analysis of mobility and stability in joint compartments and of the muscle–tendon apparatus under constant visual control.
- Aspirations, injections, and biopsies are safer and more accurate when performed with ultrasound guidance or assistance.
- The technique is rapidly available at low cost.

Weaknesses of ultrasound:
- Inability to penetrate bony or calcified structures
- Poor visualization of deeper structures
- Poorer lateral resolution than MRI, with comparable axial resolution

Ultrasound can provide the experienced examiner with a wealth of additional information within a short time, allowing for the prompt and purposeful initiation of treatment while eliminating the need for costly or invasive tests:
- It can detect and differentiate between articular or periarticular swelling, effusion or hemarthrosis, seroma or hematoma, and exudative or proliferative synovitis.
- It can determine accessibility to percutaneous aspiration or biopsy; compression and pressure-release testing with the probe.

The following can also be discerned:
- Tears of the joint capsule and ligaments: complete, partial, stability testing, measurements
- Heel pain: differentiation of lesions affecting the Achilles tendon, bursa, traction spur, exostosis, Haglund heel
- Tendon lesions: differentiation of complete, partial, tendinopathy, peritendinous changes, displacement, reparability

1.5 Bibliography

Radiography

Christman RA. Foot and Ankle Radiology. St. Louis: Churchill Livingstone; 2003

Cobey JC. Posterior roentgenogram of the foot. Clin Orthop Relat Res 1976; 118: 202–207

Coughlin MJ, Saltzman CL, Nunley JA. Angular measurements in the evaluation of hallux valgus deformities: a report of the ad hoc committee of the American Orthopaedic Foot & Ankle Society on angular measurements. Foot Ankle Int 2002; 23: 68–74

Saltzman CL, el-Khoury GY. The hindfoot alignment view. Foot Ankle Int 1995; 16: 572–576

Ultrasound

Gaulrapp H, Binder C. Grundkurs Sonografie der Bewegungsorgane. Munich: Elsevier; 2011

Gaulrapp H, Szeimies U. Diagnostik der Gelenke und Weichteile: Sonographie oder MRT. Munich: Elsevier; 2008

Chapter 2

Clinical Evaluation

2 Clinical Evaluation

R. Degwert and M. Walther

A patient with foot pain, whether due to an acute injury or a chronic cause, always presents a certain challenge. This challenge is rooted in the complex anatomy and biomechanics of the foot and in the importance of the foot for the musculoskeletal system as a whole. A detailed knowledge of biomechanics and anatomy is essential for purposeful history-taking and an effective clinical examination.

Foot complaints are often part of a more complex problem. For example, 50% of all lower limb injuries that are missed in multiply injured patients involve the foot. It is common for injuries to occur at a variety of locations in the foot and ankle, and an examination that is not thorough and systematic is likely to miss some pathology.

Pre-existing complaints or degenerative changes can hamper the search for new pathology. All of these factors call for a highly systematic and logically structured approach to clinical examination. We recommend the routine use of an algorithm as outlined below.

2.1 Diagnostic Algorithm

2.1.1 Clinical Examination

1. History
2. Inspection
3. Palpation
4. Motion tests
5. Translation tests and sensory testing
6. Muscle function tests
7. Special tests
8. Stress tests
9. Examination of other structures

2.1.2 Imaging and Other Tests

- Ultrasound
- Radiography (may include stress views)
- MRI
- CT
- Other imaging modalities (scintigraphy, etc.)
- Laboratory tests
- Analysis of stance/gait/running, 3D motion analysis

Diagnostic arthroscopy has become almost entirely obsolete owing to the excellent quality of MR images.

2.1.3 Referral for Further Evaluation

- Neurology, angiology, phlebology, rheumatology, dermatology, etc.
- Possible referral for evaluation by an alternative health care provider
- Examination for craniomandibular dysfunction

! Note

The physician should always personally examine the patient before ordering imaging studies or reviewing the findings, diagnoses, or images from other examiners to avoid compromising his or her own judgment and differential diagnosis. Clinical examination based on a standard algorithm will ensure that nothing is missed on inspection and manual examination. Even when faced with obvious pathology, the examiner should still keep to the algorithm and proceed with a systematic examination of the whole foot.

2.2 History

History-taking should cover general elements as well as specific, current details. The balance of these elements will depend on the timing of the history and the nature of the injury or complaints.

2.2.1 Relevant Questions

Take a personal history and ask specific questions regarding age, occupation, sex, family and social history, occupational and/or athletic activities, and leisure activities. If necessary, include information elicited from a third party. The following questions are particularly important:

- What? Where? When? How? How long?
- What triggers the pain?
- Risk factors, older injuries, scars, systemic underlying or accompanying diseases, medication use?
- In athletic patients, ask about activity level and any recent increase in exercise level. Ask about the intensity of training and its content. The answers may provide clues to stress fractures or other sports-related injuries.
- Trauma mechanism: It is helpful to reconstruct the trauma mechanism as accurately as possible, as this may call attention to specific patterns of injury or complaints.
- High-impact trauma? Other traumatizing forces?
- Mental status: vague or exaggerated description, constant repetition, patient claims "everything hurts," etc.
- Prior illnesses, injuries, previous and current treatments or operations?

Certain mechanisms are known to produce specific injury patterns in the foot. To a degree, this can aid in determining the extent of foot and ankle injuries and may suggest the presence of injuries to other body structures. For example, jumping or falling from a height and landing on both feet may produce injuries that include vertebral compression fractures of the lumbar spine. Thus, the whole body axis should be examined in addition to both heels.

2.2.2 Pain History

- Pain location
- Pain intensity
- Weight-bearing capabilities or limitations
- Disability in everyday activities, work, or sports
- Braces, shoe inserts, crutches, or other aids
- With chronic diseases and follow-up examinations after acute onset of complaints, ask about the patient's current complaints
- In some cases administration of a pain questionnaire may be deemed appropriate

2.3 Inspection

The goal of inspection is to detect externally visible changes and distinguish them from normal findings. It is helpful to compare the affected foot with the opposite foot as a reference. The patient should be inspected while walking, standing, and with the foot hanging over the edge of the table. Pants (trousers) should be removed for evaluating the axial skeleton and musculature.

- Surface contours, swelling, skin color (e.g., postthrombotic changes)
- Hematoma, open wounds, injuries
- Foreign bodies
- Position, deformities, malalignment, longitudinal and transverse arches
- Asymmetry, atrophy of muscles and skin
- Hematoma, swelling, visible bony landmarks
- Calluses, thickening, scars, nail bed
- Special signs (e.g., the "too many toes" sign)

2.4 Palpation

Palpation should also follow a structured protocol and documentation. This includes:

- Palpation site
- Intensity and quality of palpation
- Area of palpation
- Palpation technique

Selecting the correct palpation site is crucial for establishing contact. The examiner should not start with the area that is apparently (by history and/or inspection) affected by the injury or complaint. It is better to start by palpating structures that are less sensitive or painful. Also, beyond physiological aspects, it is important to consider that different patients will respond differently to physical contact. Thus, a firm pressure may be interpreted as pleasant, confident, or threatening, while a gentle touch may be perceived as respectful or indecisive.

Palpation of the tissues should begin with a light pressure that is carefully increased in both its area and intensity. It should be kept in mind that tactile sensation will dwindle if palpation starts with a heavy pressure and whenever the pressure is increased. Only after completing a "superficial" assessment should the examiner progress to deeper levels while gradually increasing the intensity of the palpation. Individual structures are identified while the site(s) of any pain are explored as accurately as possible.

It should also be noted that the moving hand is better for identifying shapes and structures than a stationary hand. Movement activates significantly more skin receptors in the palpating hand; this prevents or limits their adaptation while supplying more detailed sensory information. A moving-hand technique also allows proprioception to contribute more to the recognition of shapes and surfaces. It improves temperature sensation as well.

The palpable structures of the foot are listed in ▸ Table 2.1.

Another factor that should be considered when palpating the foot is that accessory tarsal bones occur as normal anatomic variants in up to 30% of the population. They have no pathologic significance in themselves, but they may easily be mistaken for fractures, and this should be considered during the interpretation of subsequent imaging studies (see 11.2 Accessory Ossicles in Chapter 11). The four most common accessory bones are:

- Os trigonum
- Os tibiale externum (accessory navicular bone)
- Os peroneum
- Os vesalianum

2.5 Motion Tests

Motion tests, whether active or passive, supply information on the mobility of specific joint compartments. As in inspection and palpation, a systematic routine should be followed because the cumulative mobility of multiple joints can occasionally mask motion deficits in a single joint. Again, the opposite side provides a useful reference standard for comparison.

To avoid the misinterpretation of limited motion, the examiner should understand that it may have both structural and functional causes:

- *Structural:*
  - Fractures, dislocations
  - Contractures due to a chronic process (e.g., rheumatoid arthritis)
  - Contractures due to chronic functional (e.g., neurologic) deficits
  - Congenital deformities
  - Growth abnormalities
  - Postoperative scarring
  - Posttraumatic deformities
- *Functional:*
  - Pain-induced
  - Neurologic
  - Caused by intra-articular effusion or hematoma

As a rule, active range of motion should be tested first, as it is reasonable to assume that the patient will not exceed the range that can be subjectively tolerated. This is then followed by passive range-of-motion testing by the examiner.

The neutral-0 method, which forms the basis of normal-value tables for various joints, has become established only for the ankle joint and first metatarsophalangeal joint when applied to the foot. Movements in the midfoot and hindfoot are described as a fraction of the normal range of motion (e.g., subtalar joint = 1/3).

Table 2.1 Palpable structures in the foot

Medial side of the foot	Lateral side of the foot	Dorsum of the foot	Sole of the foot
• Medial malleolus • Deltoid ligament • Flexor retinaculum • Posterior tibial tendon • Posterior tibial artery • Sustentaculum tali • Talonavicular joint (medial Chopart joint line) • Navicular tuberosity with insertion of the posterior tibial tendon • Tarsal joint between navicular and cuneiform • Medial cuneiform • Medial tubercle of cuneiform (insertion of tibialis anterior tendon) • Tibialis anterior tendon • First tarsometatarsal joint (Lisfranc joint line) • First metatarsal • First metatarsophalangeal joint • Proximal phalanx of the big toe • First interphalangeal joint • Distal phalanx of the big toe	• Lateral malleolus • Anterior fibulotalar ligament • Fibulocalcaneal ligament • Posterior fibulotalar ligament • Peroneal retinaculum • Anterior syndesmosis • Peroneal (calcaneal) trochlea and peroneus brevis and longus tendon • Calcaneocuboid joint (lateral Chopart joint line) • Calcaneocuboid ligament • Tuberosity of fifth metatarsal with peroneus brevis tendon insertion • Fifth metatarsal • Fifth metatarsophalangeal joint • Proximal phalanx of the small toe • Fifth proximal interphalangeal joint • Middle phalanx of the small toe • Fifth distal interphalangeal joint • Distal phalanx of the small toe	• Dorsal pedal artery • Ankle joint with anterior tibial margin • Talar head with talonavicular joint (Chopart joint line) • Extensor retinaculum • Long extensor tendon • Extensor hallucis longus tendon • Extensor digitorum brevis tendon • Articulations of talus with intermediate and lateral cuneiforms • Tarsometatarsal joints of the second through fourth toes (Lisfranc joint line) • Lisfranc ligament • Second through fourth metatarsophalangeal joints • Proximal phalanx of the second through fourth toes • Second through fourth proximal interphalangeal joints • Middle phalanx of the second through fourth toes • Distal phalanx of the second through fourth toes • Superficial peroneal nerve • Saphenous nerve	• Calcaneal tuberosity • Plantar aponeurosis and long plantar ligament • Flexor digitorum brevis • Abductor and flexor digiti minimi muscles • Abductor hallucis • Metatarsal heads • Sesamoids of flexor hallucis longus • Plantar nerve

2.5.1 Translation Tests

Translation tests are motion or stress tests that evaluate the stability of a joint. It is particularly important in the foot to test for individual joint function and corresponding range of motion. A systematic routine is followed so that crucial findings will not be missed.

2.5.2 Muscle Function Tests

The goals of muscle function tests are twofold: test the function of a muscle and assess its strength. Deficits in muscular strength or function may be attributable to disease or injury involving any of the following structures:

- Muscle
- Tendon (▶ Fig. 2.1)
- Mechanics of tendon-to-bone junction
- Innervation, as well as intra- and intermuscular coordination

The principal muscular structures in the foot are listed below.

- *Foot muscles:*
  - Plantar flexors: triceps surae, tibialis posterior, plantaris
  - Extensors: tibialis anterior, extensor hallucis longus, extensor digitorum longus, extensor hallucis brevis, extensor digitorum brevis
  - Foot evertors: peroneus longus and brevis, peroneus tertius
  - Foot invertors: tibialis posterior, tibialis anterior
- *Toe muscles:*
  - Flexors: lumbricals, flexor hallucis brevis, flexor digitorum brevis, flexor hallucis longus
  - Extensors (dorsiflexors): extensor digitorum brevis, extensor hallucis brevis, extensor digitorum longus, extensor hallucis longus

The degree of muscle strength that can be developed is generally rated on a scale of 1/5 to 5/5 (after Janda), with 5/5 signifying the highest muscle strength and 1/5 the lowest (0/5 indicates complete paralysis).
Attention should also be given to the following factors:

- Muscle tone
- Muscle shortening
- Palpable discontinuities (e.g., including the lower leg muscles)

2.6 Sensory Testing

The examiner can make a crude assessment of sensation by touching the skin. The Semmes–Weinstein monofilament can provide a more differentiated assessment of cutaneous sensation (▶ Fig. 2.2). This thin filament can detect even mild sensory disturbances. Other options are touch tests with a cotton swab or feather.

! Note

In touch tests, make sure that the patient does not compensate for sensory loss by watching the tester.

A tuning fork can be used to test vibration perception threshold. Diminished vibratory sensation may be an early sign of nerve damage.

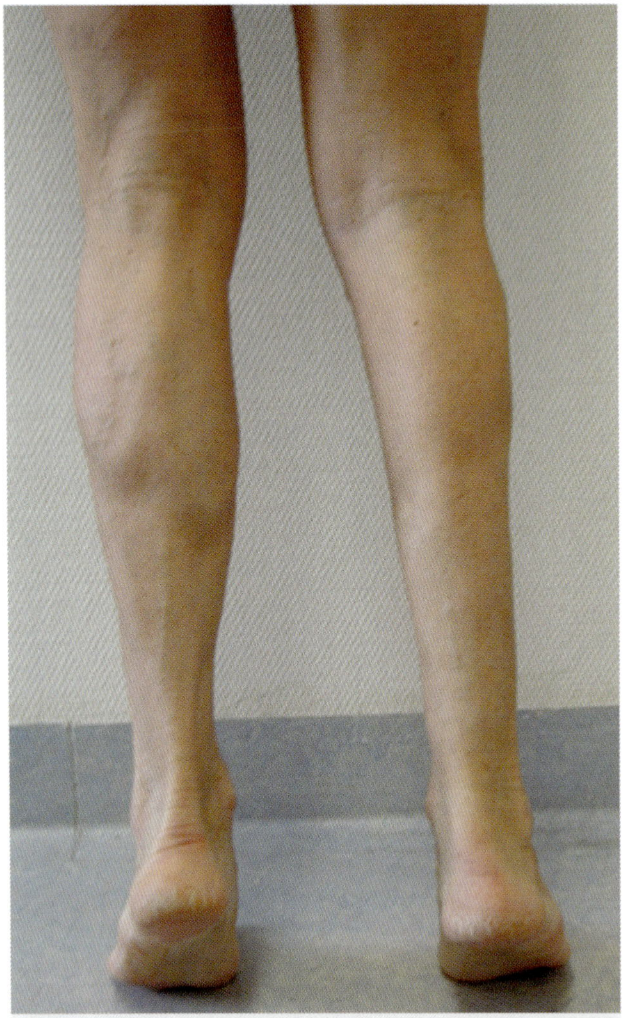

Fig. 2.1 Muscular atrophy. Atrophy of the right calf muscles has resulted from a ruptured Achilles tendon that healed in an elongated state.

2.7 Assessment of Blood Flow

The dorsal pedal artery is most easily palpated lateral to the extensor hallucis longus tendon on the dorsum of the foot. The tibial artery is palpable behind the medial malleolus (see ▶ Table 2.1). Normally, both arteries can be palpated without difficulty. Blood flow at the capillary level (in the small vessels) is assessed by the capillary refill time. This is done by pressing briefly on the ball of the toe with the finger, releasing the pressure, and measuring the time it takes the blanched area to regain its pink color. A normal refill time is < 2 seconds. Absence of the fine hairs on the toes may also signify impaired blood flow.

Other technical options for measuring blood flow are Doppler ultrasonography and angiography.

2.8 Special Tests on the Foot

2.8.1 Hindfoot

Hindfoot Inversion in Tiptoe Stance

The heel normally assumes a slight valgus position during stance. When the patient then rises up onto the toes, the heel

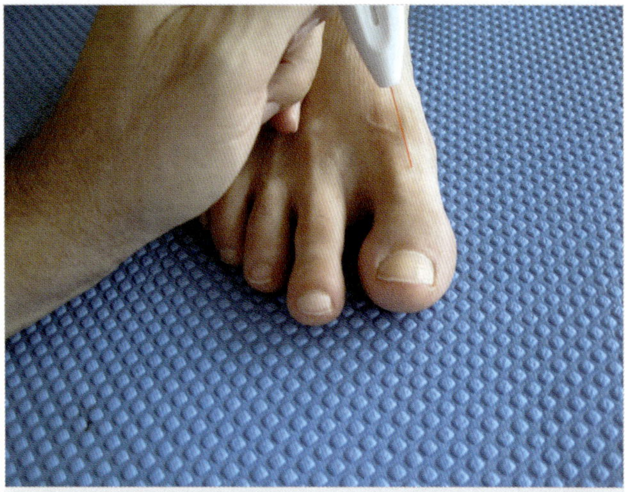

Fig. 2.2 Testing sensation with a Semmes–Weinstein monofilament.

moves to a varus position that is equal on both sides. If the heel remains in varus, this is considered an abnormal sign that may have several causes:

- Rigid pes planovalgus
- Posterior tibial tendon dysfunction
- Coalition
- Posttraumatic deformity

"Too-Many-Toes" Sign (▶ Fig. 2.3)

When the foot is inspected from behind with the patient standing, the big toe is normally visible on the medial side while one or two toes are visible lateral to the heel. If the big toe is not visible while three or more toes can be counted on the lateral side, this "too-many-toes" sign indicates increased abduction of the forefoot (e.g., due to pes planovalgus or posterior tibial insufficiency).

Thompson Squeeze Test (▶ Fig. 2.4)

With the patient lying prone, the examiner squeezes the patient's calf. This pressure will normally evoke slight plantar flexion at the ankle joint. Unilateral absence of plantar flexion indicates rupture or elongation of the Achilles tendon.

Heel Compression Test

The examiner symmetrically compresses the heel between the balls of both thumbs. With a fracture of the calcaneus, this test will elicit pain in the heel.

Single-Heel-Rise Test

The inability to rise onto the toes while standing on one leg signifies a lesion of the posterior tibial tendon.

Silfverskiöld Test (▶ Fig. 2.5)

This maneuver tests the correctibility of equinus deformity with the knee joint flexed and extended. If the deformity can be corrected with the knee flexed, the cause of the deformity is

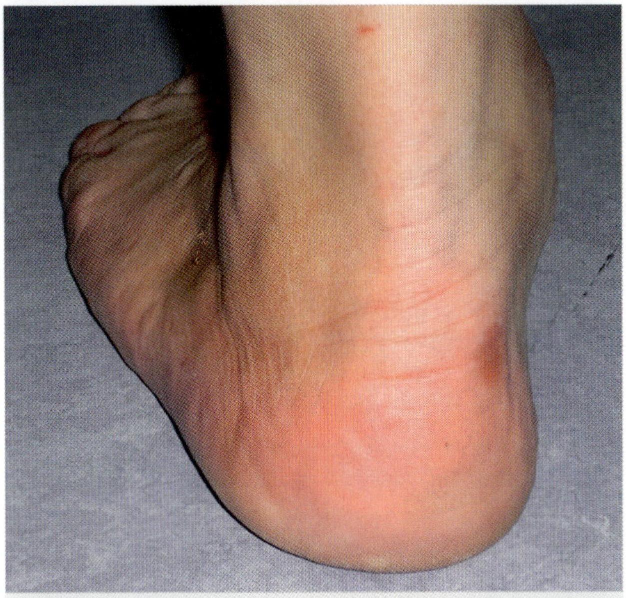

Fig. 2.3 **"Too-many-toes" sign.** With valgus deformity of the hindfoot, three or more toes are visible on the lateral side. Normally the big toe is visible medially while one or two toes are visible laterally.

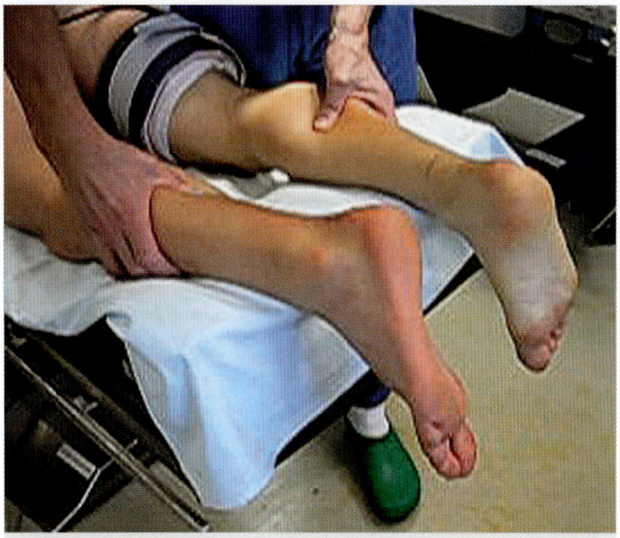

Fig. 2.4 **Thompson test.** With the patient lying prone, the examiner squeezes the calf. This normal response is slight plantar flexion at the ankle joint. Unilateral absence of this response indicates a ruptured or elongated Achilles tendon.

gastrocnemius shortening (positive Silfverskiöld test). An equinus deformity that persists in knee flexion is due to pathology of the joint, Achilles tendon, or soleus muscle.

2.8.2 Joint Stability

Coleman Block Test

This test evaluates hindfoot flexibility and pronation of the forefoot. With the patient standing, torsional deformities of the hindfoot or forefoot are temporarily corrected with wooden blocks of varying height. This test can help to localize the deformity and determine its flexibility. The Coleman block test is often used in patients with pes cavus deformity, for example.

Lateral/Medial Ankle Stability Test

This test assesses the stability of the ankle joint capsule and ligaments in a side-to-side comparison.

- *Ankle joint:* the ankle (talocrural) joint is plantar-flexed to eliminate bony stabilization of the joint.
- *Subtalar joint:* the ankle joint is flexed 90° to maximize bony stabilization of the ankle and allow a preponderance of motion in the subtalar joint.

Drawer Test

The drawer test is performed by grasping the ankle joint above the malleolar mortise. The other hand grasps the heel and pulls the foot forward. Increased translation signifies instability of the anterior fibulotalar ligament.

Drawer tests can also be performed on the metatarsophalangeal joints and tarsometatarsal joints to test capsuloligamentous stability.

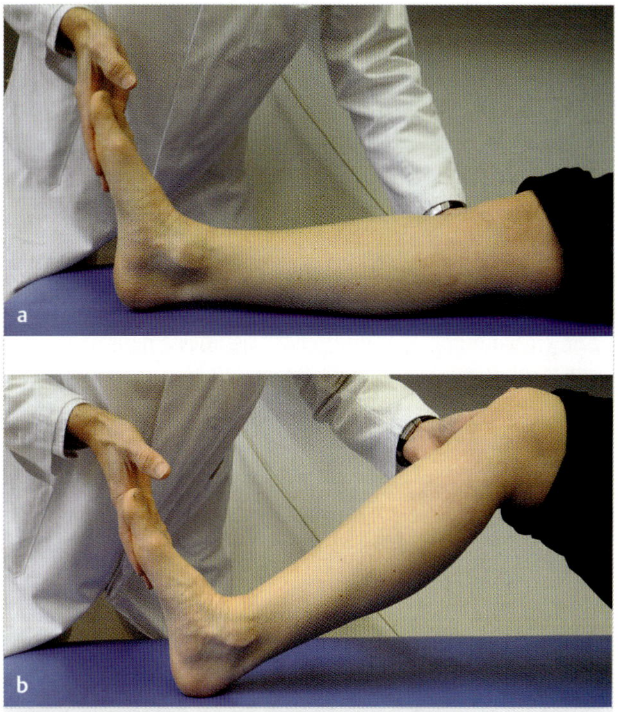

Fig. 2.5 a, b **Silfverskiöld test.** If an equinus deformity is correctible with the knee flexed, its cause is gastrocnemius shortening (positive Silfverskiöld test). If the deformity persists despite knee flexion, the cause is localized to the joint, Achilles tendon, or soleus muscle.

Pronation/Abduction Test

Pain in the syndesmosis area during pronation and abduction in the ankle joint is a sign of syndesmotic injury.

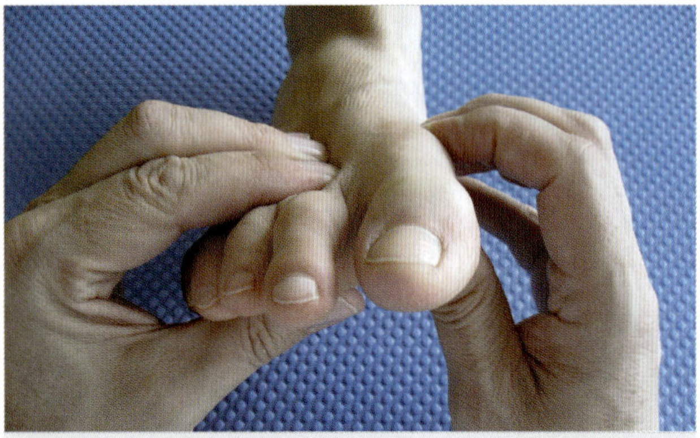

Fig. 2.6 First tarsometatarsal joint stability test.

Squeeze Test

Pain in the syndesmosis area in response to compressing the tibia against the fibula a handwidth above the syndesmosis is a sign of syndesmotic injury.

First Tarsometatarsal Joint Stability Test (▶ Fig. 2.6)

A physiologic translation of the first tarsometatarsal joint is noted when the foot hangs over the edge of the table. When the lateral border of the foot is raised (tensing the peroneus longus), the joint is stabilized. Persistent instability is abnormal.

2.8.3 Nerve Irritation

Mulder Click Test

Mediolateral compression of the forefoot exerts pressure on the intermetatarsal space and pushes the adjacent metatarsal heads against each other. A painful "click" signifies a neuroma of the plantar interdigital nerve (Morton neuroma).

"Doorbell" Sign (▶ Fig. 2.7)

Isolated plantar tenderness between the metatarsal heads (usually the third and fourth) is called the "doorbell" sign. Pain may radiate into the adjacent toes. A positive doorbell sign is indicative of a Morton neuroma.

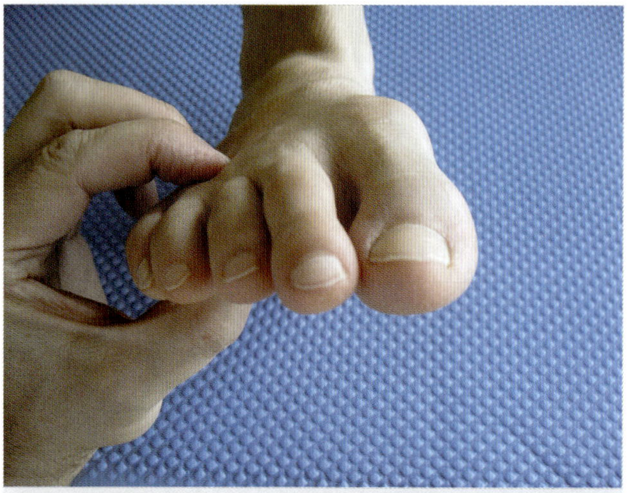

Fig. 2.7 "Doorbell" sign. Isolated plantar tenderness between the metatarsal heads (usually the third and fourth), with possible pain radiating into the toes, is a positive "doorbell" sign suggestive of Morton neuroma.

Hoffmann–Tinel Sign at the Medial Malleolus

The patient lies prone with the knee flexed 90°. If percussion of the tibial nerve behind the medial malleolus elicits an electric-shock sensation, this indicates the presence of a tarsal tunnel syndrome.

2.8.4 Forefoot

Toe Translation Test

The toe translation test evaluates dorsoplantar translation in the metatarsophalangeal joint. Increased translation and pain may signify instability, possibly associated with a tear of the plantar plate.

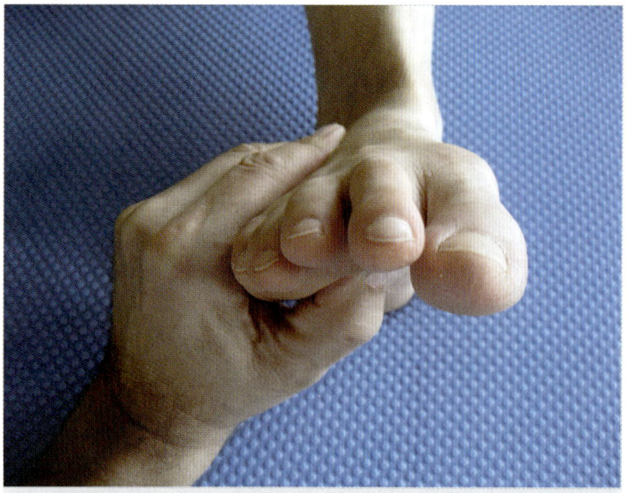

Fig. 2.8 Push-up test. Pushing up on the metatarsal head from the plantar side will reduce a flexible hammer toe into a neutral position. A positive push-up test indicates a fixed hammer toe deformity.

Gaensslen Maneuver

The metatarsal heads are immobilized between a finger placed on the plantar side of the foot and the thumb on the dorsal side. The other hand grasps the toes in a pincer grip, applying medial and lateral compression to the forefoot via the metatarsal heads of the first and fifth toes. This maneuver will elicit pain in a variety of forefoot disorders. A bilateral positive Gaensslen test may be an initial sign of rheumatoid arthritis.

Push-Up Test (▶ Fig. 2.8)

This test involves the reduction of a flexible hammer toe deformity into a neutral position when the metatarsal head is passively pushed up from the plantar side. It enables the examiner to distinguish between a flexible and fixed deformity.

2.9 Stress Tests and Provocative Testing

Stress tests are used in making a final evaluation. They can be used only in patients who have no fulminating complaints or significant instabilities. Stress tests are also capable of worsening a patient's condition. On the other hand, the very purpose of these tests is to identify symptoms and changes that were not reproducible by the other test methods described above. Stress tests may involve any of the following:

- Standing tests in which the examiner evaluates the alignment of the knee joint, ankle joint, foot, hindfoot valgus or varus, abduction or adduction
- Standing on one leg
- Walking
- Rocking
- Stair climbing
- Running
- Jumping
- Sport-specific stresses

2.10 Other Diagnostic Options

- Imaging
- Laboratory tests
- Consultation with other specialties (dermatology, neurology, angiology, rheumatology, endocrinology, osteology)
- Functional and gait analysis
- Craniomandibular evaluation

2.11 Summary

Especially in patients with foot trauma, a detailed clinical examination should be performed after the prompt exclusion of a neurovascular injury or compartment syndrome. Given the complex anatomy and biomechanics of the foot and ankle and the associated complexity of potential injuries and complaints, it is important to consider the possible coexistence of multiple entities or pathologies.

A detailed history will aid in directing the clinical examination, and a more detailed examination will aid in directing further diagnostic tests. A thorough overall work-up will enable a more precise diagnosis, which in turn will allow for more specific and effective treatment.

A systematic or algorithmic approach is strongly advised. A precise, anatomically correct topographic description of potential pathology is helpful. The site of maximum pain or tenderness often correlates with the location of the pathology.

! Note

It is important to collect and document adequate information for follow-up.

2.12 Special Case: Chronic Pain Syndrome without Objective Findings

At a large foot and ankle center it is common to see patients who present with significant, persistent, credible pain. But previous diagnostic efforts have been unable to detect a causative lesion or disorder in these patients, and previous treatment attempts have been unsuccessful. Available diagnostic options should be exhausted, because these patients are in considerable distress and are often handicapped in their ability to continue working. Even relatively unimpressive findings and a scant amount of fibrovascular granulation tissue may lead to significant disability at corresponding levels of pain perception.

The following staged approach has yielded good results, though the exact sequence may vary:

1. High-resolution MRI with IV contrast administration, giving particular attention to the painful area
2. Stress radiographs in multiple planes with a side-to-side comparison (may detect possible occult instabilities)
3. Gait analysis, pressure distribution (to exclude functional problems)
4. Post-exercise MRI—particularly recommended in patients with complaints during or after exercise to help detect overloading of the capsule and ligaments, activation tissue, or reactive synovitis. See 2.9 Stress Tests and Provocative Testing (p. 19)
5. Diagnostic infiltration with local anesthetic (helpful in diagnosing unexplained nerve compression syndromes and focal compression due to scar tissue)
6. Exclusion of proximal pain sources (referred pain) in the lower leg, thigh, or spinal column
7. Scintigraphy for the exclusion of systemic pathology

2.13 Bibliography

Coughlin MJ, Mann RA, Saltzman CL. Surgery of the Foot and Ankle. Philadelphia: Elsevier; 2007

Delcourt A, Huglo D, Prangere T et al. Comparison between Leukoscan (Sulesomab) and Gallium-67 for the diagnosis of osteomyelitis in the diabetic foot. Diabetes Metab 2005; 31: 125–133

Frisch H. Programmierte Untersuchung des Bewegungsapparates. Berlin: Springer; 2009

Gondring WH, Trepman E, Shields B. Tarsal tunnel syndrome: assessment of treatment outcome with an anatomic pain intensity scale. Foot Ankle Surg 2009; 15: 133–138

McNally EG. Ultrasound of the small joints of the hands and feet: current status. Skeletal Radiol 2008; 37: 99–113

Mondelli M, Morana P, Padua L. An electrophysiological severity scale in tarsal tunnel syndrome. Acta Neurol Scand 2004; 109: 284–289

Rammelt S, Biewener A, Grass R, Zwipp H. Foot injuries in the polytraumatized patient [Article in German]. Unfallchirurg 2005; 108: 858–865

Rohen JW. Funktionelle Anatomie des Menschen. Stuttgart: Schattauer; 1984

Rohen JW. Topographische Anatomie. Stuttgart: Schattauer; 1984

Rubello D, Casara D, Maran A, Avogaro A, Tiengo A, Muzzio PC. Role of anti-granulocyte Fab' fragment antibody scintigraphy (LeukoScan) in evaluating bone infection: acquisition protocol, interpretation criteria and clinical results. Nucl Med Commun 2004; 25: 39–47

Sarrafian SK. Anatomy of the Foot and Ankle. Philadelphia: Lippincott; 1993

Shands AR, Wentz IJ. Congenital anomalies, accessory bones, and osteochondritis in the feet of 850 children. Surg Clin North Am 1953; 33: 1643–1666

Chapter 3

Ankle and Hindfoot

3 Ankle and Hindfoot

3.1 Trauma

3.1.1 Capsule and Ligaments

M. Walther and U. Szeimies

Lateral Ligaments

Definition

Traumatic injuries to the lateral ligaments involve the partial or complete tearing of one or more lateral ligaments of the ankle joint, usually as a result of supination trauma.

Symptoms

Typical symptoms are pain and swelling about the lateral malleolus, often extending to the dorsum of the foot.

Predisposing Factors

- Previous ankle sprains
- Chronic instability
- Lax joint capsule and ligaments
- Hindfoot varus

Anatomy and Pathology

Anatomy

The lateral ligament complex of the ankle joint consists of the anterior talofibular ligament, the calcaneofibular ligament, and the posterior talofibular ligament. Numerous anatomic variants are encountered. For example, the anterior talofibular ligament may be poorly developed in the presence of a very strongly developed calcaneofibular ligament.

Pathology

The anterior talofibular ligament tears first. The injury may then progress to a concomitant partial or complete tear of the calcaneofibular ligament. The posterior talofibular ligament is very rarely affected. The most vulnerable ligament in the subtalar joint is the lateral calcaneocuboid ligament. The three grades of lateral ligament sprain are stretching (I), partial tearing (II), and complete tear or rupture (III). The most common injury in children is a proximal osteochondral avulsion of the anterior talofibular ligament. All tears do not lead to ankle instability, however.

An injury to the anterior talofibular ligament may be a proximal avulsion from the distal anterior fibula, a tear in the middle third of the ligament, or a distal avulsion from the neck of the talus. The proximal and distal injuries may have an osseous component. Bony avulsions are important because the hematoma that forms at the site of the avulsed bone flake may lead to ossification or ossicle formation. The ligament itself is not torn in these cases but attaches normally to the avulsed bone fragment. The separation of the bone flake from the distal fibula results in chronic instability and proneness to recurrent supination injuries. The origins of the anterior talofibular ligament and calcaneofibular ligament may avulse jointly from the distal fibula, with corresponding instability of both ligaments.

A complete two-ligament lateral ankle sprain may be associated with concurrent medial-side injury to the deltoid ligament. The medial malleolus "grinds" the medial ligament against the medial talus. The medial ligament lesion that may accompany lateral ankle sprains may lead to incomplete healing and persistent complaints on the medial side. This pathology has to be considered in patients with lateral instability, complaining of medial ankle pain.

Imaging

Radiographs

Stress radiographs are no longer used in the evaluation of acute injuries. If a fracture is suspected, radiographs of the ankle joint are obtained in two planes.

! Note

When ankle radiographs are obtained in two planes, the foot should be internally rotated 15° for the DP view to get a non-superimposed projection of the distal fibula and talar shoulders.

Ultrasound

The ultrasound imaging of ankle sprains should follow a systematic approach. A longitudinal scan over the anterior side of the ankle joint will demonstrate the hematoma that is typically associated with a capsuloligamentous injury. Lateral longitudinal scans over the distal fibula, anterior talofibular ligament, calcaneofibular ligament, and lateral calcaneocuboid ligament provide information on concomitant bony involvement and ligament continuity. Also, the examiner can perform a reliable, measurable assessment of joint stability in real time by watching the monitor during stress testing. With an osteochondral avulsion (of the fibula), ultrasound may show an echogenic fragment with an acoustic shadow that is often first noted on stress testing and is sometimes missed on radiographs.

MRI

Interpretation Checklist

Differentiate among the following:

- Partial ligament tear
- Complete tear
- Displaced ligament ends
- Proximal or distal avulsion fracture

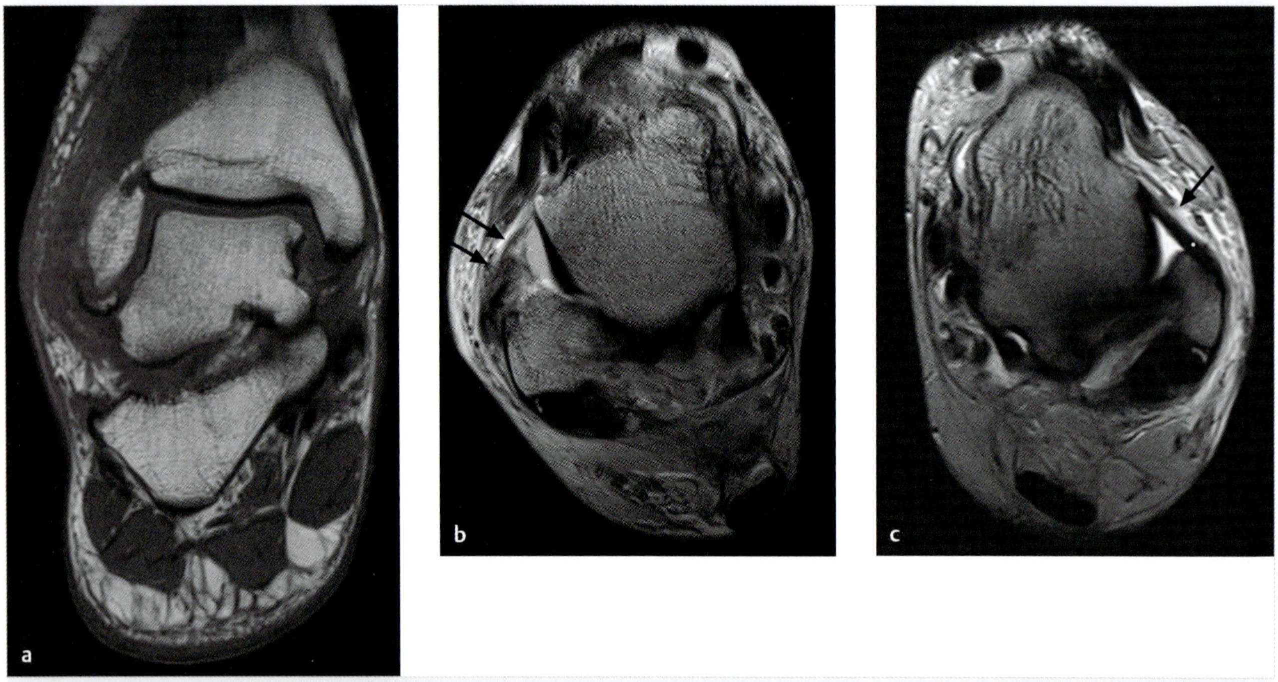

Fig. 3.1 a, b Fresh rupture of the anterior talofibular ligament, c normal anterior talofibular ligament.
a Coronal T1-weighted MRI shows a bony avulsion of the anterior talofibular ligament from the tip of the lateral malleolus. It is difficult to distinguish between an old or recent avulsion fracture in the absence of bone marrow edema, but the cortical discontinuity shown in part **b** makes the diagnosis clear. It is more difficult to interpret injuries in which the anterior talofibular ligament inserts on an ossicle fixed by fibrous tissue. It may be helpful in these cases to look for fluid signal in the slightly enlarged space between the ossicle and parent bone.
b Axial T2-weighted image shows a hemorrhagic area with fraying of the anterior talofibular ligament on the fibular side (arrows). The dehiscent bone fragment is visualized.
c Compare with axial T2-weighted image of a normal anterior talofibular ligament in a different patient (arrow).

! Note

Injury to the calcaneofibular ligament must be accurately assessed because a complete tear in a two-ligament injury can be treated surgically in competitive athletes. Quantify the percentage of the tear may be helpful for the treating physician.

Attention should also be given to frequently missed associated injuries with potentially severe consequences such as joint instability and early degenerative changes in joints.

Besides the lateral and medial ligaments (normal-appearing deltoid ligament with no evidence of crush injury, fascicle discontinuity, or hemorrhage), the MRI examination should also include an evaluation of the following structures:

- Anterior syndesmosis
- Volkmann triangle (posterior tibial margin)
- Ligaments in the sinus tarsi
- Peroneal tendon retinaculum
- Articular cartilage, including the talar shoulders, to exclude osteochondral injury
- Subtalar joint facets
- Midtarsal (Chopart) joint line

These structures should be individually assessed and noted in the report.

Examination Technique

- *Standard trauma protocol:* High-resolution multi-channel coil (in the prone position if necessary); contrast administration is not required.
- *Sequences:*
  - Coronal T1-weighted, parallel to the transverse axis of the ankle joint through the talus and malleoli
  - Sagittal and coronal PD (proton density)-weighted fat-sat (fat saturation)
  - Axial T2-weighted, angled parallel to the anterior talofibular ligament
  - If necessary: axial oblique PD-weighted fat-sat sequence in the syndesmotic plane

MRI Findings (▶ Fig. 3.1, ▶ Fig. 3.2, ▶ Fig. 3.3)

- Midsubstance tear, fibular, or talar avulsion of the anterior talofibular ligament with a visible discontinuity and wavy contours of the ligament stump
- Associated anterolateral capsule tear with edema and hemorrhage along the anterolateral soft tissues
- Interstitial hemorrhage and increased signal intensity with/without continuity disruption in the calcaneofibular ligament (the posterior talofibular ligament is generally intact)
- Frequent significant hemorrhage and marked soft-tissue hematoma encircling the ankle joint, most pronounced anterolaterally due to the disruption of subcutaneous and deeper veins
- Contusional bone edema on the medial talar border, medial malleolus, talar shoulders, etc.

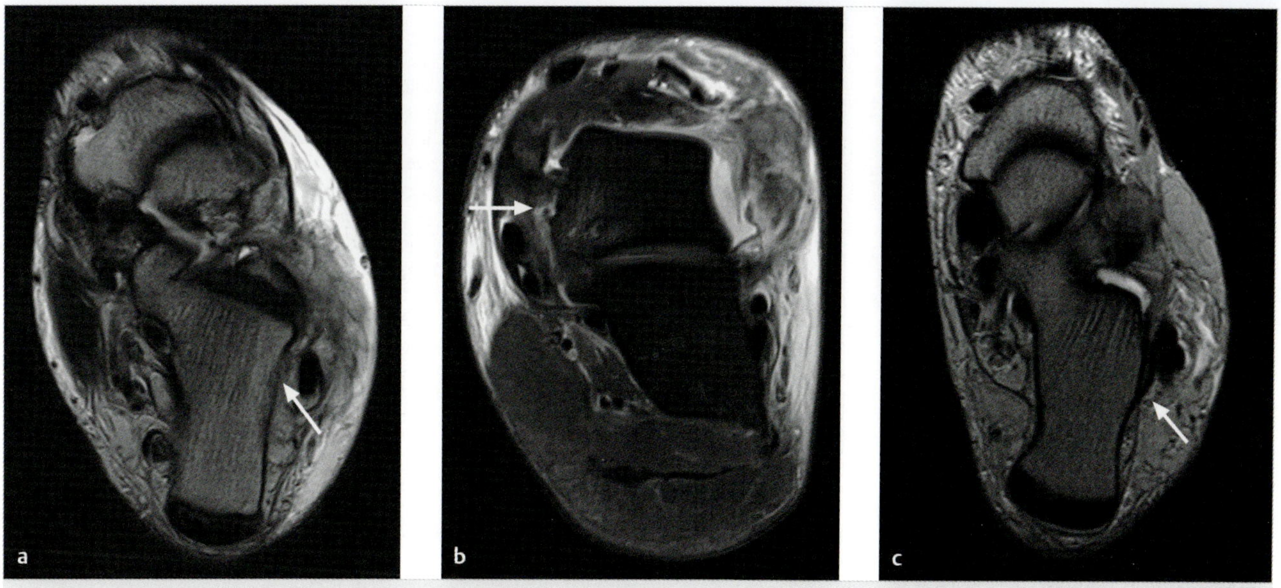

Fig. 3.2 a, b Fresh rupture of the calcaneofibular ligament, c normal calcaneofibular ligament.
a Axial T2-weighted image shows absence of the hypointense calcaneofibular ligament below the peroneal tendon with cloudy hemorrhage into the soft tissues (arrows).
b Coronal PD-weighted fat-sat image shows avulsion of the calcaneofibular ligament from the lateral border of the talus (arrow).
c Compare with axial T2-weighted image of a normal calcaneofibular ligament in a different patient (arrow).

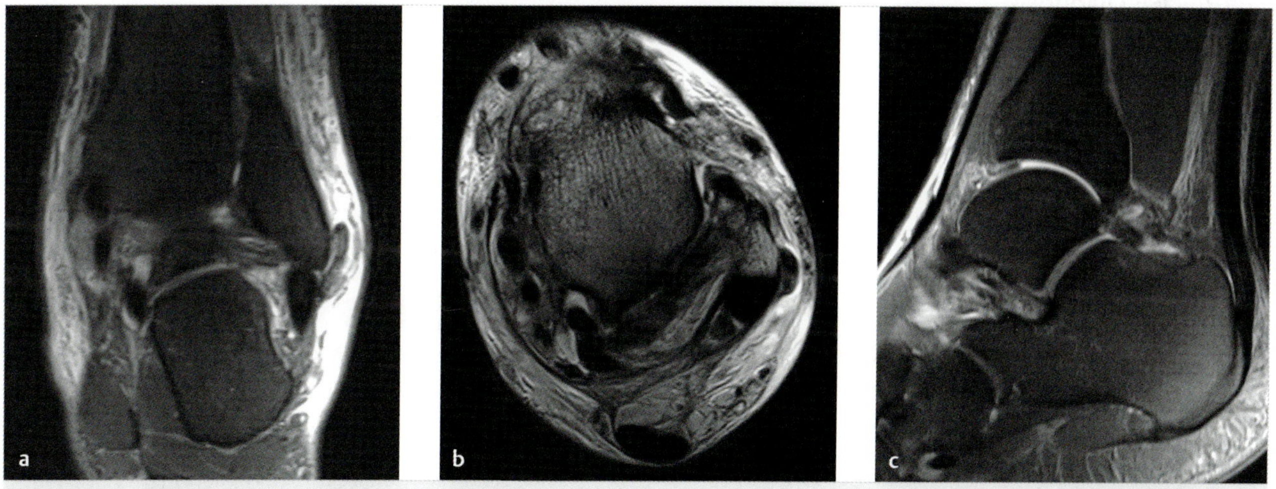

Fig. 3.3 a–c MRI in a 19-year-old male following pronation trauma and a lateral ankle sprain with unusual displacement of the torn capsule and ligaments.
a Coronal PD-weighted fat-sat image shows significant displacement of the ruptured anterior talofibular ligament. The stump is displaced upward and behind the distal fibula.
b Axial T2-weighted image shows portions of the ligament on the lateral aspect of the lateral malleolus.
c Sagittal PD-weighted fat-sat image shows that portions of the capsule have been displaced into the anterolateral part of the ankle joint space.

! Note

Special forms:

- *In children:* subperiosteal hematoma on the fibula (▶ Fig. 3.4) with patchy subperiosteal hemorrhage and an intact periosteal sleeve. Periosteal elevation usually occurs only at the metaphyseal level, proximal to the epiphyseal plate, and not on the distal fibula.
- *Repetitive trauma:* old or fresh avulsion fracture at the tip of the lateral malleolus as opposed to ossicle formation (attached by fibrous tissue) with the anterior talofibular ligament inserting on the ossicle. High-resolution imaging in three planes (T1-weighted, PD-weighted fat-sat) is necessary in these cases to differentiate among fibers inserting directly on an ossicle, an avulsion fracture, and the tip of the lateral malleolus with impending or frank instability. The calcaneofibular ligament may also arise from an avulsed fragment, indicating a high risk of (chronic) instability.

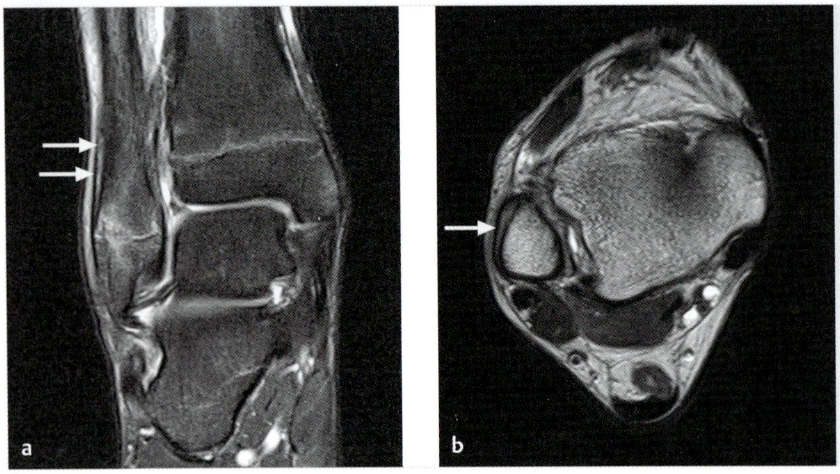

Fig. 3.4 a, b Subperiosteal hematoma in a 15-year-old boy following ankle torsion trauma with suspected syndesmotic and lateral ligament injuries.
a Coronal PD-weighted fat-sat image shows elevation of the periosteum by a subperiosteal hematoma (arrows) proximal to the epiphyseal plate of the distal fibula, which has not yet closed. Minimal edema is noted about the distal fibula with no signs of epiphyseal plate injury. The lateral ligaments are intact.
b Axial T2-weighted image shows subperiosteal hematoma along the lateral aspect of the fibula (arrow).

Imaging Recommendations

- Radiographs to exclude a fracture
- Ultrasound to evaluate for hemarthrosis, ligament continuity, and instability
- MRI for detection of associated injuries such as osteochondral lesions and other capsuloligamentous injuries

Differential Diagnosis

- Osteochondral injury of the talus or talar bony avulsion of the talonavicular joint capsule on the extensor side of the foot
- Injury of the calcaneocuboid joint
- Fracture of the calcaneus anterior process
- Peroneal tendon injury
- Fracture at the base of the fifth metatarsal
- Fracture of the distal fibula
- Fracture of the lateral process of the talus

Treatment

Conservative

- Ankle joint bracing
- Exercise therapy (conditioning the peroneal muscles and tibialis anterior, proprioception training)
- Physical therapy: ice, manual lymph drainage, compression in the acute stage
- Bracing: rapidly progressive weight bearing in the brace, according to pain tolerance

Operative

Surgery would be indicated only in exceptional cases with three-ligament tears or in competitive athletes.

Prognosis, Complications

- Chronic instability in up to 10% of cases (indication for early secondary capsuloligamentous repair)
- Ankle meniscoid lesion (poor healing of the anterior talofibular ligament with hypertrophic scarring and impingement)
- Lateral osteochondritis dissecans of the talus following an associated osteochondral lesion

Medial Ligaments

Definition

Trauma may cause injury to the superficial and/or deep portions of the deltoid ligament.

Symptoms

Pain and instability about the medial malleolus after inversion or eversion trauma.

Predisposing Factors

- Pes planovalgus
- Lateral ankle sprain

Anatomy and Pathology

The medial (deltoid) ligament complex of the ankle joint consists of both a superficial and a deep layer. Fiber bands are distributed anteriorly to the navicular bone and distally to the talus and calcaneus. The complex includes posterior and anterior tibiotalar parts, a tibiocalcaneal part, and a tibionavicular part. Deltoid ligament injuries are rare compared with lateral ankle sprains.

Imaging

Radiographs

Stress radiographs are no longer used to investigate acute medial ligament injuries. If a fracture is suspected, radiographs of the ankle joint are obtained in two planes. Stress radiographs with side-to-side comparison are justified in the evaluation of chronic instabilities.

Ultrasound

Ultrasound can detect hematoma associated with medial ligament tears. It can also detect discontinuities of individual fiber tracts. Ultrasound has not become established in the routine workup of medial ligament injuries.

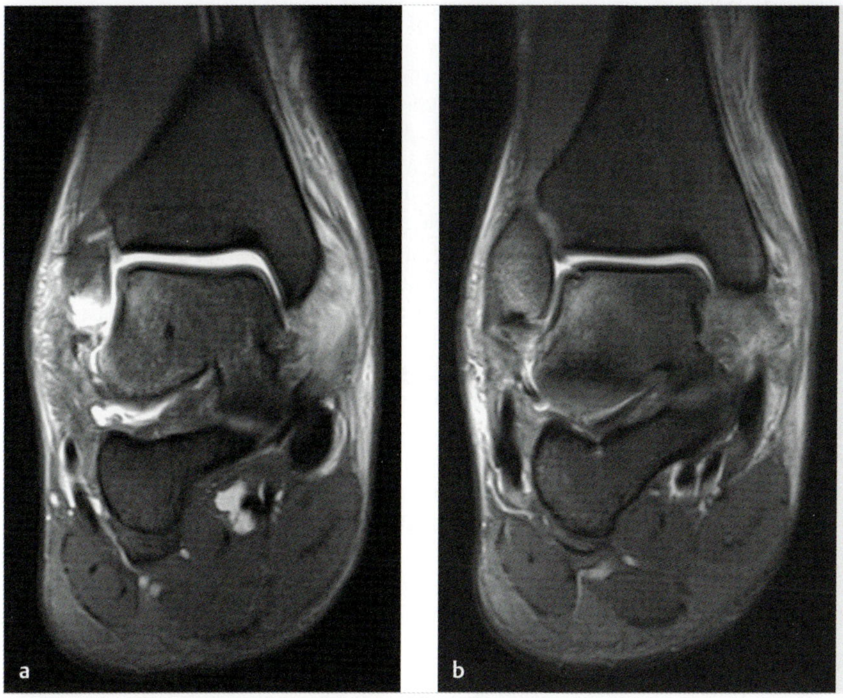

Fig. 3.5 a, b Fresh medial ligament injury in a 20-year-old male with an acute ankle sprain.
a Coronal PD-weighted fat-sat MRI shows significant deltoid ligament injury with rupture of the anterior talotibial ligament, extensive bleeding into other portions of the ligament, and elongated fibers.
b Coronal PD-weighted fat-sat image also shows bone contusion and edema on the lateral shoulder of the talus with a small osteochondral defect and tearing of the anterior talofibular ligament with a small bony avulsion from the tip of the fibula.

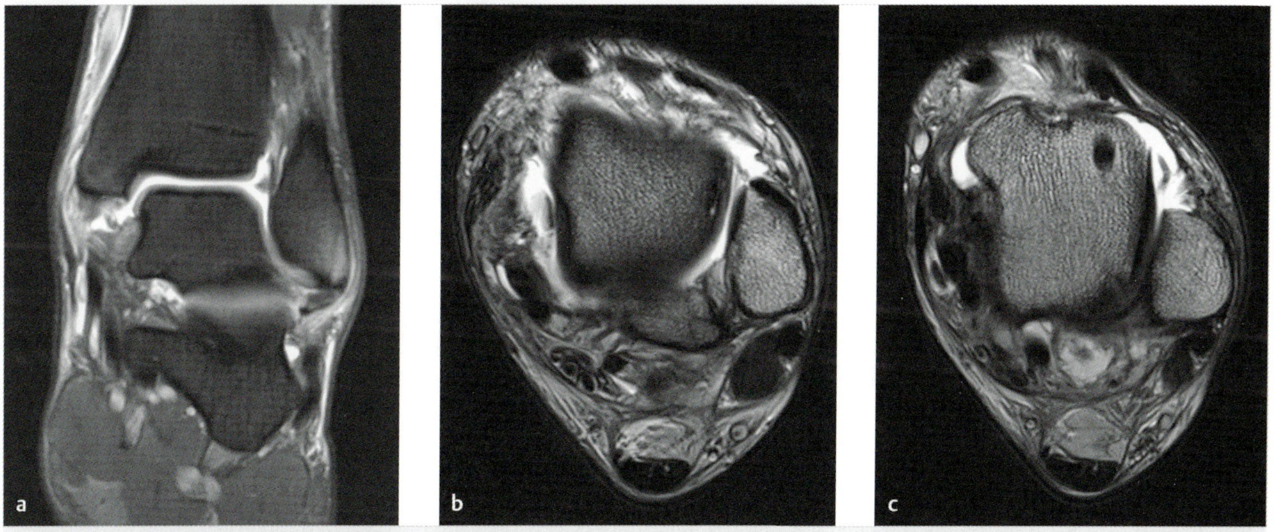

Fig. 3.6 a–c Complete tear of the deltoid ligament.
a Coronal PD-weighted fat-sat image shows a disruption of ligament continuity with a wavy contour of the fiber stumps.
b Axial T2-weighted image shows a complete tear through all portions of the medial ligament over the medial malleolus.
c Axial T2-weighted image also reveals a cortical avulsion of the anterior talofibular ligament from the distal fibula.

MRI

Interpretation Checklist

- Extent of the injury
- Which ligaments are affected (all?)
- Associated injuries (osteochondral lesions, bone contusion and edema, midtarsal joint line, etc.)

Examination Technique

- *Standard trauma protocol:* High-resolution multi-channel coil; contrast administration is not required.
- *Sequences:*
  - Coronal T1-weighted
  - Sagittal and coronal PD-weighted fat-sat
  - Axial T2-weighted, angled parallel to the anterior talofibular ligament
  - If necessary: axial oblique PD-weighted fat-sat sequence in the syndesmotic plane

MRI Findings (▶ Fig. 3.5 and ▶ Fig. 3.6)

- Patchy edema and hemorrhage along the deltoid ligament, usually sparing the strong posterior talotibial ligament
- Wavy contours
- Discontinuity of fascicles

- Joint effusion
- Associated capsular lesion
- Bone contusion and edema
- Possible cortical fragment on the lateral talar border or lateral malleolus

Imaging Recommendation

Modalities of choice: ultrasound and possibly MRI.

Differential Diagnosis

- Fracture of the medial malleolus
- Tear of the posterior tibial tendon
- Fracture of the sustentaculum tali
- Osteochondritis dissecans of the talus
- Osteochondral injury of the subtalar joint
- Talar fracture

Treatment

Conservative

- Stabilization with an ankle brace plus an orthotic insert that encompasses the hindfoot and supports the sustentaculum tali
- Alternative: taping to stabilize the medial side of the ankle

Operative

- Surgical repair is appropriate for extensive tears and chronic instability
- Augmentation of the deltoid ligament with a tendon graft for chronic insufficiency

Prognosis, Complications

Chronic medial instability causes significantly more complaints than lateral instability. It may cause varus angulation of the foot on weight bearing. Healing may be delayed due to heavy scarring.

Syndesmosis

Definition

Syndesmosis rupture is an injury affecting the ligaments connecting the distal ends of the tibia and fibula. It causes instability of the ankle mortise.

Symptoms

A syndesmosis rupture is manifested by a feeling of instability and pain at the level of the syndesmosis on weight bearing. The squeeze test (pressing the fibula and tibia together at the level of the syndesmosis) is positive. Eversion and external rotation at the ankle joint are also painful.

Predisposing Factors

A syndesmosis rupture may occur in association with an ankle sprain or a fracture of the ankle mortise. Tearing of the syndesmosis may also occur as an isolated injury.

Anatomy and Pathology

Anatomy

The tibiofibular syndesmosis is formed by various ligament systems that bind the ankle mortise together (▶ Fig. 3.7). On the anterior side of the syndesmosis, the anterior tibiofibular ligament runs obliquely downward (usually at a 45° angle) from the anterior tubercle of the distal tibia to the anterior tubercle of the fibula at a level approximately 5 mm proximal to the talocrural joint space. It consists of multiple fascicles that arise from a broad area on the tibia and converge as they pass laterally downward to the fibula. Thus the ligament presents a triangular or trapezoidal shape when imaged in an oblique axial plane of section. An accessory ligament distal and parallel to the anterior syndesmosis is called the Bassett ligament. It arises from a slightly more medial site on the tibia than the anterior tibiofibular ligament and is believed to cause syndesmotic impingement on the talus.

The posterior portion of the syndesmosis consists of several ligaments that run horizontally or obliquely between the tibia and fibula:

- *Posterior tibiofibular ligament* (posterior syndesmosis): The strong posterior tibiofibular ligament runs at an approximately 30° angle from the tibia to the fibula.
- *Transverse ligament:* This ligament runs slightly downward and forward from the edge of the fossa of the lateral malleolus along the posterior tibial margin to the posterior aspect of the medial malleolus.
- *Intermalleolar ligament:* blends medially with the transverse ligament and inserts lateral and just cranial to the posterior talofibular ligament.
- *Posterior talofibular ligament:* runs distal to the intermalleolar ligament from the posterior fibula to the talus.

The posterior syndesmosis, like the anterior portion, consists of multiple fascicles with interposed fatty tissue. It almost never tears in its substance, but it may be traumatically avulsed on a bone fragment from the posterior tibial margin (avulsion fracture of the posterior tibial margin, Volkmann triangle, fracture of the "third malleolus"). This fragment is of variable size and may involve the articular surface of the distal tibia.

The interosseous membrane thickens distally into oblique fiber tracts between the tibia and fibula, viz. the interosseous ligament, which has fatty tissue embedded among its fascicles. The syndesmosis consists of three parts: (1) an anterior syndesmosis; (2) a posterior syndesmosis with the posterior tibiofibular ligament, transverse ligament, and intermalleolar ligament; and (3) the interosseous ligament.

Pathology

Rupture of the anterior syndesmosis may occur as an avulsion from the tibia or fibula or as a midsubstance tear. Bony avulsion from the tibia tubercle may also occur (French: *tubercule de Chaput Tillaux*). See the section on Tillaux Fractures (p.48).

Most tears initially involve the oblique anterior tibiofibular ligament, and in addition the interosseous ligament may tear as instability progresses. It is extremely rare for the posterior syndesmosis to tear within its substance, but it may be traumatically avulsed from the posterior tibial margin on a bone fragment of variable size (Volkmann triangle).

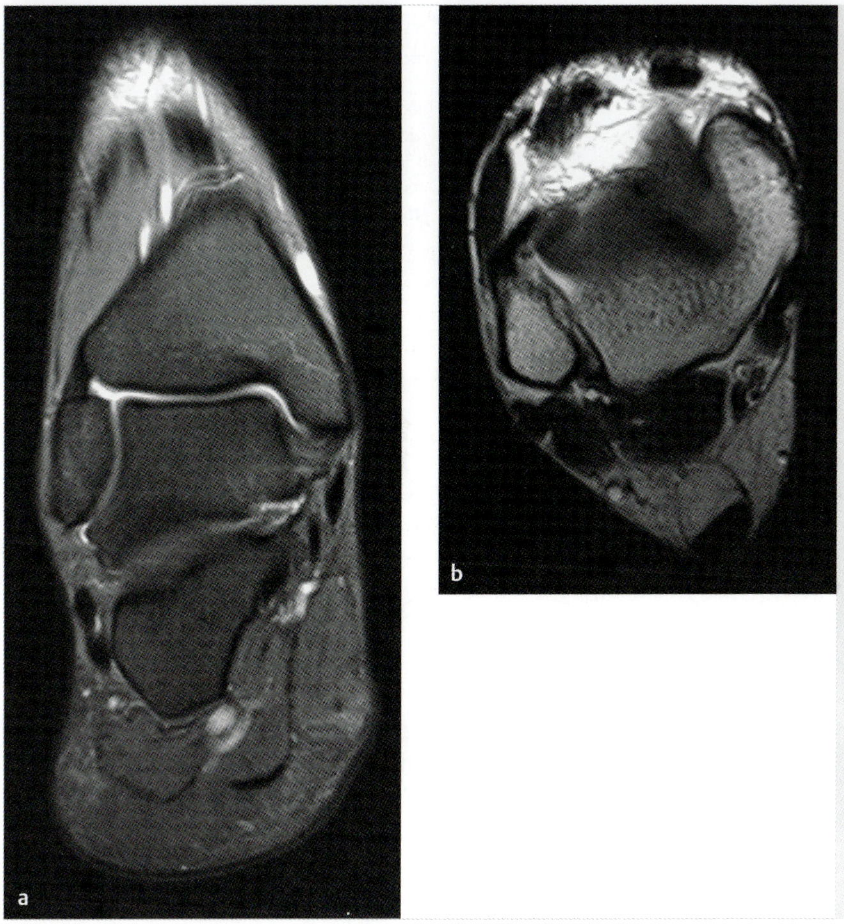

Fig. 3.7 a, b Normal MRI appearance of the anterior syndesmosis.
a Coronal PD-weighted fat-sat image. The anterior syndesmosis is intact and relatively well developed in this patient.
b Axial T2-weighted image shows an intact ligamentous connection between the distal fibula and tibia with no discontinuities.

Imaging

Radiographs

- Take an AP radiograph in 20° of internal rotation for an optimum projection of the fibulotalar joint (the width of the joint space should be equal in its medial, central, and lateral portions).
- Weight-bearing view (e.g., using image intensification fluoroscopy) adds diagnostic information.
- Contrast arthrography is obsolete.
- Visualization of avulsion fractures may be aided by a 45° oblique view with external rotation.

Ultrasound

Routine is the same as for lateral injuries:
- Longitudinal scan through the anterior part of the ankle joint: hemarthrosis?
- Longitudinal scan through the anterior talofibular ligament: continuity? hematoma?
- Rotate the probe to an anterior tibiofibular transverse scan; perform a syndesmosis stress test in maximum passive dorsiflexion and eversion.

Instability is present if the distance between the two bones is greater on the affected side than on the contralateral side.

MRI

! Note

It is important to detect a complete rupture of the anterior syndesmosis, as this is usually an indication for surgical treatment. Reporting the "suspicion" of a complete tear will not be helpful for the orthopedist.

Interpretation Checklist

Accurate image interpretation and reporting requires high-resolution oblique axial sequences with optimum image quality that can define individual fibers.
- Describe the injury to the anterior syndesmosis, interosseous ligament, and posterior tibial margin ("Volkmann triangle")
- Note associated injuries, a possible osteochondral lesion on the talar dome, bone contusion and edema (there may be a coexisting lateral ligament tear in rare cases)

Examination Technique

- *Standard trauma protocol:* High-resolution multi-channel coil; contrast administration is not required.
- *Sequences:*
  - Coronal T1-weighted
  - Sagittal and coronal PD-weighted fat-sat

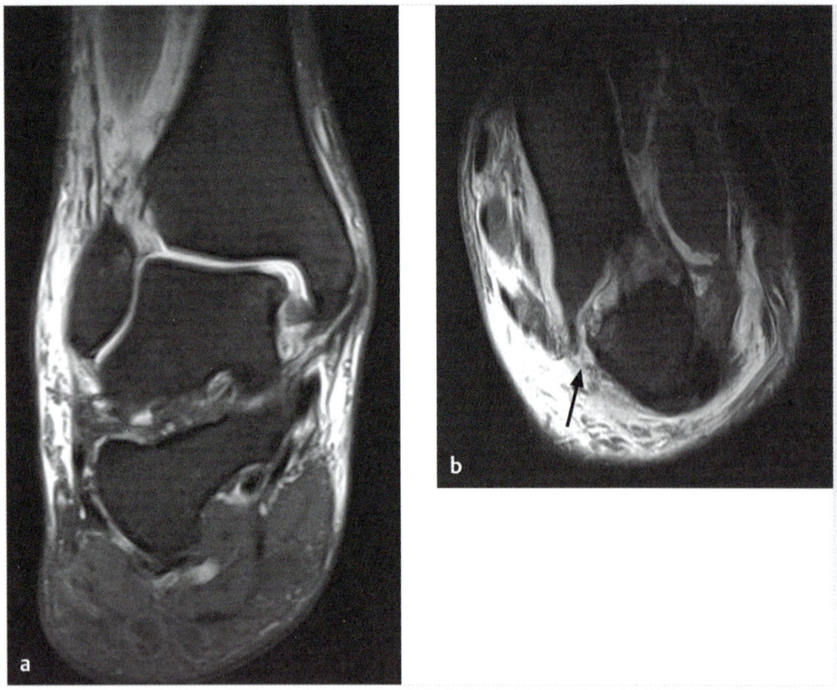

Fig. 3.8 a, b Rupture of the anterior syndesmosis.
a Coronal PD-weighted fat-sat image shows nondelineation of the syndesmotic fibers with widening of the ankle mortise.
b Oblique sagittal PD-weighted fat-sat image angled to the plane of the syndesmosis demonstrates the torn fibers (arrow) with significant associated bleeding into the soft tissues.

  - Axial T2-weighted, angled parallel to the anterior talofibular ligament
  - Axial oblique PD-weighted fat-sat sequence in the syndesmotic plane
- Optimal sequences for evaluation:
  - Coronal and sagittal PD-weighted fat-sat sequence
  - Special sequence angled to the syndesmotic plane (see ▶ Fig. 3.8 b).

MRI Findings (▶ Fig. 3.8 and ▶ Fig. 3.9)

- Wavy fibers of the anterior syndesmosis with associated edema, hemorrhage, and continuity disruption
- Detection of fluid along the interosseous membrane
- Possible avulsion fracture

! Note

A tibiofibular fluid pocket may be misinterpreted as a syndesmosis injury with fluid seepage along the interosseous membrane. A differentiating feature is that the tibiofibular pocket extends only to the tibiofibular notch.

Imaging Recommendation

Modalities of choice: standing AP radiograph (with possible side-to-side comparison) and transverse ultrasound scans over the syndesmosis with stress testing.

Given its importance for further treatment and the difficulty of treating secondary lesions, the authors perform an MRI examination whenever a syndesmosis injury is suspected.

Differential Diagnosis

- Ankle sprain
- Fracture of the ankle mortise
- Osteochondral injury of the ankle joint

Treatment

Syndesmotic injuries are surgically stabilized by screw fixation or TightRope fixation for 6 to 8 weeks. Chronic instability is treatable by an anatomic reconstruction with a peroneus longus graft.

Prognosis, Complications

Chronic instability or stabilization in a faulty position is associated with an increased incidence of degenerative joint changes.

Spring Ligament Injury

Definition

A spring ligament injury is a tear of the plantar calcaneonavicular ligament. This type of injury has a high association with injuries of the posterior tibial tendon and deltoid ligament. The spring ligament is sometimes called the "flatfoot ligament" because it stabilizes the arch and its injury may lead to flattening of the medial pedal arch.

Symptoms

The symptoms of a spring ligament tear include forefoot abduction and sagging of the longitudinal arch with pain in the medial midfoot. The single-heel-rise test is painful. The patient is unable to rise onto the toes of the affected foot in one-legged stance and employs auxiliary movements to compensate for the

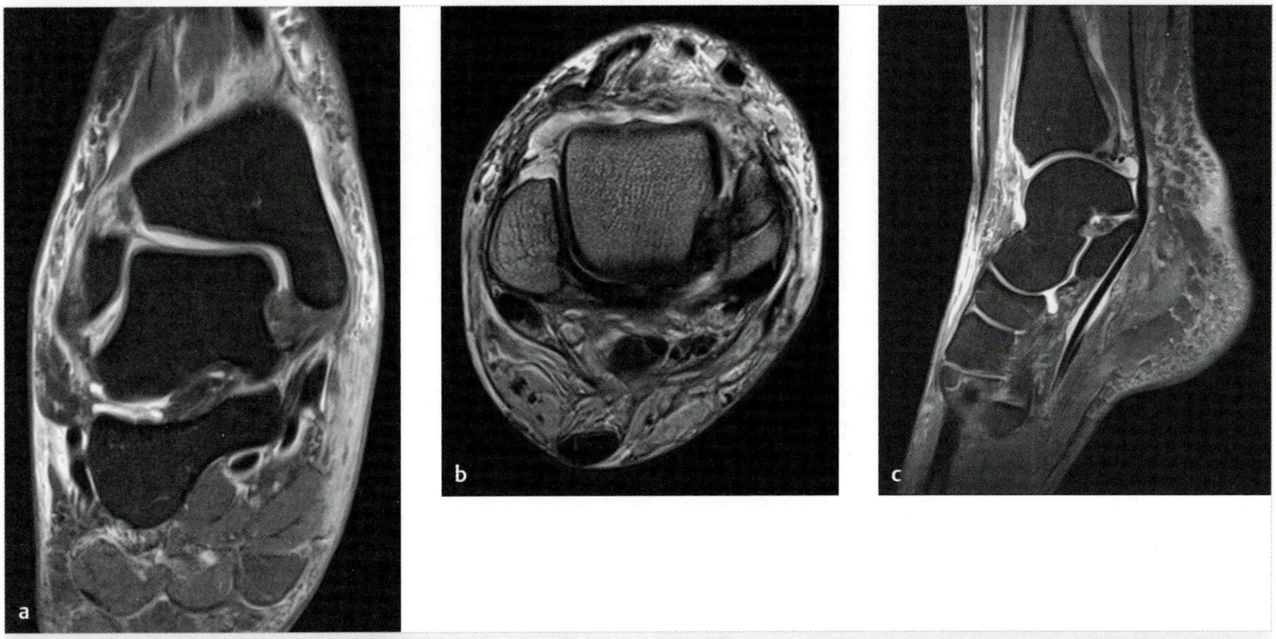

Fig. 3.9 a–c Complete syndesmosis rupture following an ankle sprain.
a Coronal PD-weighted fat-sat image shows discontinuity of the anterior syndesmosis and widening of the ankle mortise with loss of ankle joint congruity.
b Axial T2-weighted image shows a complete tear of the anterior syndesmosis with hemorrhage into the joint space.
c Sagittal PD-weighted fat-sat image shows a small posterior avulsion fracture (Volkmann triangle) and a conspicuous subperiosteal hematoma extending up the posterior tibia.

structural deficiency. Most spring ligament injuries are not diagnosed until several weeks after the trauma.

Predisposing Factors

- Pre-existing hindfoot valgus
- Posterior tibial tendon insufficiency

Anatomy and Pathology

Anatomy

The calcaneonavicular (spring) ligament complex is a key stabilizer of the longitudinal arch and hindfoot. It consists of three parts:

- Inferoplantar longitudinal component
- Oblique medioplantar component
- Superomedial component (located just below the posterior tibial tendon, blends proximally with the deltoid ligament)

The superomedial ligament has an average thickness of 4.8 mm. The thinner inferior component runs plantar and lateral to the superomedial ligament. Its origin is located between the middle and anterior facets of the subtalar joint and fans out to the navicular. The navicular insertion is lateral to the superomedial ligament, and fatty tissue is usually found between the two structures. Fat also delineates the ligament laterally from the bifurcate ligament.

Pathology

The ligament complex runs from its calcaneal origin to the navicular bone, passing like a sling beneath the talar head. With insufficiency or rupture, the talus rotates downward with valgus deviation of the calcaneus, finally corresponding to an acquired pes planovalgus. Spring ligament tears have a high association with posterior tibial insufficiency. They are most commonly seen in middle-aged or older women who sustain a twisting foot injury and have pre-existing posterior tibial insufficiency. Traumatic tears of the spring ligament are extremely rare.

Imaging

Radiographs

Stress radiographs of the foot are obtained in three planes and the two sides are compared. A Saltzman view is also obtained. Side-to-side differences in the tarsometatarsal axis in the AP and lateral views and a decreased overlap of the talar head by the navicular indicate insufficiency of the spring ligament, deltoid ligament, and/or the posterior tibial tendon. Less than a 60% overlap of the talar head is definitely abnormal.

Ultrasound

Ultrasound is not used in routine examinations.

MRI

MRI is seldom requested for investigation of an "acute isolated spring ligament injury." More commonly the tear is one component of a complex hindfoot and midfoot injury.

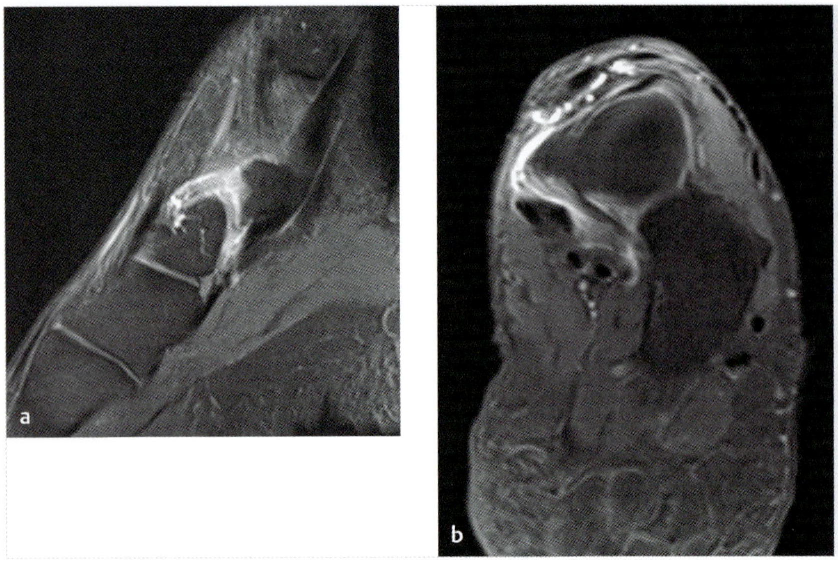

Fig. 3.10 a, b A 47-year-old woman was referred with a diagnosis of "recurrent posterior tibial syndrome."
a Sagittal T1-weighted fat-sat image after contrast administration shows intense enhancement of the plantar calcaneonavicular (spring) ligament between the navicular and calcaneus, consistent with activation in chronic insufficiency.
b Axial oblique T1-weighted fat-sat image after contrast administration. The spring ligament fibers have an expanded, wavy appearance with minimal adjacent posterior tibial peritendinitis.

! Note

It is important to identify the spring ligament and survey it in detail for pre-existing degenerative changes and injuries.

Interpretation Checklist

- Ligament continuity
- Complete or partial tear
- Bony avulsion
- Associated injuries

The MRI report should address all relevant, vulnerable structures of the hindfoot and midfoot.

Because traumatic spring ligament tears often occur in a setting of posterior tibial insufficiency with pre-existing medial instability, it is important to address the entire medial axis with its dynamic stabilizers (posterior tibial tendon) and static stabilizers (spring ligament, superficial portions of the deltoid ligament, plantar fascia, long plantar ligament) when describing the spring ligament injury.

Examination Technique

A spring ligament injury is best evaluated in axial oblique and coronal PD-weighted fat-sat MR sequences.

- *Standard trauma protocol:* High-resolution multi-channel coil; IV contrast administration is helpful due to frequent pre-existing lesions with degenerative changes and increased vascularity.
- *Sequences:*
  - Coronal T1-weighted
  - Sagittal and coronal PD-weighted fat-sat
  - T2-weighted sequence that is precisely axial to the ankle joint
  - Axial oblique PD-weighted fat-sat
  - Sagittal and axial oblique T1-weighted fat-sat perpendicular to the posterior tibial tendon after IV contrast administration

MRI Findings (▶ Fig. 3.10)

- A complete tear, which most commonly involves the superomedial component of the spring ligament ("full-thickness gap")
- Frequent inhomogeneous hyperintensity within the partially thickened ligament components
- Hematomas and other fluid collections
- Increased enhancement around the ligamentous structures
- Chronic instability, which is marked by thickening and enhancement of adjacent structures, most notably the posterior tibial tendon

! Note

Possible errors of interpretation:

- The spring ligament recess is lined by synovium, and the fluid-filled spaces communicate with the midtarsal joint. Thus, fluid detection in the recess should not be misinterpreted as a plantar tear of the spring ligament.
- Frequent inhomogeneous signal intensity in the inferior part of the spring ligament at the sustentaculum tali is caused by fatty tissue and should not be mistaken for a tear.
- All portions of the spring ligament cannot be seen at arthroscopy. The superomedial component is most easily evaluated. This may lead to discrepant findings in which arthroscopy shows an intact ligament while MRI demonstrates a tear.

Imaging Recommendation

Modality of choice: MRI.

Differential Diagnosis

- Posterior tibial tendon insufficiency
- Deltoid ligament tear
- Naviculocalcaneal or talocalcaneal coalition

Treatment

- Surgical repair of the spring ligament
- Correction of hindfoot valgus by a calcaneal sliding osteotomy
- Correction of forefoot abduction by a calcaneal sliding osteotomy

Prognosis, Complications

Prognosis

Lengthy rehabilitation for 6 to 12 months until the patient can resume sports activities.

Possible Complications

- Increasing decompensation of the hindfoot and midfoot
- Progressive hindfoot valgus deformity
- Secondary rupture of the posterior tibial tendon
- Ankle joint changes secondary to hindfoot valgus

Bifurcate Ligament

Definition

A tear of the ligament connecting the anterior process of the calcaneus to the cuboid and navicular bones is usually one component of calcaneocuboid instability (see Calcaneocuboid Joint Injuries (p. 32)).

Symptoms

- Pain over the sinus tarsi
- Possible nonspecific midfoot pain
- Increased pain in response to torsional movements

Predisposing Factors

None are known.

Anatomy and Pathology

The bifurcate ligament arises from the calcaneus and divides anterior to the sinus tarsi into a V-shaped band consisting of two parts:

- *Calcaneonavicular ligament:* runs from the calcaneus to the lateral side of the navicular
- *Calcaneocuboid ligament:* runs from the calcaneus to the medial side of the cuboid

The differential diagnosis of bifurcate ligament injuries should include an avulsion fracture of the anterior calcaneal process.

The classification of bifurcate ligament lesions is shown in ▶ Table 3.1.

Table 3.1 Classification of bifurcate ligament injuries

Grade	Description
I	Mild sprain
II	Partial tear
III	Complete tear

Imaging

Radiographs

Weight-bearing radiographs of the foot are obtained in three planes according to pain tolerance. Fractures of the anterior calcaneal process are best appreciated in the oblique view.

Ultrasound

Not indicated.

CT

CT can clearly demonstrate avulsion fractures of the anterior calcaneal process.

MRI

MRI is rarely indicated for bifurcate ligament injuries. However, MRI should be considered after complex hindfoot trauma with high rotational moments to check for ligament and cartilage injuries. MRI is more commonly used for the investigation of nonspecific midfoot pain persisting for more than about 6 weeks after trauma.

Interpretation Checklist

- Evaluate the capsuloligamentous structures of the midtarsal joint.
- Scroll through all ligament components and describe the lesion location.
- Evaluate:
  - Alignment in the midtarsal joint
  - Zones of subchondral bone contusion
  - Avulsion fracture of the anterior calcaneal process
  - Effusion
  - Hemorrhage in the calcaneocuboid joint, talonavicular joint, or anterior facet of the subtalar joint
- Address all vulnerable structures of the hindfoot and midfoot.

Examination Technique

- *Standard trauma protocol:* High-resolution multi-channel coil; contrast administration is not required
- Sequences:
  - Sagittal T1-weighted
  - Sagittal and coronal PD-weighted fat-sat
  - Axial oblique PD-weighted fat-sat sequence perpendicular to the hindfoot tendons
  - If necessary: axial T2-weighted sequence angled parallel to the anterior talofibular ligament

MRI Findings (▶ Fig. 3.11)

- Patchy hyperintensities along the ligamentous structures in fat-suppressed, water-sensitive sequences
- Wavy contours
- Circumscribed discontinuity indicating a complete tear
- Avulsion fracture of the anterior calcaneal process (T1-weighted sequences)
- Altered calcaneocuboid joint alignment with loss of joint congruity
- Subchondral bone contusion and edema on the articulating surfaces

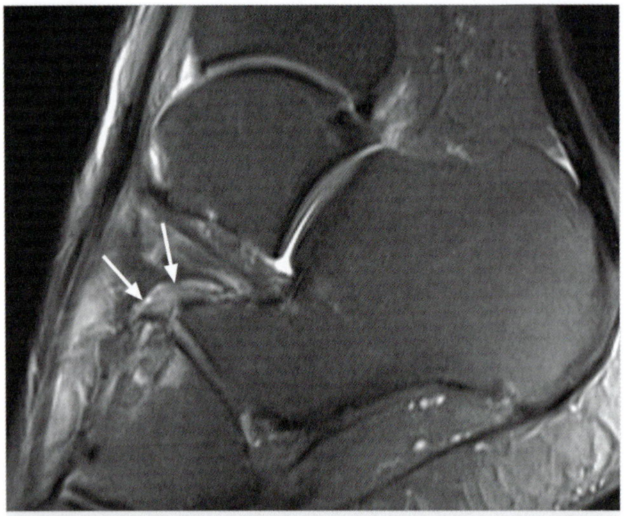

Fig. 3.11 Traumatic sprain of the bifurcate ligament. Sagittal PD-weighted fat-sat image shows moderate hemorrhage along the bifurcate ligament (calcaneocuboid part) with mild bone contusion and edema on the proximal dorsal edge of the cuboid on the articular side.

- Patchy hemorrhage in the soft tissues around the bifurcate ligament and inside the joint

Imaging Recommendation

Modalities of choice: radiography, MRI.

Differential Diagnosis

- Fracture of the anterior calcaneal process
- Tear of the calcaneocuboid ligaments
- Lisfranc ligament injury
- Subtalar joint sprain

Treatment

- *Grade I:* orthotic insert that encompasses the hindfoot and supports the longitudinal arch; partial weight bearing for 2 weeks, then progress to full weight bearing in increments
- *Grade II:* orthotic insert that encompasses the hindfoot and supports the longitudinal arch; PneumoWalker for 6 weeks; non-weight bearing for 2 weeks, then gradual progression to full weight bearing
- *Grade III:* non-weight bearing for 6 weeks in a PneumoWalker or plaster cast, then incremental weight bearing with an orthotic insert that encompasses the hindfoot and supports the longitudinal arch

Prognosis, Complications

Prognosis

The injury will heal completely in most cases. Most adverse late sequelae result from associated injuries such as cartilage lesions or fissuring of articular surfaces.

Possible Complications

- Scar adhesions in the sinus tarsi
- Secondary degenerative changes resulting from instability or the primary trauma

Calcaneocuboid Joint Injuries

Definition

Ligamentous injuries of the calcaneocuboid joint may consist of partial or complete tears.

Symptoms

- Pain and subjective instability on the lateral side of the foot
- Pain exacerbated by forefoot adduction
- With chronic instability, pain is felt while walking on uneven ground and midfoot pain is felt on side-cutting maneuvers

Initial differentiation from a lateral ankle sprain is often difficult.

Predisposing Factors

Tears of the calcaneocuboid ligament are rare. Special predisposing factors are sports that involve rapid directional changes while wearing cleats. The fixation of the forefoot on the ground combined with a high body torque over the foot is likely to cause forefoot injury. In soccer, shoes that have little midfoot stability are considered a risk factor for calcaneocuboid joint injury.

Anatomy and Pathology

Anatomy

The midtarsal joint (Chopart joint) consists of two separate articulations:

- Talonavicular joint
- Calcaneocuboid joint

When the calcaneus is everted, the axes of the talonavicular and calcaneocuboid joints assume a parallel alignment that allows motion in the midtarsal joint. When the foot is inverted, the two axes diverge in a way that restricts midtarsal joint motility. This mechanism stabilizes the foot in the push-off phase of gait.

The calcaneocuboid joint has a saddle-shaped surface and represents the functional link between the subtalar and midtarsal joints. The joint derives its ligamentous stability from the strong plantar calcaneocuboid ligament (reinforces the dorsal calcaneocuboid joint capsule) and the thinner bifurcate ligament (consisting of calcaneocuboid and calcaneonavicular parts, the key ligament of the midtarsal joint). The dorsal calcaneocuboid ligament runs from the lateral surface of the calcaneus to the dorsal surface of the cuboid.

There are many variations in the shape, number, and attachments of the calcaneocuboid ligament. The dorsal ligament is invariant. There is a somewhat narrower accessory lateral ligament, which usually runs upward from its proximal to distal end and is present in 50 to 66% of the population.

Table 3.2 Classification of calcaneocuboid joint injuries

Grade	Description
I	Joint space opening < 10°, mild sprain or partial tear with no bony injury
II	Joint space opening > 10°, complete ligament tear without bony injury or with a small flake
III	Joint space opening > 10°, ligament rupture with a large flake
IV	Joint space opening > 10°, ligament rupture with a bony joint injury (compression fracture of the cuboid)

Pathology

Mechanisms of Injury

- *Calcaneocuboid ligament:* injured by forced plantar flexion and inversion, often combined with injury to the medial column of the foot in the form of a navicular "nutcracker fracture" (see 4.1.3 Navicular Fracture in Chapter 4) or a cuneonavicular dislocation
- *Bifurcate ligament:* combined plantar flexion, supination, adduction, and inversion—after "stubbing the small toe," for example. Rarely, dorsiflexion and inversion are causative. May also be associated with an avulsion fracture of the anterior calcaneal process.

Calcaneocuboid joint injuries are classified by their degree of instability (▶ Table 3.2).

Imaging

Radiographs

Weight-bearing radiographs of the foot are obtained in three planes according to pain tolerance. Bony ligament avulsions are best appreciated in oblique and DP projections.

Stress radiographs to evaluate joint space opening in the acute stage are rewarding only when obtained under general anesthesia. In patients with chronic instability, stress radiographs will document differences in ligament constraint when the left and right sides are compared.

Ultrasound

A lateral longitudinal scan over the joint, parallel to the sole of the foot, can demonstrate increased joint space opening and small bone fragments. Ultrasound is particularly useful for narrowing the differential diagnosis (lateral ankle sprain, syndesmosis rupture).

The direct visualization of a tear of the calcaneocuboid ligament or bifurcate ligament is difficult with ultrasound. Scanning with a varus stress may be attempted, depending on complaints, and may reveal dehiscence or instability. Hematomas are indicative of an injury.

CT

CT is helpful for evaluating bone avulsions, subchondral fragments, and intra-articular fracture lines.

MRI

Interpretation Checklist

MRI is used mainly in patients with complex rotational injuries of the hindfoot and midfoot to investigate pain of unknown cause.

- Describe the location of the capsuloligamentous tear.
- Note the degree of malalignment.
- Evaluate the entire midtarsal joint line.
- Evaluate the bifurcate ligament, adjacent structures, and the status of the calcaneocuboid articular cartilage.

Examination Technique

- *Standard trauma protocol:* High-resolution multi-channel coil; contrast administration is not required.
- *Sequences:*
  - Sagittal T1-weighted
  - Sagittal and coronal PD-weighted fat-sat
  - Axial oblique PD-weighted fat-sat
  - If necessary: axial oblique T2-weighted sequence parallel to the anterior talofibular ligament

MRI Findings

- Focal hyperintensities
- Bleeding and discontinuity in the joint capsule with intra-articular effusion
- Hemorrhagic areas in periarticular soft tissues
- Possible associated injuries along the Chopart joint line
- Bony avulsion of the capsule from the anterior calcaneal process, or occasionally from the cuboid

Imaging Recommendation

Modalities of choice: radiography, CT, MRI.

Differential Diagnosis

- Bifurcate ligament tear
- Fracture of the anterior calcaneal process
- Peroneal tendon injury
- Painful os peroneum
- Lateral ankle sprain
- Distal fibular fracture
- Injury to the fifth metatarsal base
- Subtalar joint instability

Treatment

- *Grade I:* tape for 4 to 6 weeks
- *Grade II:* "boot" for 6 weeks; ligament reconstruction for chronic instability
- *Grade III:* surgical repair or reconstruction
- *Grade IV:* ligament reconstruction, possible ligament reinforcement, removal of bone fragments

Prognosis, Complications

Prognosis

Calcaneocuboid joint injuries generally have a good prognosis for return to athletic activities. Chronic instability can be treated by surgical repair of the capsuloligamentous structures by a tendon transfer (plantaris longus) or allograft reconstruction. Late changes usually result from cartilage injuries sustained in the primary trauma.

Possible Complications

- Chronic instability
- Secondary degenerative changes in the calcaneocuboid joint
- Persistent problems in 20 to 40% of patients
- Acute and chronic painful instability (approximately 33% of patients) with some degree of athletic disability

3.1.2 Fractures

A. Staebler and M. Walther

Ankle Fractures

Definition

Ankle fractures are fractures of the distal fibula that involve the talocrural joint. They are the most common fractures of the lower limb and are classified by the level of the fibular fracture in relation to the syndesmosis (Danis–Weber classification).

Symptoms

- Pain and swelling on the lateral side of the ankle and possibly over the syndesmosis
- Deformity due to lateral or posterior subluxation
- Inability or decreased ability to bear weight on the affected ankle

Predisposing Factors

- Football sports, especially soccer
- Running sports

Anatomy and Pathology

Anatomy

The ankle or talocrural joint is formed by the articulation of the distal tibia (medial malleolus), distal fibula (lateral malleolus), and talus. The ankle mortise is stabilized by powerful syndesmotic ligaments (anterior, posterior, central) and the interosseous membrane. The lateral ligaments (anterior talofibular ligament, calcaneofibular ligament, posterior talofibular ligament) and the triangular medial ligament (deltoid ligament) stabilize the position of the talus.

Pathology

Danis–Weber Classification

This classification of ankle fractures is shown in ▶ Table 3.3.

If the fibular fracture is accompanied by a fracture of the medial malleolus, the injury is classified as a bimalleolar ankle fracture. If there is also an avulsion fracture of the posterior tibial margin (Volkmann triangle), the fracture is called a trimalleolar ankle fracture, the distal tibial margin being counted as the "third malleolus."

In Weber C fractures, the interosseous membrane is torn from the level of the ankle joint line to the fibular fracture. The fracture starts at the medial malleolus and progresses laterally to the fibula, with an associated rupture of the deltoid ligament. The order of failure in a Weber C fracture is from the medial malleolus and deltoid ligament through the ankle joint space, through the syndesmosis, and finally through the fibula above the joint line.

Lauge–Hansen Classification

Ankle fractures in this system are classified according to foot position and pattern of injury (▶ Table 3.4).

The Lauge–Hansen classification is important historically but has been largely superseded by the Danis–Weber and AO/ASIF classifications.

AO/ASIF Classification

The classification of ankle fractures developed by the AO/ASIF (Arbeitsgemeinschaft für Osteosynthese and Association for the Study of Internal Fixation) follows the principle of the Weber classification (44A, 44B, 44C) by using the syndesmosis as a reference point for the fibular fracture. Concomitant fractures of the medial malleolus, such as fractures of the posterior tibial margin, cause increased instability and ankle joint disruption with an increasing danger to the joint, including long-term disability. Consequently they are assigned higher stages in the AO/ASIF classification.

- *44A injuries:* These are fibular injuries below the level of the syndesmosis, which is always intact.
  - 44A1 injuries: The lowest stage is the lateral ligament tear (44A1.1, ▶ Fig. 3.12 a) in which the ligament is injured while the fibula is intact. Avulsion fractures of the distal tip of the fibula without a medial malleolar fracture are classified as 44A1.2 (▶ Fig. 3.12 b), and transverse fibular fractures below the syndesmosis without a medial malleolar fracture as 44A1.3 (▶ Fig. 3.12 c).

Table 3.3 The Danis–Weber classification of ankle fractures

Grade	Description
Weber A	Generally horizontal avulsion fracture below the level of the syndesmosis; the syndesmosis is intact
Weber B	Oblique posterosuperior-to-anteroinferior fracture of the fibula in the coronal plane at the level of the syndesmosis; the syndesmosis may be intact or torn
Weber C	Fibular fracture above the syndesmosis; the syndesmosis is invariably torn

Table 3.4 Lauge–Hansen classification of ankle fractures based on foot position and mechanism of injury

Type of fracture	Description
Supination/adduction (SA)	• Transverse fracture of the fibula distal to the articular surface or lateral ligament injury • Vertical fracture of the medial malleolus (wedge fracture)
Supination/external-rotation (SL)	• Avulsion of the anterior tibiofibular ligament • Oblique or spiral fracture of the distal fibula • Avulsion of the posterior tibiofibular ligament or avulsion fracture of a posterior wedge • Fracture of the medial malleolus or rupture of the deltoid ligament
Pronation/abduction (PA)	• Transverse fracture of the medial malleolus • Rupture of the syndesmotic ligaments or avulsion fracture of their insertion sites • Horizontal or transverse fracture of the fibula above the plane of the articular surface
Pronation/external-rotation, including the Maisonneuve fracture	• Transverse fracture of the medial malleolus or rupture of the deltoid ligament • Rupture of the anterior tibiofibular ligament • Oblique fracture of the fibula above the plane of the articular surface • Rupture of the posterior tibiofibular ligament or avulsion fracture of the posterolateral tibial margin
Pronation/dorsiflexion fixation (vertical compression) (PD)	• Fracture of the medial malleolus • Fracture of the anterior tibial margin • Fracture of the fibula in its middle or proximal third • Wedge fracture of the posterior tibial articular surface (on a continuum with tibial pilon fractures)

 - 44A2 injuries: A concomitant fracture of the medial malleolus increases the subcategory from 1 to 2. A lateral ligament tear with a medial malleolar fracture is classified as 44A2.1 (▶ Fig. 3.12 d). An avulsion fracture of the distal tip of the fibula plus a medial malleolar fracture is 44A2.2 (▶ Fig. 3.12 e). Besides supination in the ankle joint, an adducting force acts upon the talus. A horizontal fibular fracture below the syndesmosis with an oblique or vertical fracture of the medial malleolus is classified as 44A2.3 and also involves a supination injury with an adducting force on the talus (▶ Fig. 3.12 f). In a dislocation, the medial shoulder of the talus may cause a comminuted area with impaction of the medial tibia (44A2.3 with tibial impaction, ▶ Fig. 3.12 g).
 - 44A3 injuries: In these injuries, supination at the ankle joint with an adducting force on the talus gives rise to shear forces causing posteromedial extension of the medial malleolar fracture (▶ Fig. 3.12 h).
- *44B injuries:*
 - 44B1 injuries: The most common mechanism involves maximum supination and axial compression causing an oblique fibular fracture in the coronal plane with a posterosuperior-to-anteroinferior orientation. The anterior syndesmosis may be intact (44B1.1, ▶ Fig. 3.13 a) or torn (44B1.2, ▶ Fig. 3.13 b). These injuries correspond to type B in the Weber classification and AO/ASIF classification (44B) and to stage I–II supination/external-rotation fractures in the Lauge–Hansen classification. If a third bone fragment is created by avulsion of the anterior syndesmosis from the proximal part of the fibula, a multipart fracture results (44B1.3, ▶ Fig. 3.13 c).
 - 44B2 injuries: If a displaced oblique fibular fracture at the level of the syndesmosis is accompanied by a ruptured deltoid ligament, the syndesmosis is also ruptured and instability is increased due to the added medial disruption (44B2.1, ▶ Fig. 3.13 d). The injury to the syndesmosis may be purely ligamentous or there may be an avulsion fracture of the distal fibula (Le Fort–Wagstaffe fracture) or tibia (Tillaux–Chaput fracture). A transverse or oblique fracture of the medial malleolus is classified as 44B2.2 (▶ Fig. 3.13 e). Adding a multipart fracture of the fibula makes it a 44B2.3 injury (▶ Fig. 3.13 f).
 - 44B3 injuries. An oblique fibular fracture at the level of the syndesmosis with a syndesmosis tear or bony avulsion (Le Fort–Wagstaffe or Tillaux–Chaput fracture) and medial malleolar fracture may be associated with fractures of the posterior tibial margin (44B3). These fractures may involve a small bony avulsion of the posterior syndesmosis or may include larger fragments encompassing a substantial part of the tibial articular surface. Analogous to B2 fractures, B3 fractures are subclassified as 1, 2, or 3 depending on whether the deltoid ligament is torn (44B3.1, ▶ Fig. 3.13 g), the medial malleolus is fractured (44B3.2, ▶ Fig. 3.13 h), or the fibular fracture is comminuted (44B3.3, ▶ Fig. 3.13 i).
- *44C injuries:* Type C fractures result from a pronation and external-rotation mechanism, starting with a rupture of the deltoid ligament or a fracture of the medial malleolus. This leads to anterior displacement of the talus and external rotation with a spiral fracture of the fibula as that bone rotates on its longitudinal axis. The anterior syndesmosis and interosseous ligament rupture, and the fibula fractures above the syndesmosis. 44C fractures correspond to types I–IV pronation/eversion fractures in the Lauge–Hansen classification. They are highly unstable injuries.
 - 44C1 injuries: Type 44C1.1 is a fibular fracture above the syndesmosis plus a torn deltoid ligament (▶ Fig. 3.14 a). In

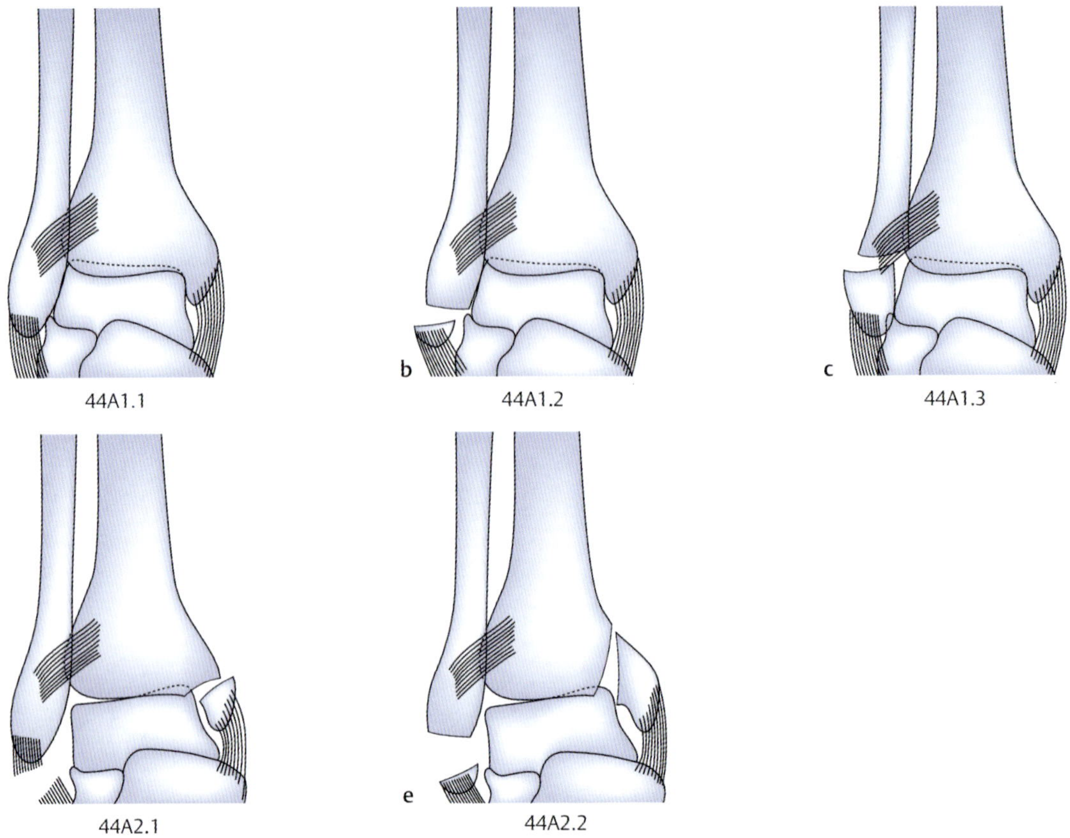

Fig. 3.12 a–h AO/ASIF classification of ankle fractures: 44A injuries. This category denotes fibular injuries below the level of the syndesmosis, which is always intact.
a Lateral ligament tear.
b Avulsion fracture of the distal tip of the fibula with an intact medial malleolus.
c Transverse fibular fracture below the syndesmosis with an intact medial malleolus.
d Lateral ligament tear with a fracture of the medial malleolus.
e Avulsion fracture of the distal tip of the fibula with a fracture of the medial malleolus.

a 44C1.2 injury, the fibular fracture is accompanied by a fracture of the medial malleolus (▶ Fig. 3.14 b). Type 44C1.3 is a fibular fracture above the syndesmosis plus a medial malleolar fracture and a fracture of the posterior tibial margin (▶ Fig. 3.14 c).

- 44C2 injuries: The fibular fracture above the syndesmosis is a wedge fracture or includes additional fragments. Subtypes are analogous to 44C1 fractures and depend on whether the deltoid ligament is torn (44C2.1, ▶ Fig. 3.14 d), the medial malleolus is fractured (44C2.2, ▶ Fig. 3.14 e), or there is an associated fracture of the posterior tibial margin (44C2.3, ▶ Fig. 3.14 f).
- 44C3 injuries: High fibular fractures that involve the ankle joint can rupture the anterior syndesmosis plus central portions of the syndesmosis and the interosseous membrane—from the ankle joint to the level of the fibular fracture—and are known as Maisonneuve fractures. Designated as 44C3.3 in the AO/ASIF classification (▶ Fig. 3.14 i), this injury is a pronation/eversion fracture in the Lauge-Hansen classification, like the other type C injuries. Subtypes 1 and 2 are distinguished by the absence (44C3.1) or presence of fibular shortening (44C3.2). There are variants with a ruptured deltoid ligament or medial malleolar fracture, both with and without an associated Volkmann triangle fracture of the posterior tibial margin. In very rare cases the proximal injury may be a ligamentous dislocation of the proximal tibiofibular joint, but generally the fracture occurs through the neck of the proximal fibula or through its proximal third.

Imaging (▶ see Figs. 3.15–3.21)

Radiographs

Radiography of the ankle joint is performed in two planes. The DP view is taken with 15 to 20° of internal rotation to display the syndesmosis and give a nonsuperimposed view of the distal fibula. Additional 45° oblique views may be helpful in some cases. Stress radiographs have been replaced by MRI.

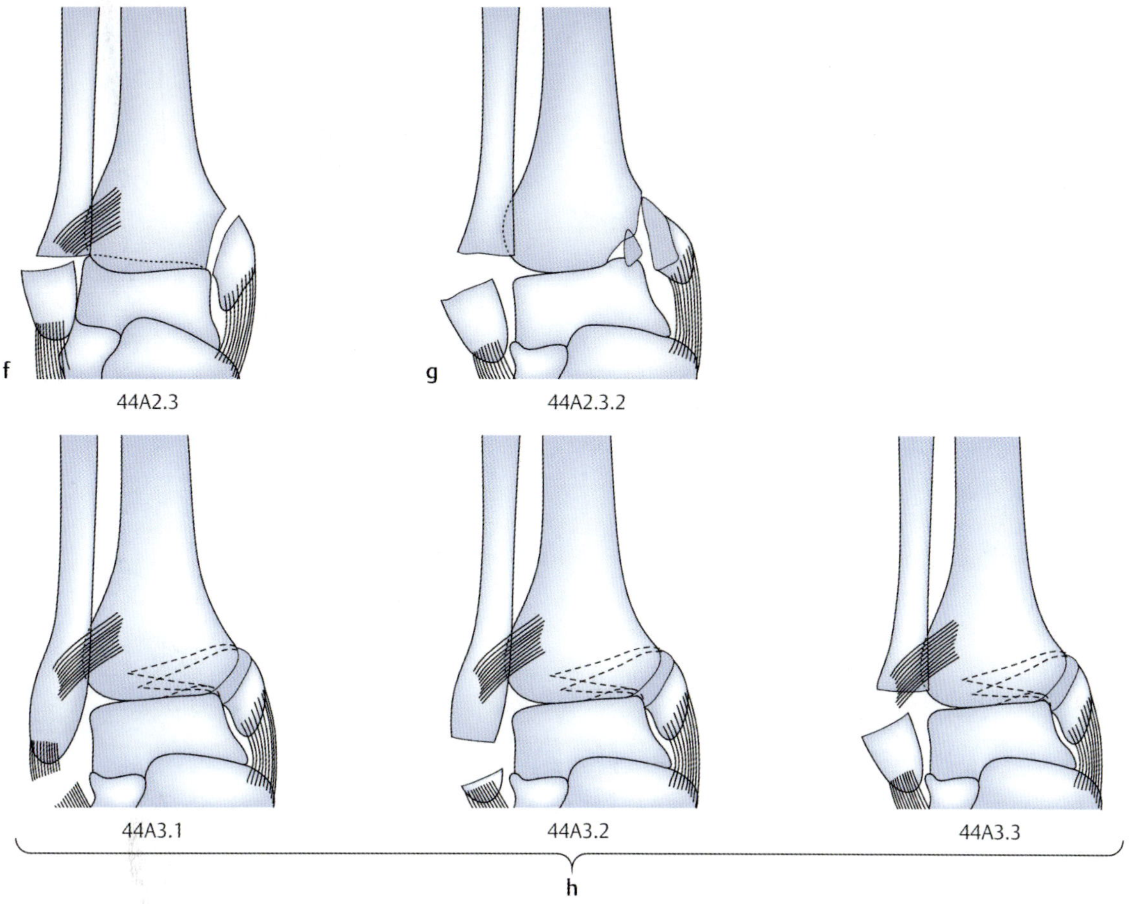

Fig. 3.12 AO/ASIF classification on ankle fractures: 44A injuries continued.
f Horizontal fibular fracture below the syndesmosis with an oblique or vertical fracture of the medial malleolus.
g Type 44A2.3 injury with tibial impaction.
h Posterior extension of the medial malleolar fracture.

! Note

Ottawa ankle rules: Patients with an ankle injury should be X-rayed if any one of the following criteria is met, indicating that a fracture is probably present:

- The patient cannot bear weight acutely or during the examination, or
- bone tenderness is noted at the tip of the lateral malleolus or the posterior edge of the fibula, or
- bone tenderness is noted at the tip of the medial malleolus or the posterior edge of the tibia.

Ultrasound

Ultrasound can detect a discontinuity in the echogenic bony surface as well as hypoechoic thickening of the periosteum (especially in pediatric fractures) caused by a hematoma.

CT

CT should employ high-resolution technique (≤ 0.5-mm slice thickness), overlapping reconstructions, and multiplanar reformatting (MPR). In patients with comminuted fractures, articular step-offs, or avulsions of the anterior syndesmosis (Le Fort–Wagstaffe fracture or Tillaux fracture), CT can accurately determine joint status and give nonsuperimposed views of bone fragments. This can supply crucial information for therapeutic decision-making and preoperative planning.

CT should be used postoperatively if there is the slightest suspicion of malalignment or articular discontinuity. Especially in the ankle joint, an anatomic reconstruction of the articular surfaces should be of primary concern.

MRI

MRI is generally unnecessary for the investigation of ankle fractures. MRI is the only modality that can evaluate the anterior syndesmosis. Occult fractures of the posterior tibial margin are clearly depicted by MRI.

Interpretation Checklist

- Articular cartilage of the ankle joint including the shoulders of the talus
- Lateral ligaments intact or torn?
- Anterior syndesmosis intact or torn?
- Fractures of the posterior tibial margin

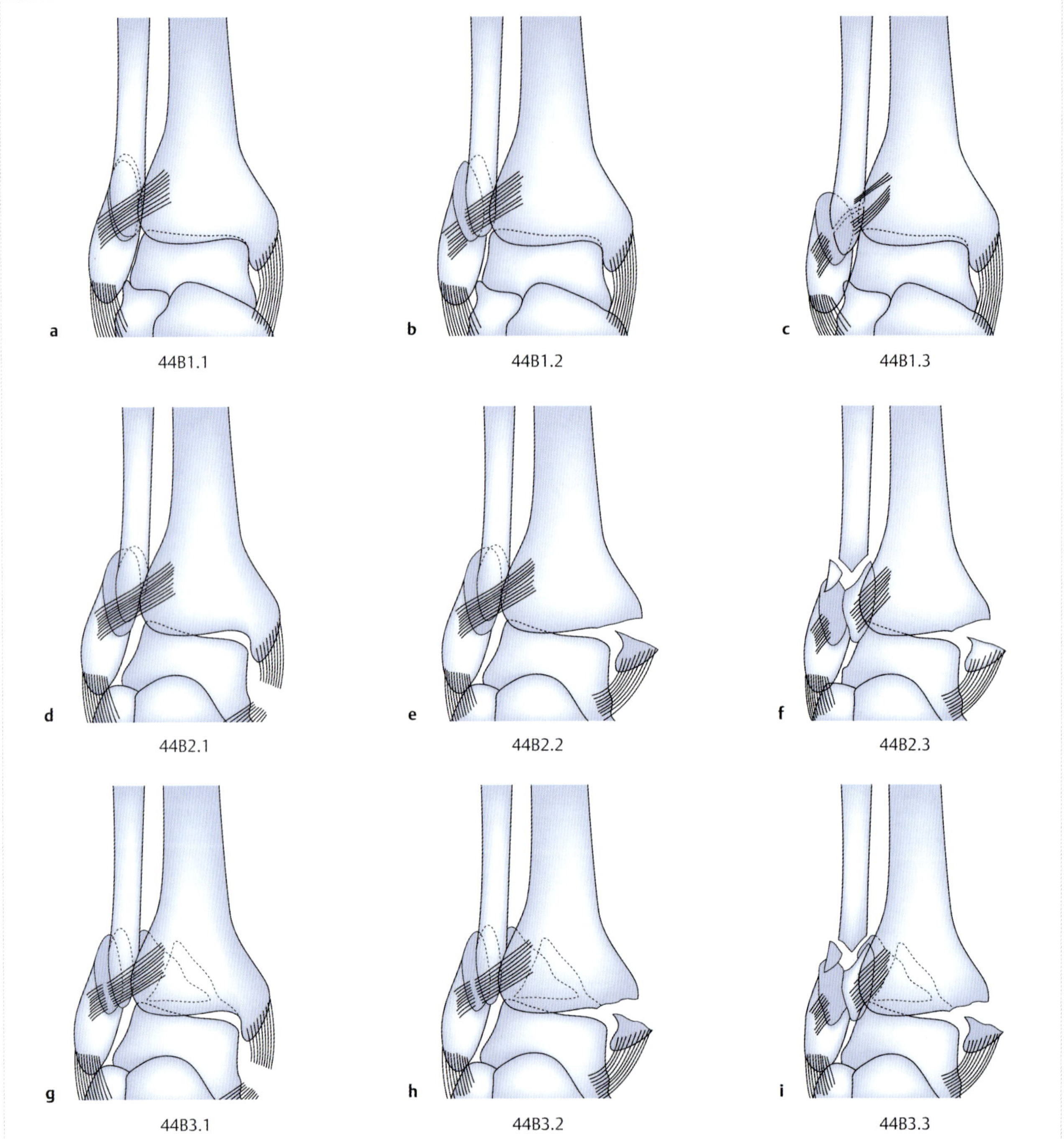

Fig. 3.13 a–i AO/ASIF classification of ankle fractures: 44B injuries. This category denotes coronal-plane fibular fractures that have a posterosuperior-to-anteroinferior orientation.
a The anterior syndesmosis is intact.
b With injury to the anterior syndesmosis.
c With a multipart fracture.
d With rupture of the deltoid ligament.
e With a transverse or oblique fracture of the medial malleolus.
f With multipart fractures of the fibula and medial malleolus.
g Oblique fibular fracture at the level of the syndesmosis with rupture of the syndesmosis plus a fracture of the posterior tibial margin.
h Oblique fibular fracture, syndesmosis rupture, fracture of the posterior tibial margin, and fracture of the medial malleolus.
i Same as **h**, but with a multipart fracture of the fibula.

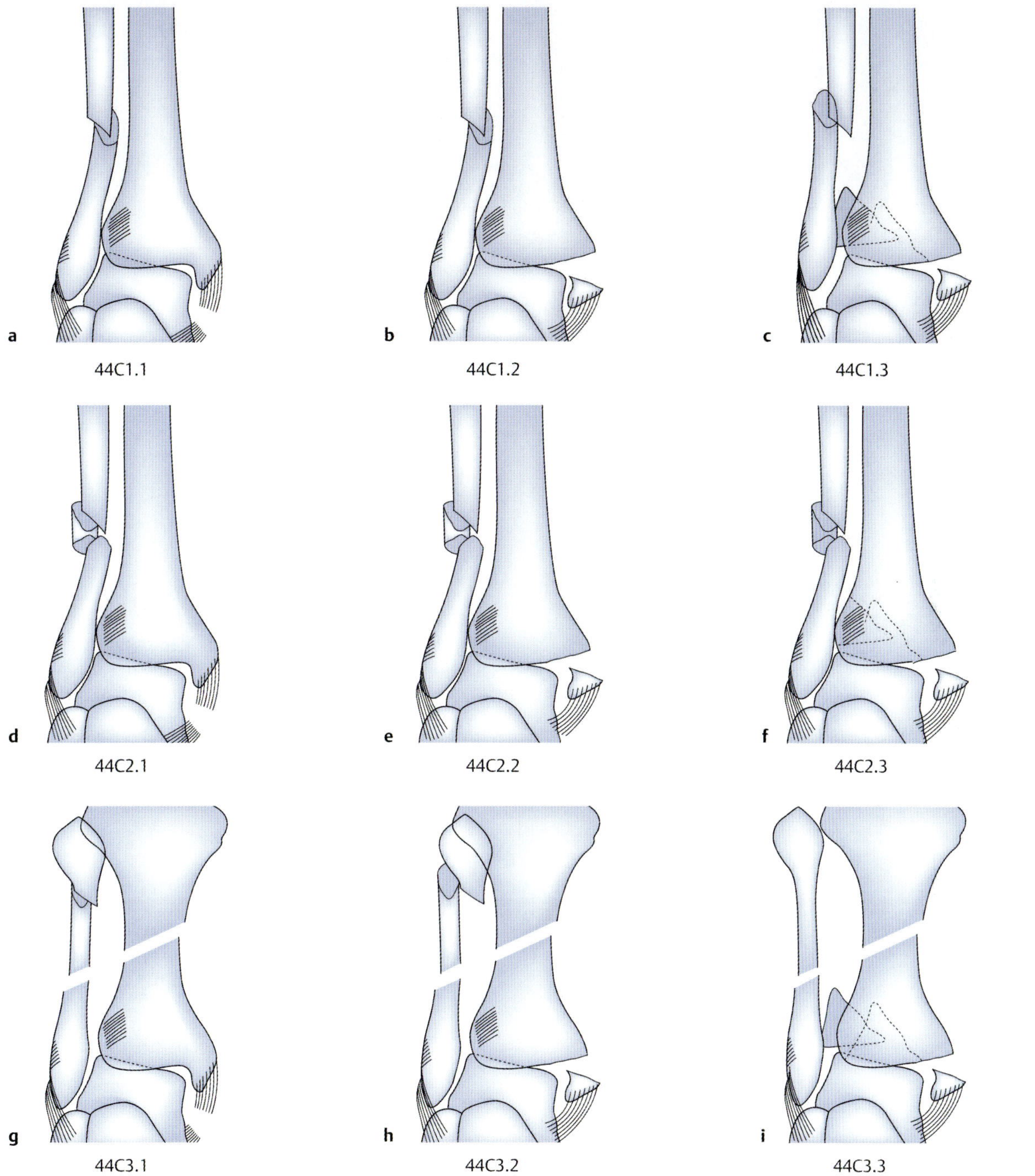

Fig. 3.14 a–i AO/ASIF classification of ankle fractures: 44C injuries. These are fibular fractures above the syndesmosis with associated tears of the anterior syndesmosis and interosseous ligaments.
a Fibular fracture above the syndesmosis with a torn deltoid ligament.
b Fibular fracture above the syndesmosis with a fracture of the medial malleolus.
c Fibular fracture above the syndesmosis with fractures of the medial malleolus and posterior tibial margin.
d Fibular fracture above the syndesmosis with a wedge or other fragments plus a torn deltoid ligament.
e Fibular fracture above the syndesmosis with a wedge or other fragments and a medial malleolar fracture.
f Fibular fracture above the syndesmosis with a wedge or other fragments, a medial malleolar fracture, and a fracture of the posterior tibial margin.
g Fracture of the proximal fibula above the syndesmosis with no shortening and no Volkmann triangle fracture.
h Fracture of the proximal fibula above the syndesmosis with shortening and no Volkmann triangle fracture.
i Fracture of the proximal fibula above the syndesmosis with a medial malleolar fracture and a Volkmann triangle fracture.

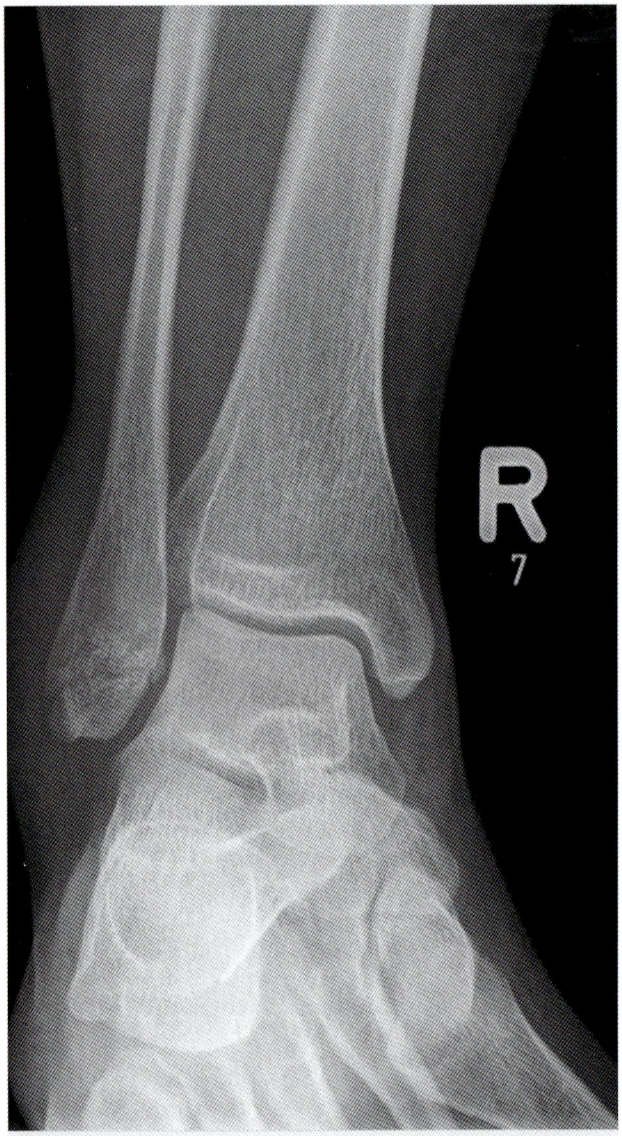

Fig. 3.15 Weber A fracture. Radiograph shows a near-horizontal avulsion fracture of the distal fibula below the syndesmosis with associated soft-tissue swelling.

Examination Technique

- *Standard trauma protocol:* High-resolution multi-channel coil; contrast administration is not required.
- *Sequences:*
  - Coronal T1-weighted sequence angled parallel to the transverse axis of the ankle joint through the talus and malleoli
  - Sagittal and coronal PD-weighted fat-sat
  - Axial T2-weighted sequence parallel to the course of the anterior talofibular ligament
  - If necessary: axial oblique PD-weighted fat-sat (2–2.5-mm slice thickness, angled to plane of syndesmosis)

MRI Findings

- Fibular fracture with or without rupture of anterior syndesmosis fascicles
- Widening of the ankle mortise with separation of the medial malleolus from the talus or a medial malleolar fracture with displacement and angulation at the fracture line
- Hematoma along the central syndesmotic ligaments and interosseous membrane, extending up the tibia and fibula
- Deltoid ligament status—thickening, increased signal intensity, fascicle discontinuity from a complete, subtotal or partial tear
- Effusion or hematoma
- Soft-tissue hematoma or edema

Imaging Recommendation

Modality of choice: radiography.

Differential Diagnosis

- Lateral ligament tear
- Peroneal tendon injury
- Syndesmosis rupture
- Subtalar joint sprain

Treatment

Nondisplaced Weber A fractures can be managed conservatively with a plaster cast or walker. All displaced fractures are treated surgically in accordance with AO/ASIF principles. Often a conventional radiograph will not reveal the full extent of the displacement, especially if there is involvement of the tibial articular surface or syndesmosis. A ruptured syndesmosis should be repaired by screw fixation in addition to the open reduction and internal fixation of fractures. The fixation screw is removed at 6 to 8 weeks.

Prognosis, Complications

Prognosis

An anatomic reconstruction is essential for a good treatment outcome. Risk factors for imperfect results are cartilage lesions and extensive, untreated instability of the syndesmosis.

Possible Complications

- Malunion
- Persistent instability of the syndesmosis
- Limited motion
- Early degenerative joint changes

Tibial Pilon Fracture

Definition

The tibial pilon is the distal end of the tibia (from the French *pilon*, meaning a ram or pestle). Tibial pilon fractures result from a vertical compression force that drives the talus into the lower end of the tibia, usually with articular involvement.

Symptoms

- Considerable soft-tissue swelling with tension blisters
- Pain
- Inability to bear weight on the affected foot
- Ankle joint deformity

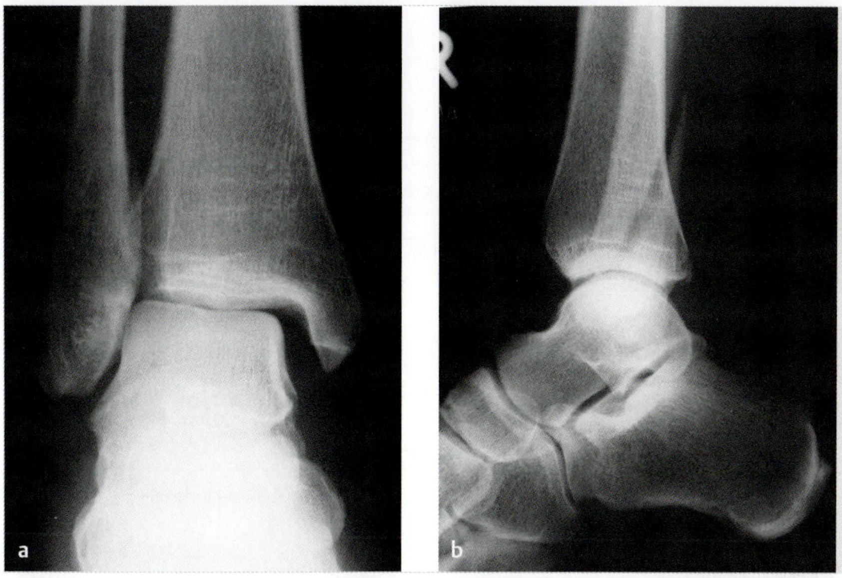

Fig. 3.16 a, b Weber B fracture.
a This injury has ruptured the anterior syndesmosis and deltoid ligament. Widening of the joint space at the medial malleolus reflects the lateral displacement of the talus relative to the tibia.
b Oblique posterosuperior-to-anteroinferior fracture of the fibula. There is an associated bony avulsion of the posterior syndesmosis from the posterior tibial margin.

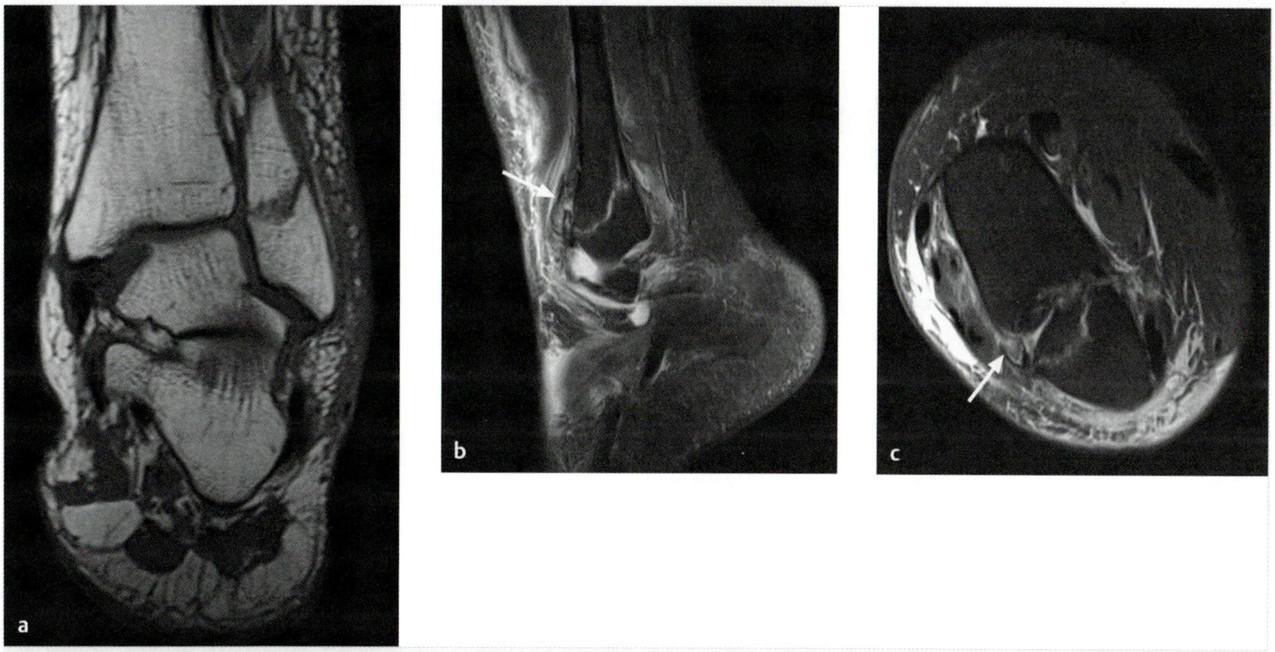

Fig. 3.17 a–c Weber B fracture.
a Coronal T1-weighted MRI shows a fibular fracture at the level of the syndesmosis.
b Sagittal PD-weighted fat-sat image. The fracture line has a posterosuperior-to-anteroinferior course. The syndesmosis is torn anteriorly. The fascicles are expanded, randomly directed, and show increased signal intensity due to bleeding (arrow).
c PD-weighted fat-sat image in the syndesmotic plane shows a rupture of the anterior syndesmosis (arrow).

Predisposing Factors

- Fall from a height
- High-impact trauma

Anatomy and Pathology

The distal metaphyseal and epiphyseal tibia may sustain extra- and intra-articular fractures. The AO/ASIF has devised a classification system for these injuries, which are designated with the number 43:

- *A43A fractures:* Type A fractures of the distal metaphyseal tibia are extra-articular noncomminuted fractures. The fractures may be oblique, transverse, or spiral, and the fibula may be intact or fractured (43A1, ▶ Fig. 3.22 a). Metaphyseal fractures with a wedge fragment comprise group 43A2 (▶ Fig. 3.22 b). Complex multipart extra-articular metaphyseal fractures are designated as 43A3 fractures (▶ Fig. 3.22 c) and may show diaphyseal extension as do 43A2 fractures.
- *A43B fractures:* Group B fractures are split fractures of the distal tibia without (43B1, ▶ Fig. 3.22 d) or with depression of

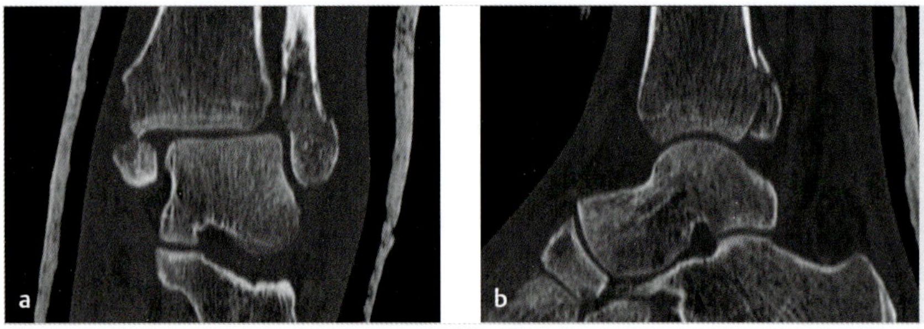

Fig. 3.18 a, b Weber type B trimalleolar ankle fracture.
a Coronal reformatted CT image shows a fibular fracture at the level of the syndesmosis associated with a fracture of the medial malleolus and lateral displacement of the talus.
b This image also shows an avulsion fracture of the posterior tibial margin with articular surface disruption. The posterior tibial fracture involves 20 to 25% of the articular surface.

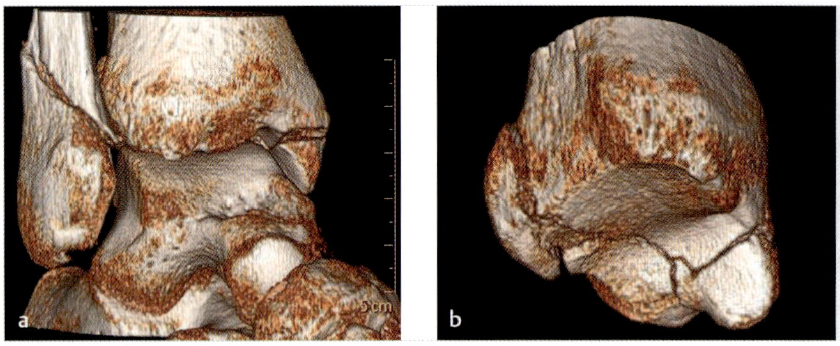

Fig. 3.19 a, b Weber type B trimalleolar ankle fracture in a different patient.
a 3D volume-rendered image of the Weber B fibular fracture at the level of the syndesmosis and the medial malleolar fracture.
b The fibula has been electronically disarticulated and removed to display the tibial articular surface of the ankle joint, showing an articular step-off caused by the fracture of the posterior tibial margin. The medial malleolar fracture is also clearly depicted.

the articular surface (43B2 and 43B3, ▸ Fig. 3.22 e, f). Each of the split fractures can be subclassified based on fracture orientation in the frontal or sagittal plane and whether multiple fragments are present. While the articular surface is not impacted or disintegrated in B1 fractures, this does occur in B2 and B3 fractures.

- *A43C fractures:* While part of the articular surface remains in contact with the tibial diaphysis in type B split fractures, there is no remaining connection between the articular surface and diaphysis in type C fractures, as the articular pillar is broken into two separate pieces. There is no remaining connection between the articular surface of the distal tibia and the diaphysis. The degree of fragmentation or disintegration and the number of metaphyseal fragments increase from C1 to C3 (▸ Fig. 3.22 g). The degree of fragmentation or disintegration and the number of metaphyseal fragments increase from C1 to C3 (▸ Fig. 3.22 g).

Imaging (▸ Fig. 3.23 and ▸ Fig. 3.24)

Radiographs

The ankle joint and lower leg is imaged in two planes. If necessary, 45° oblique views may be a helpful adjunct. CT should be performed in all cases of actual or suspected articular involvement.

Ultrasound

Ultrasound has no role in the imaging of tibial pilon fractures.

CT

CT with high-resolution scans (≤ 0.5-mm slice thickness), overlapping reconstructions, and MPRs should be performed in all distal tibial fractures with actual or suspected articular involvement. CT is crucial for preoperative planning and is used postoperatively if there is suspected deformity or articular irregularity.

MRI

MRI is generally unnecessary for the investigation of tibial pilon fractures.

Imaging Recommendation

Modalities of choice: radiography, CT.

Differential Diagnosis

- Severe capsuloligamentous injury
- Fracture of the fibula
- Fracture of the medial malleolus
- Osteochondral injury

Treatment

- Open reduction and internal fixation as soft-tissue status permits
- Surgical treatment, with arthroscopic assistance if needed
- Fractures can be temporarily stabilized by external fixation in patients with grade II or grade III soft-tissue injuries

Prognosis, Complications

Prognosis

The prognosis depends on the degree of articular surface disruption, the possibility of an anatomic reconstruction, and associated soft-tissue injuries.

Possible Complications

- Wound healing problems due to soft-tissue injury and/or tissue ischemia due to severe swelling

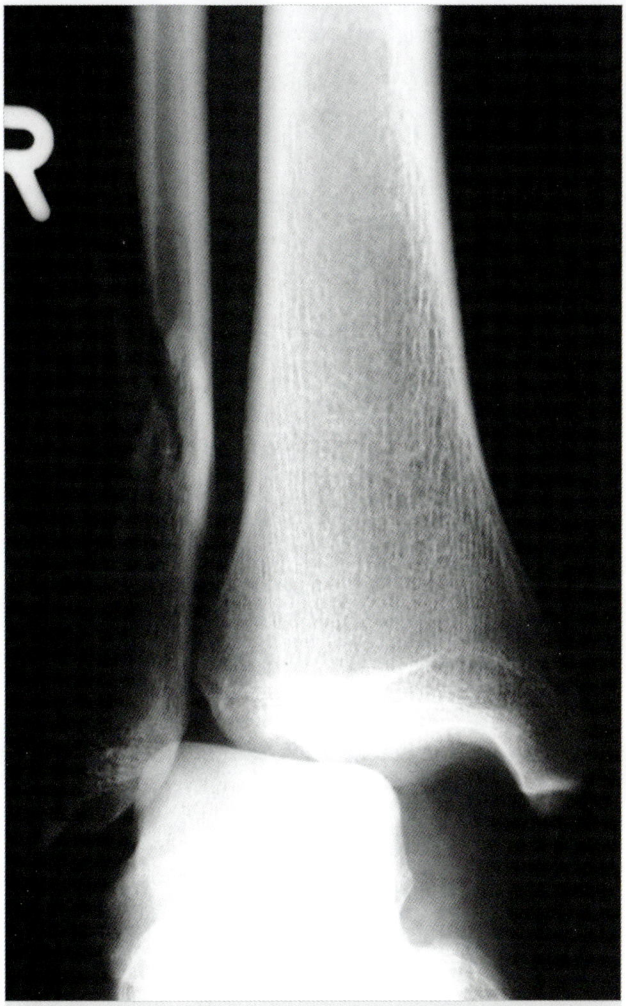

Fig. 3.20 Weber C fracture. Fibular fracture above the syndesmosis with rupture of the syndesmosis and distal interosseous membrane to the level of the fibular fracture. Disruption of the syndesmosis is evidenced by widening of the ankle mortise with separation of the medial malleolus. A fracture of the medial malleolus may be present instead of a deltoid ligament tear, as illustrated here.

- Difficult reconstruction of multipart fractures due to poor visualization of the articular surface
- Delayed union
- Nonunion
- Early degenerative changes
- Consolidation in a malaligned position

Fracture of the Posterior Tibial Margin

Definition

A fracture of the posterior tibial margin is also known as the Volkmann triangle. It is an avulsion fracture of the posterior syndesmosis, which is so sturdy that it does not tear in its substance but avulses a bone fragment from the posterior edge of the distal tibia. A fracture of the posterior tibial margin is classified as a type of ankle fracture, as described earlier under the appropriate heading and rarely occurs as an isolated injury.

Symptoms

- Swelling
- Pain
- Decreased ability to bear weight on the affected limb

Predisposing Factors

- Fibular fracture
- Rupture of the anterior syndesmosis

Anatomy and Pathology

The posterior tibial margin is fractured by posterior and superior translation of the talus leading to bony avulsion of the posterior syndesmotic ligament.

This injury reduces stability and promotes posterior subluxation of the talus. Any discontinuity in the articular surface predisposes to degenerative joint changes and should be surgically addressed. An avulsion fracture of the posterior tibial margin may occur as an isolated injury, but more commonly it occurs in the setting of a fibular or ankle fracture or combined with a medial malleolar fracture producing a "trimalleolar" injury. A fracture of the posterior tibial margin is often associated with rupture of the anterior syndesmosis.

! Note

Whenever radiographs, CT, or MRI reveal a fracture of the posterior tibial margin, a rupture of the anterior syndesmosis should be excluded or confirmed because it may destabilize the ankle mortise and require surgical stabilization.

An avulsion fracture of the posterior tibial margin is known internationally as a "Volkmanns triangle," named after Richard von Volkmann. There is evidence, however, that Volkmann did not describe this injury but actually described a different type of tibial fracture. The British surgeon Henry Earle appears to have been the first, in 1823, to publish a detailed description of an avulsed posterior tibial margin in a fracture-dislocation of the ankle. It is more accurate, then, to describe the injury as a fracture of the posterior tibial margin rather than a Volkmann triangle.

Imaging

Radiographs

Radiographs of the ankle joint are obtained in two planes. A fracture of the posterior tibial margin can be appreciated in the lateral view. It is important to determine the percentage of the distal tibial articular surface that is occupied by the fragment. A fragment that occupies 25% or more of the articular surface is an indication for surgical treatment.

Ultrasound

Ultrasound can show a discontinuity in the echogenic bony surface as well as hypoechoic thickening of the periosteum due to hematoma.

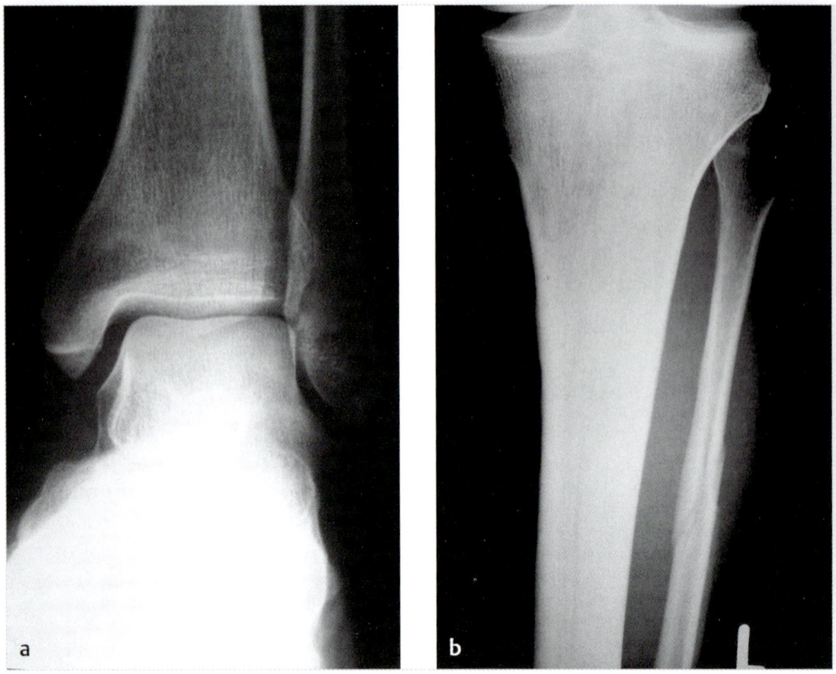

Fig. 3.21 a, b Maisonneuve fracture.
a There is no fracture at the level of the ankle joint, but the ankle joint space is widened at the medial malleolus due to rupture of the deltoid ligament and syndesmosis and disruption of the interosseous membrane.
b A supplemental view of the lower leg reveals the proximal fibular fracture. The injury is classified as a high Weber C fracture.

CT

CT with high-resolution scans (≤ 0.5-mm slice thickness), overlapping reconstructions, and MPRs should be performed in all cases with actual or suspected articular involvement. CT is essential for preoperative planning and is used postoperatively in all patients with a suspected deformity or articular discontinuity.

MRI (▶ Fig. 3.25 and ▶ Fig. 3.26)

MRI can disclose even nondisplaced fractures of the posterior tibial margin, which are often radiographically occult. It is then necessary to detect or exclude a rupture of the anterior syndesmosis.

Imaging Recommendation

Modalities of choice: radiography, CT, MRI.

Differential Diagnosis

- Pilon fracture
- Fibular fracture
- Medial malleolar fracture

Treatment

- For displaced fractures: open reduction and internal fixation with screws
- Alternative: internal fixation with an AO/ASIF anti-glide plate
- A medial or lateral approach may be used, depending on the fracture location

Prognosis, Complications

Consolidation in a malunited position or a persistent articular step-off may promote early degenerative changes. Ankle fractures with an associated avulsion fracture of the posterior tibial margin have a significantly higher association with osteoarthritis of the ankle joint than do ankle fractures with an intact posterior tibial margin.

Maisonneuve Fracture

Definition

A Maisonneuve fracture is a fracture of the proximal fibula associated with disruption of the syndesmotic ligaments and a long tear of the interosseous membrane. The Maisonneuve fracture is a type of ankle fracture that is classified as A44C3.1 to A44C3.3 in the AO/ASIF system. It is described under Ankle Fractures (p. 34).

Symptoms

- Pain from the ankle joint up to the level of the fracture
- Tenderness over the fibula
- Hematoma
- Impaired ability to bear weight on the affected ankle

Predisposing Factors

Pronation injury of the ankle joint.

Anatomy and Pathology

Differentiation is required from direct impact trauma as a cause of fibular fractures. In the case of impact trauma, the ligamentous structures of the syndesmosis are intact and the ankle joint is not injured. With a Maisonneuve fracture, on the other hand, there is always a concomitant rupture of the syndesmotic ligaments and tearing of the interosseous membrane. The fibula may be displaced cephalad (relative shortening), and the integrity of the ankle joint is disrupted.

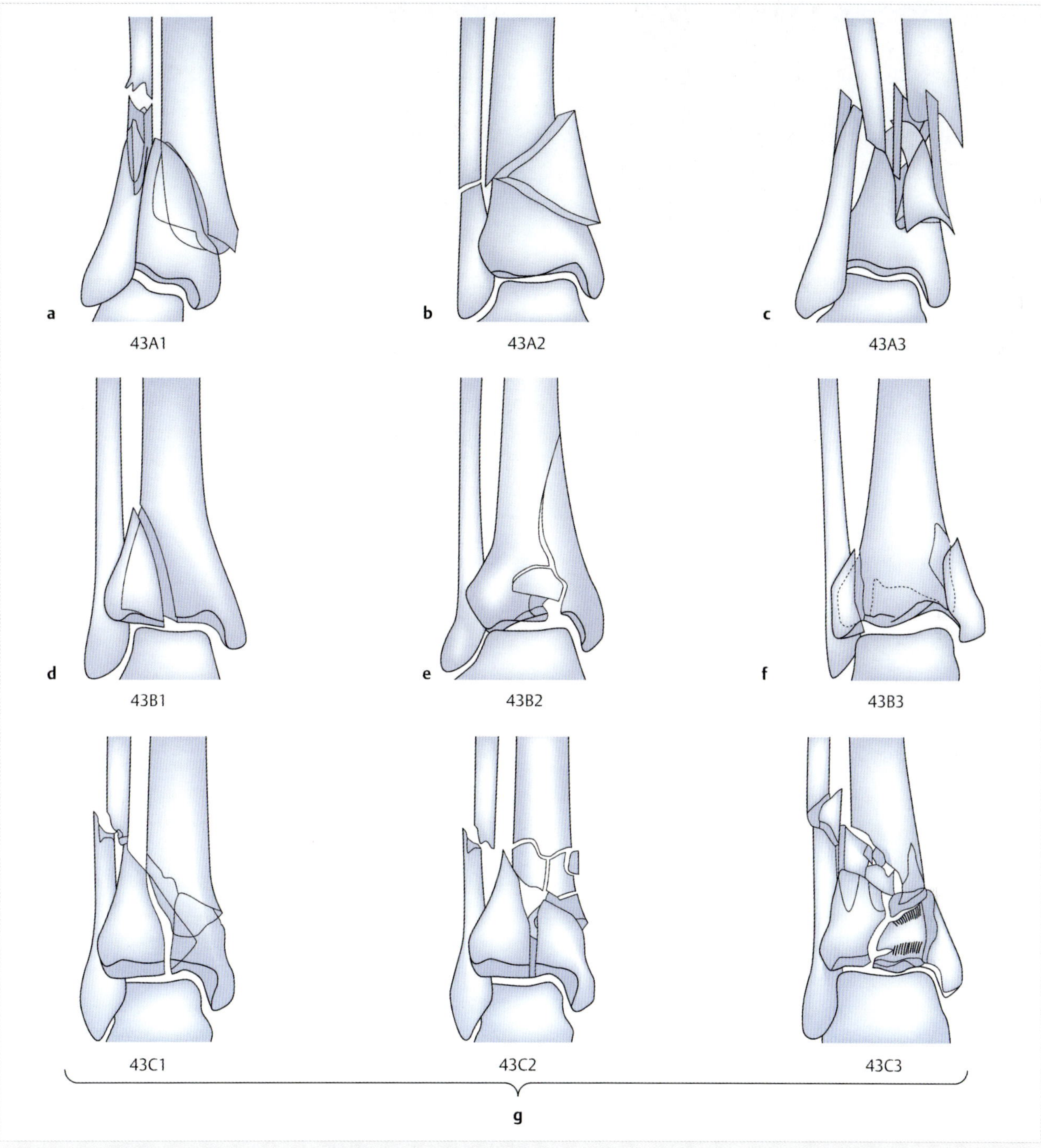

Fig. 3.22 a–g AO/ASIF classification of distal tibial fractures: 43A to 43C injuries.
a Extra-articular fractures without comminution. Fractures may be oblique, transverse, or spiral. The fibula is intact or fractured.
b With a wedge fragment.
c With comminution.
d Split fractures of the distal tibia without depression of the articular surface.
e Split fractures of the distal tibia with depression of the articular surface.
f Split fractures of the distal tibia with depression of the articular surface and comminution.
g There is no remaining connection between the articular surface of the distal tibia and the diaphysis. The degree of fragmentation or disintegration and the number of metaphyseal fragments increase from C1 to C3.

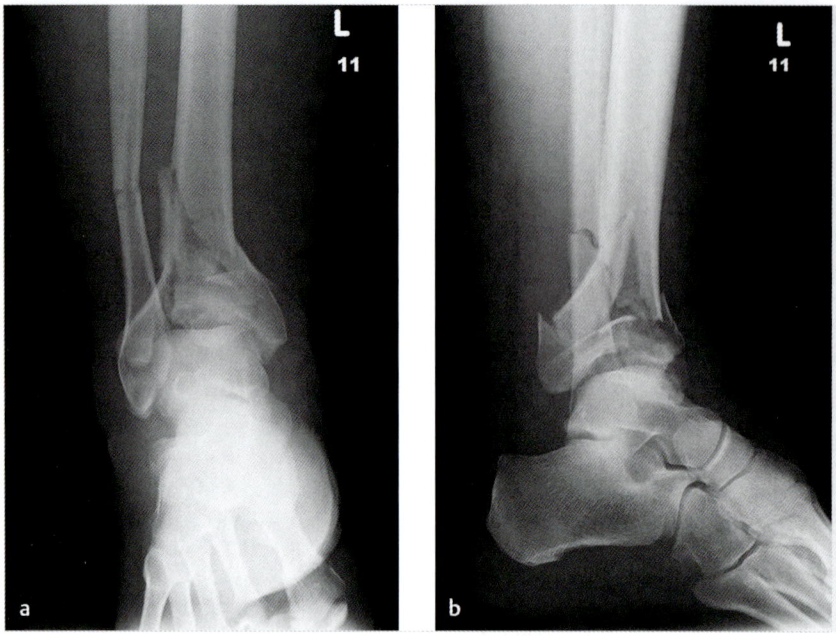

Fig. 3.23 a, b Tibial pilon fracture.
a AP radiograph shows loss of continuity between the distal tibial articular surface and the diaphysis, metaphyseal comminution, disintegration of the articular surface, and a fibular fracture.
b The disintegration of the articular surface is clearly visible on the lateral radiograph.

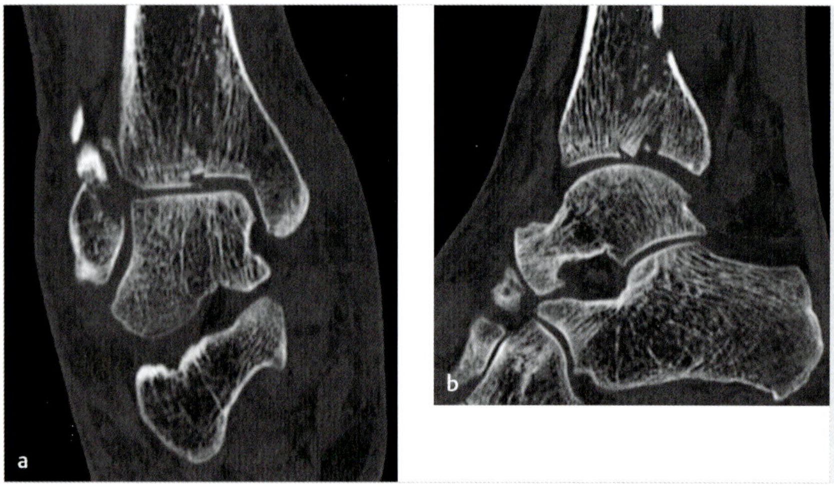

Fig. 3.24 a, b Type A43B2 tibial pilon fracture.
a CT shows a moderately displaced tibial articular surface fragment and an associated fibular fracture.
b This view shows remaining bony continuity between the distal articular surface and tibial diaphysis. The step-off in the joint and the slight rotation of one articular surface fragment are clearly demonstrated by CT.

Imaging

Radiographs

Radiographs of the ankle and lower leg are obtained in two planes. The ankle injury may be missed in patients with ligamentous disruption of the ankle joint and tears of the syndesmosis and deltoid ligament. Thus, the proximal fibula should always be imaged in suspicious cases to avoid missing a Maisonneuve fracture, which implies a significant, unstable injury of the ankle joint.

Ultrasound

Ultrasound can detect hematoma over the syndesmosis and around the deltoid ligament.

CT

Not necessary.

MRI

Interpretation Checklist

- Rupture of the anterior syndesmosis
- Fracture of the posterior tibial margin
- Joint position, lateral subluxation of the talus

Examination Technique

- *Standard trauma protocol:* High-resolution multi-channel coil; contrast administration is not required.
- *Sequences:*
  - Coronal T1-weighted sequence angled parallel to the transverse axis of the ankle joint through the talus and malleoli
  - Sagittal and coronal PD-weighted fat-sat
  - Axial T2-weighted sequence parallel to the course of the anterior talofibular ligament
  - Axial oblique PD-weighted fat-sat (2–2.5-mm slice thickness, angled to plane of syndesmosis)

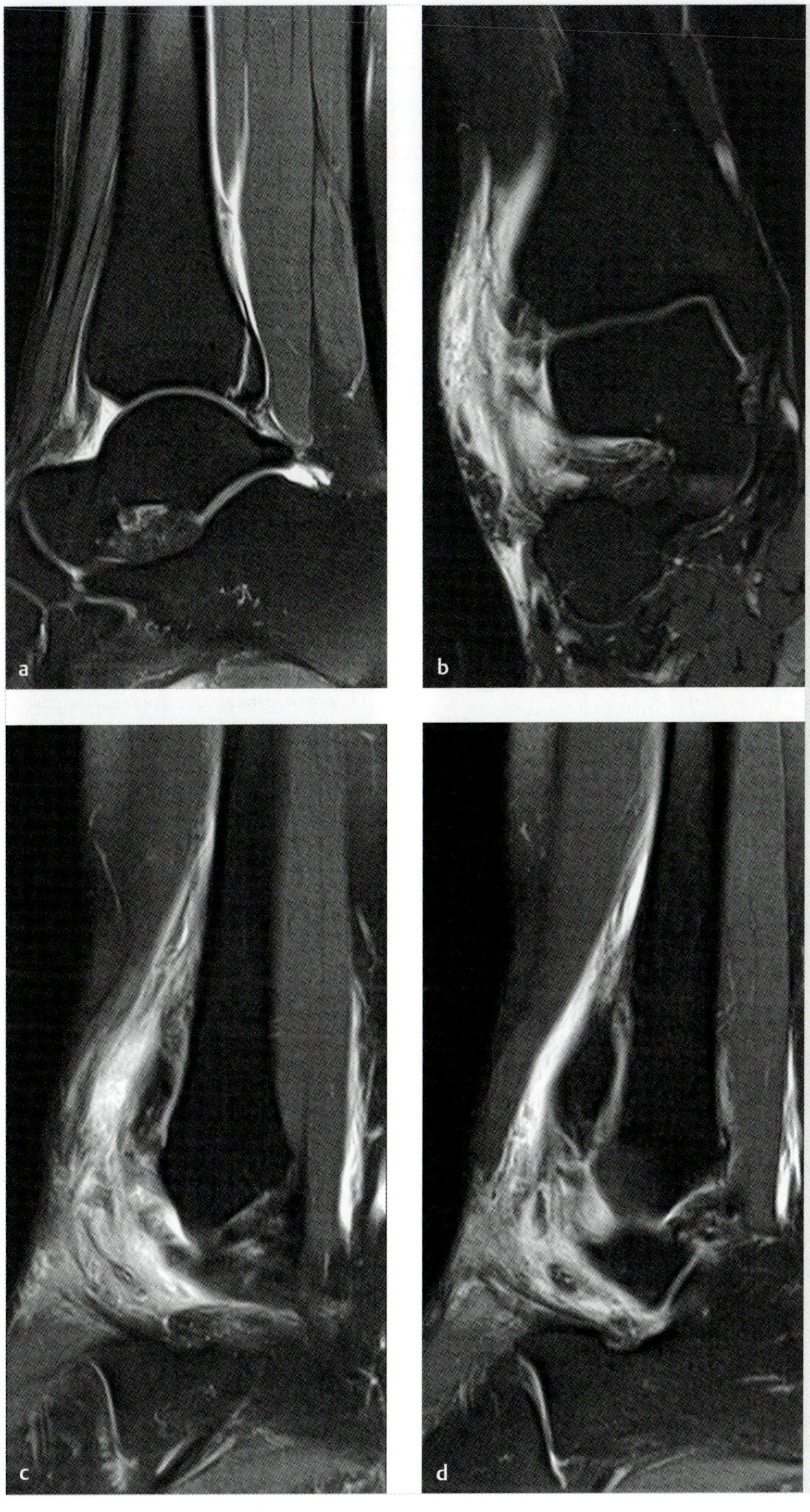

Fig. 3.25 a–d Fracture of the posterior tibial margin ("Volkmann triangle").
a Sagittal PD-weighted fat-sat MRI. The nondisplaced fracture was not visible on radiographs.
b Coronal PD-weighted fat-sat image. Conspicuous hemorrhage is noted about the anterior syndesmosis.
c Sagittal PD-weighted fat-sat image. Even consecutive slices (**c, d**) do not show continuous, intact fascicles in the anterior syndesmosis. The sagittal slice is a good projection for evaluating the anterior syndesmosis.
d Consecutive sagittal PD-weighted fat-sat image.

MRI Findings

- Discontinuity in the fascicles of a ruptured anterior syndesmosis
- Widening of the ankle mortise
- Rupture of the deltoid ligament or medial malleolar fracture
- Position of a posterior tibial edge triangle

Imaging Recommendation

Modality of choice: radiography that includes a view of the proximal fibula (see ▶ Fig. 3.21).

Differential Diagnosis

- Fibular fracture

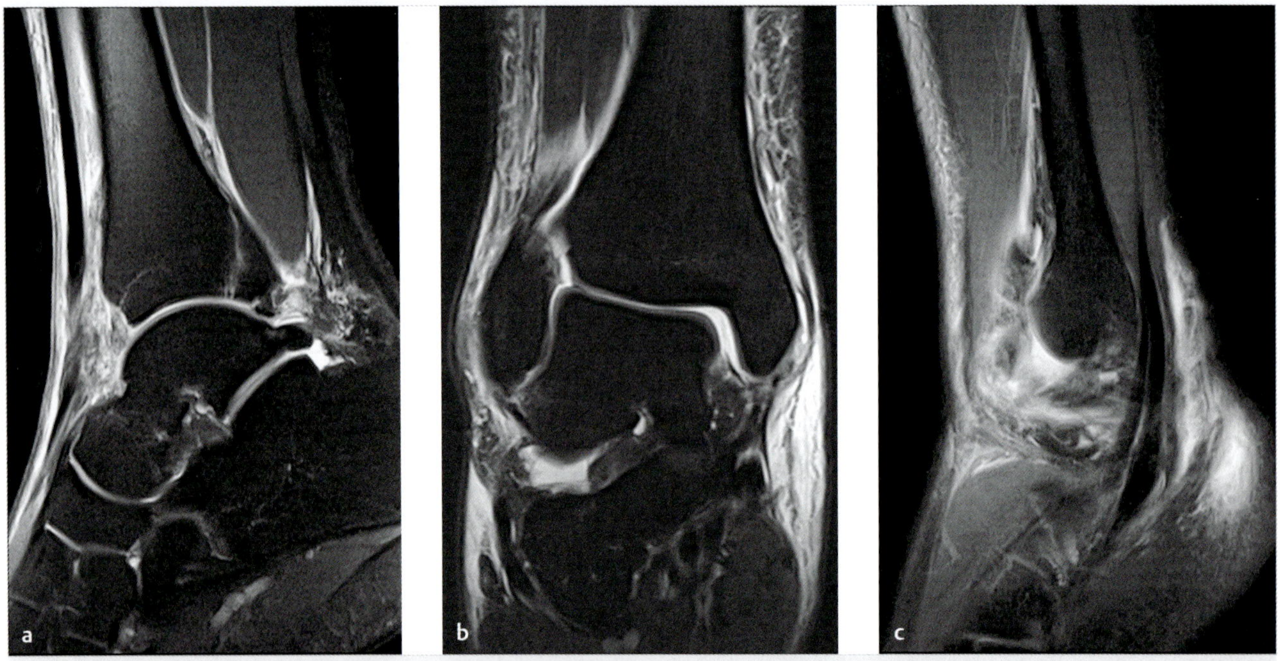

Fig. 3.26 a–c Fracture of the posterior tibial margin.
a Sagittal PD-weighted fat-sat image shows no displacement and no articular discontinuity.
b Coronal PD-weighted fat-sat image. Unlike the case in ▶ Fig. 3.25, the ankle joint space is widened at the medial malleolus indicating lateral subluxation or translation of the talus relative to the tibia.
c Sagittal PD-weighted fat-sat image. The fascicles of the anterior syndesmosis are ruptured and are not visible in continuity. Thus, the anterior syndesmosis should always be evaluated when a posterior tibial margin fracture is detected. Special angulation of the image plane may be necessary to display the syndesmosis rupture.

- Pilon fracture
- Tibial fracture

Treatment

Open reduction and internal plating by the AO/ASIF technique and screw fixation of the ruptured syndesmosis. Only CT can accurately evaluate the postoperative position of the syndesmosis. Impact trauma to the tibia with an intact syndesmosis can be treated conservatively.

Prognosis, Complications

Precise reduction of the ankle mortise will critically affect the prognosis. One possible complication is consolidation in a faulty position—especially a shortened fibula and dehiscent syndesmosis—as this will increase the risk of early degenerative osteoarthritis.

Tillaux Fracture

Definition

A Tillaux fracture is defined as a bony avulsion of the anterior syndesmotic ligament from the tibia.

Symptoms

- Tenderness over the anterolateral aspect of the ankle joint
- Pain and swelling
- Decreased weight-bearing ability on the affected leg

Predisposing Factors

None.

Anatomy and Pathology

The bony avulsion of the anterior syndesmotic ligament from the tibia is usually accompanied by a lesion of the central or occasionally the posterior syndesmotic ligament. Features may include anteroposterior displacement of the syndesmosis and rotational deformity.

Imaging (▶ Fig. 3.27)

Radiographs

The ankle joint is imaged in two planes, and a 45° oblique view may be added if required. Bony avulsions may be missed on radiographs. The external-rotation mechanism of the injury causes widening of the joint space at the medial malleolus, which will resolve after the fracture is reduced.

Ultrasound

Ultrasound shows an echogenic bone fragment separated from the bone surface and an associated local hematoma.

CT

Thin-slice CT acquisition with reformatting can provide a nonsuperimposed view of the avulsed fragment. Only CT can accurately define the epiphyseal fragments.

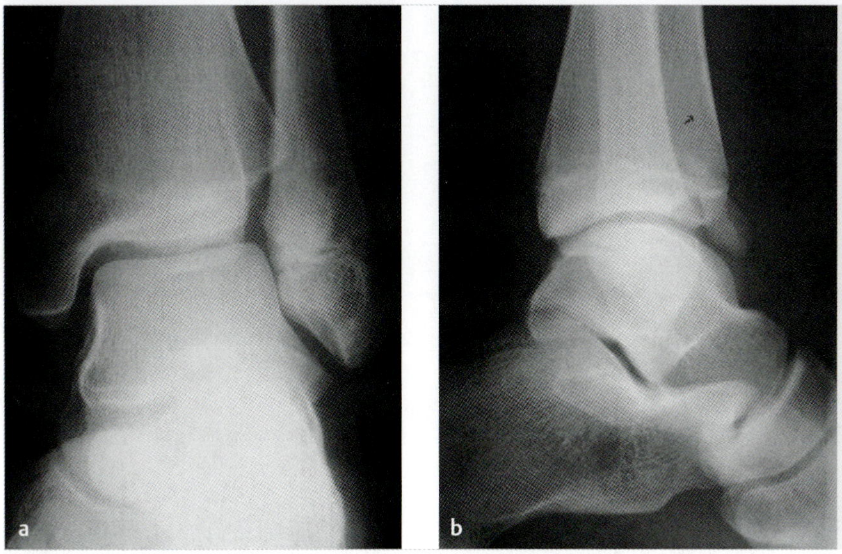

Fig. 3.27 a, b Tillaux fracture in a 14-year-old boy (transitional fracture).
a AP radiograph shows a bone fragment avulsed from the anterolateral epiphysis and located anterior to the fibula.
b The bony avulsion of the anterior syndesmosis is displaced anteriorly and slightly distally.

MRI

- *Standard trauma protocol:* High-resolution multi-channel coil; contrast administration is not required.
- *Sequences:*
  - Coronal T1-weighted sequence parallel to the transverse axis of the ankle joint through the talus and malleoli
  - Sagittal and coronal PD-weighted fat-sat
  - Axial T2-weighted angled parallel to the anterior talofibular ligament
  - Axial oblique PD-weighted fat-sat (slice thickness 2–2.5 mm, angled to the syndesmotic plane)

Imaging Recommendation

Modalities of choice: radiography, CT, MRI.

Differential Diagnosis

- Fibular fracture
- Maisonneuve fracture
- Syndesmosis rupture
- Lateral ligament tear
- Peroneal tendon injury
- Pilon fracture
- Osteochondral lesion

Treatment

- Reduction of the syndesmosis with a fixation screw
- If the size permits, open reduction and internal fixation of the Tillaux fragment with a screw
- If necessary: CT for postoperative assessment of the syndesmosis position

Prognosis, Complications

An anatomic reconstruction implies a good prognosis for recovery of ankle joint function. One possible complication is consolidation in a malunited position with widening of the syndesmosis.

Osteochondral Lesions of the Talus (p. 83)

Definition

An osteochondral lesion of the talus is a flake fracture involving the medial or lateral border of the talar dome following supination and pronation trauma.

Symptoms

- Pain in the ankle joint, often poorly localized
- Locking of the ankle joint

Predisposing Factors

None.

Anatomy and Pathology

An osteochondral lesion of the talus is a shearing injury affecting the medial border or, more commonly, the lateral border of the talar dome. It can be staged as shown in ▶ Table 3.5.

The classifications of talar osteochondral lesions originally arose from the results of radiographic studies, which focused mainly on the formation of an osteochondral fragment. Many osteochondral lesions of the talus are radiographically occult or detectable only in retrospect, with MRI showing an associated subchondral bone marrow reaction and edema. Many of these lesions do not progress to osteochondritis dissecans, and so traditional classifications are not applicable to these

Table 3.5 Staging of osteochondral lesions of the talus

Stage	Description
I	Subchondral fracture with intact cartilage
II	Partially stable fragment
III	Unstable, nondisplaced fragment
IV	Intra-articular loose body

forms. A number of MRI classifications have been developed that are based on subchondral cysts and the extent of bone edema. But these criteria show changes in follow-up scans that do not have a definite clinical correlate, and this limitation should be kept in mind whenever these criteria are applied.

Imaging

Radiographs

Radiographs of the ankle joint are obtained in two planes. Films of acute osteochondral fractures may show cortical discontinuities with or without fragmentation on one shoulder of the talus. When imaging is done in the subacute stage, the radiolucency of the subchondral bone may be increased or decreased (sclerosis).

Ultrasound

See the section on Osteochondritis Dissecans of the Talus.

CT

When intra-articular contrast administration (CT arthrography) is used, cartilage status can be accurately assessed on high-resolution scans. Today, however, this modality has been largely replaced by high-resolution multichannel MRI due to concerns about radiation exposure and invasiveness.

MRI

Interpretation Checklist

- Status of talar articular cartilage: focal thinning or circumscribed delamination; small cartilage defect, ulcer, or fissure; cartilage fully intact?
- Blood supply to the subchondral bone (contrast enhancement)
- Subchondral cysts
- Defect with decreased subchondral bone height and compensatory cartilage hypertrophy
- Fragmentation and decreased signal intensity of subchondral bone
- Bone edema in adjacent bone marrow outside the demarcated area of subchondral bone change
- Joint effusion
- Synovitis
- Formation of an osteochondral fragment: incipient or definite fluid tracking between the demarcated bone and adjacent medullary space (incipient separation) or fluid between the subchondral bone and articular cartilage (incipient delamination)

Examination Technique

- *Standard protocol for the ankle joint:* high-resolution multichannel coil and IV contrast administration
- *Sequences:*
  - Coronal T1-weighted sequence parallel to the transverse axis of the ankle joint through the talus and malleoli
  - Sagittal and coronal PD-weighted fat-sat
  - Axial T2-weighted angled parallel to the anterior talofibular ligament
  - Coronal and sagittal T1-weighted fat-sat sequence after IV contrast administration

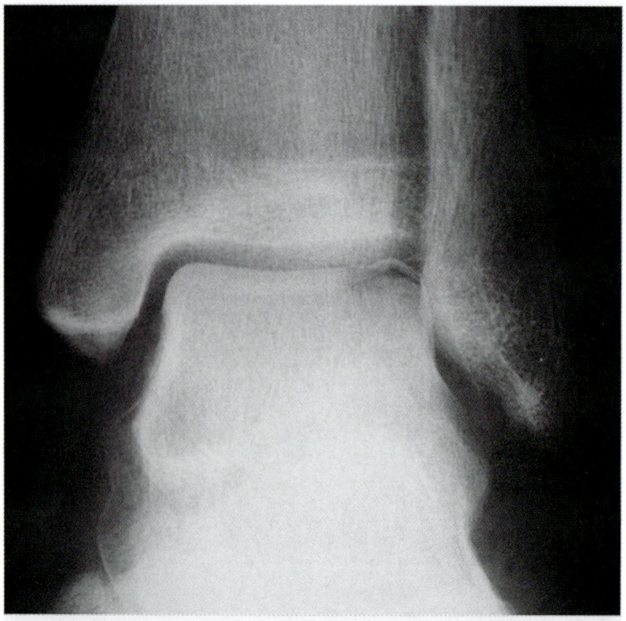

Fig. 3.28 Osteochondral lesion appears as a detached flake on the lateral shoulder of the talus following supination trauma.

MRI Findings (▶ Fig. 3.28 and ▶ Fig. 3.29)

The points listed above should be addressed. Though questionable, subchondral cysts represent zones of bone resorption and defect formation and are considered an unfavorable prognostic sign. Also, the extent of bone edema in the adjacent medullary space generally correlates with clinical complaints.

Imaging Recommendation

Modalities of choice: radiography and MRI in suspicious cases.

Differential Diagnosis

- Ankle sprain
- Talar edema
- Inflammatory joint disease
- Multiple intra-articular loose bodies

Treatment

- *Stage I:* Fresh injury is managed by non–weight bearing for 6 weeks, followed by a gradual progression to full weight bearing.
- *Stages II and III:* arthroscopy with cartilage stabilization, debridement of the lesion, and microfracturing. With larger fresh defects, reattach the fragment with absorbable pins or small screws (remove implants before weight bearing is resumed). Complete cartilage destruction can be treated by osteochondral grafting (harvested from the knee, tibiofibular joint, or lateral surfaces of the talus), autologous chondrocyte transplantation, or covering the defect with a collagen membrane.
- *Stage IV:* arthroscopic removal of the intra-articular loose body. The defect is managed as in stage III.

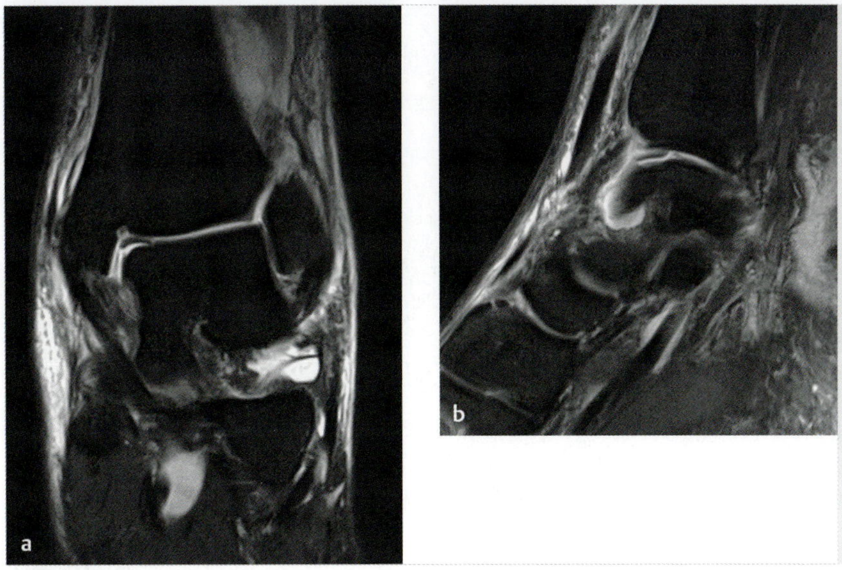

Fig. 3.29 a, b Chondral flake fragment on the medial shoulder of the talus.
a Coronal PD-weighted fat-sat MRI. A small piece of cortical bone may also be detached (osteochondral separation).
b Sagittal PD-weighted fat-sat image. A small step-off at the cortical level, consistent with an osteochondral flake fracture, is particularly well displayed in the sagittal image.

Prognosis, Complications

Prognosis

Osteochondral lesions of the talus may predispose to osteoarthritis, but this remains unclear. Good treatment results can be achieved in terms of pain relief. Most patients will have some residual functional deficit, especially during sports and high-demand activities.

Possible Complications

- Locking of the ankle joint
- Failure of consolidation
- Cyst formation
- Development of osteochondritis dissecans

Fractures of the Talus

Definition

A talar fracture may involve any of the following structures:
- Talar head
- Talar neck
- Talar body
- Posterior process of the talus
- Lateral process of the talus

Symptoms

- Pain and hematoma encircling the ankle joint
- Little or no ability to bear weight on the affected foot
- Associated injuries in up to 50% of cases

Predisposing Factors

None.

Anatomy and Pathology

Fractures of the talus (classification in ▶ Table 3.6) often result from high-energy trauma, so few patients can give details on the mechanism of the injury.

Two classifications of talar fractures have been widely used: the Weber–Marti classification and the Hawkins classification of vertical talar neck fractures. A basic distinction is drawn between peripheral fractures (flake and avulsion fractures) and central fractures of the talar body and neck. Most of the talar body and head is covered with articular cartilage, and only a few areas on the talar neck, medial and lateral talar body, and posterior process are available for blood vessels to enter the bone. Central talar fractures, especially in fracture-dislocations, are at high risk for avascular necrosis. Surgical approaches can cause further disruption of blood supply, especially on the medial aspect of the talar neck.

Imaging (▶ see Figs. 3.30–3.35)

Radiographs

Radiographs of the ankle joint are obtained in two planes. Talar fractures may be radiographically occult, especially nondisplaced fractures of the talar neck and fractures of the lateral process. If the patient cannot bear weight on the affected foot, further investigation by CT or MRI is indicated.

The Hawkins sign is a radiolucent band appearing in the subchondral talar dome 6 to 8 weeks after a displaced and reduced talar neck fracture. This is taken as a positive sign that excludes avascular necrosis, because the bone can participate in the general decalcification resulting from hyperemia. On the other hand, a relative increase of sclerosis or the absence of decalcification is considered to indicate decreased viability or necrosis.

Ultrasound

Not indicated.

CT

Thin-slice CT acquisition with MPRs can provide nonsuperimposed images of the talus.

Table 3.6 Fractures of the talus

Part of talus	Cause of fracture	Possible fractures
Head	Axial loading or forced dorsiflexion	• Flake fracture • Impaction • Subtalar displacement (possible)
Neck	Forced dorsiflexion	• Complete fracture with separation of the talar head and body • Possible associated injuries: ◦ Rupture of interosseous talocalcaneal ligament ◦ Disruption of blood supply ◦ Dislocation of talar body from the ankle mortise
Body	Axial compression during plantar flexion of the talus	• Comminuted fracture, nondisplaced or minimally displaced • Fracture with dislocation of the ankle joint and/or subtalar joint • Simple fracture
Posterior process	Forced plantar flexion	• Dorsal fragment with sharp edges
Lateral process	Snowboarder's ankle; inversion, dorsiflexion and compression	• Simple fracture, displaced or nondisplaced • Comminuted fracture

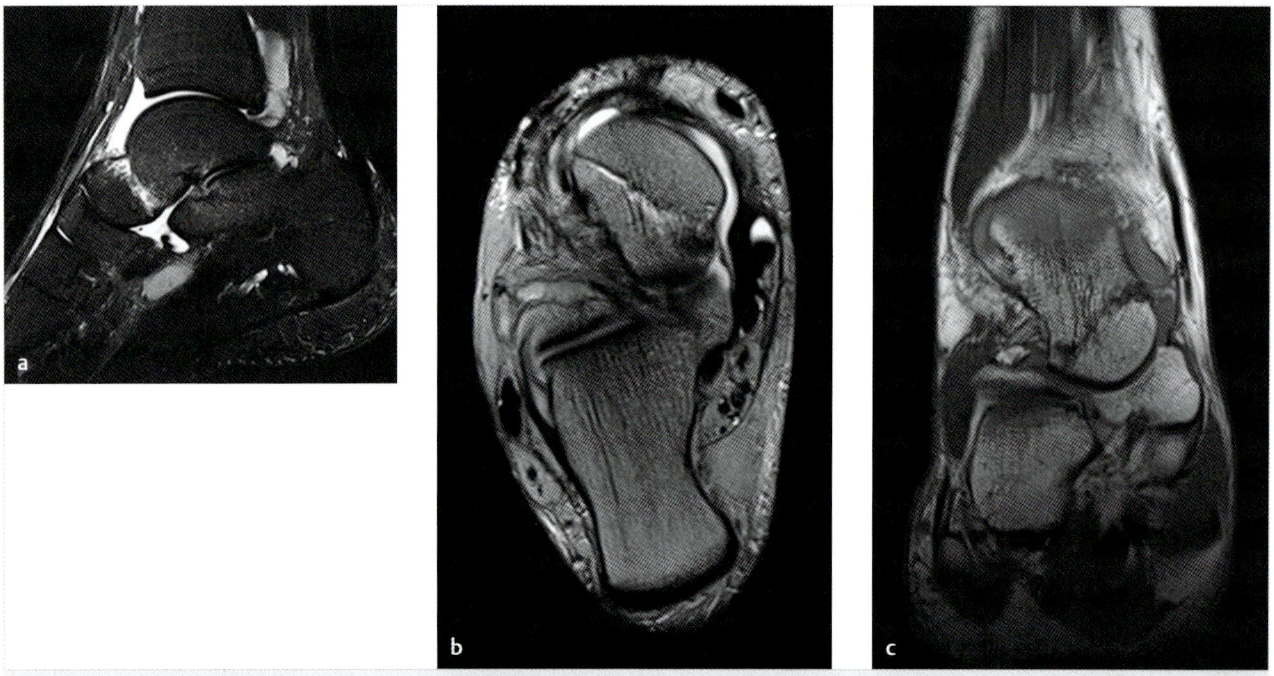

Fig. 3.30 a–c Nondisplaced fracture of the talar neck.
a Sagittal PD-weighted fat-sat image. The fracture was initially occult on radiographs. Water-sensitive image shows the fracture as a hyperintense band of fluid signal intensity.
b Axial T2-weighted image shows a small discontinuity in the anterolateral cortex.
c Coronal T1-weighted image. Fractures appear as hypointensive lines on T1-weighted images.

MRI

Interpretation Checklist

- Articular surfaces with the tibia, fibula, and calcaneus (middle and posterior compartments of the subtalar joint) and the talonavicular joint are congruent and normally visualized
- Hypointense fracture line
- Contusional bone edema
- Soft tissues
- Ligamentous and capsular structures

Examination Technique

- *Standard trauma protocol:* High-resolution multi-channel coil; contrast administration is not required.
- *Sequences:*
  - Coronal T1-weighted sequence parallel to the transverse axis of the ankle joint through the talus and malleoli
  - Sagittal and coronal PD-weighted fat-sat
  - Axial T2-weighted sequence angled parallel to the anterior talofibular ligament

- Contrast administration may be indicated following a fracture-dislocation of the talar head or body if there is evidence of vascular disruption.

MRI Findings

Talar fractures may be followed by avascular necrosis of the talar head and trochlea.

Imaging Recommendation

Modalities of choice: radiography and CT for fracture evaluation; MRI for assessing the viability of the talus.

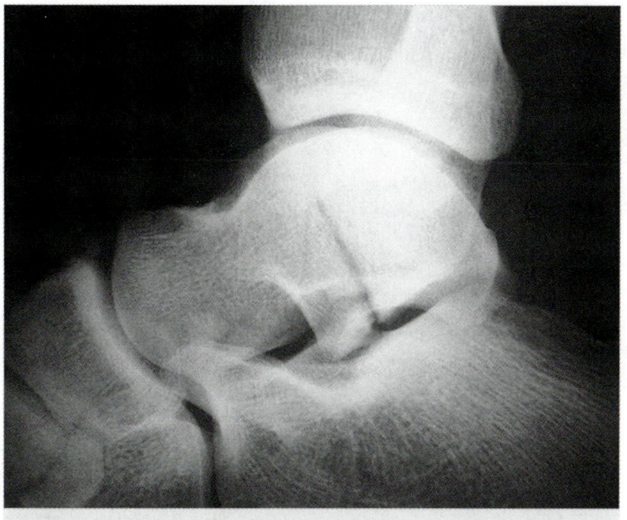

Fig. 3.31 Nondisplaced central fracture of the talar body with involvement of the subtalar joint. A small step-off is visible in the articular surface.

Differential Diagnosis

- Ankle sprain
- Os trigonum (rounded outline is different from a sharp-edged fracture line in the talar posterior process)
- Osteochondritis dissecans
- Osteochondral lesion of the talus

Treatment

- *Talar head, neck, and body:* Nondisplaced fractures can be immobilized in a plaster cast for 8 to 12 weeks, followed by gradual progression to weight bearing based on radiographic follow-ups. Displaced fractures are treated by open or percutaneous reduction and internal fixation. Avascular necrosis or delayed healing may occur in fractures with vascular disruption.
- *Posterior process:* treated conservatively. If complaints persist, the bone fragment should be resected.
- *Lateral process:* internal fixation if required. Small fragments can be resected.

Prognosis, Complications

- Avascular necrosis occurs in up to 70% of patients, depending on fracture type
- Incidence of degenerative changes is 40 to 90%, especially in the subtalar joint
- Frequent permanent limitation of motion and functional loss

Calcaneal Fractures

Definition

Fractures of the calcaneus may be extra-articular or intra-articular. Calcaneal fractures account for just 2% of all fractures, but 75% of tarsal fractures are calcaneal fractures.

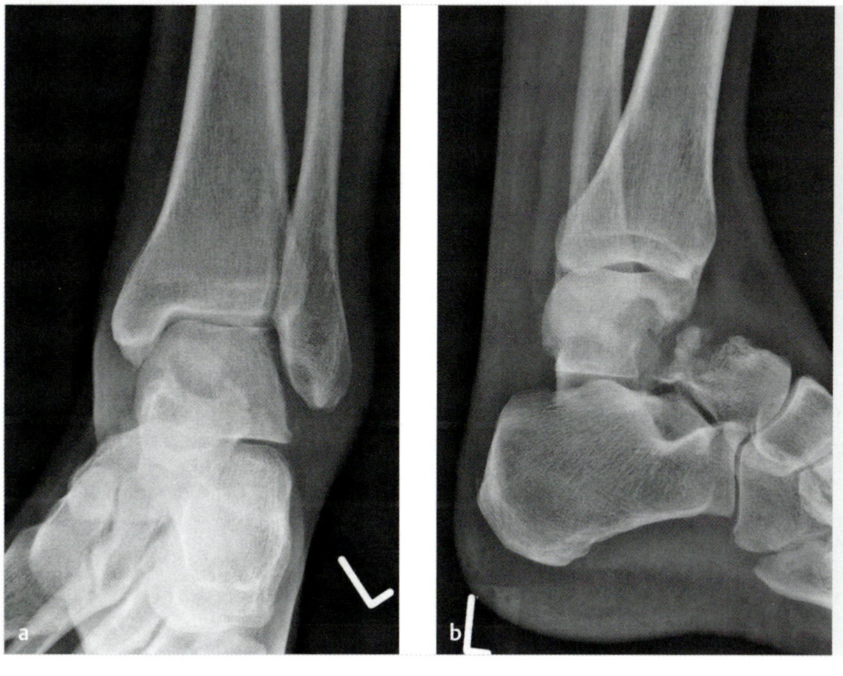

Fig. 3.32 a, b Talar neck fracture with 90° rotation of the talar body in the horizontal plane.
a On initial viewing of the AP radiograph, it is easy to miss the altered overlap of the medial malleolus and the incongruent articular surfaces with the tibia and lateral malleolus.
b The lateral radiograph shows significant displacement of the talar neck fracture with rotation of the talar body. This image gives a side view of the subtalar articular surface of the posterior compartment, which is rotated approximately 90°.

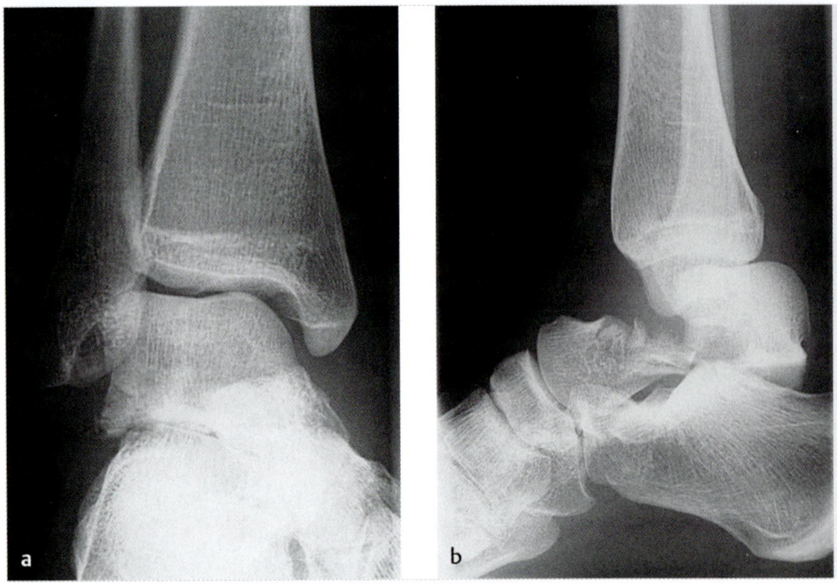

Fig. 3.33 a, b Case similar to ▶ **Fig. 3.32****: talar neck fracture with the talar body fragment rotated 90°.**
a The normal overlap of the fibula is visibly altered.
b There is associated posterior dislocation of the talar body fragment.

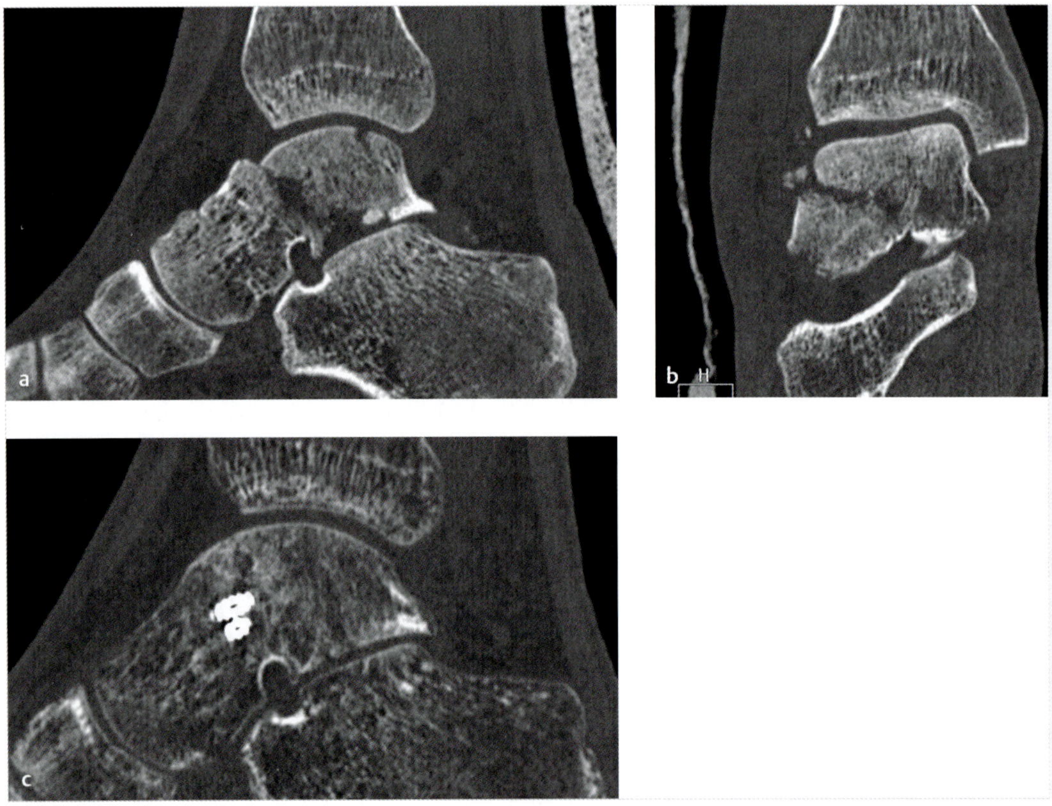

Fig. 3.34 a–c Fracture through the body of the talus.
a Sagittal reformatted CT image. The talar body fracture has sheared the posterior portion of the talus from the lateral process, causing subluxation and involvement of the posterior compartment of the subtalar joint.
b Coronal reformatted image.
c Postoperative image documents a good anatomic reconstruction.

Symptoms

- Pain with massive swelling of the hindfoot
- Extensive subcutaneous hematoma
- Inability to bear weight on the affected foot
- Flattened longitudinal arch
- Tension blisters

Predisposing Factors

None.

Anatomy and Pathology

Anatomy

The calcaneus has four articular surfaces—three with the talus and one with the cuboid—and five bony processes (the sustentaculum tali, anterior calcaneal process, peroneal trochlea or tubercle, and the medial and lateral processes of the calcaneal tuberosity).

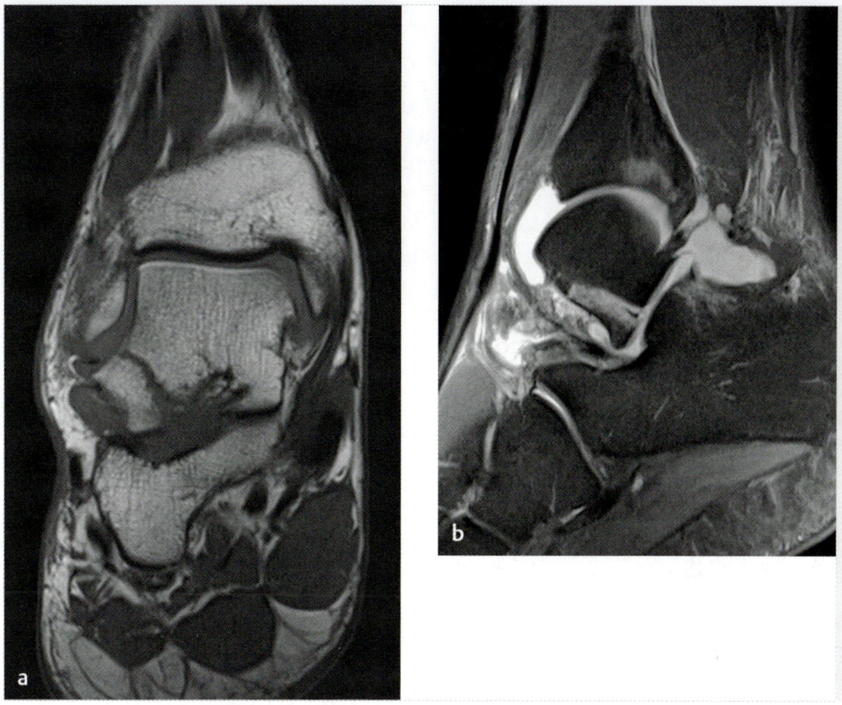

Fig. 3.35 a, b Fracture of the lateral process of the talus ("snowboarder's ankle").
a Coronal T1-weighted MRI clearly demonstrates the hypointense fracture, which is dehiscent distally.
b Sagittal PD-weighted fat-sat image shows hyperintense bleeding into the subtalar and ankle joints. An articular step-off and dehiscence are visible in the subtalar joint.

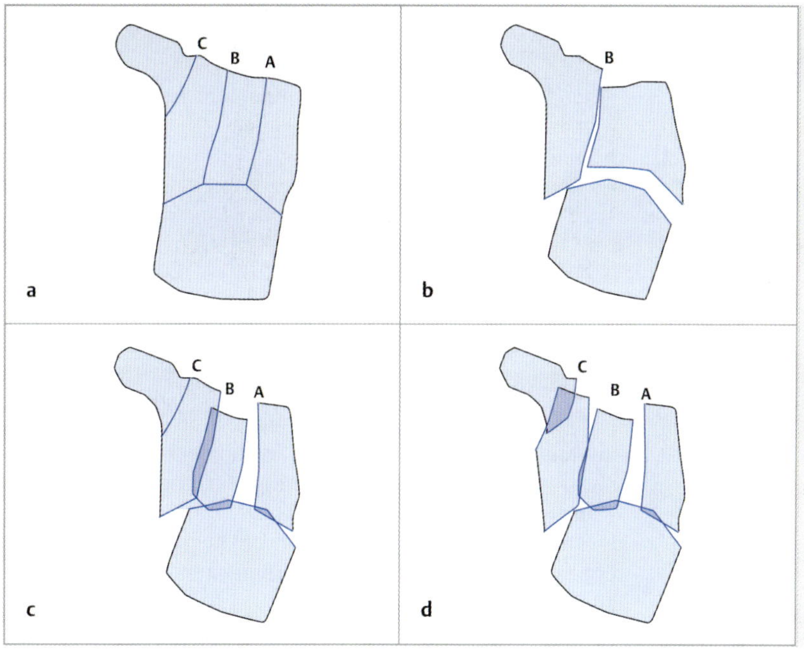

Fig. 3.36 a–d Sanders classification.
a The Sanders classification is based on the number of fragments and the position of the main fracture line (A = lateral, B = central, C = medial).
b Type 2B fracture with two articular fragments and the main fracture line passing through the center of the posterior subtalar facet of the calcaneus.
c Type 3AB fracture with three articular fragments and a lateral and central position of the main fracture lines.
d Type 4ABC fracture with four articular fragments and lateral, central, and medial fracture lines.

Pathology

Mechanism of injury

Calcaneal fractures result from axial loading of the calcaneus due to a fall from a height, motor vehicle accident, or other high-energy trauma. They may also occur as stress fractures due to repetitive loading (endurance sports).

Classifications

- *Essex–Lopresti classification:* This system divides calcaneal fractures into two main groups: intra-articular (80%) and extra-articular (20%). Intra-articular fractures are divided into two subgroups: joint-depression and tongue-type fractures. The joint-depression type involves both fracture and depression of the posterior articular facet in the extended foot. Tongue-type fractures occur in the plantar-flexed foot and involve the distraction and creation of a "tongue fragment." Two primary fragments are formed: a posterolateral fragment and an anteromedial fragment bearing the sustentaculum tali, which remains in continuity with the talus. Other main fragments are an anterior process fragment and a fragment of the anterior joint facet.
- *Sanders classification types I–IV:* Today, the best way to classify calcaneal fractures is by their CT features. The

Table 3.7 Rowe classification of calcaneal fractures.

Type	Description	Percentage of all calcaneal fractures
I	Peripheral fracture	21
Ia	Fracture of the tuberosity	
Ib	Fracture of the sustentaculum tali	
Ic	Fracture of the anterior calcaneal process	
II	Beak fracture or avulsion fracture of the Achilles tendon	3.8
IIa	Beak fracture of the posterosuperior aspect of the calcaneus	
IIb	Avulsion fracture of the Achilles tendon insertion	
III	Extra-articular fracture	19.5
IIIa	Simple fracture	
IIIb	Multipart fracture	
IV	Same as type III with involvement of the posterior facet	24.7
V	Central depression and/or comminution	31
Va	With involvement of the subtalar joint	
Vb	With involvement of the calcaneocuboid joint	

Sanders classification (▶ Fig. 3.36) is based on the degree of involvement of the posterior facet of the subtalar joint. CT images are reformatted parallel and perpendicular to the posterior facet of the subtalar joint in addition to sagittal MPRs:

- Type I: The articular fragments are displaced by less than 2 mm.
- Type II: This fracture has two articular fragments which are displaced more than 2 mm relative to each other.
- Type III: Three articular fragments are displaced more than 2 mm relative to each other.
- Type IV: Four or more articular fragments are displaced more than 2 mm relative to each other.

- *Rowe classification:* see ▶ Table 3.7.
- *Zwipp classification:* This is a CT-based, x-fragment/y-joint system that determines the number of main fragments and the number of affected joints (2–5 fragments and 0–3 joints yield a score in which additional points are assigned for open fractures, severe comminution, or associated injuries such as soft-tissue lesions and talar or cuboid involvement. The total score is from 0 to 12 points).

The severity of a calcaneal fracture is described well by quantifying the degree of disintegration and deformation. Criteria are the degree of step formation and the disintegration of the posterior articular facet of the subtalar joint, loss of height of the central calcaneus, widening of the compressed calcaneus, and axial malalignment. Brunner and his group introduced a system for the quantification of these criteria.

Imaging (▶ Fig. 3.37, ▶ Fig. 3.38, ▶ Fig. 3.39)

Radiographs

Radiographs of the foot are obtained in three planes, if possible with weight bearing. The oblique view clearly demonstrates fractures of the anterior calcaneal process. The calcaneus is imaged in lateral, axial, and Broden views. CT has largely replaced classic radiography for classification and treatment planning. Fractures of the sustentaculum tali are consistently missed on conventional radiographs.

Ultrasound

Not indicated.

CT

CT should employ thin-slice volume acquisition (0.4–0.6-mm slice thickness) and overlapping reconstructions with a high-resolution bone algorithm. MPRs are performed in three planes. The coronal slices are angled slightly anteriorly and directed perpendicular to the posterior facet (posterior compartment). Axial reconstructions are performed perpendicular to the coronal images and parallel to the posterior facet. Direct coronal scans, and even direct sagittal acquisitions, have become obsolete with modern CT systems.

MRI

- *Standard trauma protocol:* High-resolution multi-channel coil; contrast administration is not required.
- *Sequences:*
  - Coronal T1-weighted sequence parallel to the transverse axis of the ankle joint through the talus and malleoli
  - Sagittal and coronal PD-weighted fat-sat (perpendicular to the posterior compartment)
  - Axial T2-weighted sequence angled parallel to the anterior talofibular ligament

CT is superior to MRI in the evaluation of traumatic calcaneal fractures. MRI can add information only in special investigations such as suspected entrapment of the long peroneal tendon. MRI is useful for fatigue fractures of the calcaneus, which are often radiographically occult. A hypointense, incomplete fracture line that terminates in the cancellous bone can be detected within an often extensive area of bone edema.

Imaging Recommendation

Modalities of choice: radiography and CT for traumatic calcaneal fractures, MRI for fatigue fractures of the calcaneus.

Differential Diagnosis

- Ankle sprain
- Achilles tendon rupture
- Peroneal tendon dysfunction
- Sinus tarsi syndrome
- Tarsal tunnel syndrome
- Rupture of the bifurcate ligament

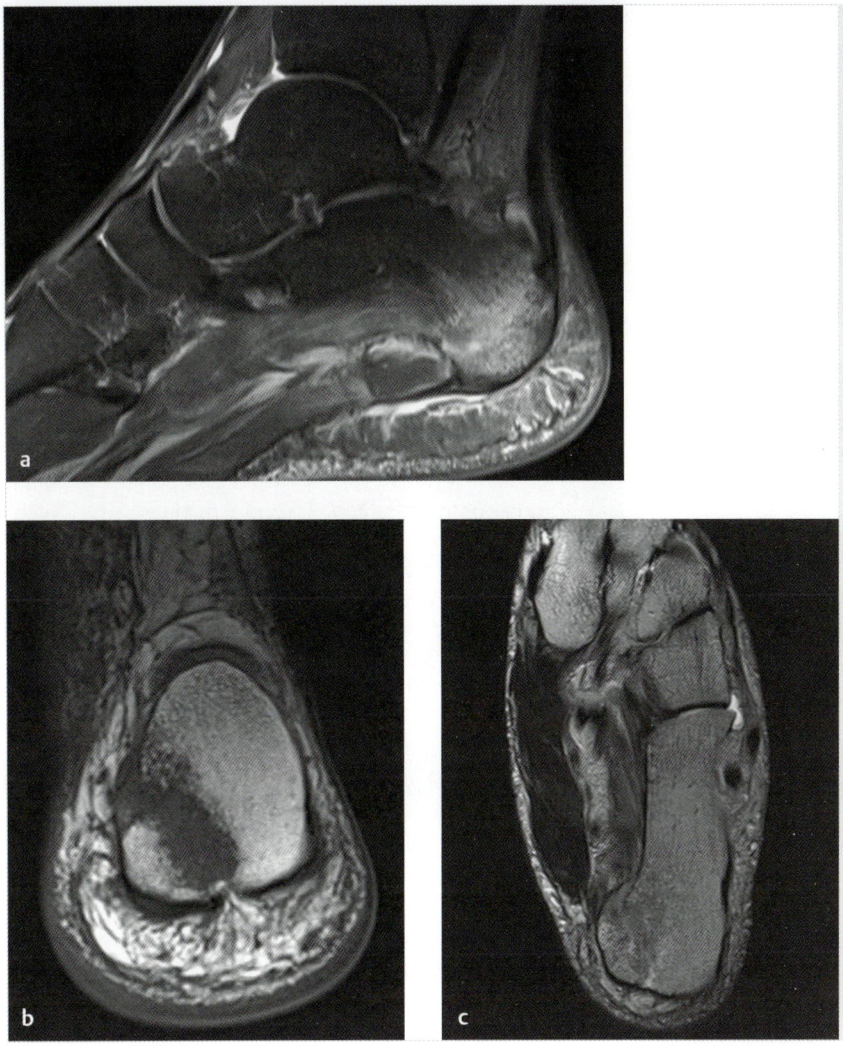

Fig. 3.37 a–c Peripheral calcaneal fracture with a fragment avulsed from the calcaneal tuberosity.
a Sagittal PD-weighted fat-sat MR image shows conspicuous muscular and subcutaneous soft-tissue edema associated with a nondisplaced calcaneal fracture. Often this type of fracture is radiographically occult.
b Coronal T1-weighted image shows slight medial widening and thickening of the calcaneal tuberosity. Incarceration of some subcutaneous fatty tissue into the slightly dehiscent cortex is noted distally and on the plantar aspect.
c Axial T2-weighted image shows slight widening of the calcaneal tuberosity.

Treatment

- Conservative treatment with early mobilization for nondisplaced or minimally displaced calcaneal fractures
- Percutaneous reduction and screw fixation of minimally displaced fractures
- Open reduction and internal screw or plate fixation of complex, markedly displaced fractures
- Exceptional cases with complete destruction of the subtalar joint can be managed by primary arthrodesis.

Prognosis, Complications

Prognosis

- *Fracture of the anterior calcaneal process:* good prognosis. With a nonunion, the loose bone fragment should be resected.
- *Extra-articular fractures:* Their prognosis depends on the size, location, and displacement of the fragments. An anatomic reconstruction of the following angles implies a good prognosis:
  - Gissane angle: 120 to 145° angle formed by the downward and upward slopes of the superior surface of the calcaneus. The angle is distal to the lateral talar process and marks the posterior boundary of the sinus tarsi.
  - Böhler angle: formed by 1) the intersection of a superior tangent to the calcaneal tuberosity and the highest point of the calcaneus in the lateral radiograph and 2) a line from that point to the highest point on the anterior calcaneal process. Normal = 20 to 40°.
- *Involvement of the subtalar joint facet:* Secondary degenerative changes occur in 16% of cases, making it necessary to perform a subtalar arthrodesis.
- *Anatomic reconstruction:* Even with an anatomic reconstruction, secondary degenerative changes may develop due to traumatic cartilage lesions.

Possible Complications

- Compartment syndrome due to swelling (clinical presentation: very severe pain that is difficult to manage even with opioids)
- Secondary skin necrosis

Pediatric Fractures

Definition

Specific pediatric fractures are injuries occurring to the epiphysis and metaphysis of the distal tibia while the growth plate is still open.

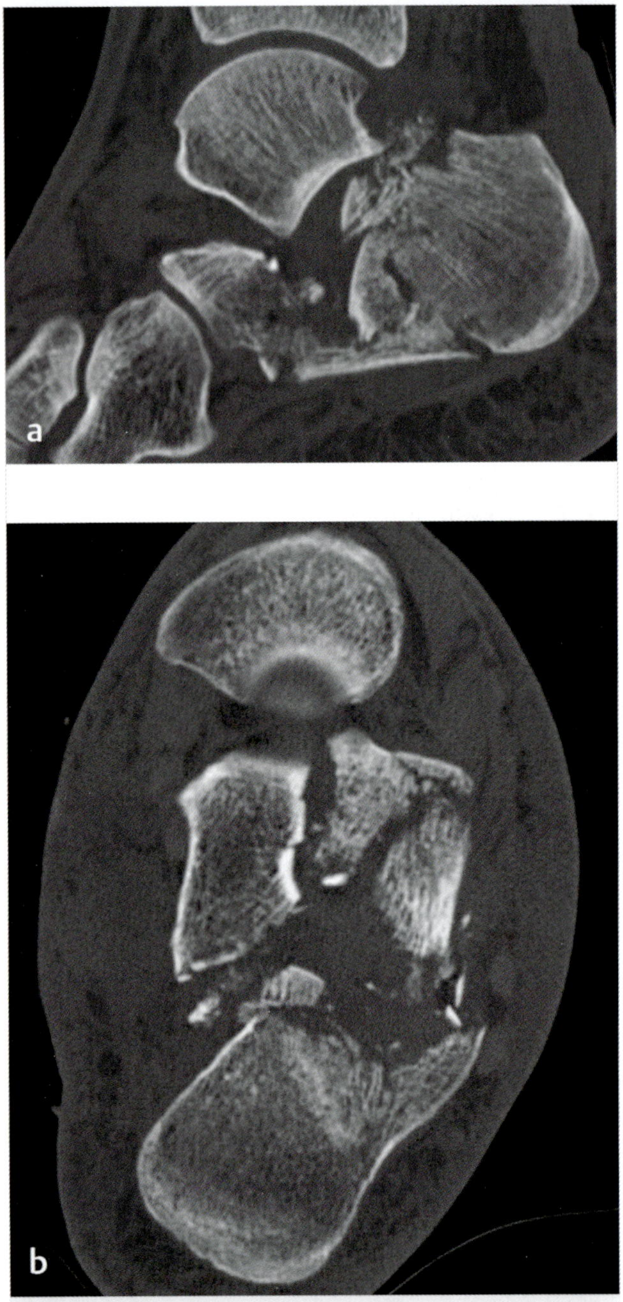

Fig. 3.38 a, b **Joint-depression-type calcaneal fracture.**
a Sagittal reformatted CT image shows deep impaction and depression of the articular surface of the posterior inferior ankle joint, creating a large defect in the cancellous bone.
b Oblique coronal reformatted image shows widening and thickening of the calcaneus and loss of calcaneal height. The main fragments can be identified.

Symptoms

Pain with decreased ability to bear weight on the affected foot.

Predisposing Factors

Open growth plates (transitional fractures occur only during the period of physeal closure from 10 to 16 years of age).

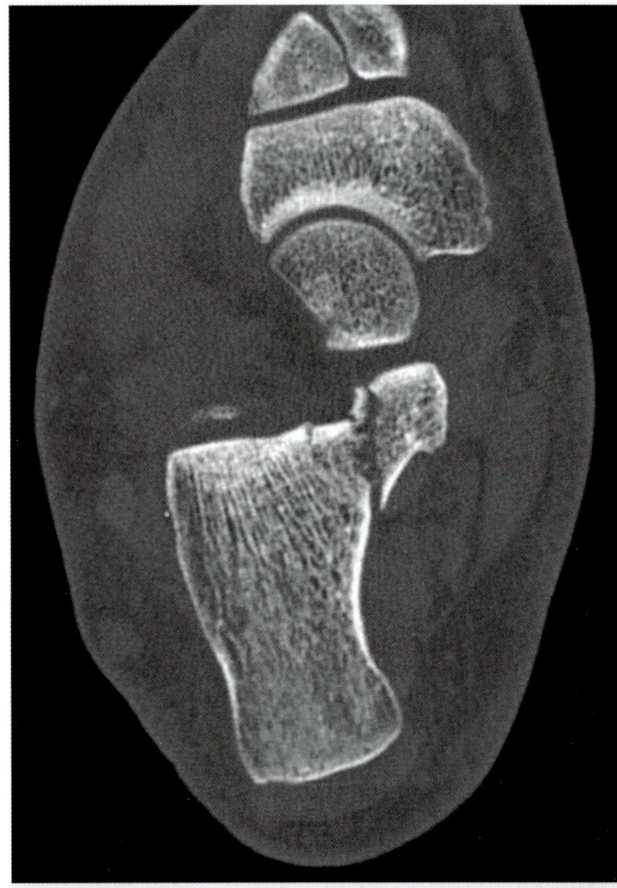

Fig. 3.39 **Fracture of the sustentaculum of the calcaneus.** Oblique coronal reformatted CT image: the flexor hallucis longus tendon runs around the sustentaculum and may be entrapped by a markedly displaced fracture.

Anatomy and Pathology

The Aitken or Salter–Harris classification can be used for fractures involving the growth plate (▶ Fig. 3.40).

Special types of transitional fracture occur only when the growth plates have already started to close:

- *Two-plane fracture:* The fragment is purely epiphyseal. When ossification begins at approximately 10 to 11 years of age, almost the entire epiphysis may be involved and the fracture line is located at a far medial site (intramalleolar). As physeal closure progresses, the typically sagittal fracture line assumes a more lateral position and generally has a sagittal orientation. Finally the injury involves only a bony avulsion of the syndesmosis with an anterolateral fragment. This last type is called a Tillaux or Kleiger fracture.
- *Type I triplane fracture:* Extending through the transverse, sagittal, and coronal planes, this injury includes an epiphyseal fracture plus a lateral metaphyseal wedge fragment. The metaphyseal fracture line does not extend through the growth plate, however.
- *Type II triplane fracture:* An additional metaphyseal wedge fracture is present as in type I, but in type II the fracture line extends into the epiphysis and creates two epiphyseal fragments. The second fragment is posterior and corresponds to a Volkmann-type fracture in adult traumatology.

Fracture pattern	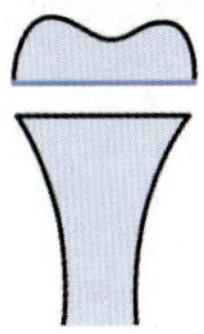	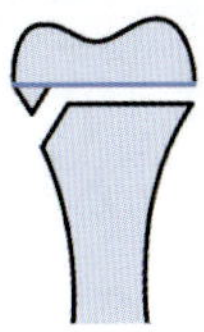	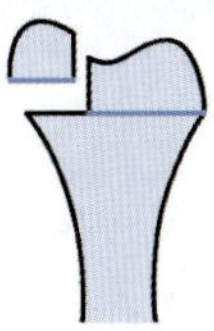	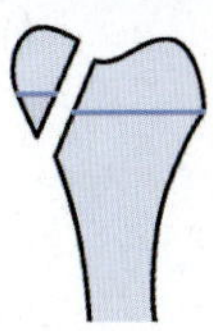
Salter–Harris	I	II	III	IV
Aitken	0	I	II	III

Fig. 3.40 Aitken and Salter–Harris classifications.

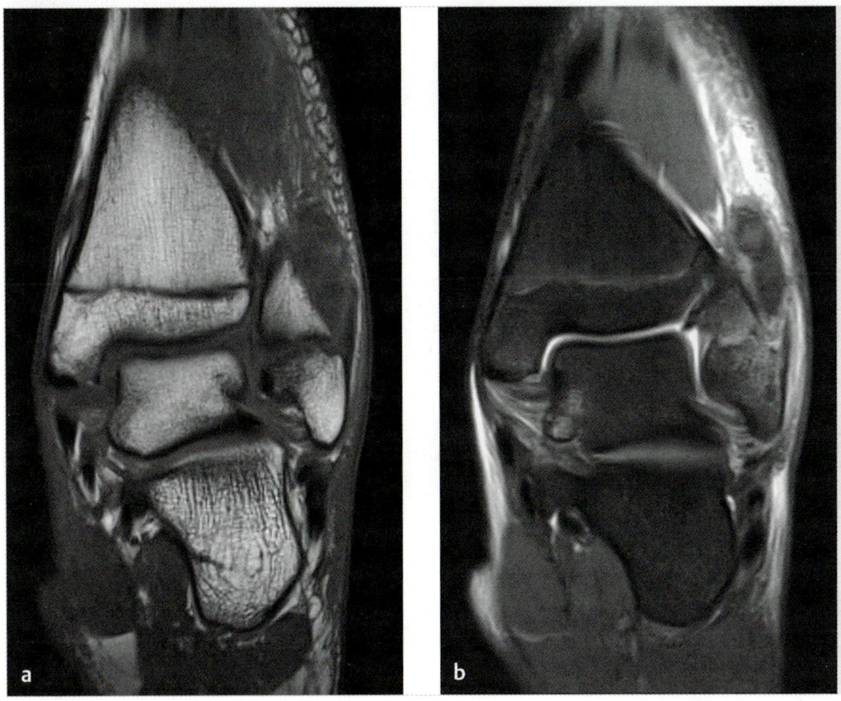

Fig. 3.41 a, b Traumatic epiphyseal separation of the fibula.
a Coronal T1-weighted MRI shows hypointense widening of the epiphyseal plate with some loss of congruity. The periosteum is greatly elevated by a large, hypointense hematoma extending up the lateral aspect of the bone.
b Coronal fat-sat PD-weighted sequence more clearly demonstrates lateral displacement of the fibular epiphysis. The very fresh, extensive hematoma is still hypointense at this early stage.

Imaging (▶ see Figs. 3.41–3.47)

Radiographs

Radiographs of the ankle joint are obtained in two planes, and oblique views are added if required. The sagittal fracture plane and rotational malalignment of the epiphyseal fragment can be difficult to evaluate on radiographs.

Ultrasound

Ultrasound can detect a discontinuity in the echogenic bone surface as well as hypoechoic thickening of the periosteum (especially in pediatric fractures) due to hematoma.

CT

CT employs thin-slice volume acquisition (0.4–0.6-mm slice thickness) and overlapping reconstructions with a high-resolution bone algorithm. MPRs are performed in three planes. Transitional fractures in particular often require a detailed analysis on nonsuperimposed sectional images. CT should be replaced by MRI whenever possible.

MRI

- *Standard trauma protocol:* High-resolution multi-channel coil; contrast administration is not required.
- *Sequences:*
  - Coronal T1-weighted and PD-weighted fat-sat sequences parallel to the transverse axis of the ankle joint through the talus and malleoli
  - Sagittal PD-weighted fat-sat
  - Axial T2-weighted and PD-weighted fat-sat sequences

Slice thicknesses of 2 to 3 mm are desirable. Particular care should be taken to assess the rotational displacement of epiphyseal fragments, the epiphyseal plate, the anterior syndesmosis, and the ligaments.

Imaging Recommendation

Modalities of choice: radiography, MRI.

Differential Diagnosis

- Fibular fracture
- Ankle sprain
- Osteochondral lesion of the talus

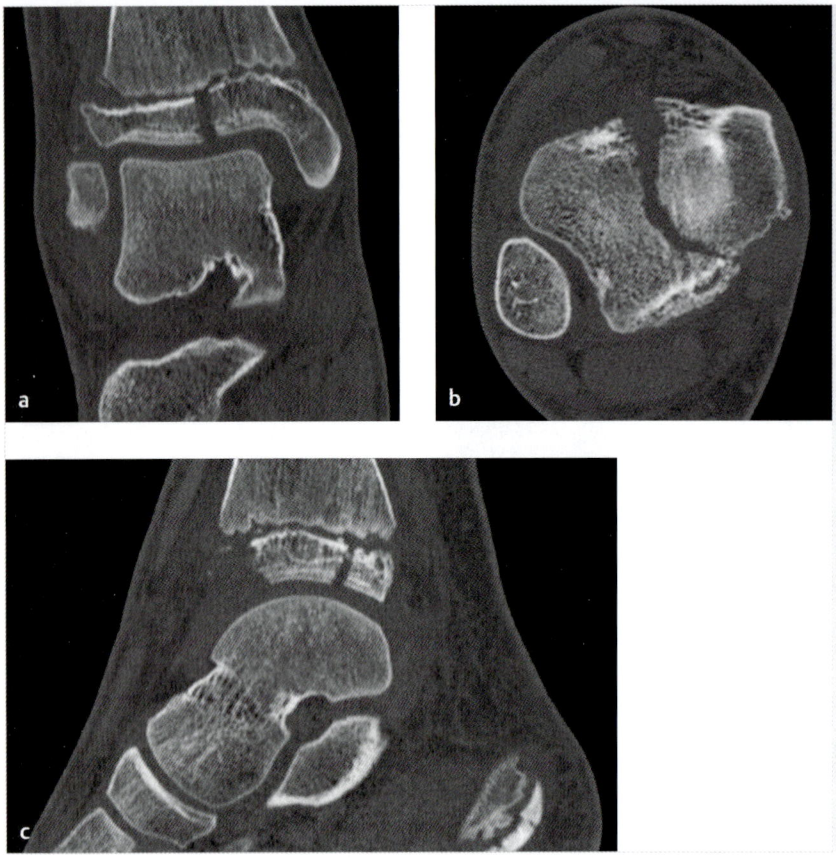

Fig. 3.42 a–c Two-plane epiphyseal fracture.
a Coronal reformatted CT image. The lateral portion of the distal tibial epiphysis is detached, and plate separation has occurred between this lateral part of the epiphysis and the metaphysis.
b Axial reformatted image shows anterior gaping of the epiphyseal fracture with lateral rotational displacement.
c Sagittal reformatted image does not show a metaphyseal wedge.

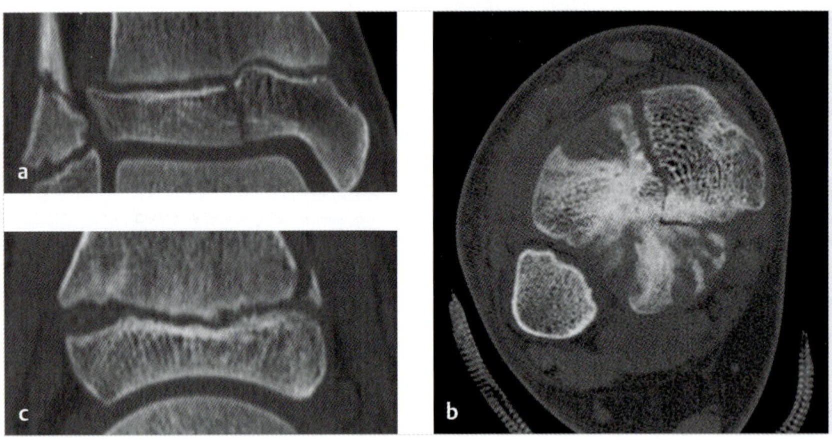

Fig. 3.43 a–c Two-plane fracture with a minimal metaphyseal wedge.
a Coronal reformatted CT image. Case similar to ▶ Fig. 3.42 involves a sagittal fracture through the epiphysis. The lateral piece is displaced laterally and shows lateral rotation. There is an associated fibular fracture.
b Axial image shows lateral rotational displacement.
c Sagittal reformatted image shows a small metaphyseal wedge.

Treatment

Immobilization is usually adequate for the simple fractures (Aitken I and Salter–Harris I and II). The more problematic forms (Aitkin II and III, Salter–Harris III and IV) are generally managed by internal fixation (e.g., with Kirschner wires).

Nondisplaced transitional fractures can be managed conservatively by 4 weeks in a short leg cast with follow-ups. Rare displaced fractures and posterior epiphyseal fragments (type II triplane) should be managed by open reduction and internal fixation. Lag screws are most commonly used for this purpose. The two-plane fracture requires a screw placed horizontally in the epiphysis, and triplane fractures in addition require a metaphyseal screw, which is usually directed anteroposteriorly.

Prognosis, Complications

The prognosis following an anatomic reconstruction is good. Problems result from fractures that are initially missed. Gaping of the fracture line by more than 2 mm poses a risk of eventual degenerative changes or instability.

Subtalar Dislocations

Definition

A subtalar dislocation, also referred to as a peritalar dislocation, involves a dislocation of the subtalar and talonavicular joints while the calcaneocuboid and tibiotalar joints remain intact. The talar neck is not fractured.

Symptoms

From 50 to 80% of subtalar dislocations are caused by high-energy trauma. The remainder result from simple inversion injuries of the foot. Approximately 40% of these injuries are associated with significant soft-tissue damage.

Predisposing Factors

None.

Anatomy and Pathology

A medial subtalar dislocation is caused by forceful inversion of the plantar-flexed foot and a lateral dislocation by forceful eversion of the plantar-flexed foot. Due to anatomic constraints, the lateral injury requires a considerably greater traumatizing force with severe associated soft-tissue disruption.

Imaging

Radiographs

Two-plane views of the ankle joint are obtained. The radiographic features of these rare injuries may be difficult to interpret.

Ultrasound

Not indicated.

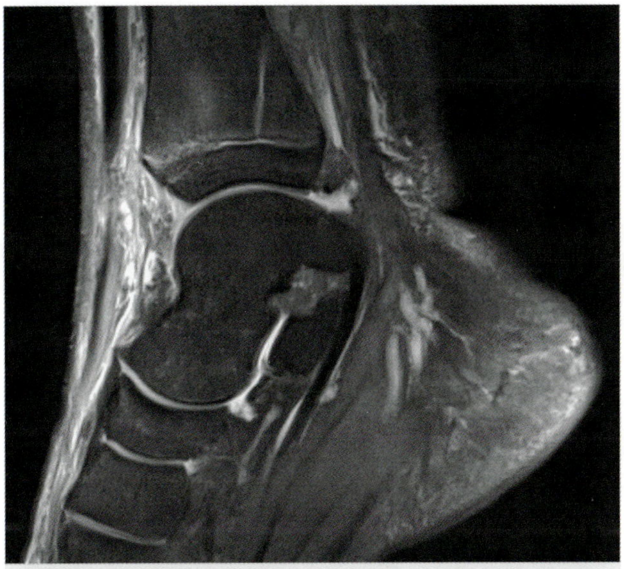

Fig. 3.44 Salter–Harris fracture type II (Aitken type I). Sagittal PD-weighted fat-sat MRI shows a transitional fracture with anterior epiphysiolysis and a posterior metaphyseal wedge.

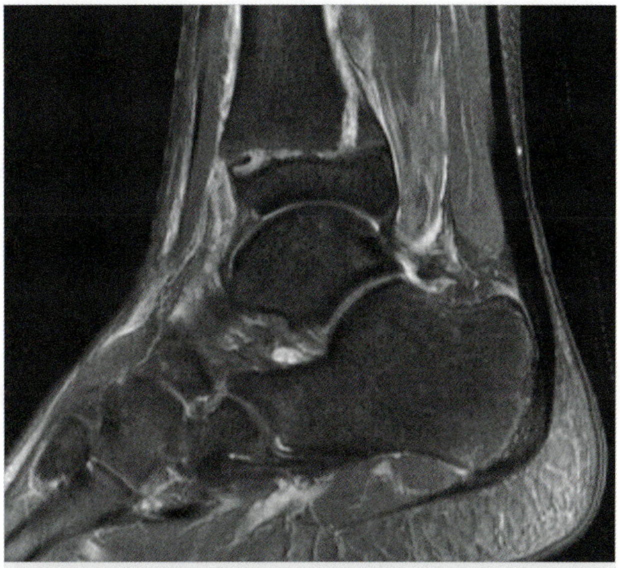

Fig. 3.45 Salter–Harris fracture type II (Aitken type I) similar to the injury in ▸ Fig. 3.44, but with greater displacement. Sagittal PD-weighted fat-sat MRI shows a transitional fracture with anterior epiphysiolysis and a posterior metaphyseal wedge. Some periosteum was avulsed from the proximal metaphysis and displaced into the front of the epiphyseal fracture site as a result of distraction during the injury and subsequent spontaneous reduction. The entrapped periosteal tag is visible in the sagittal image.

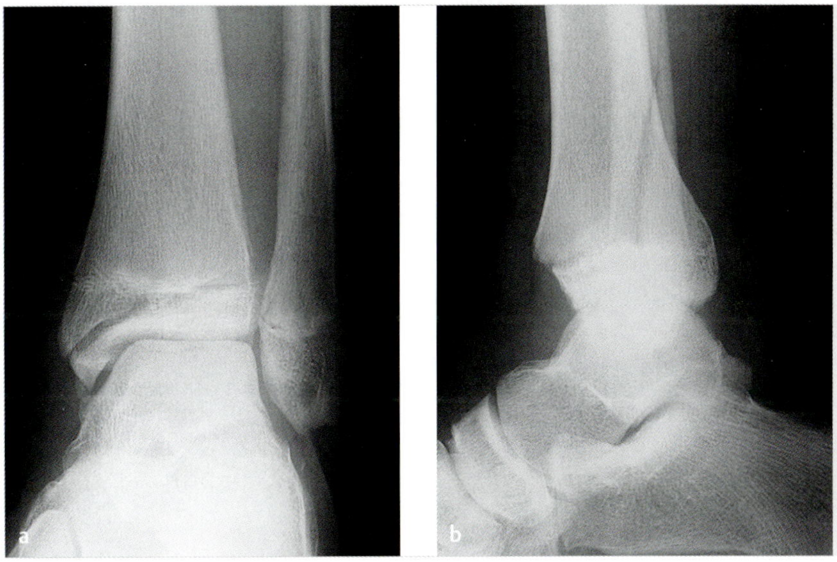

Fig. 3.46 a, b Type I triplane fracture.
a AP radiograph demonstrates a sagittal fracture of the epiphysis.
b Lateral radiograph shows anterior epiphysiolysis with posterior displacement of the distal tibial epiphysis and a metaphyseal wedge fracture. There is also a fibular fracture that directly overlies the tibial metaphyseal fracture in this projection

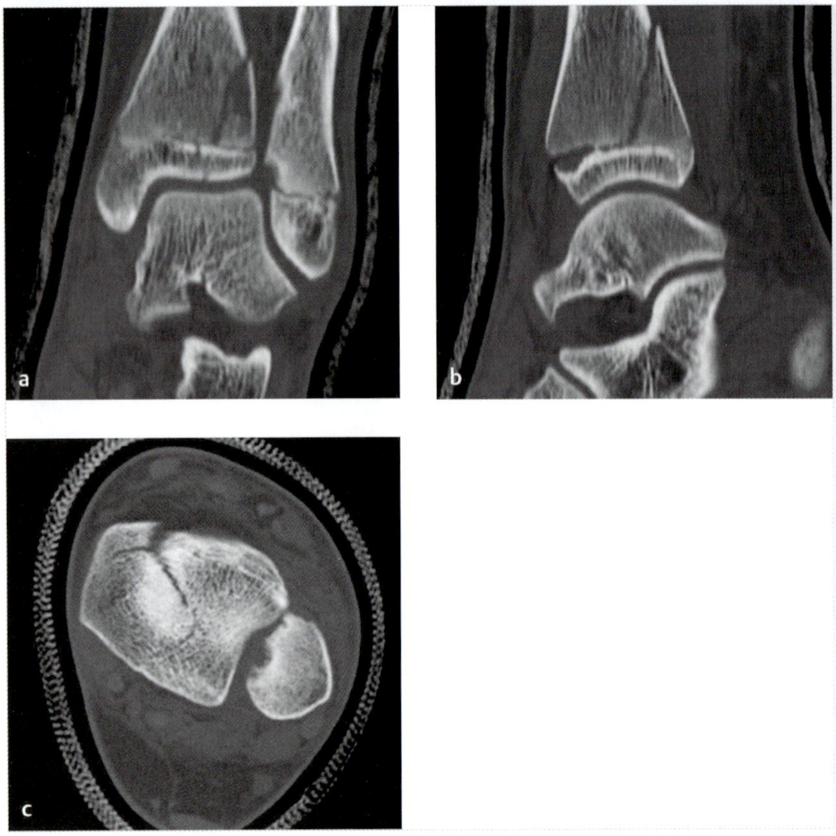

Fig. 3.47 a–c Type II triplane fracture.
a Coronal reformatted CT image shows a metaphyseal wedge fracture that extends into the epiphysis.
b Anterior epiphysiolysis is shown accompanied by a posterior metaphyseal wedge fracture.
c Axial reformatted image displays the course of the sagittal epiphyseal fracture.

CT

CT employs thin-slice volume acquisition (0.4–0.6-mm slice thickness) and overlapping reconstructions with a high-resolution bone algorithm. MPRs are performed in three planes. Reformatted CT images are best for evaluating alignment.

MRI

- *Standard trauma protocol:* High-resolution multi-channel coil; contrast administration is not required.
- *Sequences:*
  - Coronal T1-weighted and PD-weighted fat-sat sequences parallel to the transverse axis of the ankle joint through the talus and malleoli
  - Sagittal PD-weighted fat-sat
  - Axial T2-weighted

MRI can clearly depict alignment, cartilage status, soft-tissue injuries, and associated injuries. MRI with IV contrast is the modality of choice in patients with suspected talar necrosis.

Imaging Recommendation

Modalities of choice: radiography, CT; MRI if required.

Differential Diagnosis

Dislocation of the talocrural joint.

Treatment

Subtalar dislocations require prompt reduction to prevent skin necrosis. This reduction is accomplished by exerting traction on the heel while the knee is in flexion and pushing the talar head back into its physiologic position.

- *Medial dislocation:* The reduction maneuver for a medial dislocation should include plantar flexion and inversion of the foot, followed by eversion and dorsiflexion while a medial plantar pressure is simultaneously applied to reduce the posterolaterally dislocated talar head.
- *Lateral dislocation:* A lateral dislocation is reduced by inversion of the foot with simultaneous lateral pressure on the medially displaced talar head.
- *Posterior dislocation:* The reduction of a posterior dislocation begins with plantar flexion of the forefoot to separate the navicular bone from the undersurface of the talar neck. Next the heel is pushed distally while traction is applied. Finally the foot is dorsiflexed with plantar pressure to reduce the talar head.
- *Anterior dislocation:* With an anterior dislocation, sufficient traction is applied to disengage the posterosuperior edge of the posterior facet from the talar sulcus.

A closed reduction fails in up to 10% of medial dislocations and 20% of lateral dislocations, and an open reduction is indicated. Normally, the joint will be stable following a closed or open reduction.

Further treatment includes a short leg cast worn for 1 to 3 months, depending on the degree of instability.

Prognosis, Complications

The prognosis depends particularly on soft-tissue trauma and cartilage injuries. A prompt reduction also appears to have a favorable effect on outcome. Avascular necrosis of the talus occurs in approximately 5% of cases. Posttraumatic degenerative changes in the subtalar joint are described in up to 40% of cases. This rises to more than 80% in patients with a concomitant fracture. For this reason, CT of the hindfoot is recommended after the reduction of a subtalar dislocation, so that associated osteochondral lesions can be positively identified.

Midtarsal Dislocation

Definition

This is a dislocation injury involving the midtarsal joint (also called the transverse tarsal or Chopart joint).

Symptoms

Midtarsal dislocations most commonly result from high-energy trauma. They rarely result from a simple midfoot sprain. The cardinal symptoms are swelling, tenderness, pain, and subcutaneous hemorrhage. Midtarsal dislocations may be combined with significant soft-tissue injury, depending on the magnitude of the traumatizing force.

Predisposing Factors

None.

Anatomy and Pathology

The midtarsal joint includes the talonavicular and calcaneocuboid joints, which are oriented transversely to the longitudinal arch of the foot and combine with the subtalar joint to allow for coupled, multidimensional movements.

The talonavicular and calcaneocuboid joints are incorporated into the medial and lateral columns of the foot in accordance with their function. The talonavicular joint is part of the medial column and is supported by the talonavicular ligament. The very rigid calcaneocuboid joint is part of the lateral column and has a saddle-shaped structure. The calcaneocuboid joint is stabilized by the calcaneocuboid ligaments.

Imaging

Radiographs

Radiographs of the ankle joint are taken in two planes. The radiographic features of these rare injuries may be difficult to interpret.

Ultrasound

Not indicated.

CT

CT employs thin-slice volume acquisition (0.4–0.6-mm slice thickness) and overlapping reconstructions with a high-resolution bone algorithm. MPRs are generated in three planes. Reformatted CT images are best for evaluating alignment.

MRI

- *Standard trauma protocol:* High-resolution multi-channel coil; contrast administration is not required.
- *Sequences:*
  - Coronal T1-weighted and PD-weighted fat-sat sequences parallel to the transverse axis of the ankle joint through the talus and malleoli
  - Sagittal PD-weighted fat-sat
  - Axial T2-weighted

MRI is good for assessing alignment, cartilage status, soft-tissue injuries, and associated injuries. Contrast-enhanced MRI is the modality of choice in cases with suspected talar necrosis.

Imaging Recommendation

Modalities of choice: radiography, CT; MRI if required.

Differential Diagnosis

- Achilles tendon rupture
- Ankle sprain
- Talar fracture
- Tarsometatarsal joint injuries

Treatment

Treatment options include closed reduction, primary arthrodesis, and open reduction with or without transfixation of the affected joints. An external Ilisarov frame can be used in patients with extensive soft-tissue injuries. Primary arthrodesis is very rarely practiced today owing to improved diagnostic and treatment options. The goal of acute treatment is an anatomic reduction secured by internal or external fixation. Arthrodesis is appropriate only in patients with posttraumatic osteoarthritis that cannot be successfully managed by other means.

Prognosis, Complications

Prognosis

The prognosis of the injury depends greatly on the extent of the primary injury, the degree of dislocation, and possible associated fractures. A concomitant injury of the tarsometatarsal (Lisfranc) joint line is an unfavorable prognostic factor. Midtarsal dislocations are very serious foot injuries that often cause permanent functional impairment, even with optimum treatment.

Possible Complications

- Compartment syndrome in the foot
- Soft-tissue necrosis
- Avascular necrosis of the talus
- Avascular necrosis of the navicular

3.2 Chronic, Posttraumatic, and Degenerative Changes

3.2.1 Axial Malalignment of the Hindfoot

M. Walther and A. Staebler

Osteoarthritis of the Ankle Joint with Varus or Valgus Deformity

Definition

Osteoarthritis of an ankle joint with varus or valgus deformity consists of degenerative changes resulting from ankle malalignment.

Symptoms

Small degrees of malalignment can often be tolerated for decades without complaints. But there is a long-term risk for the development of degenerative changes (osteoarthritis) due to abnormal loading of the ankle joint.

Predisposing Factors

Malalignment of the hindfoot may eventually lead to secondary deformities about the ankle joint (grade IV posterior tibial insufficiency, varus deformity in pes cavus). The axial malalignment of the hindfoot is aggravated by a lack of muscular stabilization. When a varus or valgus deformity of the ankle joint is diagnosed, pathology should be excluded in the following additional structures:

- Varus deformity:
  - Peroneal tendons
  - Lateral ligaments
- Valgus deformity:
  - Posterior tibial tendon
  - Deltoid ligament

Anatomy and Pathology

A varus or valgus malalignment of the ankle joint very rarely represents an isolated problem. Usually it is secondary to one of the disorders listed below:

- Epiphyseal fracture with a secondary growth abnormality
- Neuromuscular disease
- Axial malalignment after a tibial or pilon fracture
- Angular deformity at the level of the knee joint
- Pes cavus
- Chronic lateral ligamentous instability
- Peroneal tendon rupture
- Pes planovalgus
- Rupture of the posterior tibial tendon
- Rupture of the deltoid ligament
- Instability of the talonavicular, naviculocuneiform, or tarsometatarsal joint

Imaging

Radiographs (▶ Fig. 3.48)

- *Single-leg stance radiograph:* used for determining the axial alignment of the femur and tibia (normal femorotibial angle = 174°) and the mechanical axis of the leg (Mikulicz line). The center of the femoral head, the center of the knee joint, and the center of the talar dome should all be located on one line called the mechanical limb axis. Varus or valgus malalignment is measured as the deviation of the center of the knee joint from the mechanical limb axis.
- *Ankle joint in two planes, weight bearing:* used for evaluating cartilage status and ankle alignment.
- *Foot in three planes, weight bearing:* longitudinal arch, forefoot abduction, position of the talonavicular joint.
- *Saltzman view:* for evaluating the position of the calcaneus.
- *Special views in patients with pes cavovarus:* weight-bearing AP and lateral views of the foot using the Colman block test with no weight on the plantar-flexed first metatarsal.

Ultrasound

Not indicated.

CT

Thin-slice CT (0.4–0.6-mm slice thickness, overlapping reconstructions) with MPRs is used to evaluate the joint space width and subchondral bone for possible sclerosis, defects, subchondral cysts, osteophytes, or bony intra-articular loose bodies.

MRI

Interpretation Checklist

Assess the articular cartilage status and describe any cartilage lesions present as focal defects or more diffuse changes. Cartilage lesions should be graded on the Outerbridge scale. It is important to describe the morphology and location of cartilage injuries.

Examination Technique

- *Standard protocol:* High-resolution multi-channel coil; IV contrast administration
- *Sequences:*
  - Coronal T1-weighted sequences parallel to the transverse axis of the ankle joint through the talus and malleoli
  - Sagittal and coronal PD-weighted fat-sat
  - Axial T2-weighted, angled parallel to the anterior talofibular ligament
  - Coronal and sagittal T1-weighted fat-sat sequences after IV contrast administration

MRI Findings

- Joint effusion
- Articular cartilage
- Synovitis (contrast enhancement)
- Fibrovascular granulation tissue in the capsule and ligaments
- Foci of activation, including the ankle joint capsule and talonavicular joint

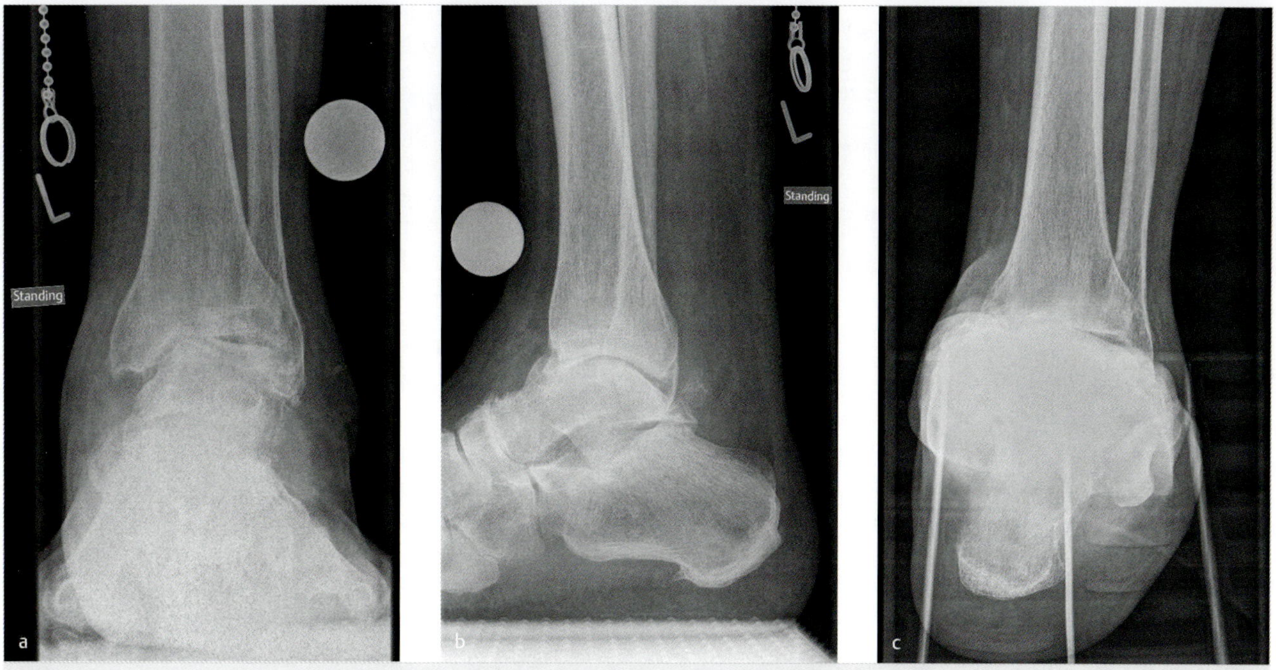

Fig. 3.48 a–c Osteoarthritis with varus deformity. Grade IV osteoarthritis of the ankle joint with predominantly medial joint space narrowing and varus deformity of the entire hindfoot.
a DP view.
b Lateral view.
c Saltzman view: varus angulation of the calcaneus.

Imaging Recommendation

Modality of choice: radiographs, CT, or MRI should be used as needed for further investigation.

Differential Diagnosis

- Epiphyseal fracture with secondary growth abnormality
- Neuromuscular disease
- Axial malalignment after a tibial or pilon fracture
- Axial malalignment at the level of the knee joint
- Pes cavus
- Chronic lateral ligament instability
- Rupture of the peroneal tendons
- Pes planovalgus
- Rupture of the posterior tibial tendon
- Rupture of the deltoid ligament
- Instability of the talonavicular, naviculocuneiform, or tarsometatarsal joint

Treatment

Treatment depends on the underlying disease. With otherwise normal anatomic relationships, angular deformities of the distal tibia can be corrected by an opening- or closing-wedge osteotomy.

Prognosis, Complications

In patients with intact articular cartilage, restoring a physiologic axis can significantly improve joint function. Frequent limiting factors are underlying diseases and pre-existing degenerative changes in the talocrural and subtalar joints.

Pes planovalgus

Definition

Pes planovalgus is a flatfoot deformity with the following components, which may vary considerably in their degree:

- Hindfoot valgus
- Flattened longitudinal arch
- Abduction of the forefoot
- Supination of the forefoot
- Shortening of the gastrocnemius

Symptoms

Symptoms depend on the underlying pathology. Patients may be largely asymptomatic or may have complaints ranging to significant functional disability of the foot. Typical complaints are as follows:

- Medial ankle pain due to a rupture of the posterior tibial tendon or deltoid ligament
- Lateral ankle pain due to impingement between a valgus calcaneus and the distal tip of the fibula

Predisposing Factors

- Talocalcaneal or calcaneonavicular coalition
- Congenital short lateral column
- Rupture of the posterior tibial tendon
- Rupture of the deltoid ligament
- Congenital valgus calcaneus

Anatomy and Pathology

Patients with congenital pes planovalgus are often free of complaints for many years. Typical pathologies tend to occur in certain age groups:

- *Children:* flexible pes planovalgus with no pathologic significance; congenital short lateral column
- *Adolescents:* talocalcaneal or calcaneonavicular coalition
- *Young adults:* traumatic lesions
- *Older adults:* rupture of the posterior tibial tendon

Imaging

Radiographs (▶ Fig. 3.49)

- *Weight-bearing radiographs of the foot in three planes:* longitudinal arch, forefoot abduction, position of the talonavicular joint
- *Saltzman view:* to evaluate the position of the calcaneus

Ultrasound

In patients with posterior tibial insufficiency:

- Thickening of the posterior tibial tendon
- Loss of function

MRI

Interpretation Checklist

- Cause of flatfoot
- Alignment of the tarsal bones
- Exclude a fibrocartilaginous or bony coalition (complete or partial)
- Signs of posterior tibial insufficiency

Examination Technique

- *Standard protocol:* Scan in the prone position using a high-resolution multi-channel coil and IV contrast administration.
- *Sequences:*
  - Coronal T1-weighted sequences parallel to the transverse axis of the ankle joint through the talus and malleoli
  - Sagittal and coronal PD-weighted fat-sat
  - Axial T2-weighted, angled parallel to the anterior talofibular ligament
  - Axial oblique and sagittal T1-weighted fat-sat sequences after contrast administration

MRI Findings

- Fluid around the posterior tibial tendon
- Tendon diameter is thickened (tendinopathy) or thinned (partial tear)
- Peritendinous fluid collection
- Synovitic contrast uptake in the tendon sheath or fibrovascular tissue with increased vascularity in the tendon substance
- Possible bone reaction at fibro-osseous junctions
- Position and possible irritation of the talonavicular joint in patients with forefoot abduction
- Possible signs of stress in the posterior capsule of the subtalar joint and/or in the sinus tarsi
- Possible infiltration of enhancing fibrotic tissue into the sinus tarsi (sinus tarsi syndrome)
- Possible signs of bony or fibrocartilaginous coalition—especially calcaneonavicular or talocalcaneal

! Note

Give particular attention to bone edema, cyst formation, and irregularities in the "subchondral" plate. Do not miss possible sites of fibrous or bony coalition.

Imaging Recommendation

Modalities of choice: radiography, MRI.

Differential Diagnosis

- Neuromuscular disease
- Posterior tibial tendon rupture
- Fibrous or bony coalition
- Axial malalignment after a tibial or pilon fracture
- Deltoid ligament injuries

Treatment

Treatment depends on the underlying pathology:

- Flexible pes planovalgus in children > 10 years old who have failed conservative treatment: arthroereisis (subtalar implant), Evans osteotomy
- Coalition: resection of the bone bridge; arthroereisis may be added if necessary. Corrective arthrodesis of the subtalar joint is rarely performed.
- Rupture of the posterior tibial tendon: possible options are a flexor digitorum longus transfer, calcaneal sliding or lengthening osteotomy, plantar flexion osteotomy of the first cuneiform, and Achilles tendon lengthening.

Prognosis, Complications

The pediatric foot tolerates three-dimensional corrections relatively well. The prognosis after the resection of a coalition depends greatly on the size of the bone bridge and the condition of the joints. Rupture of the posterior tibial tendon can be effectively treated as noted above, but it will take at least 6 months before the foot can tolerate full weight bearing. Patients may have residual deficits of strength, range of motion, and weight-bearing ability.

Pes cavus

Definition

Pes cavus is a foot deformity characterized by increased height of the plantar arch, a high instep, and excessive plantar flexion of the first ray.

Symptoms

- Limited dorsiflexion of the ankle joint
- Pressure points on the lateral border of the foot and over the metatarsal heads
- Giving-way episodes

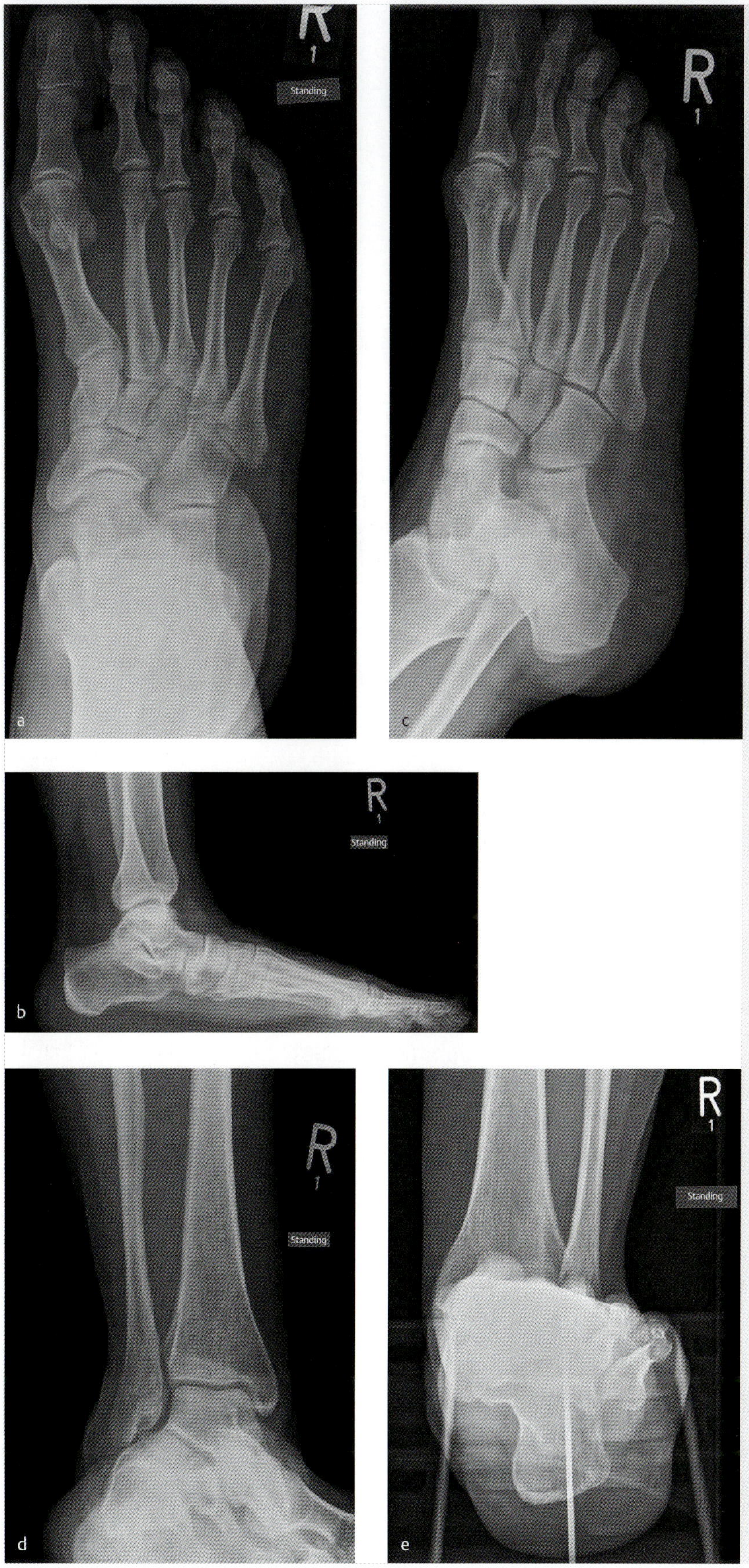

Fig. 3.49 a–e Pes planovalgus. Congenital pes planovalgus deformity with only a mild forefoot abduction component. The deformity is caused chiefly by the varus position of the calcaneus.
a DP view.
b Lateral view.
c Oblique view.
d AP projection.
e Saltzman view shows impingement between the calcaneus and the distal tip of the fibula.

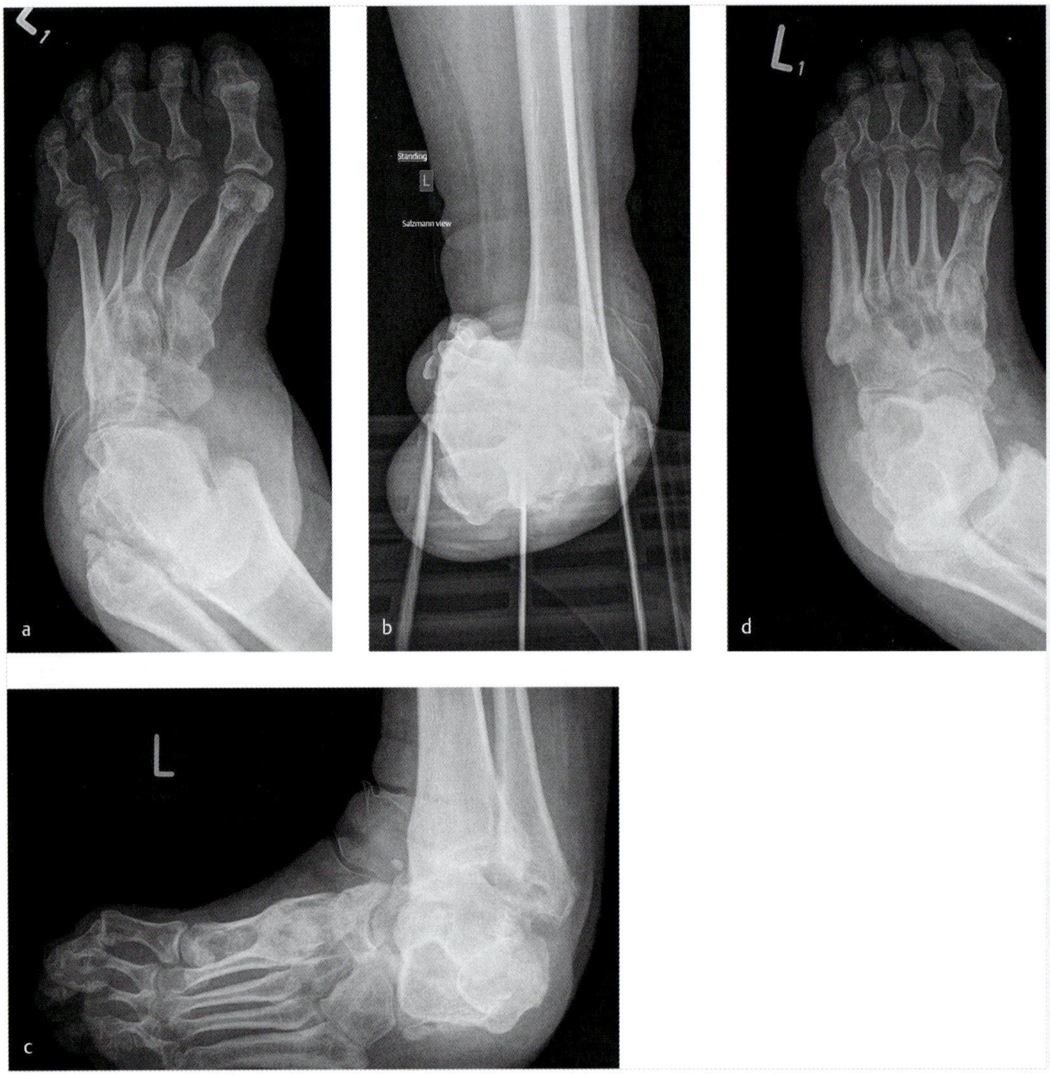

Fig. 3.50 a–d Neurogenic pes cavus. This patient has a severe pes cavus deformity based on a hereditary sensorimotor neuropathy.
a DP view.
b Oblique view. The inversion deformity of the foot is so pronounced that the oblique view gives a DP projection of the forefoot.
c Lateral view.
d Saltzman view.

- Toeing-in gait with weight shifted to the lateral side of the foot
- Achillodynia
- Overextension of the knee and rapid fatigability

Predisposing Factors

Predisposing factors include neurologic diseases such as Charcot–Marie–Tooth disease, Friedreich ataxia, and Roussy–Levy syndrome. Pes cavovarus (see paragraph below) is often the initial sign of a neurologic disease.

Anatomy and Pathology

The two main types of pes cavus are pes calcaneocavus and pes cavovarus. Pes cavovarus, characterized by an increased arch of the forefoot, develops only after the child has started walking; the foot is still normal in infancy. Pes calcaneocavus is characterized by a steep upward tilt of the calcaneus. Pes cavovarus features a muscular imbalance caused by neuromuscular disease (spastic, flaccid paralysis, abnormal interaction of the intrinsic foot muscles) or a non-neuromuscular cause (in a setting of congenital clubfoot or other idiopathic deformities).

Imaging

Radiographs (▶ Fig. 3.50)

- *Weight-bearing radiographs of the foot in two planes:*
  - Lateral view:
    - Ankle mortise is rotated and displaced posteriorly
    - Parallel alignment of the talar and calcaneal axes
    - Sinus tarsi window
    - Shortened longitudinal dimension of the calcaneus due to varus angulation
    - Decreased distance between the medial malleolus and navicular
    - Horizontal projection of the posterior facet of the subtalar joint
    - Lack of overlap between the navicular and cuboid
    - Plantar prominence of the fifth metatarsal parallel to the contact surface of the foot
    - Plantar flexion of the first metatarsal
    - Hammer toes
  - DP view:
    - Parallel axes of the talus and calcaneus
    - Adduction of the forefoot

  - Relative shortening of the first metatarsal due to its plantar-flexed position
  - Overlapping of the metatarsal bones
- *Weight-bearing radiographs of the foot in two planes using the Coleman block test:* Relieving pressure on the plantar-flexed first metatarsal can differentiate between a fixed and flexible hindfoot deformity. A flexible hindfoot will correct on the block.
- *Saltzman view:* The axial weight-bearing view of the calcaneus documents hindfoot varus.

MRI, CT

MRI: secondary degenerative joint changes?
CT: 3D position of the foot?

Imaging Recommendation

Modality of choice: radiography.

Treatment

Flexible deformities can be corrected by tendon transfers if muscle function is intact. Fixed deformities can be corrected by osteotomies or corrective arthrodesis. The goal is to perform the correction at the point of greatest deformity. Correction typically involves a wedge resection in the midfoot and a calcaneal osteotomy for the correction of hindfoot valgus.

Prognosis, Complications

The prognosis and possible complications depend on the underlying disease.

3.2.2 Impingement

U. Szeimies

Anterolateral Impingement

Definition

In anterolateral impingement, soft tissues are entrapped due to causes such as heavy scarring, a thickened ankle joint capsule, or chronic inflammatory irritation of the anterior talofibular ligament. Anterolateral impingement is the most common form of impingement and usually occurs after trauma.

Symptoms

Typical signs are tenderness to pressure and load-dependent anterolateral pain that is worsened by dorsiflexion.

Predisposing Factors

The patient may describe a history of an ankle twist with capsuloligamentous injuries weeks or months before presentation.

Anatomy and Pathology

Scarring or synovitis leads to soft-tissue impingement in the anterolateral corner of the ankle joint. A thick band of scar tissue forms along the anterior talofibular ligament. Histology reveals fibrovascular reactive tissue, synovitis, and meniscoid scar tissue in the triangle between the tibia, fibula, and talus.

Imaging

Radiographs

Radiographs show no abnormalities.

Ultrasound

- Thickening of the anterolateral capsule
- Chronic soft-tissue proliferation
- Possible echogenic synovitis with mild-to-moderate joint effusion
- Vascular engorgement on Duplex scans

MRI

Interpretation Checklist

- Degree of scarring
- Activity
- Evaluate the structure of the anterior talofibular ligament and nearby structures (peroneal tendons, distal tip of the fibula)
- Other posttraumatic changes (e.g., posttraumatic osteochondritis dissecans)
- Signs of ankle instability
- Cartilage quality
- Cartilage lesions

Examination Technique

- *Standard protocol:* prone position, high-resolution multichannel coil
- *Sequences:*
  - Coronal and sagittal PD-weighted fat-sat
  - Coronal T1-weighted
  - Axial T2-weighted
  - T1-weighted fat-sat, true axial (angled to joint plane) and sagittal after IV contrast administration; add coronal images if needed

MRI Findings (▶ Fig. 3.51)

MRI typically shows enhancing fibrovascular scar tissue along the anterolateral capsule and ligaments, usually with an ill-defined anterior talofibular ligament that is markedly thickened due to scarring.

Imaging Recommendation

Modality of choice: contrast-enhanced MRI of the ankle joint.

Differential Diagnosis

- Chronic instability
- Pigmented villonodular synovitis
- Ganglion
- Chondromatosis
- Osteochondral lesion of the talus

Treatment

- Physical therapy
- Nonsteroidal anti-inflammatory drugs

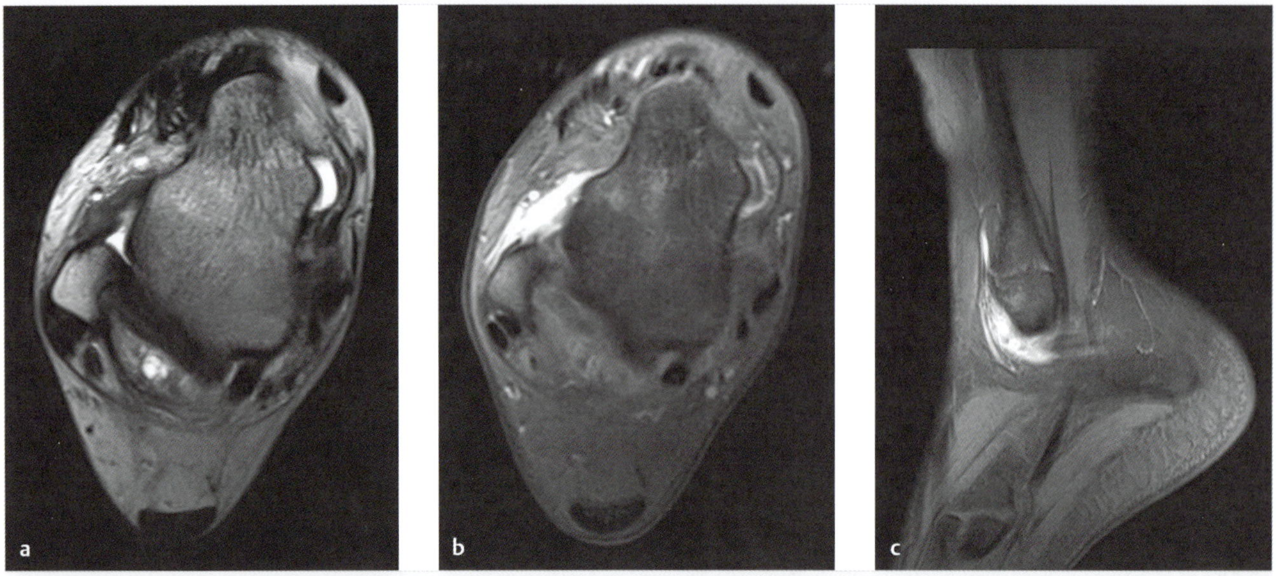

Fig. 3.51 a–c Anterolateral impingement. Increasing pain and swelling developed over the lateral malleolus several months after the patient suffered a lateral ankle sprain.
a Axial T2-weighted image shows marked thickening and scarring of the anterior talofibular ligament.
b Axial T1-weighted fat-sat image after contrast administration shows intense enhancement of the fibrovascular tissue along the course of the anterior talofibular ligament.
c Sagittal T1-weighted fat-sat image after contrast administration.

- Local steroid injections
- Arthroscopic debridement of scar tissue
- With instability: ankle ligament reconstruction

Prognosis, Complications

Possible complications:
- Heterotopic ossification of the capsule
- Osteophyte formation on the anterior tibial margin and talar neck
- Chronic lateral ankle pain
- Chronic lateral synovitis of the ankle joint

Anterior Impingement, Anteromedial Impingement, Posteromedial Impingement

Definition

These conditions refer to the anterior or medial entrapment of bone or soft tissue between the tibial border and the neck of the talus.
- *Anterior impingement:* common type of bony impingement caused by osteophytes and bony outgrowths on the anterior tibial margin. Common on the anterior talar neck in soccer players (repetitive dorsiflexion with bone irritation). Synonym: soccer ankle.
- *Anteromedial impingement:* rare type caused by posttraumatic scarring of the anterior part of the deltoid ligament, marked by soft-tissue proliferation on the joint capsule and possible osteophytes. Usually results from supination trauma.
- *Posteromedial impingement:* rare type caused by scar build-up after posterior deltoid ligament injuries with impingement occurring between the medial malleolus and talus.

Symptoms

- Anterior ankle pain that is increased by dorsiflexion or eccentric loading (e.g., kicking a football in soccer)
- Limitation of dorsiflexion
- Occasional palpable osteophyte on the talar neck or anterior tibial margin

Predisposing Factors

- Ball sports and jumping sports, especially soccer (shooting leg)
- Ballet dancers
- Prior history of multiple ankle sprains

Anatomy and Pathology

Bony outgrowth and/or scar build-up on the anterior tibial margin and talar neck results from multiple sprain injuries with overloading of the capsular attachment. Soft-tissue impingement is distinguished from bony impingement with a normal talocrural joint. Differentiation is required from osteophyte formation in the setting of ankle osteoarthritis.

Imaging

Radiographs

Radiographs show osteophytes on the medial talar neck and anterior tibial margin, or less commonly at a central or lateral site. Standard views may be supplemented by oblique views in 30° of internal and external rotation to help demonstrate marginal osteophytes about the ankle joint.

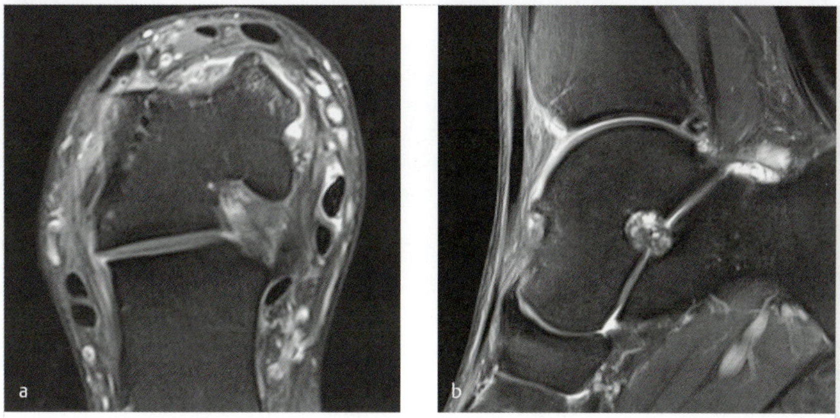

Fig. 3.52 a, b A 37-year-old athletically active (soccer) man presented with increasing anterior and anteromedial ankle pain on maximum dorsiflexion. Anteromedial ankle impingement on the right side is caused by circumscribed bony osteophytes on the anteromedial talus. Local bone and soft-tissue activation with associated synovitis is noted at the junction of the talar neck and trochlea.
a Axial T1-weighted fat-sat image after contrast administration shows bone activation with associated osteophytes and adjacent fibrovascular reaction in the soft tissues.
b Sagittal T1-weighted fat-sat image after contrast administration shows the osteophytes with predominantly anterior synovitis in the ankle joint.

Ultrasound

Ultrasound shows an echogenic bulge on the bony talar surface in the course of the anterior tibiotalar part of the deltoid ligament. Scans may show a medial, echogenic intracapsular or intraligamentous change in the periarticular bone structure with an associated acoustic shadow. Thickening of the echogenic synovium and a small joint effusion are occasionally noted. Real-time impingement dynamics can sometimes be seen on the monitor. An ultrasound stress test of the anterior talofibular ligament may be positive in patients with ankle instability.

MRI

Interpretation Checklist

- Degree of bone or soft-tissue activation and osteophyte formation on the adjacent talar neck and anterior tibial margin
- Synovitis of the ankle joint
- Cartilage status
- Anterior degenerative changes in the ankle joint
- Involvement of extensor tendon sheaths

Examination Technique

- *Standard protocol:* prone position, high-resolution multichannel coil
- *Sequences:*
  - Coronal and sagittal PD-weighted fat-sat
  - Coronal T1-weighted
  - Axial T2-weighted
  - T1-weighted fat-sat, true axial (angled to joint plane) and sagittal after IV contrast administration; add coronal images if needed

MRI Findings (▸ Fig. 3.52)

- Intracapsular or intra-articular osteophytes, usually found on the medial side of the anterior tibia and at corresponding sites on the talus in the ankle joint
- Extra-articular enthesiophytes, usually found on the lateral side of the capsule and ligaments
- Bone activation with associated osteophytes on the anterior side of the ankle joint
- Enhancing synovitis in the anterior part of the ankle joint
- Reactive fibrovascular tissue around the osteophytes
- Visualization of detached bone fragments, ossicles, or intra-articular loose bodies

Imaging Recommendation

Modalities of choice: clinical examination and radiography. MRI is recommended for a precise evaluation of ankle joint status (incipient osteoarthritis) and degree of activation.

Differential Diagnosis

- Generalized osteoarthritis of the ankle joint
- Talar fracture
- Ankle joint synovitis
- Intra-articular loose bodies

Treatment

Conservative

- Nonsteroidal anti-inflammatory drugs
- Steroid injections
- Physical therapy (conservative therapy can reduce inflammatory irritation but cannot eliminate the mechanical cause)

Operative

- Arthroscopic removal of osteophytes
- Local synovectomy and debridement of scar tissue
- With large osteophytes: arthrotomy with open removal is an option

Prognosis, Complications

Prognosis

The prognosis depends on the condition of the articular cartilage. Arthroscopic removal of osteophytes can provide significant symptom relief. Higher grades of chondropathy pose a risk of progressive degenerative changes in the ankle joint, limited motion, and the development of equinus deformity.

Possible Complications

- Synovitis
- Fracture of osteophytes
- Development of intra-articular loose bodies

Posterior Impingement

Definition

Posterior impingement is the posterior entrapment of soft tissues or scar tissue between the posterior talus and the tibia due, for example, to scar thickening of the posterior joint capsule, synovitis, a prominent talar posterior process, or a large os trigonum. Concomitant involvement of the flexor hallucis longus tendon sheath may occur. Posterior impingement is on a continuum with os trigonum syndrome.

Symptoms

- Posterior ankle pain, load-dependent
- Local tenderness over the posterior tibial margin
- Pain on forced plantar flexion

Predisposing Factors

- Large talar posterior process
- Large os trigonum (congenital) or posterior labrum
- Sports involving repetitive forced plantar flexion such as gymnastics and ballet, occasionally soccer or basketball

Anatomy and Pathology

Soft tissues are entrapped between the posterior tibial margin and talus, giving rise to local synovitis, capsulitis, or fibrositis. Histology reveals fibrovascular reactive tissue or synovitis. Complaints may arise from a large talar posterior process or mobile os trigonum.

Imaging

Radiographs

With bony impingement in the ankle joint, lateral radiographs may show an extended, prominent, or perhaps separated talar posterior process, which should not be confused with a rounded os trigonum or posterior osteophytes.

Ultrasound

Ultrasound shows echogenic lengthening and bulging of periarticular bone structures in osteophytosis and acoustic shadowing from posterior intra-articular loose bodies.

MRI

Interpretation Checklist

- Extent of inflammatory reaction
- Bone involvement
- Cause of the posterior impingement: anatomical shape of the posterior talus (projecting osteophytes, prominent posterior process, os trigonum, thickened ligaments, scar tissue)
- Evaluation of the flexor hallucis longus tendon sheath
- Evaluation of tendon sheath involvement by the inflammatory process

Examination Technique

- *Standard protocol:* prone position, high-resolution multichannel coil
- *Sequences:*
  - Coronal and sagittal PD-weighted fat-sat
  - Coronal T1-weighted
  - Axial T2-weighted
  - Sagittal T1-weighted (if required)
  - T1-weighted fat-sat, true axial (angled to joint plane) and sagittal after IV contrast administration

MRI Findings (▶ Fig. 3.53)

- Fluid collection and soft-tissue edema in the posterior recess of the ankle joint
- Enhancing fibrovascular reactive tissue
- Thickened posterior ligamentous structures
- Enlarged transverse ligament (posterior labrum)
- Bone marrow edema with periostitis
- Ganglion cysts
- Increased enhancement of the synovium and adjacent capsule and soft tissue

Imaging Recommendation

Modalities of choice: radiography (bone shape) and MRI (soft tissues, bone edema).

Differential Diagnosis

- Fracture of the talar posterior process
- Mobile os trigonum
- Intra-articular loose body in the posterior compartment
- Degenerative changes in the posterior ankle or subtalar joint
- Peroneal tendon lesions
- Tarsal coalition

Treatment

Conservative

- Activity modification
- Nonsteroidal anti-inflammatory drugs
- Steroid injections

Operative

- Arthroscopic or open removal of osteophytes
- Resection of the posterior joint capsule
- Resection of a thickened posterior labrum

Prognosis, Complications

The prognosis is good after complete removal of the mechanical obstruction. Any cartilage lesions already present will compromise the clinical result. They may lead to chronic thickening of the posterior joint capsule with limitation of ankle dorsiflexion and chronic joint pain.

Os Trigonum Syndrome

Definition

Os trigonum syndrome is a special form of posterior impingement caused by mechanical irritation of the ankle joint by an os trigonum. The syndrome is caused by repetitive impingement

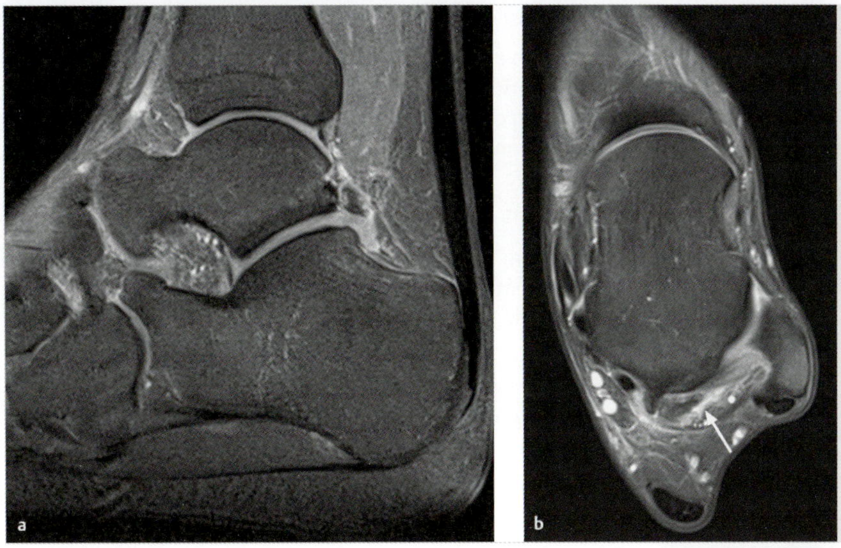

Fig. 3.53 a, b Posterior impingement due to chronic synovitis with an activated os trigonum. A 25-year-old man with posterior ankle pain which is worsened by dorsiflexion.
a Sagittal T1-weighted fat-sat image after contrast administration shows a small os trigonum fixed by fibrous tissue and surrounded by increased activity.
b Axial T1-weighted fat-sat image after contrast administration shows increased enhancement in the posterior joint recess due to chronic synovitis around the os trigonum (arrow).

of the accessory os against the structures of the posterior ankle joint during plantar flexion.

Symptoms

- Posterior and posterolateral ankle pain behind the lateral malleolus, with pain worsened by maximum plantar flexion or dorsiflexion of the big toe
- Medial retromalleolar pain may result from flexor hallucis longus irritation
- Painful, tender swelling on the back of the ankle joint
- Pain on walking downhill

Predisposing Factors

- Acute injury
- Repetitive microtrauma and ankle sprains
- Ball sports and dance sports, especially ballet

Anatomy and Pathology

The os trigonum, along with the accessory navicular (os tibiale externum), is the most common and important accessory bone in the foot (prevalence in adults: 3–15%). The os trigonum is connected anatomically to the flexor hallucis longus tendon, deltoid ligament, and posterior talofibular ligament as one component of a kinetic chain. Increased tension loads on the tendon or repetitive stretching of the ligaments may lead to entrapment between the posterior tibial margin and calcaneus or increased friction with impingement.

Imaging

Radiographs (▶ Fig. 3.54)

The lateral radiograph shows a triangular, round or oval bony structure on the posterior border of the talus.

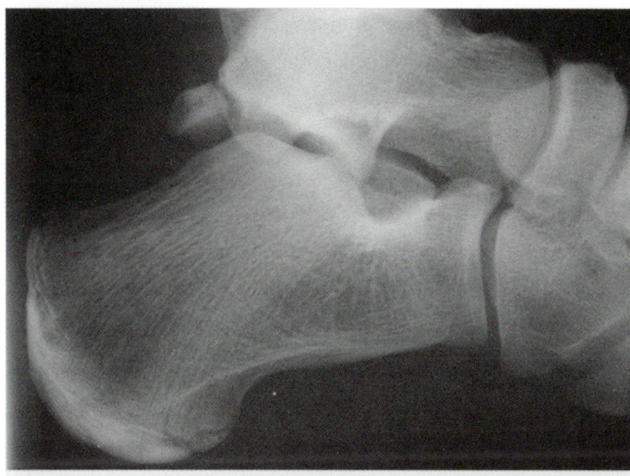

Fig. 3.54 Os trigonum syndrome. Lateral radiograph of the calcaneus shows a relatively prominent os trigonum in an adolescent male with chronic posterior ankle pain.

Ultrasound

Ultrasound scans show a bony structure at the typical site associated with echogenic intracapsular reactive tissue.

MRI

Interpretation Checklist

- Degree of bone activation adjacent to the os trigonum, tibial border, and calcaneal border
- Degree of synovitis
- Concomitant involvement of the flexor hallucis longus tendon sheath, deltoid ligament, and posterior talofibular ligament
- Exclude differential diagnoses (activated osteoarthritis, nonunion, ganglion cyst)

Examination Technique

- *Standard protocol:* prone position, high-resolution multichannel coil
- *Sequences:*
  - Coronal and sagittal PD-weighted fat-sat
  - Coronal T1-weighted
  - Axial T2-weighted
  - Sagittal T1-weighted (if required)
  - T1-weighted fat-sat, true axial (angled to joint plane) and sagittal after IV contrast administration

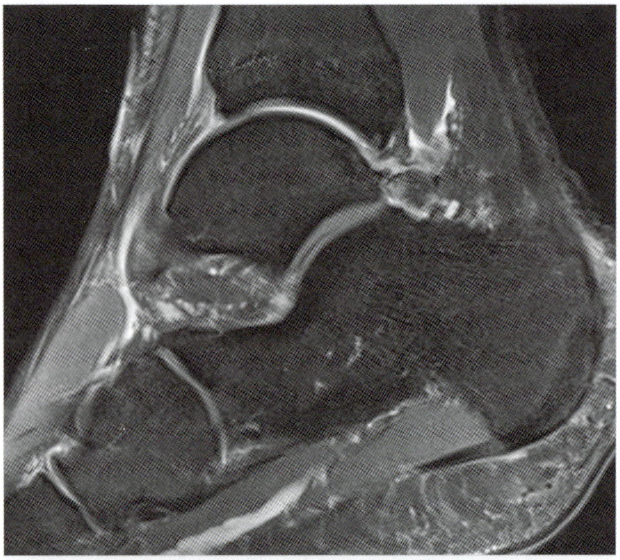

Fig. 3.55 **Activated os trigonum in a 20-year-old soccer player.** Sagittal PD-weighted fat-sat image shows the os trigonum with its fibrous attachment to the talus, bone marrow edema, and associated irritation.

MRI Findings (▸ Fig. 3.55)

- Os trigonum—free or bound to the talus by a fibrous or bony attachment—with bone marrow edema and increased enhancement
- Adjacent enhancing fibrovascular reactive tissue
- Posterior synovitis in the ankle joint
- Posterior effusion in the joint recess
- Flexor hallucis longus peritendinitis
- Fibrovascular activation in posterolateral and posteromedial ligaments
- Cartilage quality in the posterior ankle joint

Imaging Recommendation

Modalities of choice: clinical examination and lateral radiograph.

Differential Diagnosis

- Intra-articular loose body
- Periarticular osteophytes
- Achillodynia
- Achilles tendon injury
- Ankle sprain
- Talar fracture
- Degenerative changes in the ankle or subtalar joint
- Flexor hallucis longus peritendinitis
- Tarsal tunnel syndrome

Treatment

Conservative

- Immobilization in a brace
- Nonsteroidal anti-inflammatory drugs
- Local anti-inflammatory injections
- Steroid injections

Operative

- Resection of the os trigonum, usually arthroscopic, combined with debridement of the flexor hallucis longus tendon
- Resection of the posterior joint capsule and posterior synovectomy

Prognosis, Complications

Os trigonum syndrome is a highly treatable disease. Fragmentation with entrapment of the intra-articular loose bodies is rare. It is possible for flexor hallucis longus dysfunction or rupture to occur.

3.2.3 Instability

U. Szeimies

Syndesmotic Instability

Definition

This condition is defined as persistent instability of the ankle syndesmosis after a fibular fracture with syndesmotic involvement or after an isolated syndesmosis tear.

Symptoms

- Diffuse ankle pain and subjective instability with no clinically detectable increase in joint space opening
- Complaints aggravated by physical activity
- Possible local tenderness over the syndesmosis
- Pain on external rotation of the foot
- Diagnosis confirmed by trial infiltration of the syndesmosis with local anesthetic

Predisposing Factors

Prior history of ankle trauma with an unrecognized or inadequately treated syndesmosis injury.

Anatomy and Pathology

The syndesmotic instability can range from weakness to a complete loss of function. The tibiofibular space may be occupied by scar tissue, or there may elongation of the anterior, central, and posterior syndesmotic ligaments.

Imaging

Radiographs

A widening of the syndesmosis up to more than 4–6 mm in the AP view is suspicious of a syndesmotic injury. Due to the high variability further imaging is recommended. Stress radiographs with rotation may show abnormal widening of the tibiofibular clear space.

Ultrasound

Color duplex ultrasound scanning may show increased soft tissue in the anterior tibiofibular space. A dynamic examination can be performed with rotation and weight bearing. Stress testing of the syndesmosis consists of maximum passive dorsiflexion

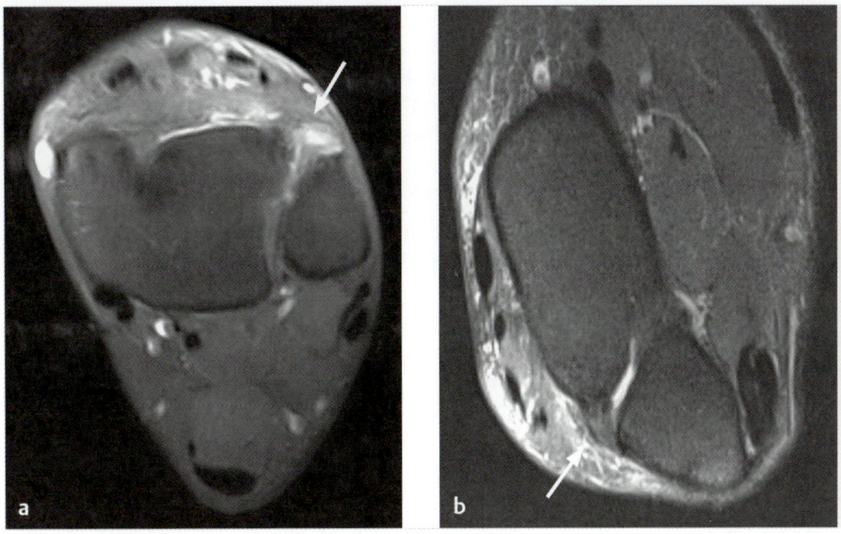

Fig. 3.56 a, b Injury of the anterior syndesmosis following an ankle sprain in a 42-year-old woman. The patient presented 6 months after conservative therapy with persistent focal complaints over the anterior syndesmosis, especially on weight bearing.
a Axial T1-weighted fat-sat image after contrast administration shows intense focal enhancement of fibrovascular scar tissue in the anterior syndesmosis consistent with chronic irritation and instability (arrow).
b Oblique sagittal PD-weighted fat-sat image in the plane of the syndesmosis shows overall continuity of the syndesmotic fibers. Individual fiber bands are thickened, especially on the fibular side, and are poorly delineated (arrow).

and eversion. Instability is present if the tibiofibular gap is greater on the affected side than on the opposite side.

CT

CT can define the precise width of the anterior syndesmosis, and ankle joint congruity can be accurately assessed. Normal CT findings do not exclude syndesmosis instability, however. CT cannot evaluate fiber structures, scarring, activation around the syndesmosis, or initial secondary degenerative changes.

MRI

Interpretation Checklist

- Continuity and quality of the anterior syndesmosis fibers
- Complete disruption
- Elongation
- Old avulsion
- Extent of scarring and fibrovascular activation
- Possible scar impingement
- Secondary degenerative changes in the ankle joint
- Evaluation of cartilage quality
- Signs of chronic instability with synovitis
- Evaluation of ligament structures about the lateral and medial malleolus

Examination Technique

- *Standard protocol:* prone position, high-resolution multichannel coil
- *Sequences:*
  - Coronal and sagittal PD-weighted fat-sat
  - Coronal T1-weighted
  - Axial T2-weighted
  - Oblique sagittal PD-weighted fat-sat, angled parallel to the syndesmosis fibers in the anterior superior corner of the ankle joint
  - T1-weighted fat-sat, true axial (angled to joint plane) and sagittal after IV contrast administration

MRI Findings (▶ Fig. 3.56)

- Absence of well-defined, hypointense fiber structure in the anterior syndesmosis
- Thickened, enhancing fibrovascular scar tissue in the syndesmosis with reactive synovitis in the ankle joint, predominantly on the anterior side
- Evidence of syndesmotic impingement
- Coronal projection may show incongruity with joint-space widening on the medial side
- Possible cartilage lesions due to chronic instability, most pronounced on the anterior side

Imaging Recommendation

Modality of choice: MRI for direct visualization of the syndesmosis and secondary changes.

Differential Diagnosis

- Lateral ankle instability
- Fibular fracture
- Osteoarthritis of the ankle joint
- Anterolateral ankle impingement

Treatment

Conservative

- For functional instability without frank dehiscence: steroid injections
- For persistent complaints: injection of platelet-derived growth factor plus TightRope or screw fixation of the syndesmosis

Operative

Syndesmoplasty in cases where imaging shows definite diastasis of the syndesmosis.

Prognosis, Complications

Even with surgical reconstruction of the syndesmosis, functional deficits of the ankle joint may persist in young, athletically active patients. A chronic ankle pain syndrome may develop. Persistent instability may lead to early degenerative changes in the ankle joint.

Ankle Instability

Definition

This condition is defined as mechanical instability of the ankle joint due to insufficiency of the lateral ligaments and/or deltoid ligament, usually as a result of trauma.

Symptoms

- Subjective instability
- Increased lateral joint-space opening
- Anterior translation of the tibia
- Unsteadiness on weight bearing and when walking on uneven ground
- Nonspecific ankle pain

Predisposing Factors

- General laxity of capsule and ligaments
- Prior history of ankle sprains
- Pes cavus
- Hindfoot varus
- Peroneal tendon pathology

Anatomy and Pathology

Mechanical insufficiency of the lateral capsule and ligaments leads to increased joint-space opening and anteroposterior translation of the tibia in the ankle mortise.

Imaging

Radiographs

AP stress radiographs may be taken and evaluated in a side-to-side comparison. Lateral views may also be obtained. The radiographs may show joint incongruity, and a side-to-side comparison may show increased opening of the ankle joint space on the affected side.

Ultrasound

A dynamic ultrasound examination can be performed. A longitudinal scan over the anterior talofibular ligament will show a ligament defect with associated instability on stress testing. The examiner can measure translational motion between the posterior tibia and calcaneal tuberosity by performing a longitudinal scan of the posterosuperior quadrant of the ankle joint in the prone position and watching the monitor while heel pressure is applied. The advantage of this method is that it allows for very brief, precisely controlled stress testing of the ankle joint.

MRI

Interpretation Checklist

- Direct evaluation of the capsule and ligaments
- Scar tissue in older injuries
- Signs of impingement
- Excessive scar formation
- Assessment of cartilage quality
- Degree of effusion and synovitis
- Accurate localization of capsule and ligament pathology
- Early secondary degenerative changes
- Bone marrow edema
- Condition of the subtalar joint
- Overloading of hindfoot tendons
- Sinus tarsi ligaments

Examination Technique

- *Standard protocol:* prone position, high-resolution multichannel coil
- *Sequences:*
  - Coronal and sagittal PD-weighted fat-sat
  - Coronal T1-weighted
  - Axial T2-weighted
  - T1-weighted fat-sat, true axial (angled to joint plane) and sagittal after IV contrast administration

MRI Findings (▶ Fig. 3.57, ▶ Fig. 3.58)

MRI cannot supply an accurate diagnosis, which must rely on a combination of subjective complaints (feeling of instability, nonspecific pain), clinical findings (increased laxity of capsule and ligaments, especially in a side-to-side comparison), and MRI findings (effusion and synovitis in the ankle joint with little or no associated pathology). The capsule and ligaments may appear fully intact on MRI.

! Note

The detection of pre-existing secondary degenerative changes and impending cartilage defects is important for treatment planning.

Imaging Recommendation

Modalities of choice: radiography and ultrasound. MRI is a useful adjunct for planning treatment and narrowing the differential diagnosis.

Differential Diagnosis

- Osteochondral lesion of the talus
- Peroneal tendon lesion
- Arthritis
- Ankle joint impingement
- Subtalar joint disease
- Pes supinatus/varus
- Palsy

Treatment

Conservative

- Proprioception exercises
- Strengthening of the peroneus longus and brevis
- Ankle brace
- High-top shoes

Surgical

- Anatomic reconstruction of damaged ligaments (Broström)

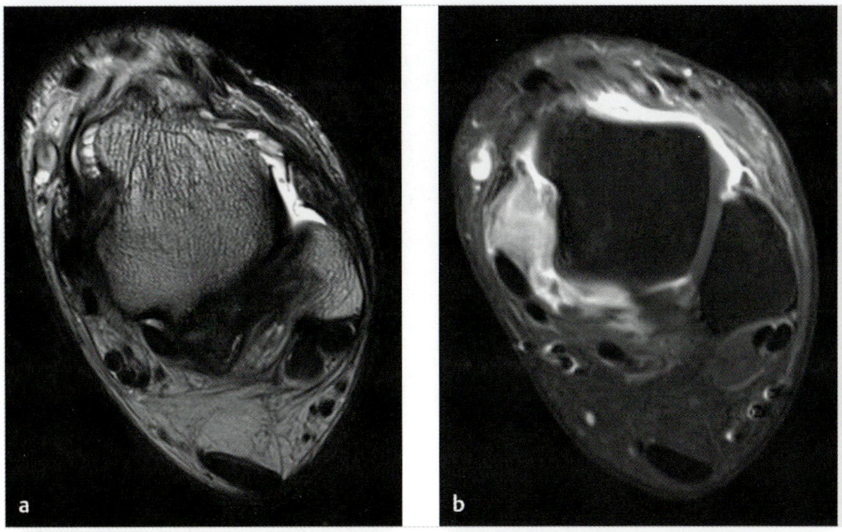

Fig. 3.57 a, b Ankle instability in a 26-year-old man who had a prior ankle sprain with rupture of the anterior talofibular ligament. He presented with ankle pain and swelling, aggravated by exercise, and subjective ankle instability.
a Axial T2-weighted MRI (angled to the joint plane) shows moderate effusion and a complete tear of the anterior talofibular ligament.
b Axial T1-weighted fat-sat image after contrast administration shows intense synovitic enhancement encircling the ankle joint due to chronic ankle instability with fibrovascular activation along the deltoid ligament.

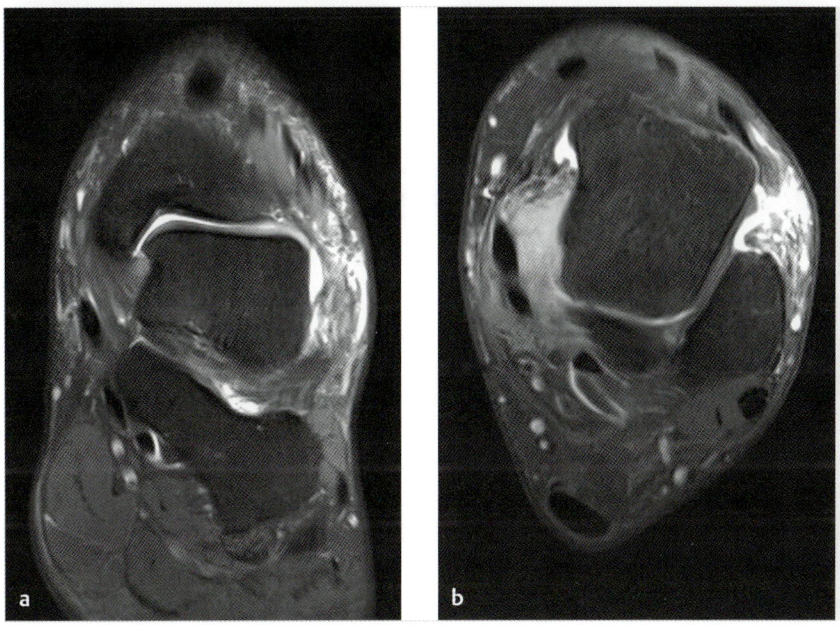

Fig. 3.58 a, b Ankle instability in a 37-year-old man 3 months after a pronation injury. He complained now of increasing pain on weight bearing, predominantly on the medial side.
a Coronal PD-weighted fat-sat image. The deltoid ligament is seen to be structurally intact, but all portions of the ligament are thickened and expanded.
b Axial T1-weighted fat-sat image after contrast administration shows marked fibrovascular activation along the deltoid ligament associated with severe ligament dysfunction. Soft-tissue activation is seen anterolaterally over the lateral malleolus.

- If tissue quality is deficient: augmentation with plantaris longus tendon or an allograft
- Tenodesis (Watson–Jones and similar procedures have poorer long-term results than an anatomic reconstruction)

Prognosis, Complications

Prognosis

Patients who respond well to conservative therapy have a good prognosis. In cases that require surgical treatment, possible complications include adhesion formation, scar impingement, and limited motion. Recurrent sprains may give rise to secondary degenerative changes.

Possible Complications

- Osteochondral lesion of the talus
- Peroneal tendon overload
- Rupture of the peroneus brevis tendon

Subtalar Joint Instability

Definition

Instability of the subtalar joint is manifested as hypermobility of the joint.

Symptoms

- Nonspecific pain at the level of the subtalar joint
- Subjective ankle instability
- Pain relieved by diagnostic local anesthesia
- With a stable ankle: increased joint-space opening in the subtalar joint (tested with the ankle joint in dorsiflexion)
- Increased mediolateral translation in the subtalar joint

Predisposing Factors

Subtalar joint instability may develop after a sprain injury that tears the interosseous talocalcaneal ligament and calcaneofibular ligament.

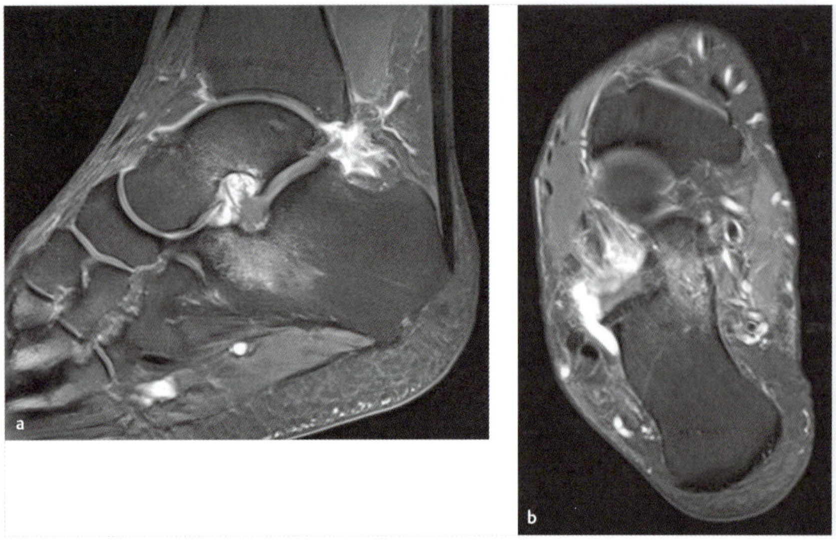

Fig. 3.59 a, b Significant chronic subtalar instability in a 40-year-old active soccer player. Findings include massive fibrovascular tissue in the sinus tarsi, adjacent bone edema in the calcaneus and, to a lesser degree, in the talus with no significant degenerative changes.
a Sagittal T1-weighted fat-sat image after contrast administration shows marked synovitic enhancement, most notably in the posterior recess of the subtalar joint. There is no evidence of deep cartilage lesions in the posterior facet of the subtalar joint.
b Axial T1-weighted fat-sat image after contrast administration shows fibrovascular enhancement along the interosseous ligament with bone marrow edema in the anterior process of the calcaneus.

Anatomy and Pathology

A sprain of the subtalar joint causes elongation or tearing of the interosseous talocalcaneal ligament and calcaneofibular ligament, resulting in increased joint laxity with complaints related to overloading of the joint capsule.

Imaging

Radiographs

The Broden view with 45° of internal rotation and a varus stress shows abnormal passive opening of the subtalar joint space.

Ultrasound

Not indicated.

MRI

Interpretation Checklist

- Carefully evaluate the subtalar ligament structures and the ligaments in the sinus tarsi, giving particular attention to the interosseous ligament and calcaneofibular ligament (elongation, discontinuity, thickening due to scarring).
- Evaluate the articular cartilage in the subtalar joint, the joint capsule, and subchondral bone.
- Edema
- Enhancing reactive tissue
- Synovitis
- Transition to degenerative arthritis
- Evaluation of the tendons of the hindfoot and midfoot

Examination Technique

- *Standard protocol:* prone position, high-resolution multichannel coil
- *Sequences:*
  - Coronal and sagittal PD-weighted fat-sat
  - Coronal T1-weighted
  - Axial T2-weighted
  - T1-weighted fat-sat, true axial (angled to the joint plane) and sagittal after IV contrast administration

MRI Findings (▶ Fig. 3.59)

- Effusion and synovitis in the subtalar joint
- Signs of overload
- Thickened joint capsule
- Poor delineation, thickening, and possible enhancement of the fibers of the interosseous ligament and calcaneofibular ligament
- Possible wavy contours (like the findings in sinus tarsi syndrome). See 3.2.10 Subtalar Joint: Sinus Tarsi Syndrome (p. 120)
- Complete tear of the interosseous ligament (extremely rare)

! Note

Instability may be present, even if the ligament structures appear morphologically normal! Subtalar instability is often difficult to recognize and may have equivocal clinical findings. Be alert for subtle changes, especially in the sinus tarsi.

An early sign is a fibrovascular reaction in the sinus tarsi, which is sometimes accompanied by mild irritative synovitis in the subtalar joint. Cartilage involvement is found only in advanced stages. A helpful study is post-exercise MRI (imaging after strenuous treadmill exercise), which will usually demonstrate subtalar effusion and synovitis.

! Note

Sinus tarsi syndrome should not be offered as an interpretation. It is not a diagnosis in the strict sense, but describes a fibrovascular activation chiefly involving the ligaments in the presence of subtalar instability.

Imaging Recommendation

Modality of choice: MRI is useful for evaluating secondary degenerative joint changes and for narrowing the differential diagnosis.

Differential Diagnosis

- Primary osteoarthritis of the subtalar joint
- Osteochondral injury in the subtalar joint
- Coalition
- Instability of the ankle joint

Treatment

Conservative

- Exercises to improve active stabilization
- Proprioception exercises
- Shoe inserts and ankle brace

Operative

- Plication of the calcaneofibular ligament and lateral joint capsule
- Plus augmentation of the interosseous talocalcaneal ligament, if required

Prognosis, Complications

Secondary degenerative changes may develop in the subtalar joint, and a chronic pain syndrome may develop. To date, few data have been published on the clinical results of surgical stabilization of the subtalar joint.

3.2.4 Chronic Disorders of Cartilage and Bone

U. Szeimies

Osteoarthritis of the Ankle Joint or Subtalar Joint

Definition

Osteoarthritis is marked by patchy degenerative changes affecting the cartilage on both articular surfaces.

Symptoms

- Morning stiffness
- Pain after periods of inactivity
- Pain during exercise
- Pain at rest
- Limitation of motion
- Swelling
- Local warmth and redness over the joint
- Diffuse ankle or subtalar joint pain

Predisposing Factors

- Large, repetitive loads with inadequate recovery periods (competitive athletes)
- Strenuous exercise or exertion
- High body weight
- Trauma (unhealed capsuloligamentous injury with instability, step-off caused by an intra-articular fracture, such as a subtalar injury in snowboarder's ankle)
- Inflammatory joint disease
- Congenital factors
- Genetic disposition
- Disorders of cartilage metabolism (ochronosis, chondrocalcinosis)

Anatomy and Pathology

Osteoarthritis is the most common disease process affecting the joints. Its incidence increases as the population ages.

Under normal conditions a balance exists between the breakdown and synthesis of articular cartilage matrix. The capacity for matrix synthesis declines with ageing, however. When high loads are placed upon the joint, synovial fluid is expressed from the joint space; this increases the friction between the cartilage surfaces, causing mechanical wear of the articular cartilage with delamination of the superficial cartilage layer, loss of cartilage thickness, subchondral sclerosis due to an abnormal pressure distribution, osteophyte formation, and fluid penetration of the subchondral bone layer causing cyst formation. The wear-and-tear process initiates a kind of inflammatory response.

! Note

Cartilage status is not the only concern. Associated structures (joint capsule, ligaments, tendons, articulating bone ends, bursa) are also important, and changes in these structures may contribute to osteoarthritis.

Imaging

Radiographs

Typical radiographic findings in osteoarthritis are sclerosis of the subchondral cancellous bone, subchondral cysts, marginal osteophytes, joint space narrowing, articular surface remodeling after cartilage loss (surface grinding), subluxation, capsular chondromas, and intra-articular loose bodies.

Ultrasound

A longitudinal scan through the anterior ankle joint will show effusion due to activated osteoarthritis, irregular thickening of the joint capsule, and an irregular, echogenic bone surface.

CT (▸ Fig. 3.60)

CT with submillimeter isotropic voxels and MPRs in three planes are recommended for the optimum evaluation of bony structures. Findings may include osteophytes, subchondral cysts, erosion of the subchondral plate, joint space narrowing or bone-on-bone contact, and intra-articular loose bodies.

MRI

Imaging technology is particularly important in evaluations of articular cartilage, and the poor correlation between MRI and arthroscopy often reported in the literature most likely results from less-than-optimal imaging equipment. A high field intensity (at least 1.5 T) should be combined with the use of dedicated high-resolution joint coils, thin slice acquisition (2–3 mm), increased phase-encoding steps, and an increased image matrix. Unfortunately, the longer scan time and higher procurement costs of these systems are difficult to justify economically in most office settings.

Interpretation Checklist

- Carefully evaluate the articular cartilage; possible findings range from early signal changes and superficial fibrillations and ulcerations to deep ulcers or cartilage defects with exposed subchondral bone.
- Describe the extent of changes in millimeters and in at least two planes.
- Look for associated phenomena such as effusion, subchondral bone marrow edema, or synovitis as an expression of activated osteoarthritis.

Examination Technique

- *Standard protocol:* prone position, high-resolution multichannel coil

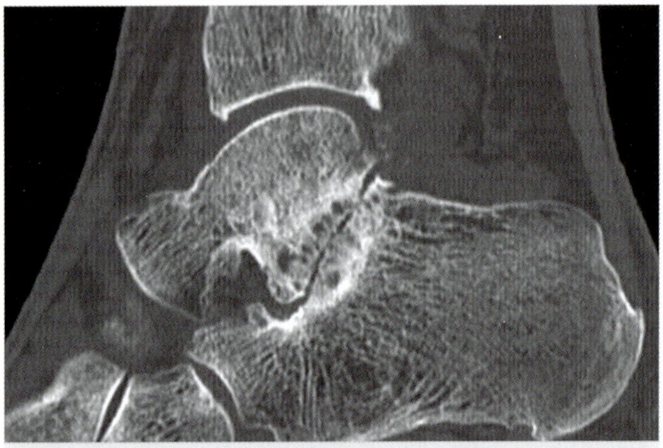

Fig. 3.60 Sagittal reformatted CT image of subtalar osteoarthritis. The image shows complete loss of the subtalar joint space with subchondral sclerosis and multiple subchondral cysts.

- *Sequences:*
  - Coronal and sagittal PD-weighted fat-sat
  - Coronal T1-weighted
  - Axial T2-weighted
  - T1-weighted fat-sat, true axial (angled to the joint plane) and sagittal after IV contrast administration

MRI Findings (▶ Fig. 3.61)

- *Cartilage evaluation:*
  - Areas of increased signal intensity
  - Cartilage swelling
  - Chondromalacia
  - Fibrillations
  - Fissures
  - Erosions
  - Ulcerations
  - Indicate extent (superficial, deep, extending to subchondral bone, patchy cartilage defects)
  - Measure the defect
  - Exposed subchondral bone
- *Evaluation/description of the subchondral bone:*
  - Edema formation
  - Softening
  - Chondromalacia
  - Cortical fissures
  - Cyst formation
  - Subchondral cysts
  - Marginal osteophytes
  - Sclerosis
  - Articular surface deformity
  - Joint congruity
  - Subluxation (degenerative arthritis)
  - Measure subchondral defects and cysts
- *Description of repair mechanisms:*
  - Intra-articular osteophytes
  - Regenerative cartilage
- *Evaluation of the synovium:*
  - Effusion
  - Synovitis

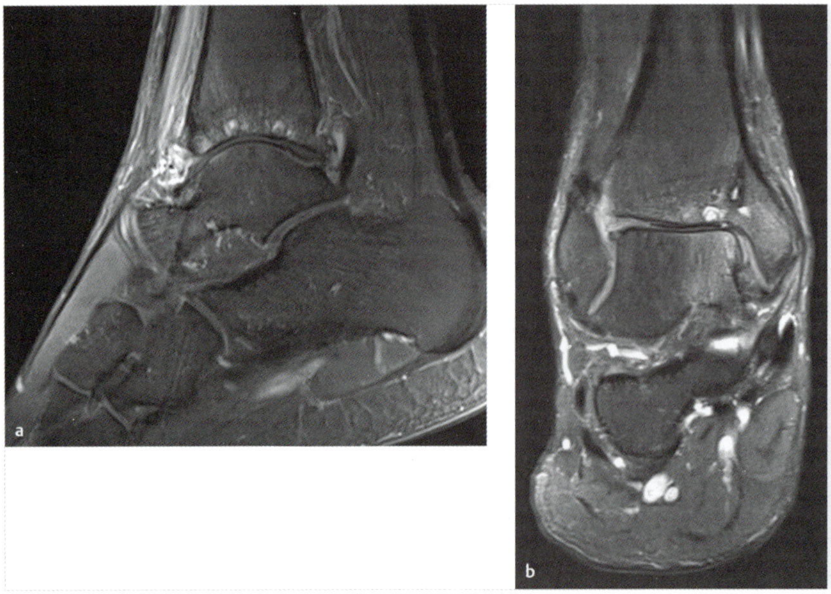

Fig. 3.61 a, b Activated osteoarthritis of the ankle joint.
a Sagittal T1-weighted fat-sat image after contrast administration demonstrates synovitis with subchondral bone marrow edema and the development of subchondral cysts.
b Coronal T1-weighted fat-sat image after contrast administration shows joint incongruity resulting from cartilage loss with exposure of subchondral bone. The linear signal void in the joint space is caused by a vacuum phenomenon.

Table 3.8 Outerbridge classification of cartilage lesions

Grade	Description
I	MRI signal changes with no loss of cartilage thickness
II	Superficial cartilage lesions affecting no more than 50% of the cartilage thickness
III	Cartilage lesions affecting more than 50% of the cartilage thickness but without exposure of subchondral bone
IV	Full-thickness cartilage defect with exposure of subchondral bone

  - Synovial villi
- *Evaluation of the capsule and ligaments:*
  - Thickened joint capsule
  - Capsular chondromas
  - Osteomas
  - Intra-articular loose bodies
  - Adjacent ligament structures
- *Sequelae of osteoarthritis:*
  - Degenerative changes in neighboring joints
  - Signs of overload in tendons and in adjacent ligaments and capsule-ligament attachments

Chondropathy can be classified, but there is no uniform system for grading cartilage lesions. The best approach is to give a precise description of the cartilage lesion in the radiology report. The Outerbridge system is widely used for the classification of cartilage lesions (▸ Table 3.8).

Imaging Recommendation

Modality of choice: varies with the treatment approach. The initial study is radiography. MRI is used to evaluate early forms of osteoarthritis and determine degree of activation, while CT is used to exclude ossified intra-articular loose bodies.

Differential Diagnosis

- Osteochondritis dissecans
- Arthritis
- Hemarthrosis
- Chondromatosis
- Pigmented villonodular synovitis

Treatment

Conservative

- Nonsteroidal anti-inflammatory drugs
- Physical therapy
- Ankle brace
- Intra-articular injection of steroids or hyaluronic acid

Operative

- *Grades I and II:* arthroscopic debridement, synovectomy, osteophyte removal, cartilage stabilization; with > 5° malalignment: axial correction
- *Grade III or higher:* arthrodesis of the ankle joint or endoprosthesis

Prognosis, Complications

Prognosis

Secondary axial malalignment may result from local wear. The rate of progression of the disease cannot be predicted. Moreover, the complaints do not always correlate with the degree of joint damage revealed by imaging.

Possible Complications

- Chronic activated osteoarthritis
- Subluxation
- Dislocation
- Complete destruction of the joint and adjacent structures

Chondromatosis, Multiple Intra-Articular Loose Bodies

Definition

Chondromatosis is characterized by the formation of benign cartilage neoplasms (chondromas) within the joint capsule and in tendon sheaths and bursae. The chondromas may ossify, creating a condition known as synovial osteochondromatosis. Synonyms for chondromatosis are articular chondromatosis, synovial chondromatosis, and Reichel disease.

Symptoms

- Locking of the joint
- Limited motion
- Pain
- Joint swelling
- Palpable intra-articular bodies
- Crepitation

Predisposing Factors

- Poorly understood
- Recurrent microtrauma
- Genetic disposition is known (familial synovial chondromatosis with dwarfism)

Anatomy and Pathology

- Chondromatosis: rare in the ankle joint; most common in the hip, knee, and elbow. The precise cause is unknown. It is characterized by multiple calcified or ossified sites of cartilage proliferation and by metaplasia of the synovial membrane in joints, tendon sheaths, and bursae.
  - Primary chondromatosis: synovial metaplasia
  - Secondary chondromatosis: small, loose cartilage fragments detached from the synovial membrane in a setting of joint degeneration, trauma, or an osteochondral fracture
- *Isolated intra-articular loose bodies:* posttraumatic or, more commonly, in a setting of degenerative joint disease

Imaging

Radiographs

Classic findings of multiple calcifications and isolated intra-articular loose bodies are not always seen and may be obscured by superimposed bony structures. Cartilage fragments are not visible unless calcified or ossified.

CT

CT can accurately define and localize calcified intra-articular loose bodies for preoperative planning.

Ultrasound

Sonography is useful for evaluating effusion and synovitis. A dynamic examination is performed. The location and mobility of intra-articular bodies can be determined by their acoustic shadows, depending on their density.

MRI

Interpretation Checklist

- Chondromatosis:
  - Evaluate extent
  - Associated synovitis
  - Early cartilage lesions
  - Preosteoarthritic changes
  - Secondary osteoarthritis
  - Evaluate tendon sheaths and bursae
  - Exclude malignant change
- Intra-articular loose bodies:
  - Extent of synovitic irritation
  - Evaluate cartilage quality
  - Exclude osteochondritis dissecans
  - Accurate preoperative localization

Examination Technique

- *Standard protocol:* prone position, high-resolution multichannel coil
- *Sequences:*
  - Coronal and sagittal PD-weighted fat-sat
  - Coronal T1-weighted
  - Axial T2-weighted
  - T1-weighted fat-sat, true axial (angled to the joint plane) and sagittal after IV contrast administration

MRI Findings (▸ Fig. 3.62)

- Marked effusion.
- Signal characteristics of chondromas vary depending on degree of calcification.
- Noncalcified lesions have high signal intensity in the proton-density image (interactive window!); they may appear, for example, as myriad small, scattered, bright nodules floating in the effusion.
- Calcified chondromas have low signal intensity in T1- and T2-weighted sequences.
- Ossified lesions may be hyperintense in T1- and T2-weighted sequences due to fatty bone marrow.
- Synovitis enhances on postcontrast images.

Imaging Recommendation

Modalities of choice: initial study is radiography. If x-rays are equivocal, MRI is performed. MRI gives an excellent view of noncalcified chondromas.

! Note

Bone erosion without marginal sclerosis on radiographs is suspicious for a malignant process.

Differential Diagnosis

Osteoarthritis with capsular chondromas and osteomas or ossified foci. Differentiating feature: capsular chondromas are usually isolated, unlike the multiple tiny spheres in synovial chondromatosis. Intra-articular loose bodies and capsular chondromas always occur in an advanced stage of degenerative joint disease.

Treatment

Intra-articular loose bodies are removed at surgical synovectomy. This can be done arthroscopically in the ankle joint. An open procedure may be indicated for the smaller joints.

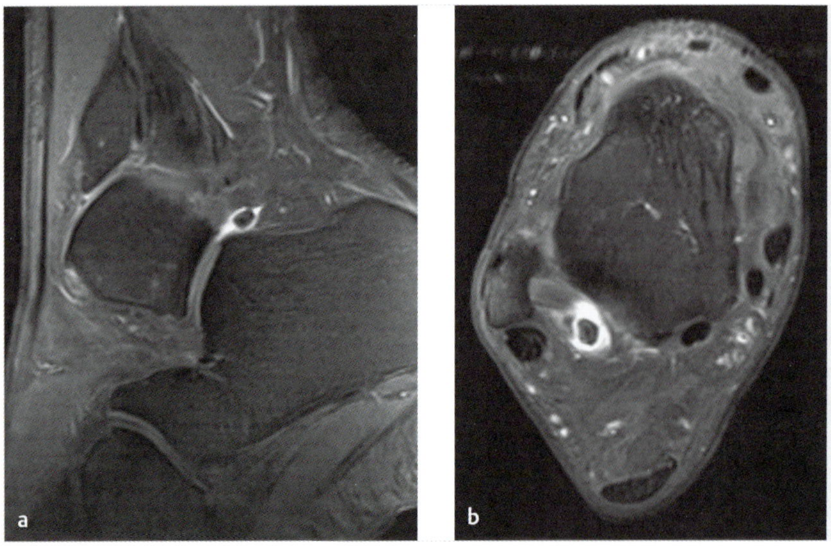

Fig. 3.62 a, b A 41-year-old man with locking and pain in the posterior ankle joint.
a Sagittal T1-weighted fat-sat image after contrast administration reveals an intra-articular loose body in the posterior joint recess with surrounding synovitic enhancement.
b Axial T1-weighted fat-sat image after contrast administration. Contrast imaging can distinguish between a sessile and loose or symptomatic intra-articular body, with increased enhancement in the adjacent tissue.

Prognosis, Complications

Pressure from the synovial chondromas may damage the bone and cartilage, giving rise to secondary osteoarthritis. Malignant transformation to low-grade chondrosarcoma rarely occurs. A large percentage of noncalcified synovial chondromas signify an active proliferative process, associated with an increased risk of malignant degeneration. The incidence of recurrence is 3 to 23%.

Osteochondral Lesions of the Talus

It is common to find posttraumatic osteochondral lesions on the talar dome as the result of a sprain (talar rim lesion, osteochondritis dissecans, flake fracture) as well as ischemic osteonecrosis of the talar trochlea. Lesions of the cartilage and bone located on the medial or lateral shoulder of the talus are currently referred to as osteochondral lesions of the talus. Increasingly, this term is replacing the older blanket term "osteochondritis dissecans."

A somewhat less common entity is epiphyseal developmental disorder or maturation disorder of the talus (abnormal ossification of the talar rim). A small portion of the epiphysis remains separate and does not undergo further maturation with the rest of the epiphysis. This leads to the formation of an intra-articular loose body with a bony defect in the talar shoulder with possible remodeling of the articular surface and fibrocartilage formation.

Definition

An osteochondral lesion is an ischemic condition that progresses in stages culminating in osteonecrosis of the subchondral bone and adjacent cartilage. It is a chronic, persistent lesion of the talar rim that typically develops after an ankle sprain. A subtype is ischemic osteonecrosis, a circumscribed fragmentation of cartilage and bone that predominantly affects convex articular surfaces in adolescents.

Symptoms

- Activated lesions cause persistent joint pain, which is often independent of the lesion site
- Pain
- Locking (joint mouse)
- Recurrent effusions
- Limited motion

Differentiation is required from silent lesions that are detected incidentally, especially in children. Even higher-grade lesions may be completely asymptomatic.

Predisposing Factors

- Prior history of a single lateral ankle sprain, recurrent medial sprains, high level of athletic activity, high body weight
- Most lateral lesions result from osteochondral flake fractures
- Up to 30% of patients with a medial lesion have bilateral lesions
- Genetic predisposition has been postulated; hemoglobinopathies, Gaucher disease

Males are predominantly affected.

Anatomy and Pathology

- *Posttraumatic osteochondral lesion:* Direct trauma and repetitive microtrauma may cause lesions of the bone and overlying cartilage. Repetitive shear forces are also considered a risk factor in patients with joint instability. The activated stage is marked by the development of extensive bone edema ranging to osteonecrosis. Subchondral sclerosis develops around the necrotic zone, resulting in dissection. Joint pressures force synovial fluid through the damaged cartilage surface into the subchondral bone, leading to the cystic form of osteochondritis dissecans. The devitalized fragment may increasingly separate from its base and become an intra-articular loose body.
- *Ischemic osteonecrosis:* According to the prevailing theory of pathogenesis, ischemic osteonecrosis results from a subchondral fatigue fracture causing diminished blood flow at the end-artery level.

Traumatic osteochondral lesions are most commonly located on the lateral border of the talus, while ischemic lesions predominantly affect the medial talar shoulder and central portion of the trochlea. Often it is difficult to distinguish between a traumatic and ischemic cause, and both forms exist on a continuum.

Classification is based on intraoperative assessment of cartilage and bone lesions (Outerbridge, Cheng-Ferkel, International Cartilage Research Society [ICRS] Classification; ▶ Table 3.9).

Imaging

Radiographs

The Berndt and Harty classification is most commonly used for lesion classification on conventional radiographs. The Arcq grading system is less widely used (▶ Table 3.10).

Table 3.9 Classification of osteochondral lesions of the talus

Grade	Description
I	Smooth and intact, soft
II	Rough surface
III	Fissures
IV	Flaplike detachment with exposed bone
V	Loose bone fragment, not displaced
VI	Loose fragment displaced within the joint

Table 3.10 Radiographic grading system for osteochondral lesions of the talus

Grade	Description
I	Subchondral lucent zone
II	Sclerotic focus with a peripheral lucent line and sclerotic rim
III	Partial separation of the fragment
IV	Complete separation of the fragment

Radiographs are often negative in the early stage. Later they show a faint lucency with ill-defined central density in the shoulder or trochlear surface of the talus. The end stage is marked by an intra-articular loose body and an associated subchondral defect with sclerotic margins.

Ultrasound

Not indicated. At most, sonography may show a nonspecific reactive effusion.

MRI

Before the advent of MRI, very little was known about the pathophysiology of osteochondral lesions of the talus. Conventional radiographs could depict only the end-stage features of a crater base and loose body. With its capability for water-sensitive imaging of the subchondral bone, MRI can now demonstrate all stages from early bone marrow edema to necrosis, sclerosis, and cartilage disruption.

Interpretation Checklist

- Evaluation of the subchondral region
- Bone marrow edema
- Demarcation
- Viability of the osteochondral fragment
- Cartilage quality
- Differentiation between a stable or unstable lesion
- Extent of necrosis
- Associated changes
- Synovitis
- Effusion
- Evaluation of progression
- Comparison with prior images

Examination technique

Contrast administration is not strictly necessary; necrosis can also be evaluated with fat-suppressed water-sensitive sequences and unenhanced T1-weighted images. Contrast administration is helpful for evaluating synovitis, however.

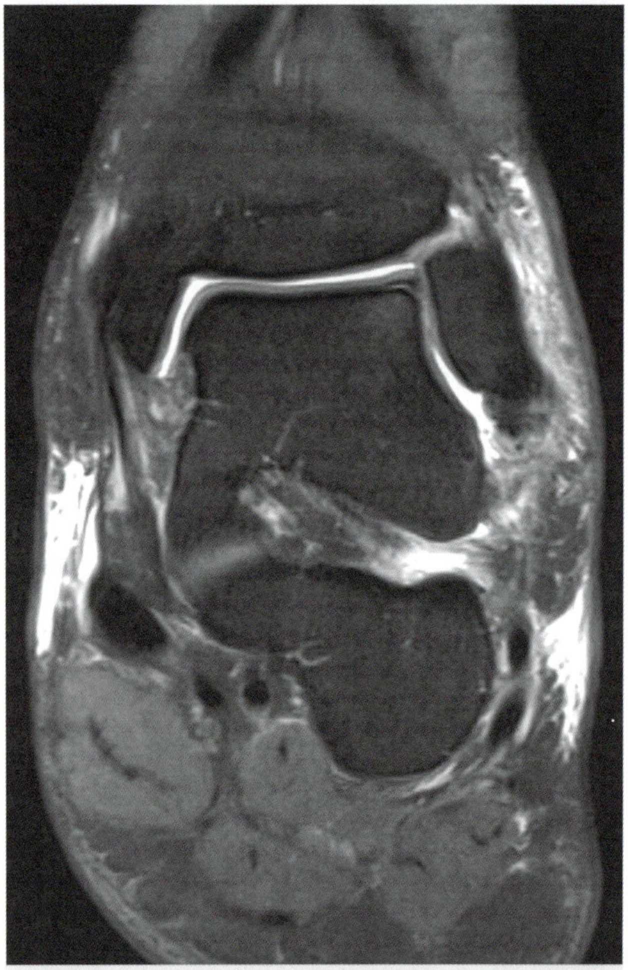

Fig. 3.63 Chondral flake fracture on the lateral shoulder of the talus following an acute ankle sprain. The 44-year-old woman presented with a lateral ankle sprain and patchy hematoma in the soft tissues. Coronal PD-weighted fat-sat MR image shows a faint zone of bone contusion on the lateral talar shoulder with fresh delamination of the overlying articular cartilage.

MRI Findings (▶ Fig. 3.63, ▶ Fig. 3.64, ▶ Fig. 3.65, ▶ Fig. 3.66)

Various classifications have been developed, most of which are based on radiographic features. At present there is no uniform MRI classification system, so reporting must rely on an accurate description of findings:

- Early stage: diffuse, faint, subchondral bone marrow edema in the lateral or medial talar dome, an intact cortical layer, normal hyaline articular cartilage; measure extent of edema, effusion, and reactive synovitis.
- Edema zone is demarcated by a fairly well-defined "jump" in intensity from normal fatty marrow signal to bone marrow edema with no fluid detection. T1-weighted sequence shows preservation of fatty marrow signal without necrosis (= stable lesion), which is important for directing transchondral drilling.
- Incipient separation: water image shows hyperintense fluid around the osteochondral lesion indicating the development of a crater base; fragment undergoes necrosis with loss of T1-weighted fatty marrow signal, often with continued detection of edema (= unstable lesion).
- Separation: the detached fragment may be whole or fragmented, with cyst formation deep to the base.
- Assessment of cartilage surface: initial signal changes, fibrillation and fissuring; look for undermining cartilage lesions, followed later by fibrocartilage formation and articular surface remodeling.
- Associated changes: effusion, reactive synovitis, cartilage lesions at other sites caused by the osteochondral fragment.
- Two sites of predilection: ischemic osteonecrosis is usually located on the medial side and produces deeper lesions; posttraumatic osteochondritis dissecans usually affects the anterolateral dome and is more superficial.

Imaging Recommendation

Modality of choice: MRI for early detection, follow-up, assessment of cartilage quality, assessment of stability, and determining the degree of activation.

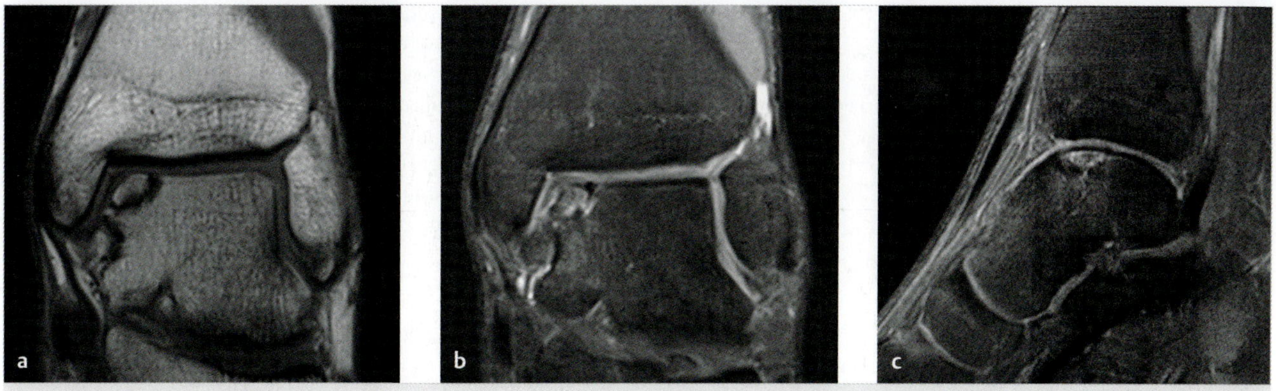

Fig. 3.64 a–c Osteochondral lesion on the medial talar dome.
a Coronal T1-weighted image shows preservation of fatty marrow signal in the osteochondral fragment with no evidence of necrosis.
b Coronal T1-weighted fat-sat image after contrast administration shows enhancement in the fragment with no signs of necrosis. Even if the overlying articular cartilage appears sound, it is important to describe even the slightest signal changes in the cartilage since it is common to find compromised (soft) cartilage adjacent to an osteochondral lesion.
c Sagittal T1-weighted fat-sat image after contrast administration shows an intact cortical layer with no subchondral fissures.

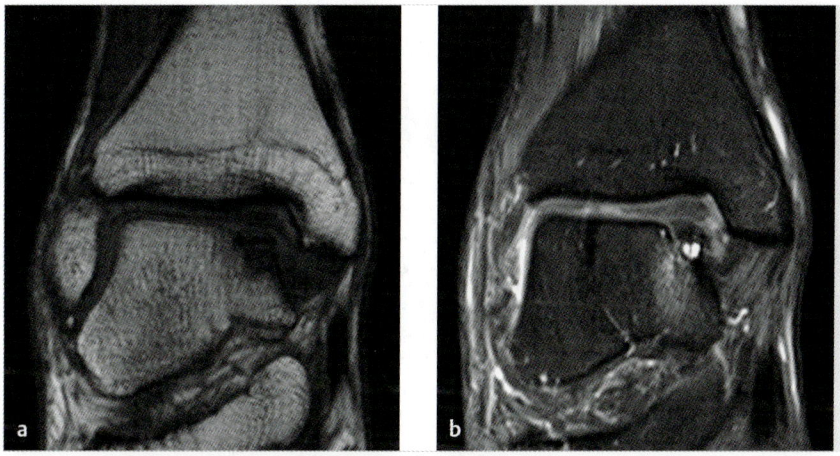

Fig. 3.65 a, b Osteochondral lesion on the medial talar dome in a woman with chronic complaints and pain that is aggravated by physical activity.
a Coronal T1-weighted image shows flattening of the medial talar dome with joint incongruity. Absence of fatty marrow signal indicates necrosis of the osteochondral fragment.
b Coronal T1-weighted fat-sat image after contrast administration shows no enhancement of the fragment. Adjacent mild bone marrow edema indicates chronic activation.

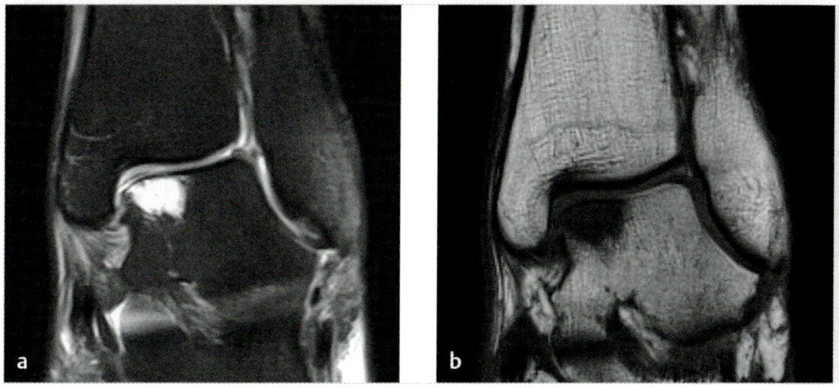

Fig. 3.66 a, b Osteonecrosis of the medial talar dome.
a Coronal PD-weighted fat-sat image shows a relatively large subchondral lesion in the medial shoulder of the talus.
b Unenhanced coronal T1-weighted image shows a large necrotic area with absence of fatty marrow signal.

Differential Diagnosis (▶ Fig. 3.67)

- Osteochondral lesion of the tibial articular surface
- Talar fracture
- Inflammatory joint disease
- Transient bone marrow edema syndrome
- Ossification disturbance of the talar dome

Treatment

Conservative

- Grades I–III: activity modification, stress reduction
- Fresh injuries: immobilization

Operative

- Arthroscopic debridement of unstable cartilage
- Microfracturing

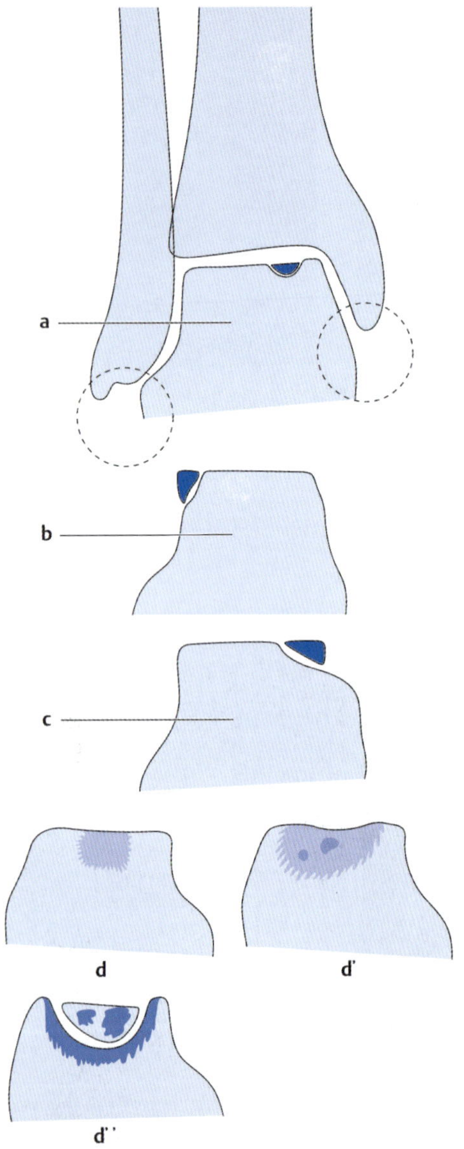

Fig. 3.67 a–d Differentiation of osteochondritis dissecans from a developmental disturbance and partial ischemic osteonecrosis of the talar dome (source: Dihlmann and Stäbler 2010).
a Osteochondritis dissecans, osteochondral lesion of the talus: dissection is close to the medial edge of the trochlea.
b Dissection is on the lateral edge of the trochlea.
c Developmental disturbance of the talar dome.
d–d" Ischemic osteonecrosis of the talar trochlea (early stage, necrosis trochlear fragment, demarcation, fibrocartilage repair).

- For larger defects: cancellous bone grafting
- Autologous chondrocyte transplantation
- Coverage with a membrane or repair with an osteochondral autograft taken from the knee

Prognosis, Complications

Stable, viable fragments may gain reattachment, whereas unstable fragments usually undergo sequestration. It is unclear whether osteochondritis dissecans represents a preosteoarthritic condition of the ankle joint, but the high rate of incidentally detected lesions suggests that osteochondritis dissecans does not inevitably progress to osteoarthritis of the ankle. Progressive cyst formation may occur in activated lesions with unstable cartilage. Unstable cartilage leads to functional impairment of the ankle joint with painful weight bearing. All surgical options yield good results in terms of pain reduction, but some functional limitation usually remains and may be disabling for young, athletically active patients.

Avascular Necrosis of the Talus

Definition

Avascular necrosis (AVN) of the talus is bone death due to ischemia.

Symptoms

- *Early stage:* diffuse bone marrow edema, pain on weight bearing, limited motion, effusion
- *Demarcation stage:* usually less painful or even asymptomatic
- *End stage with articular surface collapse:* return of mechanically induced symptoms, similar to those of activated osteoarthritis

Predisposing Factors

- Approximately three-quarters of cases are posttraumatic, resulting from fractures or dislocations of the talar neck or body and developing over a period of weeks to 3 months.
- Atraumatic AVN due to vascular disease (vasculitis, lupus erythematosus, diabetes mellitus) may occur in patients on corticosteroid therapy, or may be due to embolism.
- AVN is a possible complication of high-dose immunosuppression in organ transplant recipients.
- AVN may be bilateral.

Anatomy and Pathology

The talus has a tenuous extra- and intraosseous vascular network with relatively poor blood flow to its lateral portion. Most of the talar blood supply is medial, derived from the artery of the tarsal canal—a branch of the anterior tibial artery—and from the deltoid artery, which is protected by the medial ligament (▶ Fig. 3.68).

Imaging

Radiographs

Radiographs demonstrate subchondral sclerosis, an irregular trabecular structure with osteolytic foci and marginal sclerosis, and articular surface deformity in the late stage. The Hawkins sign is useful for excluding posttraumatic AVN. If the talar blood supply is intact, fracture healing at approximately 6 to 8 weeks will produce a subchondral radiolucent band in the talar dome caused by hyperemic decalcification of the bone. This radiographic sign is very sensitive but relatively nonspecific.

Ultrasound

Ultrasound does not contribute to the diagnosis of AVN. It may detect joint effusion in some cases.

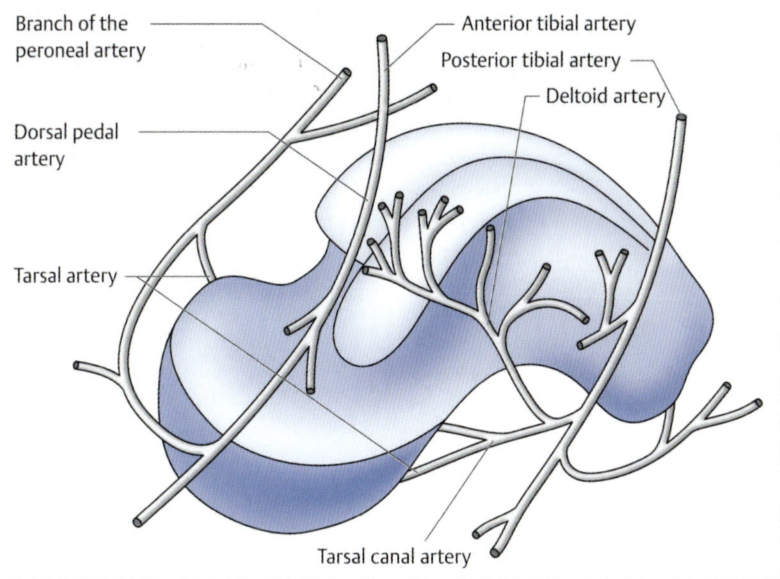

Fig. 3.68 Arterial supply to the talus.

CT

CT may initially show irregular diffuse sclerosis, depending on the duration of edema and the degree of perfusion. Later scans show sharply demarcated sclerosis, cortical fissuring, articular surface deformity, and loose fragments.

MRI

Interpretation Checklist

There is no generally valid staging system for AVN of the talus. The following points should be addressed:

- Describe the stage.
- Evaluate reversible or irreversible perfusion deficits.
- Evaluate extent.
- Evaluate the articular surface.
- Determine the cartilage status.
- Evaluate progression (revascularization).

Examination Technique

Contrast administration is not essential. Necrosis can also be evaluated with fat-suppressed, water-sensitive sequences and unenhanced T1-weighted images.

- *Standard protocol:* prone position, high-resolution multi-channel coil
- *Sequences:*
  - PD-weighted fat-sat coronal (may use short-tau inversion recovery [STIR] sequence) and sagittal
  - Coronal T1-weighted
  - Axial T2-weighted
  - If necessary: T1-weighted fat-sat, true axial (angled to the joint plane) and sagittal after IV contrast administration

MRI Findings (▶ Fig. 3.69)

MRI ultimately shows a pattern that is typical of AVN in any bone:

- Early stage: bone marrow edema without demarcation.
- Later, T1-weighted images show a hypointense line or circumscribed necrotic area with absence of fatty marrow signal.

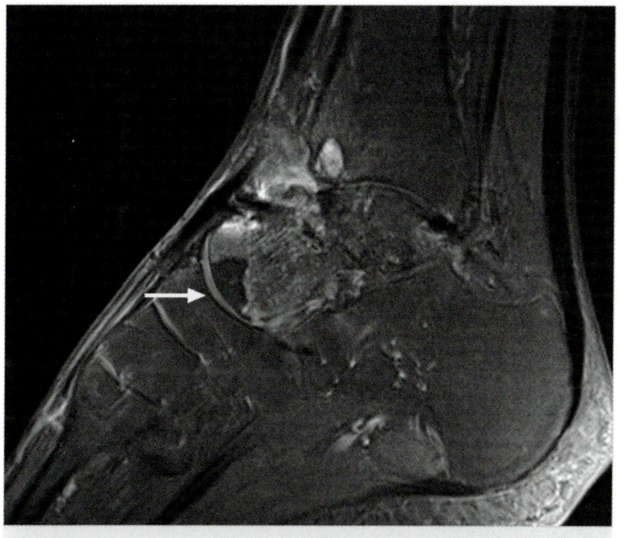

Fig. 3.69 Focal avascular necrosis of the talus following a comminuted fracture of the talus with marked deformity and flattening of the talar dome. Sagittal T1-weighted fat-sat image after contrast administration. A necrotic area (arrow) is demarcated in the distal talar head. There is no evidence of articular surface collapse.

- Diffuse bone marrow edema.
- Large central necrotic areas are sharply demarcated by a serpiginous hypointense line.
- Double-line sign: a hypointense outer line caused by sclerosis and fibrosis, and an inner line of higher signal intensity caused by granulation tissue.
- Late stage is characterized by articular surface collapse, fragmentation, and secondary degenerative changes.

Imaging Recommendation

Modality of choice: MRI for evaluating extent and staging, follow-up, and evaluating the articular cartilage surface.

Differential Diagnosis

- Osteochondral lesion of the talus
- Osteochondritis dissecans
- Activated osteoarthritis
- Transient bone marrow edema syndrome

Treatment

Conservative

- Activity modification in the early stage
- Nonsteroidal anti-inflammatory drugs

Operative

- *Necrotic stage:* necrosectomy, debridement, bone grafting, and remodeling of the articular surface
- *Osteoarthritic stage:* arthrodesis

Prognosis, Complications

Possible complications are early osteoarthritis, degenerative changes due to articular surface collapse, chronic synovitis, effusion, and the development of a pain syndrome.

Avascular Necrosis of the Navicular

Definition

AVN of the navicular bone is an ossification disturbance that occurs in children and has a favorable prognosis (ischemia of the navicular, Köhler disease type I).

Symptoms

- Load-dependent pain in the talonavicular joint and midfoot
- Swelling
- Tenderness

Predisposing Factors

- Occurs spontaneously during the first decade of life (3 to 10 years, predominantly affecting males)
- Can occur posttraumatically at any age

Anatomy and Pathology

The blood supply to the navicular is relatively poor, especially in its central portion. In children, differentiation is required from transient opacities or developmental variants of the navicular.

Imaging

Radiographs

Radiographs show increased density and apparent dissolution of the ossification center of the navicular. If a lateral view is obtained, it may show increased radiodensity of the navicular with no discernible subchondral plate, alteration of bone shape, and possible fragmentation.

Ultrasound

In a side-to-side comparison, ultrasound scans show an irregular surface of the ossification center with a thickened, echo-free hyaline cartilage layer.

MRI

Interpretation Checklist

- Describe the anatomy
- Note shape abnormalities
- Determine extent of edema and decreased blood flow
- Reversible/irreversible
- Metatarsal alignment
- Midtarsal joint line

Examination Technique

Contrast administration is not essential. Necrosis with loss of fatty marrow signal can also be evaluated with fat-suppressed, water-sensitive sequences and unenhanced T1-weighted images.

- *Standard protocol:* prone position, high-resolution multichannel coil
- *Sequences:*
  - Coronal and sagittal PD-weighted fat-sat
  - Coronal T1-weighted
  - Axial T2-weighted
  - If necessary: T1-weighted fat-sat, true axial (angled to the joint plane) and sagittal after IV contrast administration

MRI Findings

- Patchy bone marrow edema in the early stage
- Effusion in neighboring joints
- Subcutaneous soft-tissue edema, most conspicuous on the dorsum of the foot
- Hypointense subchondral zone in all pulse sequences
- Larger necrotic areas appear as signal voids without fatty marrow in proton-density and T1-weighted images
- Shape abnormalities
- Collapse
- Fragmentation

Imaging Recommendation

Modality of choice: radiography. MRI is useful for evaluating extent and staging, follow-up, and evaluating the articular cartilage surface.

Differential Diagnosis

- Two-part or multi-part navicular bone as an anatomic variant
- Old fractures
- Abnormally large accessory bones
- Transient bone marrow edema syndrome
- Activated osteoarthritis
- Rheumatoid arthritis
- Activated coalition
- Osteomyelitis
- Stress fracture

Treatment

- *Initially:* rest the affected foot for several weeks
- *For osteoarthritis:* arthrodesis

Prognosis, Complications

Possible complications are fragmentation, subluxation, and osteoarthritic changes. Navicular deformity may occur despite revascularization, creating a risk of osteoarthritis.

Calcaneal Apophysitis

Definition

Calcaneal apophysitis, known also as Sever disease, is an inflammationlike irritation of the apophysis of the heel bone.

Symptoms

- Heel pain over the calcaneal apophysis, aggravated by physical activity
- Predominantly affects adolescent males

Predisposing Factors

- Overweight
- Endurance sports
- Growth spurt with relative shortening of the muscular sling composed of the Achilles tendon and plantar fascia, exerting pressure on the calcaneal tuberosity
- Accentuated by pes cavus and decreased flexibility of the hindfoot and tarsus
- Risk particularly high in soccer players who undergo rigorous training during the adolescent growth spurt

Anatomy and Pathology

An inflammationlike irritation of the still-unossified apophysis occurs in a setting of overexertion and repetitive microtrauma due to increased Achilles tendon traction. Osteonecrosis does not occur.

Imaging

Radiographs

Radiographs generally do not show a correlative structural abnormality. Films may show sclerosis and increased radiopacity of the apophysis, followed later by fragmentation. (The apophysis is radiographically visible after about 5 years of age, and ossification can be seen after about 11 years of age.)

Ultrasound

Ultrasound shows irregular, fragmented ossification centers at the Achilles tendon insertion that form a bulge on the calcaneal tuberosity.

MRI

Interpretation Checklist

- Exclusion of other causes
- Extent of edema
- Fibro-osseous junction of the Achilles tendon
- Quality of the Achilles tendon
- Initial internal degeneration in young competitive athletes

Examination Technique

- *Standard protocol:* Prone position, high-resolution multichannel coil; contrast administration is not required.
- *Sequences:*
  - Sagittal T1-weighted and STIR sequences
  - Coronal PD-weighted fat-sat
  - Axial T2-weighted

MRI Findings (▶ Fig. 3.70)

- Bone marrow edema in the apophysis (may be very faint in some cases)
- Possible fluid accumulation between the calcaneus and apophysis
- Mild edema of adjacent soft tissues, around the Achilles tendon, and around the apophysis

Imaging Recommendation

The diagnosis is made clinically. Imaging is used to exclude other causes.

Differential Diagnosis

- "Growing pains"
- Bony stress reaction or stress fracture of the calcaneus
- Symptomatic bone cyst
- Bursitis
- Reiter syndrome

Treatment

- Rest
- Analgesics as needed
- Orthotic with a heel lift

Prognosis, Complications

Calcaneal apophysitis is a self-limiting disease that generally resolves completely within a few weeks. The incidence of recurrence is approximately 30%.

Coalition

Definition

Coalition is a congenital fibrous (syndesmotic), cartilaginous (synchondrotic) or bony (synostotic) fusion with an absence of joint development.

The condition is not a fusion but a failure of normal segmentation within a common cartilaginous rudiment.

Symptoms

- Rigid valgus angulation of the hindfoot
- Limitation of motion
- Pain during or after physical activity
- Bilateral in 50% of cases
- Onset of complaints in adolescence or early adulthood
- Complaints often begin after trauma

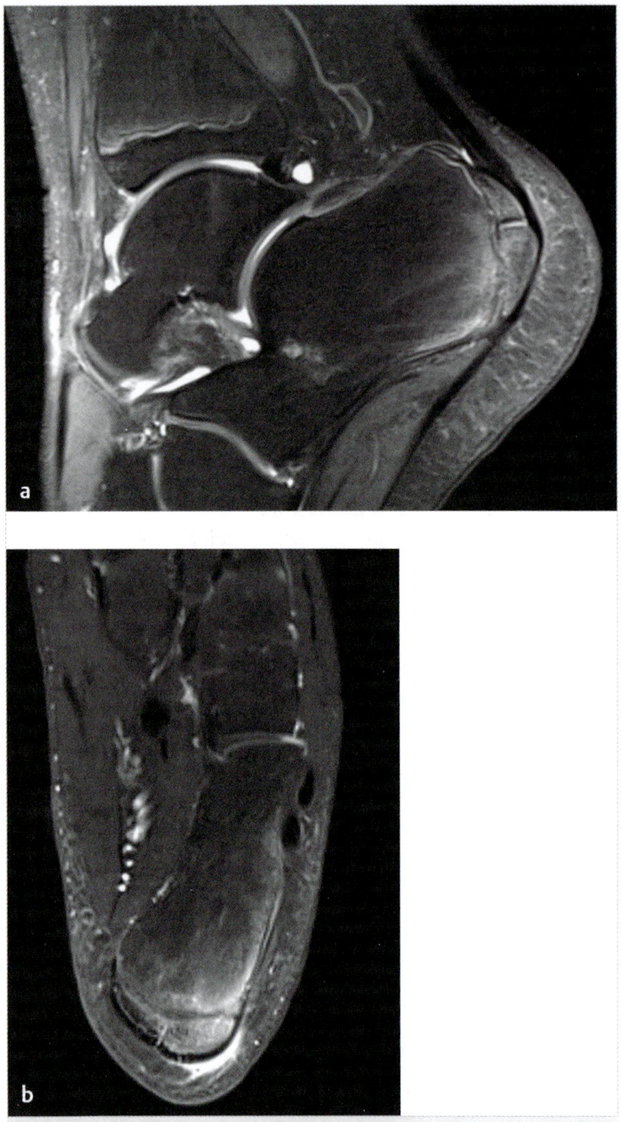

Fig. 3.70 a, b **Calcaneal apophysitis** in a 12-year-old girl referred with a diagnosis of "unexplained refractory heel pain."
a Sagittal PD-weighted fat-sat image shows the typical appearance of apophysitis with edema formation in the still-unossified apophysis of the calcaneus.
b Axial T1-weighted fat-sat image after contrast administration shows increased enhancement of the bone and adjacent fibro-osseous junction on the medial side of the Achilles tendon. Contrast administration is unnecessary for diagnosing calcaneal apophysitis but was used in this case owing to the unexplained nature of the pain symptoms.

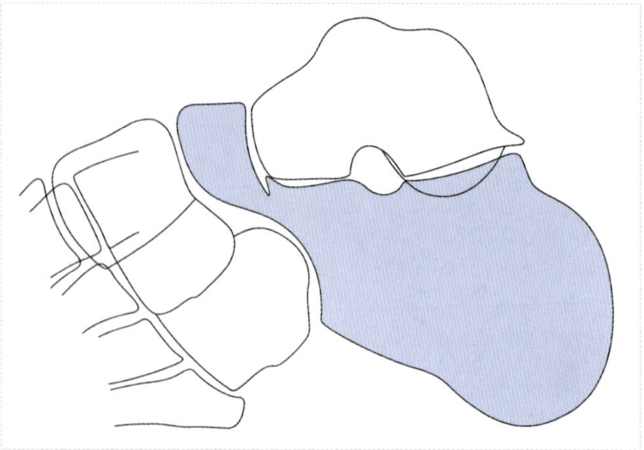

Fig. 3.71 **Congenital bony coalition: calcaneonavicular coalition** (source: Dihlmann and Stäbler 2010). This coalition is already apparent on oblique radiographs. Note the hypoplasia of the talar head and the deformity (narrowing, beaking) of the anterosuperior calcaneus to form an "anteater snout." With a fibrous or cartilaginous coalition, CT shows an irregular, narrowed joint space with incipient trabecular sclerosis (axial scan in the long calcaneal axis or in the sagittal plane).

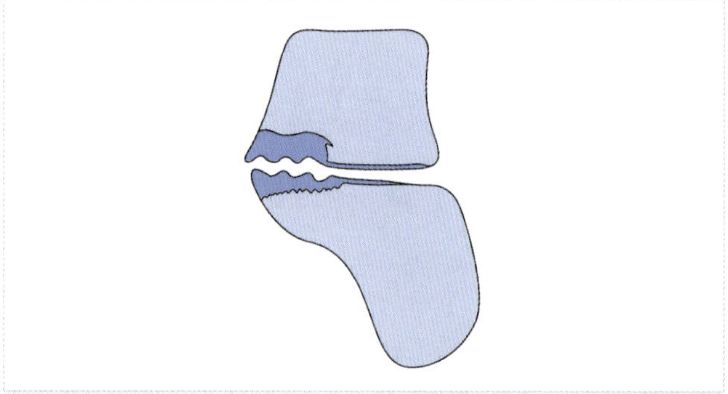

Fig. 3.72 **CT appearance of a fibrous coalition** (source: Dihlmann and Stäbler 2010). The irregular, eroded-looking contours of the talocalcaneal articular surfaces and the adjacent trabecular sclerosis are strongly suspicious for a nonbony coalition on CT, but these signs are not always present.

Predisposing Factors

None. Coalition is a development anomaly, which is frequently activated by trauma.

Anatomy and Pathology

Incidence of coalitions in the foot is approximately 1 to 2%, the most common forms being talocalcaneal and calcaneonavicular. Talonavicular coalition is less common. Coalitions may place unphysiologic loads on the ankle ligaments, making them more susceptible to injury.

Imaging (▶ see Figs. 3.71–3.75)

Radiographs

Indirect radiographic signs may be found, but they are not very specific and are unrewarding in fibrous coalitions.
Possible radiographic signs:

- Dorsal talar beak
- Ball-and-socket deformity of the talocrural joint
- Broadening and flattening of the talar lateral process
- Narrowing or absence of the subtalar joint space
- Talocalcaneal C sign (C-shaped bony contour from the posterior talar dome to the sustentaculum tali)

CT

We recommend at least 1-mm slice acquisitions with MPRs. CT provides an excellent view of bony coalitions in which neighboring bones are fused together. It is difficult to diagnose a

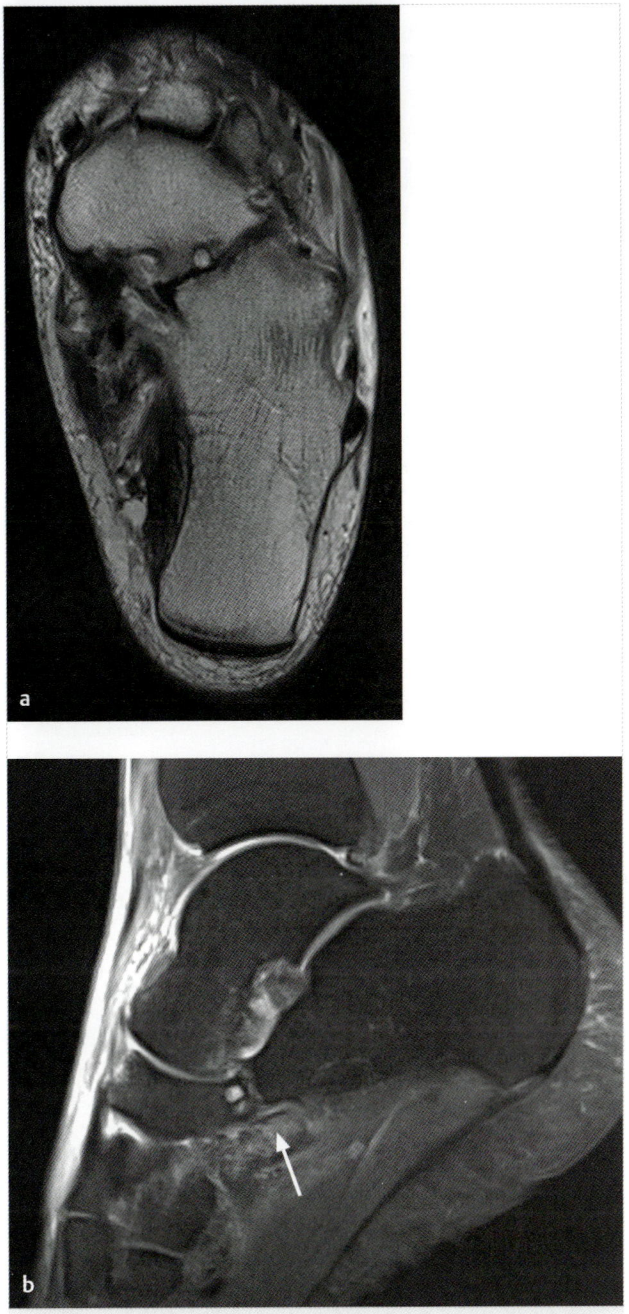

Fig. 3.73 a, b **Fibrous calcaneonavicular coalition** in a 41-year-old woman with increasing nonspecific hindfoot and midfoot pain, more severe on the lateral side and aggravated by physical activity.
a Axial T2-weighted image (angled to the joint plane) shows an irregular bony protrusion from the anterior process of the calcaneus to the navicular bone on the plantar side.
b Sagittal PD-weighted fat-sat image shows the typical appearance of a fibrous coalition with small subchondral cysts and an irregular bone contour (arrow).

fibrous coalition, although detection may be aided by noting subcortical or subchondral irregularities in the articular surfaces.

Ultrasound

Ultrasound does not contribute to the diagnosis, although it may demonstrate secondary changes such as a hypoechoic mass on the talar neck, intra-articular osteophytes, or secondary joint instability.

MRI

The most frequent use of MRI is for excluding other potential causes of unexplained hindfoot pain.

> **! Note**
>
> Coalition of the medial facet of the subtalar joint is difficult to detect on radiographs. Thus MRI is a very important study, especially for the diagnosis of fibrous coalition.

Interpretation Checklist

- State the precise anatomic location
- Evaluate the extent of the coalition
- Estimate the percentage of intact articular surface (> or < 50%)
- Degree of activation
- Differentiate between fibrous and bony coalition
- Evaluate neighboring joints
- Initial degeneration
- Cartilage quality

Examination Technique

Contrast administration is unnecessary. The degree of activation in a coalition is investigated with fat-suppressed sequences.

- *Standard protocol:* prone position, high-resolution multichannel coil
- *Sequences:*
  - Coronal and sagittal PD-weighted fat-sat
  - Coronal T1-weighted
  - Axial T2-weighted

MRI Findings

MRI can show the activated component of a fibrous coalition with bony reactive edema, adjacent soft-tissue edema, and overload signs in adjacent joints associated with a bony coalition. A fibrous coalition is sometimes difficult to detect but may be suggested by deficient articular cartilage with subchondral irregularities. Bony coalitions are usually easy to detect in multiple imaging planes (talocalcaneal: coronal and sagittal; calcaneonavicular: axial and coronal to the midfoot).
Associated findings:

- Early degenerative changes in neighboring joints
- Tendon overload (especially the peroneal tendons)
- Bony irritation from exostoses on tendon sheaths

Imaging Recommendation

Modality of choice: radiography. MRI is used to investigate equivocal findings and assess the degree of activation and adjoining segments. CT should be used in equivocal cases with a suspected fibrous coalition.

Differential Diagnosis

- Too-long anterior process
- Osteoarthritis
- Arthritis

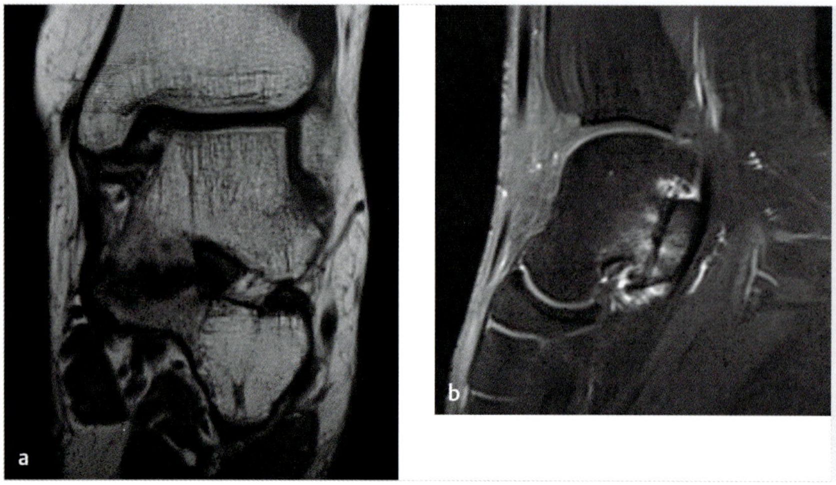

Fig. 3.74 a, b Activated fibrous coalition of the medial facet of the subtalar joint in a 48-year-old woman with a very long history of hindfoot complaints.
a Coronal T1-weighted image shows a widened, expanded medial compartment of the subtalar joint with irregular bone contours.
b Sagittal T1-weighted fat-sat image after contrast administration shows signs of an activated coalition with bone marrow edema and adjacent synovitis.

- Osteochondral lesion of the talus/osteochondritis dissecans
- Impingement

Treatment

Conservative

- Bracing
- Shoe inserts to relieve mechanical stresses

Operative

- Resection with interposition of muscle or fatty tissue; collagen membranes may also be used
- Concomitant correction of the hindfoot axis by calcaneal osteotomy or sinus tarsi spacer
- Primary arthrodesis is indicated only if the subtalar joint is largely absent. If complaints persist, arthrodesis may be carried out secondarily after resection of the coalition.

Prognosis, Complications

Prognosis

The smaller the bone bridge and the younger the patient at the time of diagnosis, the better the prognosis in terms of functional joint recovery after resection of the bone bridge.

Possible Complications

The treatment of large bone bridges is often followed by secondary degenerative changes in adjacent joints. Other potential late problems include increased laxity of the ankle and metatarsal ligaments and tendons (especially the peroneal tendons) and bony impingement with exostoses and soft-tissue pressure injury from bony prominences, especially on the talus.

3.2.5 Achilles Tendon Pathology

M. Walther and U. Szeimies

Achillodynia

Definition

Several forms of achillodynia are distinguished:

- Peritendinitis with inflammation limited to the paratenon (surrounding tissue that allows tendon gliding)
- Peritendinitis with Achilles tendinosis
- Tendinosis as an isolated degenerative lesion of the Achilles tendon

Degenerative tendon disease may be associated with partial tearing.

Symptoms

- Pain, especially before and after physical activity
- Complaints are often less severe during physical activity
- Local tenderness
- Palpable nodular thickening of the paratenon
- Fusiform thickening of the tendon
- Insidious onset of complaints
- Normal resting tension of the tendon

Predisposing Factors

- Dancers
- Runners (approximately 10% prevalence in runners, with a male preponderance)
- Improper training (excessive concentric loads without rest periods, too-rapid progression of training intensity)
- Repetitive sprinting (acceleration) and stopping (deceleration)
- Training in a cold environment
- Human leukocyte antigen type B27 (HLA-B27)
- Rheumatoid arthritis
- Hindfoot valgus
- Use of steroids or fluoroquinolones (e.g., Tarivid, Tavanic, Ciprobay)
- Supinated forefoot

Anatomy and Pathology

The Achilles tendon has a paratenon instead of a tendon sheath. Focal or diffuse tendon thickening most commonly occurs in the middle third. A "watershed" zone of relative hypovascularity is located 2–6 cm proximal to the fibro-osseous junction on the calcaneus; this is a site of possible calcifications and poor healing after microtrauma.

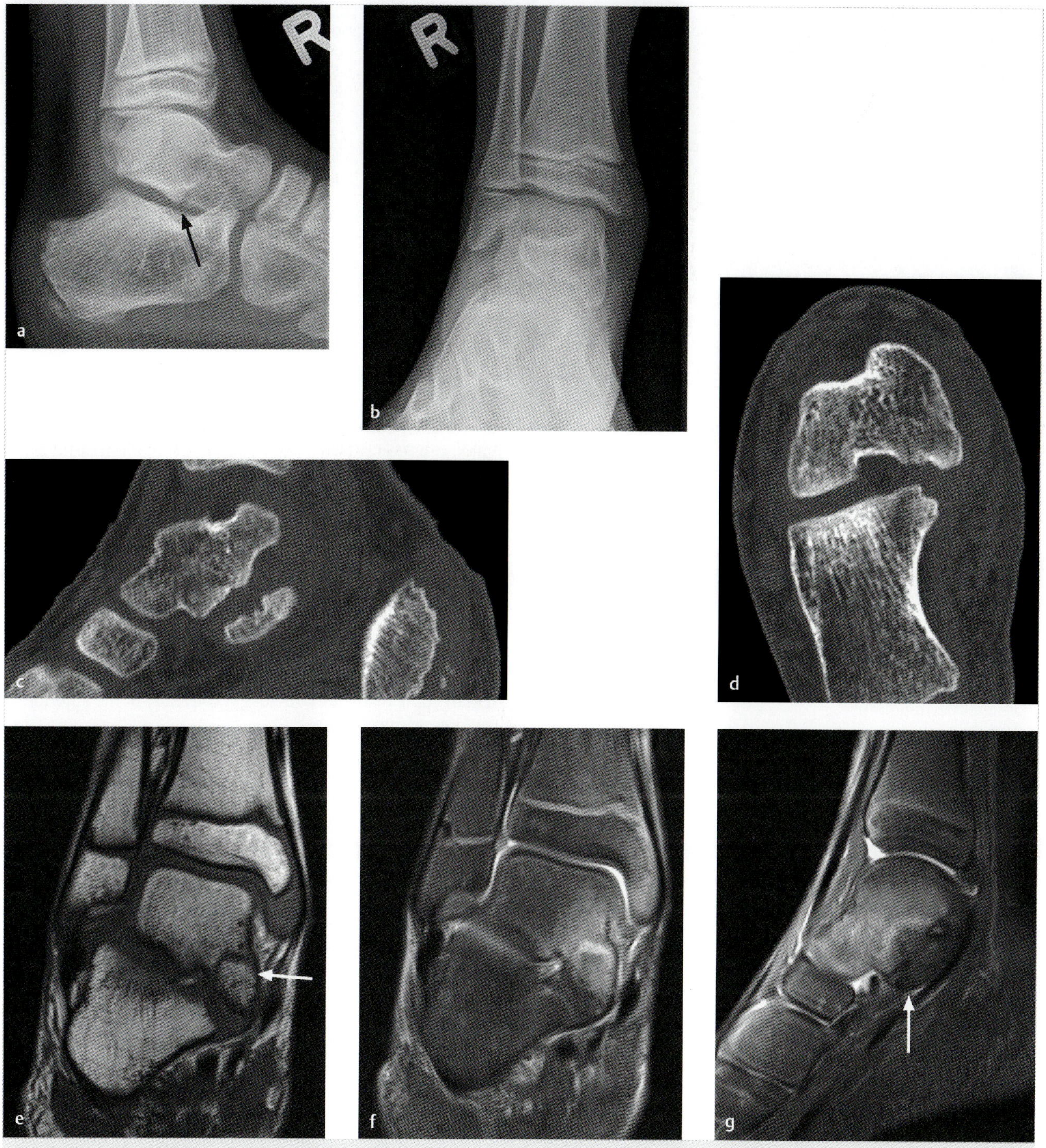

Fig. 3.75 a–g Acute ankle sprain in a 9-year-old boy. This patient sustained a fresh fracture of the medial distal talar body at the level of the sustentaculum tali with intensive fracture edema. There is a pre-existing, clinically silent fibrous coalition of the medial facet. The trauma-induced bending forces acted mainly on the medial talar rim instead of the medial articular facet.

a Lateral radiograph of the right ankle joint. The fracture itself is not visualized, and this poorly positioned view does not clearly demonstrate the coalition. The only obvious findings are small bony irregularities on the plantar aspect of the talar neck (arrow).

b AP radiograph of the right ankle joint shows no evidence of a talar fracture.

c Sagittal reformatted CT image displays the irregular shape of the bony joint contour.

d Axial oblique reformatted image. Compare with the smooth bony surface of the lateral subtalar articular surface.

e Coronal T1-weighted MRI demonstrates the fracture line (arrow).

f Coronal PD-weighted fat-sat image.

g Sagittal PD-weighted fat-sat image displays the fibrous coalition (arrow).

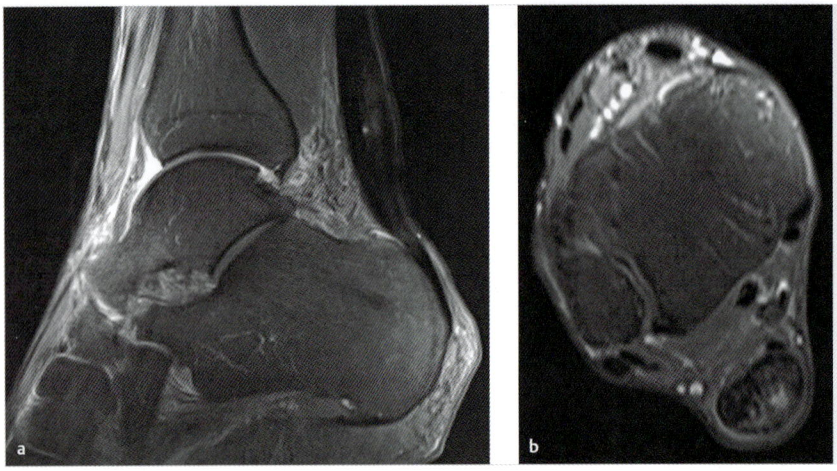

Fig. 3.76 a, b Chronic achillodynia with tendinosis in the middle third of the Achilles tendon.
a Sagittal PD-weighted fat-sat image shows fusiform thickening of the Achilles tendon in its middle and distal thirds.
b Axial T1-weighted fat-sat image after contrast administration shows increased intratendinous enhancement consistent with degenerative tendon vascularity. A semicircular enhancement pattern is noted in the paratenon in the painful area.

Imaging

Radiographs

Radiographs show obliteration of the fat stripe in the Kager triangle, an enlarged Achilles tendon due to soft-tissue proliferation, and calcifications. Radiographic imaging is not indicated as a primary study.

Ultrasound

- *Acute tendinopathy:* thickened tendon with homogeneous low echogenicity; echo-free fluid may be detected in the paratenon (peritendinitis)
- *Chronic tendinopathy:* increasingly echogenic, inhomogeneous change, caliber variations, possible fiber disruption by a partial tear (transverse scans important), degenerative cystic components, calcifications

The sonographic differential diagnosis includes a hypoechoic mass in the subachilles bursa ("subachilles bursitis"), echogenic inclusions at the tendon insertion on the calcaneal tuberosity (high heel spur), and a bony protuberance on the back of the calcaneus (Haglund exostosis).

MRI

Interpretation Checklist

- Exact location of tendon degeneration, measured up from the fibro-osseous junction on the calcaneus with determination of craniocaudal and AP dimensions
- Description of mucoid degeneration and tendon vascularity
- Evaluation of inflammation in the paratenon
- Location and intensity of contrast enhancement
- Associated subachilles bursitis
- Evaluation of any Haglund exostosis
- Concomitant involvement of the fibro-osseous junction
- Fibro-osteitis
- Bone marrow edema in the calcaneus
- Always address other hindfoot structures including the joints and tendons.

Examination Technique

Except in the case of an acute rupture, IV contrast administration is recommended to aid evaluation of the acute and chronic inflammatory component with tendon vascularization, peritendinitis, and fibro-osteitis; and to exclude necrotic areas.

- *Standard protocol:* prone position, high-resolution multichannel coil
- *Sequences:*
  - Sagittal T1- and PD-weighted fat-sat
  - Axial T2- and PD-weighted fat-sat
  - Sagittal and axial T1-weighted fat-sat after contrast administration

MRI Findings (▶ Fig. 3.76)

- Enlarged AP diameter with loss of convexity of the anterior tendon margin
- Fusiform tendon thickening
- Zones of mucoid degeneration, which are hyperintense in T2- and PD-weighted fat-sat sequences
- Increased intratendinous enhancement due to degenerative vascularization
- With peritendinitis: edema and increased enhancement in the paratenon
- Fluid detection and enhancement in the subachilles bursa due to associated bursitis
- Edema and increased enhancement at the fibro-osseous junction with bone marrow edema in the calcaneus due to fibro-ostosis
- Possible cyst formation and zones of bone softening in the advanced stage

Imaging Recommendation

Modalities of choice: ultrasound; postcontrast MRI for investigation of refractory complaints, for accurate evaluation of internal degeneration, and perhaps to exclude a partial tear.

Differential Diagnosis

- Spondyloarthropathy
- Enthesopathy
- Xanthomatosis
- Rheumatoid arthritis
- Crystal arthropathy
- Partial tear
- Haglund exostosis

- Subachilles bursitis
- Preachilles bursitis

Treatment

Conservative

- Rest
- Eccentric stretching exercises
- Anti-inflammatory medication
- Brace
- X-ray therapy (low-energy irradiation)
- Shockwave therapy
- Injection of platelet-derived growth factor
- High-volume injection therapy for paratenon adhesions; a large-volume mixture of local anesthetic and 0.9% NaCl solution is injected to dilate the space between the tendon and paratenon
- Hyaluronic acid

Operative

- Debridement (open or endoscopic)
- Augmentation with flexor hallucis longus tendon (only in cases with severe destruction of tendon tissue)

Prognosis, Complications

Possible complications:

- Persistent pain
- Partial tear
- Complete tear (rupture)
- Fibro-osteitis
- Associated bursitis
- Recurrent tear due to poor healing

Partial Tear

Definition

A partial tear is a partial-thickness disruption of the Achilles tendon in which some of the fibers are still intact and the tendon retains a degree of tension.

Symptoms

- Achilles tendon pain during physical activity
- Often the patient can point to the exact site of the injury
- Possible tendon thickening due to scarring
- Definite onset of complaints
- Preservation of tendon function
- Negative Thompson test

Predisposing Factors

- Age (loss of tendon compliance)
- Pre-existing degenerative changes in the tendon
- HLA-B27
- Rheumatoid arthritis
- Hindfoot valgus
- Use of steroids or fluoroquinolones (e.g., Tarivid, Tavanic, Ciprobay)
- Sports that involve jumping

Anatomy and Pathology

Partial tears may occur anywhere in the tendon and over time may lead to extensive scarring. Repeated partial tears may lead to a complete loss of tendon integrity.

Imaging

Radiographs

There is no primary indication for radiography.

Ultrasound

It is important to examine the tendon in transverse sections. A partial tear appears as a hypoechoic zone with associated hematoma and echogenic, partially intact tear edges. Separation and reapproximation of the torn edges can be assessed dynamically on the monitor while the foot is moved through maximum dorsiflexion and plantar flexion.

MRI

See also the section on Achillodynia (p. 92).

Interpretation Checklist

- Determine the precise level and extent of the partial tear; if possible, state the percentage disruption relative to the total tendon cross section in axial scans.
- Describe the condition of the rest of the tendon including the fibro-osseous junction and paratenon.

Examination Technique

A partial tear is best evaluated in axial T2-weighted sequences (hyperintense area) and after contrast administration.

- *Standard protocol:* prone position, high-resolution multichannel coil
- *Sequences:*
  - Sagittal T1- and PD-weighted fat-sat
  - Axial T2- and PD-weighted fat-sat
  - Sagittal and axial T1-weighted fat-sat after contrast administration

MRI Findings (▶ Fig. 3.77)

- Partial tears are hyperintense in T2-weighted images; most are longitudinal and located at a peripheral site.
- A central, intratendinous partial tear is sometimes seen.

Imaging Recommendation

Modalities of choice: ultrasound; MRI with IV contrast administration is used for special investigations.

Differential Diagnosis

- Achillodynia
- Spondyloarthropathy
- Enthesopathy
- Xanthomatosis
- Rheumatoid arthritis
- Crystal arthropathy
- Haglund exostosis

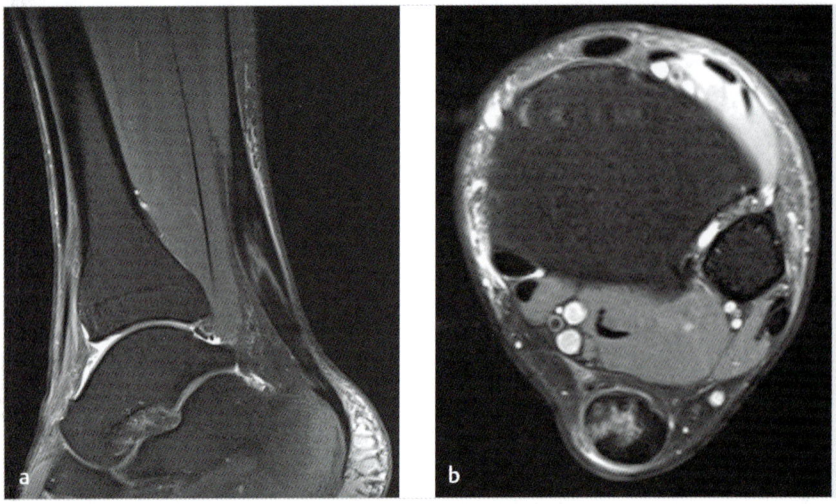

Fig. 3.77 a, b Acute increase of Achilles tendon pain in an athletically active 58-year-old man.
a Sagittal PD-weighted fat-sat image shows Achilles tendinosis with advanced internal degeneration and a longitudinal tear.
b Axial PD-weighted fat-sat image shows the partial tear entering the tendon from the medial side, with associated peritendinitis.

- Subachilles bursitis
- Preachilles bursitis

Treatment

Conservative

- Initial therapy is conservative
- Immobilization
- Rest
- Anti-inflammatory medication
- Eccentric stretching exercises after the acute injury has healed
- Injection of platelet-derived growth factor

Operative

- Surgical debridement (open or arthroscopic)
- Augmentation with plantaris longus tendon if required
- For extensive tendon lesions: augmentation with flexor hallucis longus tendon
- In patients with pre-existing shortening: gastrocnemius release

Prognosis, Complications

Possible complications:

- Persistent pain and irritation
- Chronic Achilles tendon thickening due to scarring
- Tendon rupture
- Secondary complaints in the lower limb and spinal column due to postural guarding

Rupture

Definition

An Achilles tendon rupture is defined as a full-thickness tear of the Achilles tendon with a complete loss of tendon tension.

Symptoms

- Possible popping sound or sensation
- Often the patient can point to the exact site of the injury
- Palpable depression in the course of the tendon

Table 3.11 Myerson classification of Achilles tendon ruptures

Grade	Description
I	< 2 cm
II	2–5 cm
III	> 5 cm

- Loss of tendon function
- Positive Thompson test
- Patient cannot perform a heel rise

Predisposing Factors

- Age and gender (6:1 ratio of males to females, peak incidence between 30 and 50 years of age)
- Frequent pre-existing degenerative tendon changes
- Sports that involve concentric loading (tennis, basketball, volleyball, alpine skiing)

Anatomy and Pathology

Most ruptures occur in the hypovascular middle third of the tendon. Defects often form in cases of delayed diagnosis or rerupture.

The Myerson scheme is used for classifying Achilles tendon ruptures (▶ Table 3.11).

Imaging

Radiographs

Not indicated as an initial study.

Ultrasound

A longitudinal scan over the Achilles tendon will demonstrate the echogenic torn ends, which are surrounded by hypoechoic hematoma. Ultrasound is used to evaluate gapping and reapproximation of the ruptured tendon ends in real time during passive dorsiflexion and plantar flexion of the foot.

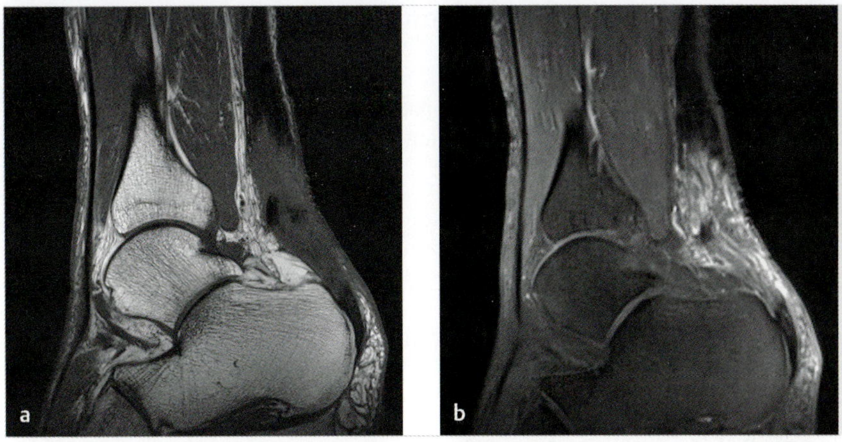

Fig. 3.78 a, b Complete, middle-third rupture of the Achilles tendon with retracted ends in a patient with pre-existing tendinosis.
a Sagittal T1-weighted image defines the extent of mucoid degeneration of the tendon ends, which show increased signal intensity. Individual tendon fragments are visible at the rupture site.
b Sagittal T1-weighted fat-sat image after contrast administration shows intense enhancement along the rupture site with elongated tendon fibers.

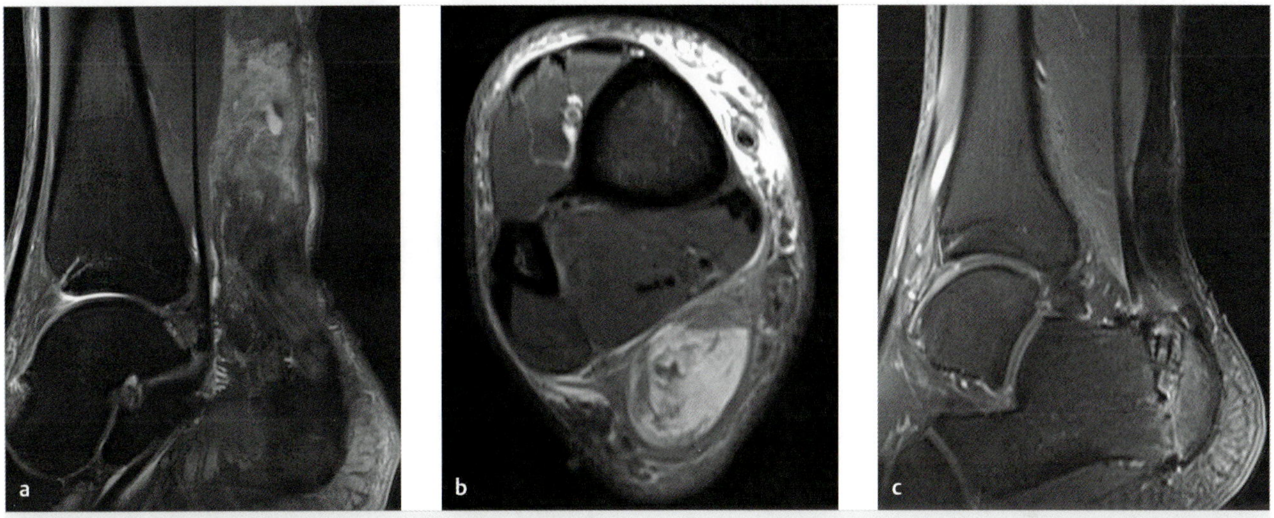

Fig. 3.79 a–c Rerupture in the proximal third of the right Achilles tendon in a 31-year-old man. There were significant pre-existing changes in the tendon substance following a previous longitudinal tear.
a Sagittal PD-weighted fat-sat image shows markedly increased signal intensity along the Achilles tendon, whose sagittal diameter is greatly enlarged. No continuous fibers are visible anywhere along the course of the tendon.
b Axial PD-weighted fat-sat image shows a fluid-filled defect that is devoid of all tendon material.
c Sagittal T1-weighted fat-sat image after contrast administration 9 months after a flexor hallucis longus transfer documents progressive hardening of the original Achilles tendon and a fully intact graft. The patient had an excellent functional result with occasional heel pain after playing soccer.

MRI

See also the section on Achillodynia (p. 92).

Interpretation Checklist

- Describe the exact location, measured up from the calcaneal insertion.
- Note the extent and direction of the tear (longitudinal, transverse, oblique).
- Evaluate the separation of the tendon ends.
- Note the quality of the rupture site.
- Describe advanced mucoid degeneration and fraying of the tendon ends (important for surgical planning).
- With distal tears, describe the calcaneal insertion.

Examination Technique

Contrast administration is not absolutely necessary for acute ruptures but is helpful for evaluating the tendon ends in patients with known achillodynia and chronic tendon degeneration.

- *Standard protocol:* prone position, high-resolution multichannel coil
- *Sequences:*
  - Sagittal T1- and PD-weighted fat-sat
  - Axial T2- and PD-weighted fat-sat
  - Sagittal and axial T1-weighted fat-sat after contrast administration (only if the rupture site is uncertain)

MRI Findings (▶ Fig. 3.78 and ▶ Fig. 3.79)

- Complete disruption of tendon continuity by a longitudinal or horizontal tear
- Frayed, hyperintense tendon ends in patients with pre-existing tendinosis
- Marked fluid accumulation in the paratenon along the course of the tendon and in adjacent soft tissues

- Retracted, tortuous tendon ends with a visible gap
- Axial T2-weighted sequence shows hypointense tendon material within tendon that is still intact
- Increased signal intensity about the frayed tendon ends
- Fluid only in the gap between the tendon ends

Imaging Recommendation

Modality of choice: ultrasound; contrast-enhanced MRI is used only for special investigations.

Differential Diagnosis

- Achillodynia
- Rupture of the plantaris longus tendon
- Partial tear
- Bony avulsion of the Achilles tendon
- Spondyloarthropathy
- Enthesopathy
- Xanthomatosis
- Rheumatoid arthritis
- Crystal arthropathy
- Haglund exostosis
- Subachilles bursitis
- Preachilles bursitis

Treatment

Conservative

- If the tendon fibers are reapproximated in plantar flexion (as determined by ultrasound)
- Brace for 8 weeks in a plantar-flexed position that is gradually reduced to neutral

Operative

- Indicated for repair of retracted tendon ends in young and athletically active patients
- Primary suture repair of an acute rupture may employ minimally invasive or open technique
- When treatment is delayed, reconstruction is tailored to the size of the defect:
  - Grade I: secondary open reconstruction
  - Grade II: open reconstruction using a VY plasty or turndown flap
  - Grade III: augmentation with the flexor hallucis longus or peroneus brevis tendon

Prognosis, Complications

Possible complications:

- Persistent pain and loss of strength
- Heavy scarring
- Loss of elasticity in the gastrocnemius–soleus complex
- Rerupture or absence of healing occurs in up to 20% of patients managed conservatively
- Incidence of rerupture after surgical treatment is 1 to 2% of patients
- Wound healing problems after surgical treatment
- Sural nerve damage during surgical treatment

Insertional Tendinopathy, Traction Spur

Definition

Insertional tendinopathy is an inflammation occurring at the junction of the tendon and bone.

Symptoms

- Pain at the Achilles tendon insertion
- Pain is often relieved during physical activity, then returns with rest
- Local tenderness, sometimes combined with bony excrescences
- Insidious onset of complaints
- Pain is increased by pressure from footwear

Predisposing Factors

- Poorly fitting shoes
- Runners
- Improper training (excessive concentric loads without rest breaks, too-rapid progression of training intensity)
- Repetitive sprinting (acceleration) and stopping (deceleration)
- Training in a cold environment
- Spondyloarthropathies

Anatomy and Pathology

Insertional tendinopathy is sometimes associated with a traction spur and Haglund exostosis. The lateral border of the calcaneus is commonly affected.

Imaging

Radiographs

A lateral radiograph of the calcaneus is supplemented by views in 30° of internal and external rotation. It is common to find no radiographic abnormalities. A traction spur may be present, and the bone may exhibit cystic changes in patients with inflammatory joint disease or a chronic course.

Ultrasound

Acoustic shadowing from a traction spur can be evaluated at the Achilles tendon insertion, but only superficially. Hypoechoic thickening and partial tearing of the Achilles tendon are sometimes observed. Periosteal insertional tendinopathy cannot be visualized with ultrasound.

MRI

Interpretation Checklist

- Accurate evaluation of tendon quality at the fibro-osseous junction
- Degree of bone marrow edema
- Associated inflammation in the paratenon
- Subachilles bursitis
- Partial tear
- Zones of mucoid softening
- Bony activation of the traction spur

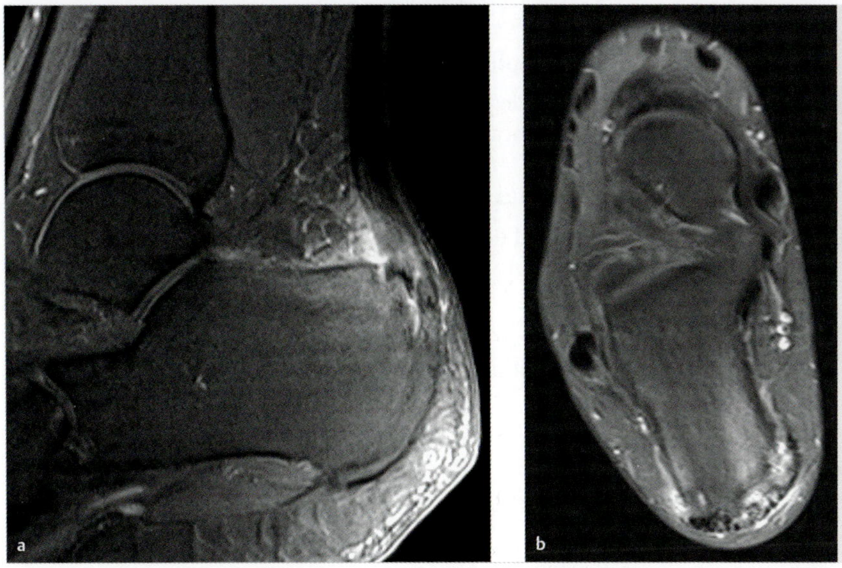

Fig. 3.80 a, b Insertional tendinopathy at the fibro-osseous junction with a small partial tear. The patient presented clinically with heel pain and footwear issues (could no longer wear a shoe with a closed heel).
a Sagittal T1-weighted fat-sat image after contrast administration shows insertional tendinopathy with increased enhancement within the tendon: at the calcaneal insertion, and in the subachilles bursa.
b Axial T1-weighted fat-sat image after contrast administration shows, in addition, peritendinitis around the back of the heel.

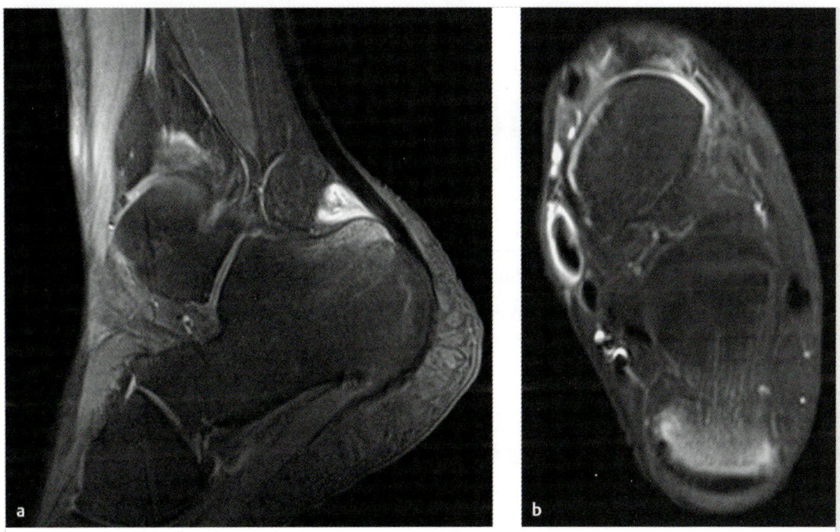

Fig. 3.81 a, b Differential diagnosis of insertional tendinopathy. The 40-year-old woman had a long history of complaints including recurrent heel and medial foot pain and nonspecific polyarticular complaints. Compared to the case in ▶ Fig. 3.80, the Achilles tendon appears intact with no internal degeneration or partial tearing. The dominant findings in this case are fibro-osteitis and bursitis, accompanied by definite peritendinitis of the posterior tibial tendon. Ultimately the patient was diagnosed with seronegative spondylarthropathy. Her complaints resolved completely with appropriate therapy.
a Sagittal T1-weighted fat-sat image after contrast administration shows marked bursitis and bone marrow edema in the calcaneus with a normal-appearing Achilles tendon.
b Axial T1-weighted fat-sat image after contrast administration shows marked bone marrow edema at the calcaneal insertion with a normal appearance of the Achilles tendon. Peritendinitis of the posterior tibial tendon is also noted.

Examination Technique

- *Standard protocol:* prone position, high-resolution multichannel coil
- *Sequences:*
  - Sagittal T1- and PD-weighted fat-sat
  - Axial T2- and PD-weighted fat-sat
  - Sagittal and axial T1-weighted fat-sat after contrast administration

MRI Findings (▶ Fig. 3.80 and ▶ Fig. 3.81)

- Unenhanced sagittal T1-weighted sequence is useful for evaluating the traction spur with bone marrow edema due to chronic activation
- Increased enhancement in the paratenon at the fibro-osseous junction with bone marrow edema in the calcaneus
- Fluid detection and contrast enhancement in the subachilles bursa
- Enhancing vascularity is detectable inside the tendon
- Small subchondral cysts may be found where the tendon fibers insert on the bone

Imaging Recommendation

Modalities of choice: radiology, ultrasound; preoperative MRI if required.

Differential Diagnosis

- Distal achillodynia
- Spondyloarthropathy (especially in patients with bilateral complaints)
- Xanthomatosis

- Rheumatoid arthritis
- Crystal arthropathy
- Haglund exostosis
- Subachilles bursitis
- Preachilles bursitis

Treatment

Conservative

- Initial therapy is conservative
- Immobilization
- Rest
- Shoe corrections for local pressure relief
- Anti-inflammatory medication
- Eccentric stretching exercises after the acute injury has healed
- Injection of platelet-derived growth factor
- Shockwave therapy
- Deep X-ray therapy

Operative

- Surgical debridement with removal of the spur
- Reattachment of the Achilles tendon with an anchor

Prognosis, Complications

Possible complications:

- Persistent pain and irritation
- Bone edema at the insertion site
- Scarring and chronic thickening of the Achilles tendon
- Tendon rupture
- Secondary complaints in the lower limb and spinal column due to postural guarding

Haglund Exostosis

Definition

Haglund exostosis refers to a bony protuberance on the posterosuperior aspect of the calcaneus.

Symptoms

- Tenderness at the superior border of the calcaneus
- Possible palpable subachilles bursa
- Pain increased by dorsiflexion of the ankle

Predisposing Factors

- Bony configuration of the calcaneus
- Poorly fitting shoes
- Running sports

Anatomy and Pathology

Bony protuberances on the posterosuperior aspect of the calcaneus (Haglund exostosis) cause irritation of the Achilles tendon resulting in inflammation and chronic enlargement of the subachilles bursa. A partial tear of the Achilles tendon may develop over time.

Imaging

Radiographs

Lateral radiograph of the foot shows a prominent hump on the back of the calcaneus.

Ultrasound

Ultrasound demonstrates a prominent posterosuperior rim on the calcaneus that may slightly displace the Achilles tendon.

MRI

Interpretation Checklist

- Degree of activation of the Haglund exostosis
- Degree of distal Achilles tendinosis
- Partial tear
- Subachilles bursitis

Examination Technique

- *Standard protocol:* prone position, high-resolution multichannel coil
- *Sequences:*
  - Sagittal T1- and PD-weighted fat-sat
  - Axial T2- and PD-weighted fat-sat
  - Sagittal and axial T1-weighted fat-sat after contrast administration

MRI Findings (▶ Fig. 3.82)

Haglund exostosis causes chronic damage to the distal anterior fibers at the fibro-osseous junction with an adjacent zone of mucoid degeneration and a possible partial tear just cranial to the fibro-osseous junction. MRI usually reveals concomitant subachilles bursitis with fluid detection and contrast uptake in the bursa, sometimes accompanied by patchy edema of adjacent tissue in the Kager triangle.

Imaging Recommendation

Modalities of choice: radiography and ultrasound; MRI is used for special investigations.

Differential Diagnosis

- Partial tear
- Bony Achilles tendon avulsion
- Insertional tendinopathy
- Achillodynia
- Posterior impingement
- Flexor hallucis longus tendinosis
- Activated os trigonum

Treatment

Conservative

- Heel wedge and padded footwear
- Steroid injection into the subachilles bursa
- Nonsteroidal anti-inflammatory drugs
- Therapeutic ultrasound
- Activity modification

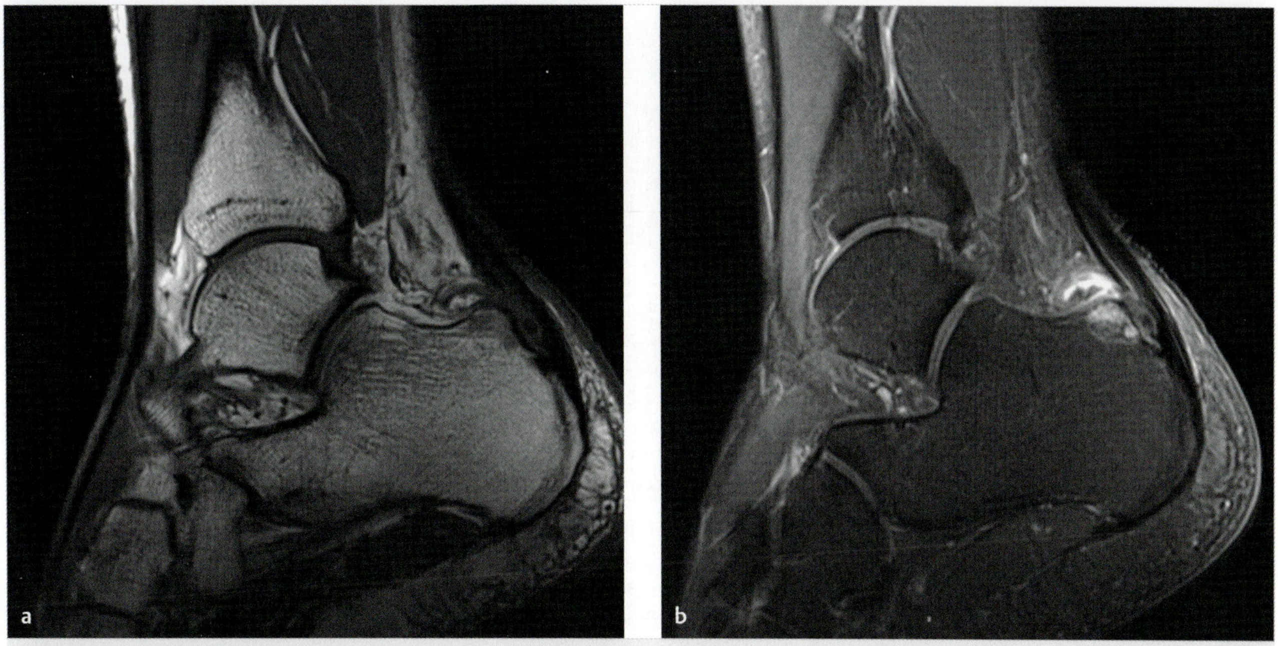

Fig. 3.82 a, b Activated Haglund exostosis.
a Sagittal T1-weighted image shows a bony prominence over the calcaneal tuberosity with bone marrow edema.
b Sagittal T1-weighted fat-sat image after contrast administration shows increased enhancement of the exostosis with adjacent activation in the sub-achilles bursa and mucoid degeneration of anterior Achilles tendon fibers at the fibro-osseous junction.

! Note

Intratendinous steroid injection is strictly contraindicated due to the risk of tendon necrosis!

Surgical

- Endoscopic removal is an option for isolated Haglund exostosis
- With associated pathology of the tendon insertion or a partial tear: open removal of the Haglund exostosis, resection of the subachilles bursa, and debridement of the tendon insertion

Prognosis, Complications

Possible complications:
- Persistent pain due to residual bony edges
- Overresection of bone
- Heavy scarring
- Persistent irritation of the fibro-osseous junction

Tennis Leg

Definition

Tennis leg is defined as a tear in the tendon aponeurosis of the medial head of the gastrocnemius muscle, causing the medial head to separate from the soleus fascia at the musculotendinous junction.

Symptoms

The cardinal symptom is an acute stabbing pain, usually felt at the upper to mid-calf level on the medial side, in response to loading and stretching.

Predisposing Factors

- Loss of elasticity in the gastrocnemius–soleus complex
- Shortening of the medial gastrocnemius muscle
- More common in sports that involve explosive acceleration such as sprinting, jumping, alpine skiing, and tennis

Anatomy and Pathology

It is common to find a more or less extensive partial tear in the aponeurosis of the medial head of the gastrocnemius. The medial head is stripped from the soleus fascia with associated hematoma formation between the fascial layers and in the subcutaneous soft tissues.

Imaging

Radiographs

Unrewarding.

Ultrasound

Ultrasound cannot detect calf strains but can demonstrate muscle tears on at least a secondary-bundle scale (▶ Table 3.12).

Table 3.12 Sonographic classification of tennis leg lesions

Grade	Description
I	Loss of parallel markings from echogenic fibrofatty septa at the triangular insertion of the gastrocnemius medial head over the soleus muscle
II	Decreased echogenicity due to interstitial hematoma; visible defect
III	Intramuscular echo-free hematoma, becoming hyperechoic after several days; decreased muscle excursion on contraction
IV	Intermuscular hematoma due to tearing of the gastrocnemius fascia, spreading distally between the gastrocnemius and soleus muscles

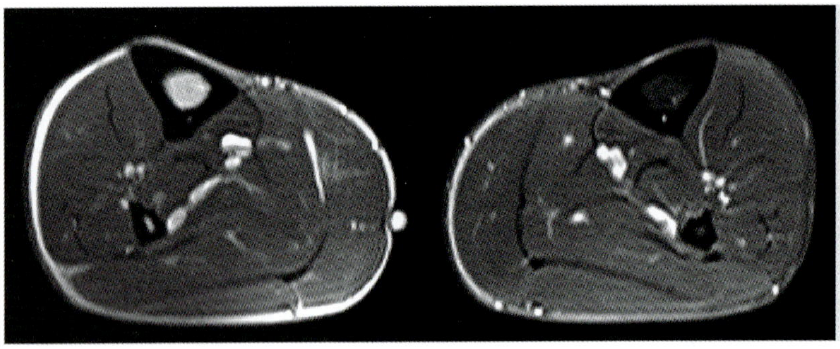

Fig. 3.83 A 24-year-old man experienced acute lancinating calf pain while playing sports. The painful site was labeled with a nitro capsule. Axial PD-weighted fat-sat MRI shows partial separation of the musculotendinous junction of the right gastrocnemius medial head from the soleus fascia, consistent with a diagnosis of "tennis leg."

MRI

Interpretation Checklist

- Precise craniocaudal visualization of the lesion
- Evaluation of the aponeurosis
- Determination of approximate percentage avulsion of the fascia from the aponeurosis
- Evaluation for possible intramuscular hematomas and fiber tears

Examination Technique

! Note

Patients are often referred with suspicion of an acute Achilles tendon tear. In some cases the image field may be too low to display the pathology in patients who describe pain at a more proximal level. After an initial assessment of the Achilles tendon displaying the leg to mid-calf, repositioning may be necessary to display the actual pathology.

- *Standard protocol:* prone position, high-resolution multichannel coil
- *Sequences:*
  - Sagittal T1- and PD-weighted fat-sat
  - Axial T2- and PD-weighted fat-sat
  - Coronal STIR sequence if needed
  - Contrast administration is not required

MRI Findings (▶ Fig. 3.83 and ▶ Fig. 3.84)

Typical findings are best appreciated in axial PD-weighted fat-sat sequences:

- Streaky fluid collection along the gastrocnemius aponeurosis, which is separated from the soleus fascia
- Severe injuries may show lengthy separation of the aponeurosis with adjacent intermuscular hematoma

! Note

Attention should be given to relatively subtle findings (scant fluid detection), which almost always cause complaints.

Imaging Recommendation

Modality of choice: ultrasonography.

Differential Diagnosis

- Muscle fiber tear
- Achilles tendon rupture
- Chronic compartment syndrome

Treatment

Conservative

- Most cases are managed conservatively
- Compression to reduce hematoma
- Physical therapy with lymph drainage
- Ultrasound
- Taping
- Immobilization in a lower leg brace for extensive tears
- Percutaneous needle aspiration of large hematomas

Operative

Indicated for extensive tears, especially in high-performance athletes.

Prognosis, Complications

Heavy scarring of the musculotendinous junction may lead to persistent complaints.

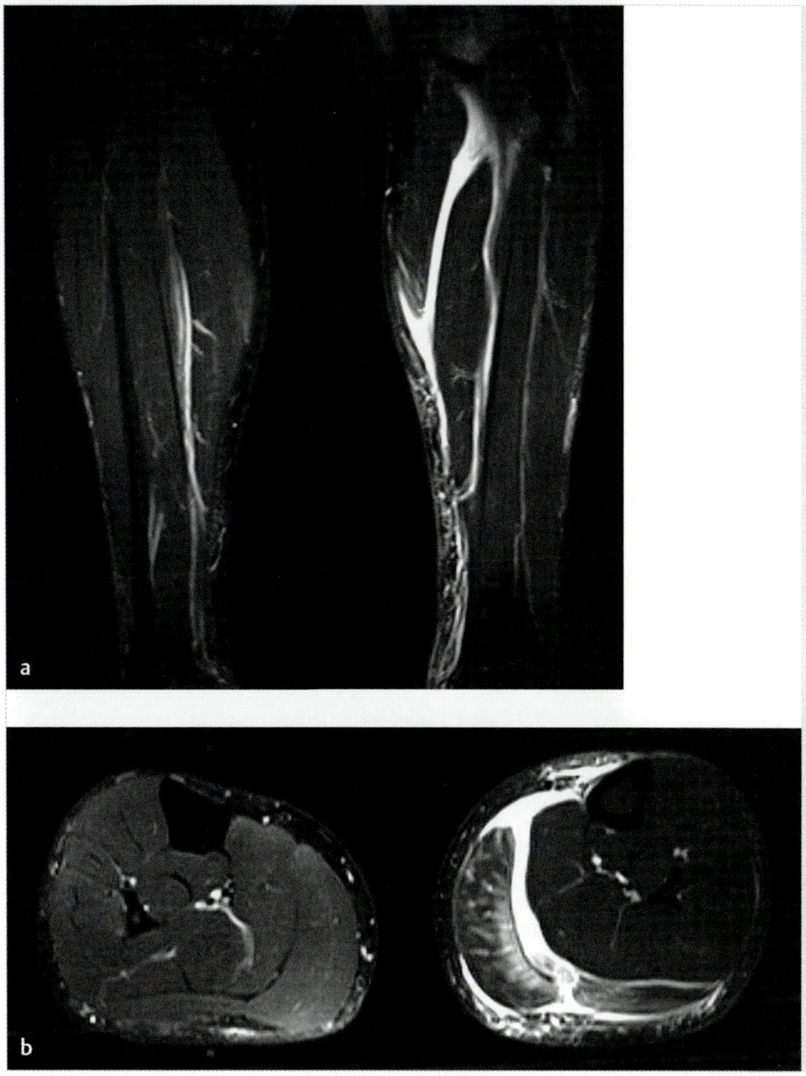

Fig. 3.84 a, b Tennis leg injury: acute pain with a "cracking whip" sound and sensation in the calf. The injury occurred during minor exertion (loading the trunk [boot] of a car).
a Coronal STIR sequence demonstrates a long, complete separation.
b Axial STIR sequence shows extensive separation of the gastrocnemius medial head from the fascia with bleeding into the muscles.

3.2.6 Disorders of the Flexor Hallucis Longus Tendon (Posterior Impingement, Os Trigonum Syndrome, Partial Tear)

U. Szeimies

Definition

Disorders of the flexor hallucis longus tendon include diseases ranging from peritendinitis and partial tearing to a complete rupture.

Symptoms

- Painful swelling about the medial malleolus
- Pain aggravated by plantar flexion

Predisposing Factors

- Pathologic findings are rare
- Dancers (repetitive plantar flexion and dorsiflexion) are commonly affected due to chronic overuse of the tendon without allowing adequate recovery
- Fracture of the sustentaculum tali

Anatomy and Pathology

- *Entrapment syndrome (stenosing tenosynovitis):* bony narrowing of the flexor hallucis longus tendon groove between the lateral and medial tubercles of the talar posterior process on the hindfoot, or within a fibro-osseous tunnel beneath the flexor retinaculum
- *Crossover phenomenon:* The flexor hallucis longus tendon crosses over the flexor digitorum tendon while passing below the sustentaculum tali to the sole of the foot.
- *Impingement:* low-lying muscle belly, accessory tendon (flexor digitorum accessorius longus); complete rupture is much rarer than peritendinitis in the fibro-osseous tunnel in a setting of stenosing tenosynovitis, under the flexor retinaculum or at the level of the sesamoids
- *Traumatic rupture:* at the distal tendon insertion on the big toe

- *Rare normal variants:* "false flexor hallucis longus" at the back of the ankle: internal peroneocalcaneal muscle

A flexor hallucis longus tendon transfer is often used for reconstruction of a chronic Achilles tendon rupture.

Imaging

Radiographs

Radiographs show intra-articular loose bodies or an os trigonum as well as ossifications in the tendon substance.

Ultrasound

Changes are rarely detectable with ultrasound. Scans may initially show a halo due to fluid collection in the tendon sheath with hyperechoic expansion, followed later by increasingly inhomogeneous changes or even a partial tear.

MRI

Interpretation Checklist

- Assess tendon quality
- Intratendinous vascularization
- Partial tear
- Complete tear
- Degree of tendon retraction
- Evaluation of tendon ends (advanced degeneration?)
- Exact location of tendon changes
- Extent of peritendinitis
- Causes of peritendinitis (entrapment syndrome, crossover phenomenon, low-lying muscle belly, os trigonum, bony or soft-tissue impingement)
- Assess muscle quality prior to reconstruction (fatty degenerative, atrophy?)

Examination Technique

- *Standard protocol:* prone position, high-resolution multichannel coil
- *Sequences:*
  - Coronal and sagittal PD-weighted fat-sat
  - Coronal T1-weighted
  - Axial T2-weighted
  - T1-weighted fat-sat sequence after IV contrast administration, axial oblique (angled to the tendon plane) and sagittal

MRI Findings (▶ Fig. 3.85)

The basic pattern is like that found with any tendinosis or peritendinitis:

- Tendon thickening
- Fluid detection and contrast enhancement along the tendon sheath
- Zones of mucoid degeneration within the tendon
- Partial tear
- Degenerative tendon vascularity
- Complete rupture with an empty, fluid-filled tendon sheath and retracted tendon ends
- Possible bony activation edema bordering on the inflammation

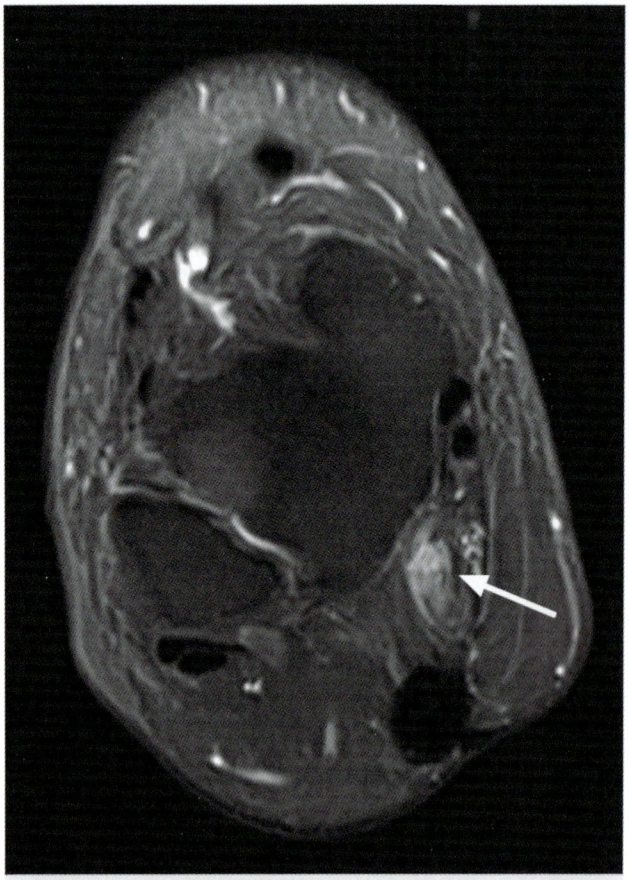

Fig. 3.85 A 46-year-old woman with status post-Achilles tendon elongation in childhood. The patient complained of chronic Achilles tendon pain and a recent acute exacerbation of pain. Axial oblique T1-weighted fat-sat MRI after contrast administration shows a normal-appearing Achilles tendon and a complete rupture of the flexor hallucis longus tendon. The image shows absence of flexor hallucis longus tendon substance with enhancing fibrovascular tissue occupying the tendon sheath (arrow).

! Note

In itself, the presence of fluid along the flexor hallucis longus tendon sheath does not usually have pathologic significance. The tendon sheath communicates with the ankle joint in more than 70% of cases. It is abnormal to find increased enhancement along the tendon sheath or increased septation (differential diagnosis: stenosing tenosynovitis).

Imaging Recommendation

Modality of choice: MRI to evaluate the degree of tendon degeneration and especially to identify the cause.

Differential Diagnosis

- Abnormalities of the posterior tibial tendon
- Achillodynia
- Os trigonum syndrome

Treatment

Conservative

- Nonsteroidal anti-inflammatory drugs
- Immobilization

Operative

Tendon impingement can be treated surgically by open or endoscopic resection of the stenosing soft tissue or bony outgrowths.

Prognosis, Complications

Chronic peritendinitis and tendinosis increase the risk of a complete tendon rupture and chronic pain syndrome.

3.2.7 Peroneal Tendon Pathology

U. Szeimies

Definition

Disorders of the peroneus longus and brevis tendons occurring from the distal lower leg to the tendon insertions are classified by the location of the tendon pathology. Peroneal split syndrome and peroneal tendon subluxation are special disorders that are discussed below under separate headings.

Symptoms

- Chronic pain about the lateral malleolus, sometimes with palpable thickening along the malleolus
- Possible painful click or snap on eversion of the foot
- Positive peroneal compression test on physical examination (compression of the peroneus longus tendon against the peroneus brevis tendon)
- Partial tears, which are more common in trauma cases, complete tears less common
- Complete rupture may occur in patients with pes cavus deformities

Predisposing Factors

- Overuse
- Repetitive trauma with incomplete healing
- Acute injuries
- Chronic irritation in sports involving frequent direction changes (tennis, ball sports such as soccer, handball, and basketball)
- Anatomic factors (accessory muscle, accessory bone, friction against the calcaneus)
- Hindfoot varus
- Chronic lateral instability

Anatomy and Pathology

The peroneus longus and brevis tendons (lateral ankle stabilizers) have sites of predilection for painful overload injuries in their course from the lateral malleolus to the midfoot. It is important, therefore, to have a precise knowledge of their anatomy and function.

Anatomy

Function of the peroneal tendons

Both tendons contribute to plantar flexion of the foot. As a powerful pronator, the peroneus longus muscle actively stabilizes the plantar vault, giving particular support to the transverse arch. The peroneal muscles are innervated by the superficial peroneal nerve (L5 and S1). Paralysis of the peroneal muscles causes a weakening of pronation, allowing the flexors to pull the foot into a supinated position (hindfoot varus) that is initially flexible but gradually progresses over time to a fixed deformity. Concomitant extensor paralysis leads to pes equinovarus.

Peroneal tendon anatomy (▶ Fig. 3.86).

Both tendons are held in place by the superior peroneal retinaculum as they pass through a bony groove behind the lateral

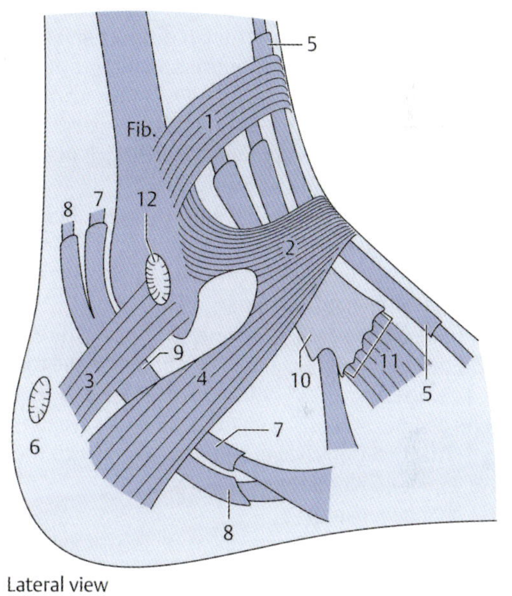

Fig. 3.86 Anatomy and relationships of the peroneal tendons (source: Dihlmann and Stäbler 2010).
Fib. = fibula
1 Superior extensor retinaculum
2 Inferior extensor retinaculum; structures 1 and 2 are bands that hold the extensor tendons (tibialis anterior, extensor digitorum longus, extensor hallucis longus) in place
3 Superior peroneal retinaculum
4 Inferior peroneal retinaculum; structures 3 and 4 are bands that hold the two peroneal muscles (peroneus longus and brevis) in place
5 Extensor hallucis longus tendon sheath
6 Retrocalcaneal bursa
7 Peroneus brevis tendon sheath
8 Peroneus longus tendon sheath
9 Short common synovial sheath for the peroneus longus and brevis tendons (starts just proximal to the superior peroneal retinaculum and extends to the cuboid)
10 Peroneus tertius tendon sheath
11 Extensor digitorum longus tendon sheath
12 Subcutaneous bursa of the lateral malleolus
The tibialis anterior tendon and its sheath (not pictured) run medial to structure 5, next to the anterior tibial margin

malleolus; they are bound to the lateral aspect of the calcaneus by the inferior peroneal retinaculum. At this level the tendons share a common fibro-osseous sheath in which they are placed not side by side but one above the other, the peroneus longus being superficial to the peroneus brevis. The common tendon sheath bifurcates at the level of the peroneal tubercle, giving rise to separate sheaths. The peroneus brevis tendon inserts on the base of the fifth metatarsal. The peroneus longus tendon runs around the cuboid tuberosity at the inferior edge of the cuboid; the tuberosity creates a fulcrum for redirecting the tendon along the pedal arch through a fibro-osseous tunnel to the medial side of the foot. Finally, the peroneus longus tendon inserts by multiple slips on the medial cuneiform, the base of the first metatarsal, and occasionally the base of the second metatarsal.

Pathology

- *Distal tip of the fibula:* The direction change at the tip of the fibula can cause mechanical irritation that may lead to a peroneal split syndrome.
- *Peroneal retinaculum:* Subluxation or dislocation of the peroneal tendons may result from injuries relating to an old ankle sprain.
- *Peroneal tubercle:* A prominent tubercle on the lateral calcaneus may cause increased frictional forces with mechanical irritation and peritendinitis or tendinosis.
- *Os peroneum:* This is a sesamoid bone in the peroneus longus tendon, located laterally on the plantar side of the cuboid. Possible disorders include fractures, osteonecrosis, and lesions of the tendon attachments.
- *Cuboid tunnel:* The peroneus longus tendon is redirected medially in this fibro-osseous tunnel. Tightness in the tunnel may cause an entrapment syndrome with tendon degeneration and osseous stenosis. Longitudinal tears have been described. The direction change and passage through the tunnel lead to increased biomechanical loads.
- *Insertional tendinopathy:*
  - Peroneus longus tendon: medial cuneiform and base of the first metatarsal. Activation at the fibro-osseous junction, especially at the lateral base of the first metatarsal, may lead to tendon thickening, fibrovascular reaction, subchondral cysts at the metatarsal base, ganglion cysts, associated bone marrow edema, fibro-osteitis, degenerative tendon vascularity, and partial tearing.
  - Peroneus brevis tendon: insertion on the tuberosity of the fifth metatarsal.
  - Another normal variant: presence of an accessory muscle, the peroneus quartus.
- *Complete rupture:* Acute ruptures of the peroneus brevis tendon most commonly occur at the level of the distal tip of the fibula or peroneal tubercle. The entrance to the cuboid tunnel is a site of predilection for tears of the peroneus longus tendon. Ruptures of both tendons are rare and are mainly found in association with severe hindfoot varus deformities.

Imaging

Radiographs

Radiographic imaging is helpful for identifying bony structures that can cause tendon degeneration (prominent peroneal tubercle, os peroneum, ossification at the distal tip of the fibula). Weight-bearing views of the foot are obtained in three planes to evaluate foot position (pes cavovarus deformity). A Saltzman view is obtained to evaluate hindfoot alignment. Weight-bearing views of the ankle joint in two planes can exclude a supramalleolar deformity.

Ultrasound

Ultrasound can display the peroneal tendons in longitudinal and transverse sections by scanning from the lower third of the tibia distally around the lateral malleolus to the fifth metatarsal (peroneus brevis muscle). A short linear-array transducer will yield better results (7.5–15 MHz). A stand-off should be used if coupling is poor. In cases of suspected dislocation, provocative testing should be done under monitor control to allow dynamic assessment of stability. A degenerative tear produces an "asparagus tip" sign.

MRI

Interpretation Checklist

- Describe the location and extent of tendon pathology
- Evaluate the cause (e.g., os peroneum, old retinacular injury)
- Evaluate tendon quality (intratendinous mucoid degeneration, partial tear)
- Evaluate bony structures (adjacent bone reaction)
- Look for secondary changes (joint overload, bony stress edema, other tendon pathology)

Examination Technique

- *Standard tendon protocol:* prone position, high-resolution multi-channel coil
- *Sequences:*
  - Coronal and sagittal PD-weighted fat-sat
  - Coronal T1-weighted
  - Axial T2-weighted (angled to joint plane)
  - T1-weighted fat-sat after contrast administration, axial oblique (angled to tendon plane), and sagittal

MRI Findings (▶ see Figs. 3.87–3.93)

- Early signs: peritendinitis with increased enhancement along the tendon sheath (more frequently involves the peroneus brevis at the lateral malleolus than the peroneus longus)
- Tendinosis: thickening of the tendon, possible degenerative tendon vascularity with increased intratendinous enhancement, sometimes localized to one point; enhancing zone of advanced mucoid degeneration within the tendon
- Longitudinal partial tear, usually affecting the peroneus brevis tendon at the lateral malleolus
- Accompanying bone irritation with bone marrow edema in the lateral malleolus, lateral calcaneus, and cuboid
- Insertional tendinopathy with increased enhancement at the fibro-osseous junction on the fifth metatarsal, medial cuneiform or base of the first metatarsal
- Possible activation of the os peroneum (bipartite ossicles and fractures are also described)
- With a complete rupture: empty, enhancing fluid-filled tendon sheath, frayed tendon ends, possible reaction of tendon ends

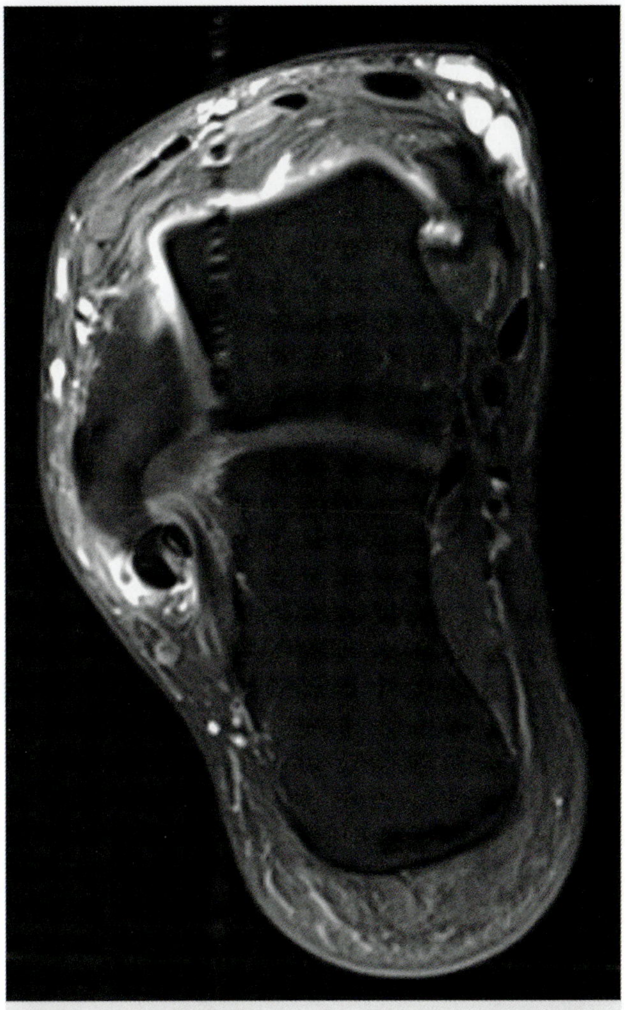

Fig. 3.87 Peritendinitis due to chronic mechanical irritation of the peroneal tendons at the distal tip of the fibula. Axial oblique T1-weighted fat-sat image after contrast administration shows increased enhancement in the common tendon sheath of the peroneus longus and brevis tendons with an incipient partial tear in the peroneus brevis at the tip of the fibula.

Imaging Recommendation

Modality of choice: MRI to evaluate the extent of pathology, for localization, for determining the cause, and evaluating associated changes.

Differential Diagnosis

- Anterolateral impingement
- Ankle instability with synovitis
- Fractures involving the lateral ankle joint or pedal border

Treatment

- Rupture of the peroneus brevis tendon: surgical reconstruction
- Rupture of the peroneus longus tendon: conservative treatment or debridement and tenodesis
- Ruptures of both tendons: surgical reconstruction
- Tendon transfer of peroneus longus to peroneus brevis, if required

Prognosis, Complications

Possible complications:

- Complete rupture due to chronic tendinosis
- Chronic pain syndrome

Peroneal Tendon Subluxation or Dislocation

Definition

Peroneal tendon subluxation or dislocation is an acute (traumatic) or chronic displacement of one or both peroneal tendons from their anatomic position along the retromalleolar groove behind the lateral malleolus.

Symptoms

- Pain posterior to the lateral malleolus
- Tendon snap provoked by dorsiflexion and eversion
- Possible painful swelling

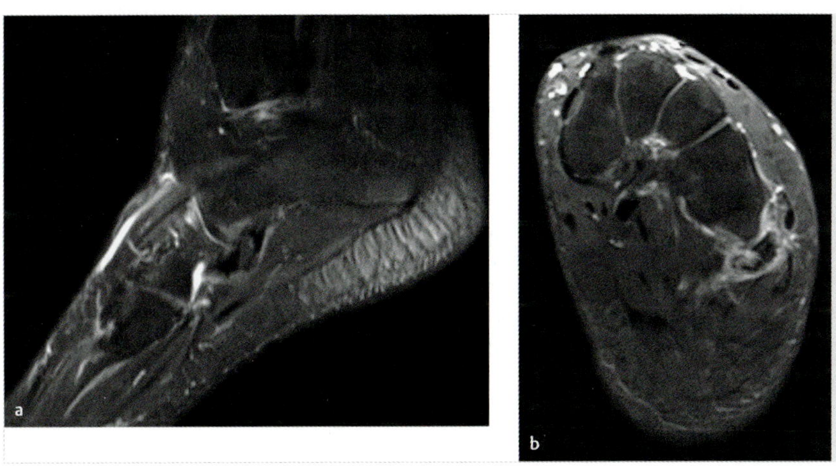

Fig. 3.88 a, b Os peroneum. Activated sesamoid bone in the peroneus longus tendon on MRI.
a Oblique sagittal PD-weighted fat-sat image shows two hypointense segments from the peroneus longus tendon at the level of the calcaneocuboid joint. A small, intratendinous bony structure is visible.
b Oblique axial T1-weighted fat-sat image after contrast administration. The marked activation process is visualized after IV contrast administration.

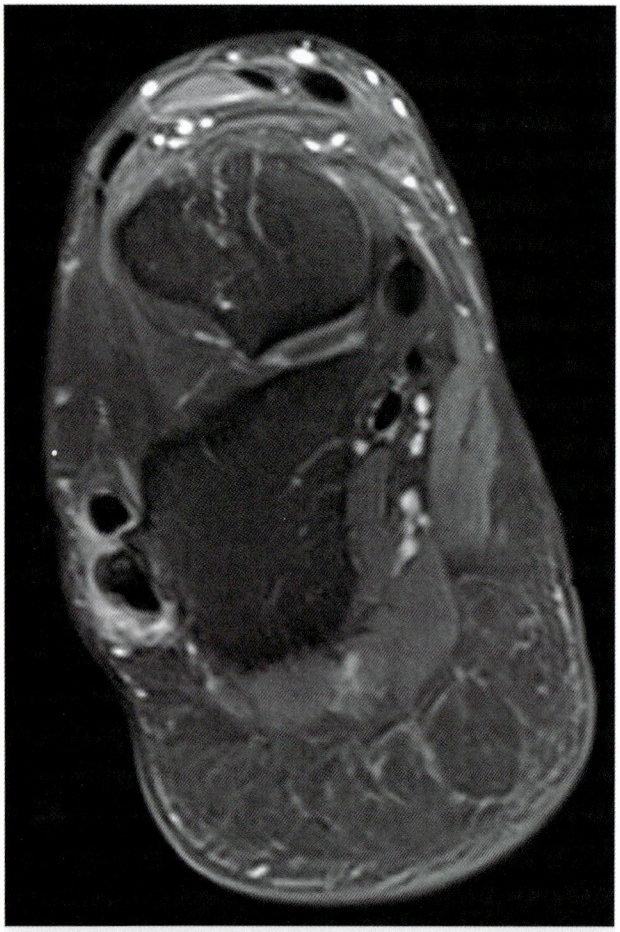

Fig. 3.89 **Peroneal tubercle.** A prominent peroneal tubercle on the lateral calcaneus. Axial oblique T1-weighted fat-sat MRI after contrast administration shows activated bony excrescences on the peroneal tubercle with associated mechanical irritation and peritendinitis, predominantly affecting the peroneus longus tendon.

Predisposing Factors

- Acute injury
- Congenital shallow retromalleolar groove
- Old lateral ankle sprain with injury to the peroneal tendon sheath and retinaculum leading to functional impairment and instability
- Lateral calcaneal fracture with injury to the superior peroneal retinaculum

! Note

There may be an associated injury of the calcaneofibular ligament.

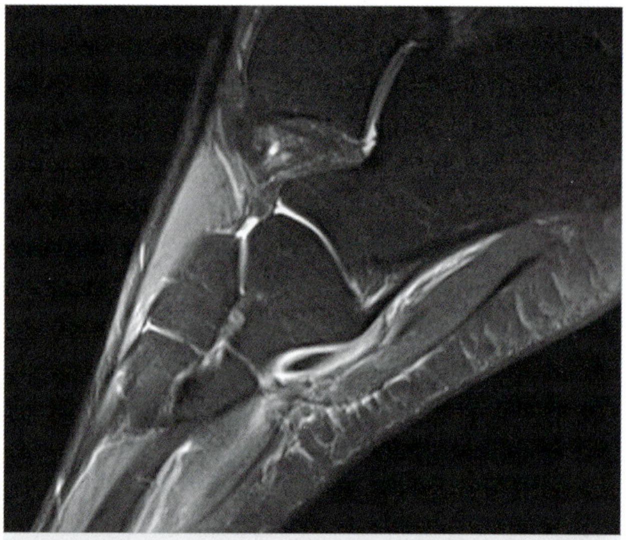

Fig. 3.91 **Cuboid tunnel.** Peritendinitis at the entrance to the cuboid tunnel. Sagittal T1-weighted fat-sat image after contrast administration shows activation of the peroneus longus tendon at the level where it turns sharply into the fibro-osseous tunnel at the cuboid bone.

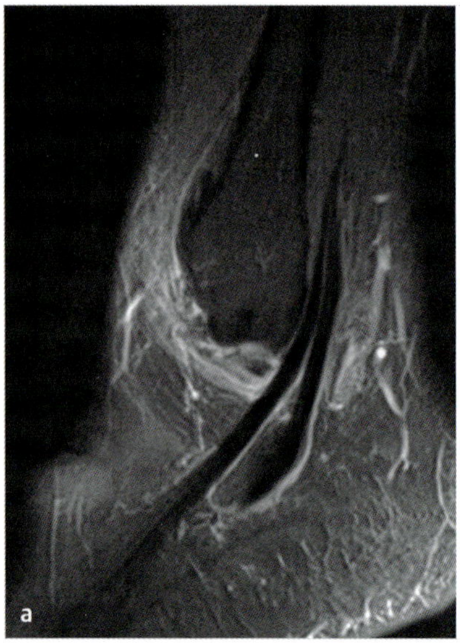

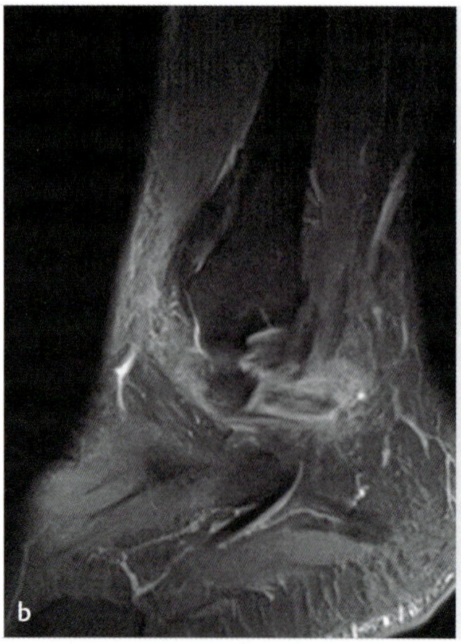

Fig. 3.90 **a, b Retinaculum.** Activation of the peroneal retinaculum in a 47-year-old muscular, athletically active man following multiple superficial injuries, the most recent occurring 4 weeks ago. The patient had a known history of peroneal tendon subluxation for years. He was investigated now for lateral ankle pain.
a Sagittal T1-weighted image after contrast administration. Both images (**a, b**) show an intense soft-tissue reaction that is most pronounced in the course of the peroneal retinaculum and calcaneofibular ligament.
b Another sagittal T1-weighted image after contrast administration.

Anatomy and Pathology

Redirection of the tendon at the lateral malleolus from a craniocaudal to anterior distal course makes it more susceptible to traumatic subluxation in response to dorsiflexion and forcible eversion of the foot.

A chronic peroneal tendon dislocation is present when an injury of the superior retinaculum allows the tendon to slip out of its groove and dislocate forward over the lateral malleolus. A painful, recurrent snapping takes place over the lateral malleolus in response to dorsiflexion and pronation. A shallow fibular groove can predispose to peroneal tendon dislocation, with stripping of the proximal retinaculum and periosteum from the lateral malleolus; isolated tearing of the retinaculum is rare. The stripped periosteum creates a "false pouch" over the lateral malleolus into which the tendon is displaced.

A special form is intratendinous subluxation with an intact retinaculum and a normal anatomic course in the retromalleolar groove. This form occurs when the peroneus longus tendon slips beneath the peroneus brevis.

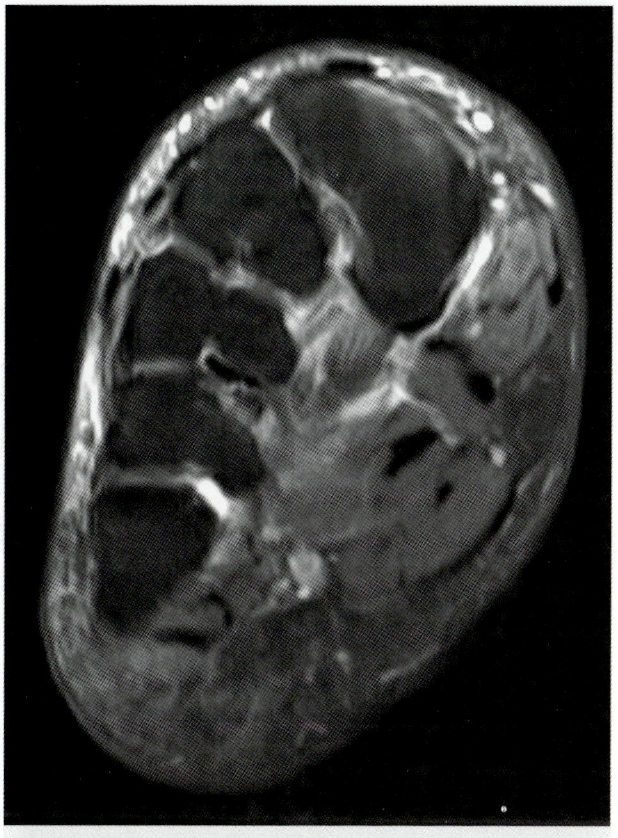

Fig. 3.92 Insertional tendinopathy of the peroneus longus tendon. Axial oblique T1-weighted fat-sat image after contrast administration documents peritendinitis and enhancing tendon fibers at the fibro-osseous junction on the lateral base of the first metatarsal.

Imaging

Radiographs

Radiography is not indicated as an initial study. When necessary, it can be used to exclude a bony injury and to identify bony structures as the cause of an abnormal retromalleolar groove. It permits differentiation from tendon degeneration (osteophytes).

Ultrasound

A transverse scan is performed behind the lateral malleolus. Dynamic ultrasound imaging can be used to evaluate tendon dislocation and intratendinous subluxation. Ultrasonography is better than MRI for documenting tendon instability.

MRI

Interpretation Checklist

The retromalleolar groove can be evaluated by MRI:

- Chronic subluxation due to a shallow groove

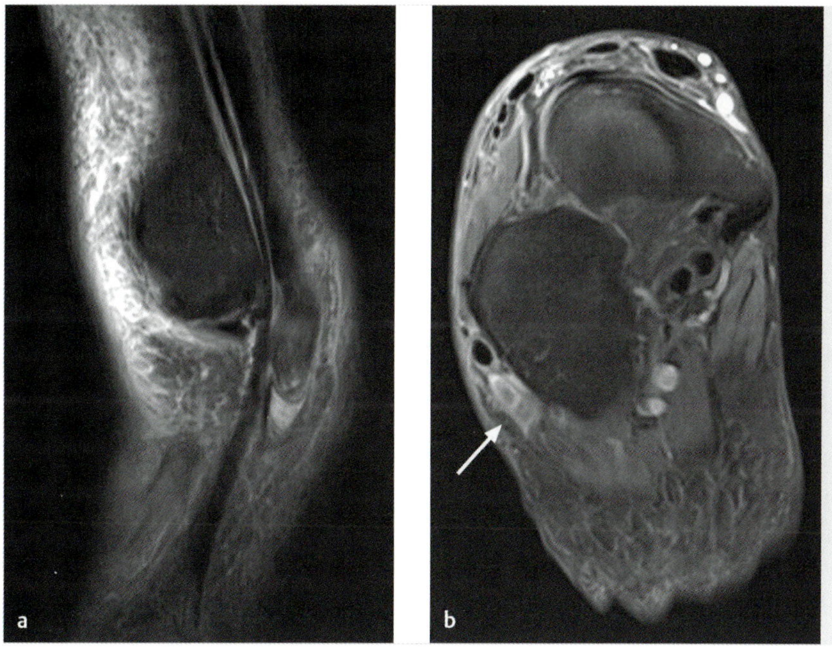

Fig. 3.93 a, b Peroneal tendon rupture.
a Sagittal PD-weighted fat-sat image shows a complete rupture of the peroneus longus tendon with mucoid degeneration and retraction of the tendon end. The peroneus brevis tendon appears intact.
b Axial oblique T1-weighted fat-sat image after contrast administration shows an absence of normal tendon structure posterior to the peroneus brevis. The tendon sheath is occupied by fibrovascular reactive tissue and degenerative residual fiber stumps (arrow).

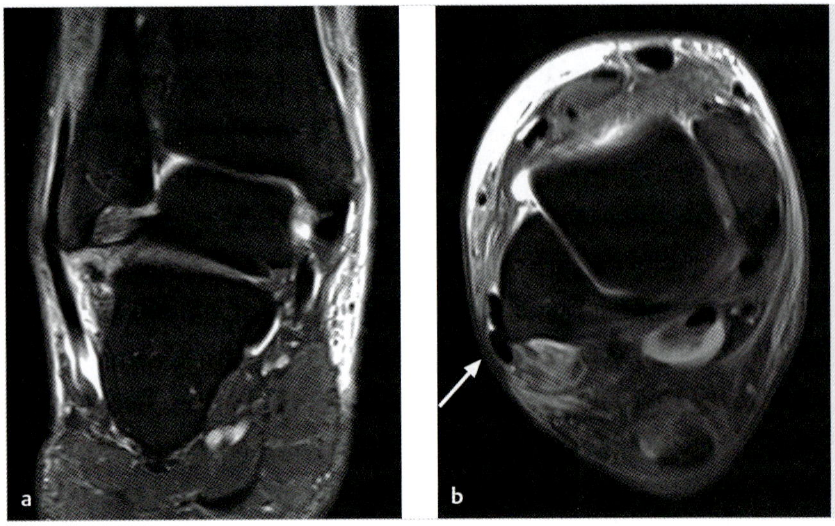

Fig. 3.94 a, b Acute traumatic dislocation of the peroneal tendons.
a Coronal PD-weighted fat-sat image (coronal section through the lateral malleolus) shows rupture of the retinaculum with anterior dislocation of the peroneus longus and brevis tendons. The peroneus longus tendon courses over the fibula.
b Axial PD-weighted fat-sat image shows the peroneal tendons dislocated from the retromalleolar groove (arrow) with conspicuous hemorrhage along the retinaculum and a patchy hematoma in the soft tissues of the ankle joint.

- Quality of the superior retinaculum
- Signs of activation
- Quality of the peroneal tendons
- Extent of peritendinitis and tendinosis
- Bone marrow edema at the fibular border
- Possible ganglion cysts, osteophytes

Examination Technique

- *Standard tendon protocol:* prone position, high-resolution multi-channel coil
- *Sequences:*
  - Sagittal and coronal PD-weighted fat-sat
  - Coronal T1-weighted
  - Axial T2-weighted (angled to joint plane)
  - T1-weighted fat-sat after contrast administration, axial oblique (angled to tendon plane) and sagittal

MRI Findings (▶ Fig. 3.94)

- Peroneal tendons do not follow their normal retromalleolar course but run over or anterior to the fibula.
- With an acute dislocation: hemorrhage along the retinaculum, possible rupture of the calcaneofibular ligament, possible fracture of the lateral calcaneal border.
- With a chronic dislocation or subluxation: fibrovascular enhancement around the peroneal tendons including the retinaculum and calcaneofibular ligament.
- Possible bone marrow edema and osteophytes along the tip of the fibula.
- The tendons themselves are usually intact; tendinosis develops only with long-standing subluxation.

! Note

The tendons may reduce spontaneously, creating problems of MRI interpretation. A dynamic ultrasound study has definite advantages in cases of this kind.

Imaging Recommendation

Modalities of choice: ultrasound for evaluating tendon stability and for dynamic examination. MRI is advantageous for detailed visualization of the peroneal tendons and establishing the cause of the dislocation.

Differential Diagnosis

- Acute lateral ankle sprain
- Chronic instability
- Lateral impingement
- Chronic synovitis
- Early osteoarthritis

Treatment

Conservative treatment with 6 weeks' immobilization should be considered only for a fresh, spontaneously reducing injury. The redislocation rate with conservative therapy is up to 50%. The treatment of choice is surgical and involves deepening the tendon groove and/or reconstructing the retinaculum.

Prognosis, Complications

The prognosis with surgical intervention is good. Chronic dislocation carries a risk of tendon rupture.

Peroneal Split Syndrome

Definition

Peroneal split syndrome refers to longitudinal tearing or splitting of the peroneus brevis tendon in the malleolar region with migration of the peroneus longus tendon into the tear.

Symptoms

- Chronic lateral ankle pain
- Painful swelling
- Tenderness to pressure

Predisposing Factors

- Overuse
- Repetitive injuries
- Torsional trauma with injury to the calcaneofibular ligament

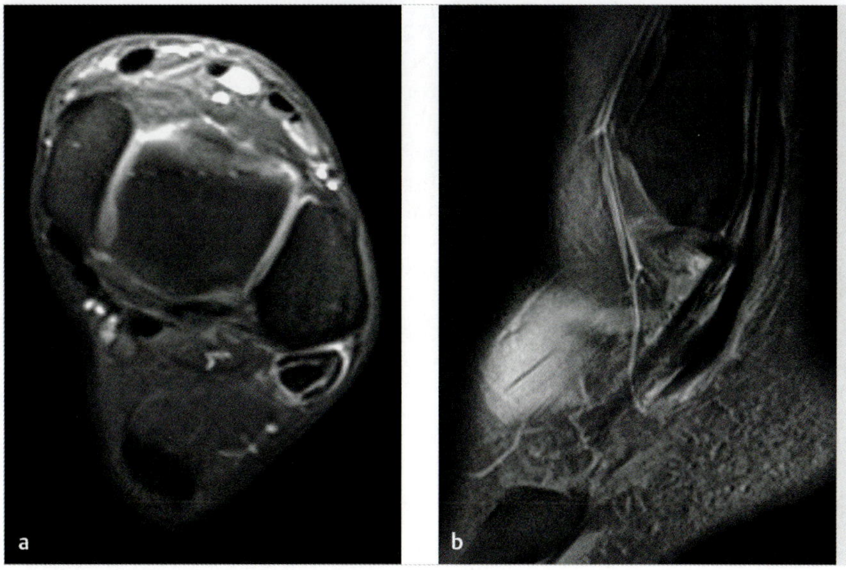

Fig. 3.95 a, b Peroneal split syndrome.
a Axial oblique T1-weighted fat-sat image after contrast administration shows a peroneal split syndrome with a long longitudinal tear of the left peroneus brevis tendon and signs of peritendinitis. The peroneus longus tendon is intact. Note the U-shaped arrangement of the torn peroneus brevis fibers partially enveloping the peroneus longus tendon.
b Sagittal T1-weighted fat-sat image after contrast administration. The sagittal slice displays three subtendons formed by longitudinal splitting of the peroneus brevis tendon.

- Shallow retromalleolar groove
- Injury to the superior retinaculum with increased tendon play and friction
- Peroneus quartus muscle
- Low-lying short peroneal muscle belly
- Secondary changes in adjacent joints

Anatomy and Pathology

At the distal tip of the fibula, the peroneus longus tendon lies deep to the peroneus brevis tendon and is compressed against the short tendon with increasing dorsiflexion. This may cause fraying and longitudinal splitting of the peroneus brevis tendon, which partially envelops the peroneus longus tendon in a U-shaped configuration. There are also asymptomatic normal variants with a short duplicated segment of the peroneus brevis tendon.

Imaging

Radiographs

Radiographic imaging is performed to exclude associated bony injuries. The ankle is imaged in two planes. Stress radiographs may be obtained in patients with suspected chronic instability of the talocrural or subtalar joint.

Ultrasound

Ultrasound can demonstrate fluid and synovitis in the peroneal tendon sheath.

MRI

Interpretation Checklist

- Extent of tendon degeneration and activated inflammation
- Evaluate anatomy (retromalleolar groove, accessory muscle, ossifications)
- Evaluate nearby structures (superior retinaculum and calcaneofibular ligament)
- Bone marrow edema in the fibula

Examination Technique

- *Standard tendon protocol:* prone position, high-resolution multi-channel coil
- *Sequences:*
  - Sagittal and coronal PD-weighted fat-sat
  - Coronal T1-weighted
  - Axial T2-weighted (angled to joint plane)
  - T1-weighted fat-sat after contrast administration, axial oblique (angled to tendon plane) and sagittal

MRI Findings (▶ Fig. 3.95)

- Differentiation from the normal variant of a bipartite peroneus brevis tendon by contrast administration
- Chronic inflammation with tendinosis: increased enhancement along the tendon sheath
- Splitting of the peroneus brevis tendon into two tendons (at the center is the peroneus longus tendon, best demonstrated in axial oblique T1-weighted fat-sat images after contrast administration)
- Possible degenerative intratendinous changes, even in the peroneus longus tendon (signal inhomogeneities, mucoid degeneration, increased vascularity in the tendon with associated enhancement)
- With chronic instability: extensive, enhancing irritative process that includes the superior retinaculum and fluid collection, which show a blurry, ill-defined structure

Imaging Recommendation

Modality of choice: MRI to define the extent of the tear and perhaps identify its precipitating causes and secondary effects.

Differential Diagnosis

- Rheumatoid arthritis
- Chronic ankle instability

Treatment

- *Acute injury:* conservative treatment with 6 weeks' immobilization in a walker boot is an option
- *Chronic lesion:* surgical treatment of the tear by intratendinous side-to-side suture repair

Prognosis, Complications

There is a risk of complete rupture of the peroneus brevis tendon.

3.2.8 Posterior Tibial Tendon Dysfunction

U. Szeimies

Insufficiency, Tendinosis, Partial Tear, Complete Rupture

Definition

Posterior tibial tendon dysfunction is a relatively common and often underestimated pathologic condition based on degenerative tendon changes in the tibialis posterior. The disorders range from peritendinitis, tendinosis, and insertional tendinopathy to chronic insufficiency with or without tendon rupture. A traumatic spontaneous rupture without prior degeneration is rare.

Symptoms

- Medial ankle pain
- Swelling
- Medial metatarsal tenderness
- Decreased strength on one-legged stance and supination
- Increasing adult planovalgus deformity
- Heel valgus viewed from behind
- Flattened plantar arch and forefoot abduction

Predisposing Factors

- Women in the fifth to sixth decade with pre-existing pes planovalgus deformity
- Rheumatoid arthritis
- Seronegative spondylarthropathy
- Abnormal insertion on an accessory or cornuate navicular bone
- Diabetes
- Obesity
- Rare iatrogenic injury of the posterior tibial tendon during the internal fixation of a medial malleolar fracture

Anatomy and Pathology

The posterior tibial tendon inserts on the navicular and cuneiform bones and at the base of the second through fourth metatarsals. These insertions are subject to numerous variants that include insertion on Accessory Navicular (p. 115). Tendon dysfunction weakens the support of the plantar arch, leading to pes planus. Tendon degeneration develops at the level of the medial malleolus, corresponding to the hypovascular zone. A complete rupture most commonly occurs at the level where the tendon makes a sharp turn at the medial malleolus.

The stages of posterior tibial tendon dysfunction are reviewed in ▶ Table 3.13.

Imaging

Radiographs

Radiographs show a decrease in the naviculocuneiform overlap index and decentering in the talonavicular joint with an increased downward tilt of the talar head, increased talocalcaneal divergence, and a supinated or abducted position of the forefoot.

Ultrasound

The tendon is imaged in longitudinal and transverse scans from the lower third of the tibia around the medial malleolus and distally to the medial cuneiform. A short linear-array transducer will yield better results (7.5–15 MHz). A stand-off should be used if acoustic coupling is poor. A degenerative tear produces an "asparagus tip" sign.

- *Acute tendinopathy:*
  - Thickened tendon with uniformly decreased echogenicity
  - Possible echo-free fluid in the tendon sheath (halo phenomenon)
- *Chronic tendinosis:*
  - Increasingly echogenic, inhomogeneous change
  - Caliber variations
  - Fiber pattern disruption by a partial tear (transverse scans important)
  - Evaluation of degenerative tendon vascularity by power Doppler: intratendinous signals

MRI

Interpretation Checklist

- Evaluate the extent of degenerative changes
- Fibro-osseous junction at the tendon insertion
- Fibro-osteitis
- Evaluate for peritendinitis, partial tear, complete rupture, and their location

Table 3.13 Johnson and Storm stages of posterior tibial tendon dysfunction, modified by Bluman and Myerson

Stage	Description
I	Tendon degeneration with an increase in cross section; no planovalgus deformity
II	Tendon degeneration with elongation or rupture; flexible planovalgus deformity
III	Tendon elongation or rupture; fixed planovalgus deformity
IV	Tendon rupture; more pronounced fixed planovalgus deformity with associated valgus tilt of the talus in the ankle mortise

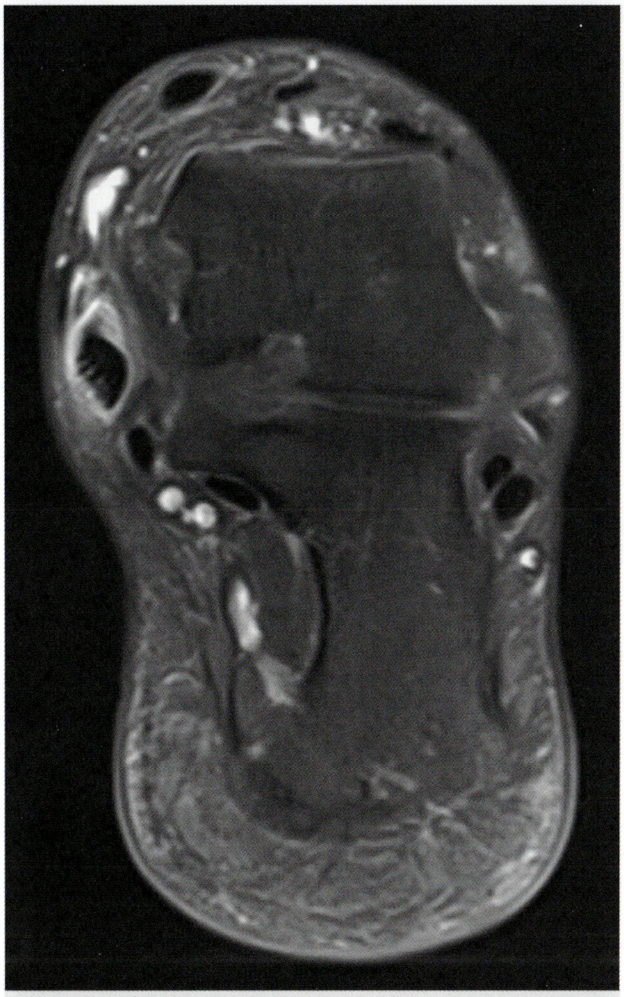

Fig. 3.96 Peritendinitis and incipient posterior tibial tendinosis. Axial oblique T1-weighted fat-sat image after contrast administration shows increased enhancement around the posterior tibial tendon with initial degenerative vascularization noted on the medial side.

- With advanced tendon dysfunction: evaluate alignment in the midtarsal joint line and plantar arch
- Secondary degenerative changes in the metatarsal joints
- With a complete rupture: evaluate retraction and quality of the tendon ends

Examination Technique

- *Standard tendon protocol:* prone position, high-resolution multi-channel coil
- *Sequences:*
  - Sagittal and coronal PD-weighted fat-sat
  - Coronal T1-weighted
  - Axial T2-weighted (angled to joint plane)
  - T1-weighted fat-sat after contrast administration, axial oblique (angled to tendon plane) and sagittal

MRI Findings (► see Figs. 3.96–3.100)

! Note

As a rule of thumb, the cross-sectional diameter of the normal posterior tibial tendon should measure twice that of the flexor digitorum longus tendon.

- *Tenosynovitis:* water-sensitive sequences show hyperintense fluid in the tendon sheath, and increased enhancement is seen after contrast administration. Degenerative changes are marked by fusiform thickening and an enlarged cross-section with enhancing areas (degenerative tendon vascularity). Mucoid degeneration within the tendon appears as foci of tendon softening (hyperintense in T2-weighted images). MRI may show progression to focal partial-thickness tears and partial longitudinal tears that reduce the cross-sectional diameter of the tendon.
- *Insertional tendinopathy:* edema and contrast enhancement at the fibro-osseous junction on the navicular, with or without bone marrow edema

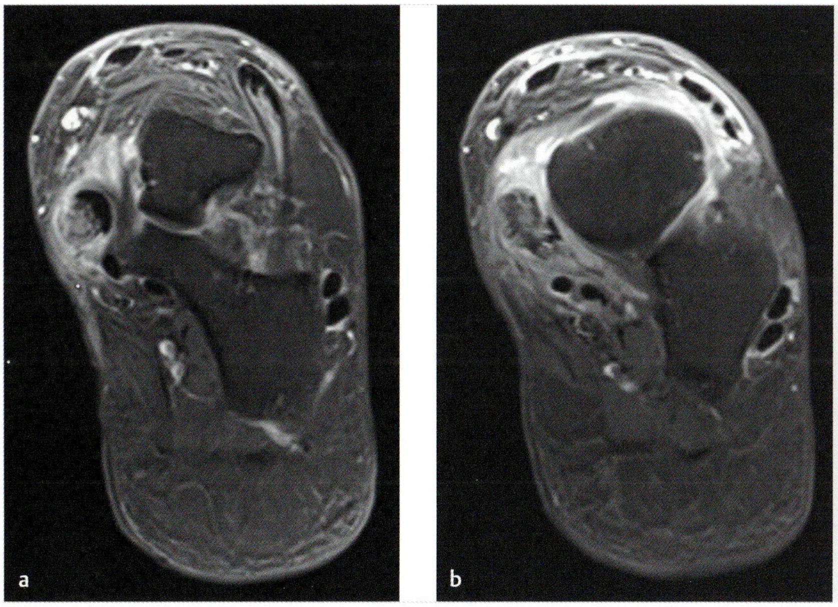

Fig. 3.97 a, b A 76-year-old woman with increasing diffuse pain in the hindfoot and plantar arch. The clinical picture was one of advanced posterior tibial insufficiency.
a Axial oblique T1-weighted fat-sat image after contrast administration shows definite features of left posterior tibial insufficiency with marked tendinosis of the distal posterior tibial tendon and fibrovascular peritendinous enhancement.
b Axial oblique T1-weighted fat-sat image after contrast administration also shows signs of activated planovalgus deformity with instability in the subtalar joint and especially in the talonavicular joint.

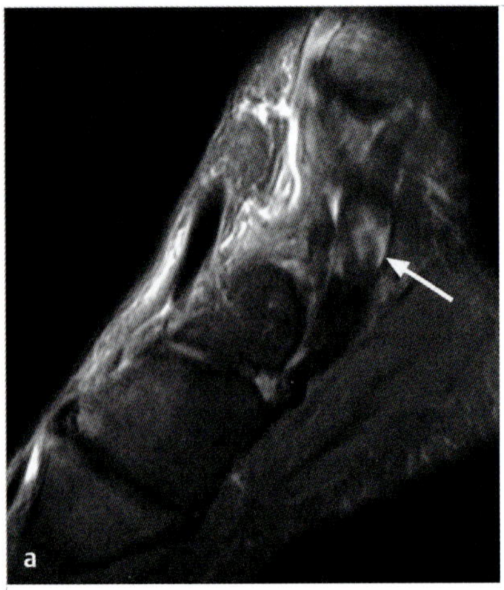
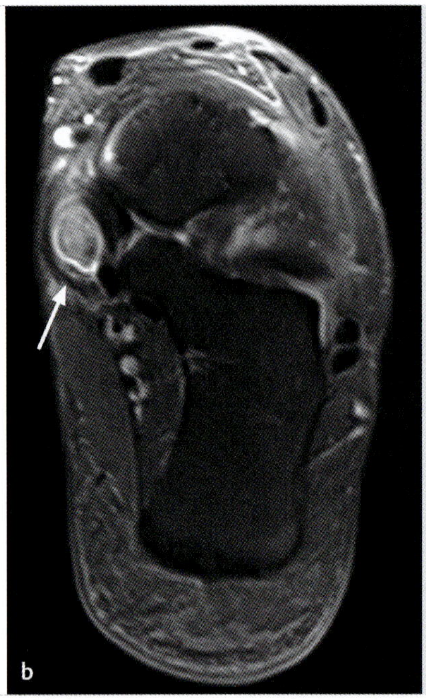

Fig. 3.98 a, b Chronic load-dependent complaints, more pronounced on the medial side. A 60-year-old woman with no history of acute pain event presented clinically with pes planovalgus and a posterior tibial tendon rupture.
a Sagittal T1-weighted fat-sat image after contrast administration shows a complete rupture of the left posterior tibial tendon at the level where the tendon changes direction at the medial malleolus (arrow). Distally the posterior tibial tendon shows pronounced tendinosis with vascularization and a tortuous course; the tendon stump has retracted proximally.
b Axial oblique T1-weighted fat-sat image after contrast administration shows absence of the ruptured and retracted posterior tibial tendon at this level (arrow).

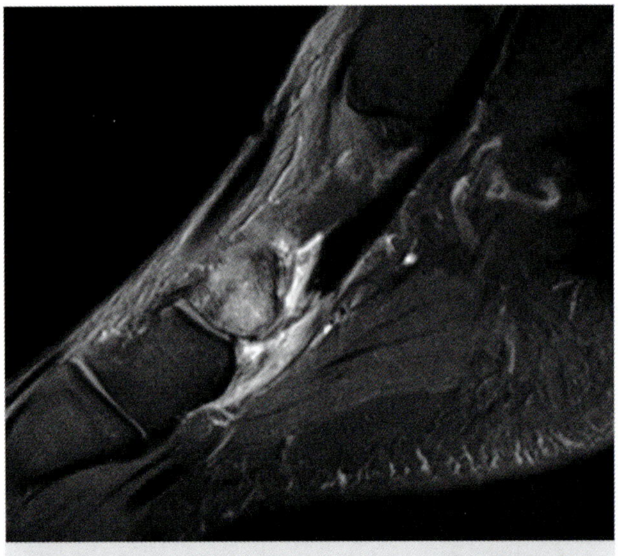

Fig. 3.99 Insertional tendinopathy of the posterior tibial tendon. Sagittal T1-weighted fat-sat image after contrast administration shows marked tendinosis, peritendinitis, and insertional tendinopathy of the posterior tibial tendon on the navicular with bone marrow edema and a partial tear of the tendon itself.

- *Complete rupture:* full-thickness disruption of continuity with a tendon gap, empty fluid-filled tendon sheath, and visualization of the retracted tendon ends
- *Additional findings:* prominent medial tuberosity of the navicular, abnormal talonavicular alignment, accessory navicular bone, flattening of the plantar arch, osteophytes and focal bone activation on the medial malleolus, thickened flexor retinaculum
- *Chronic insufficiency:* elongated spring ligament, tendinosis and peritendinitis, activation of the calcaneonavicular ligament complex, spring ligament and sinus tarsi; deformity in

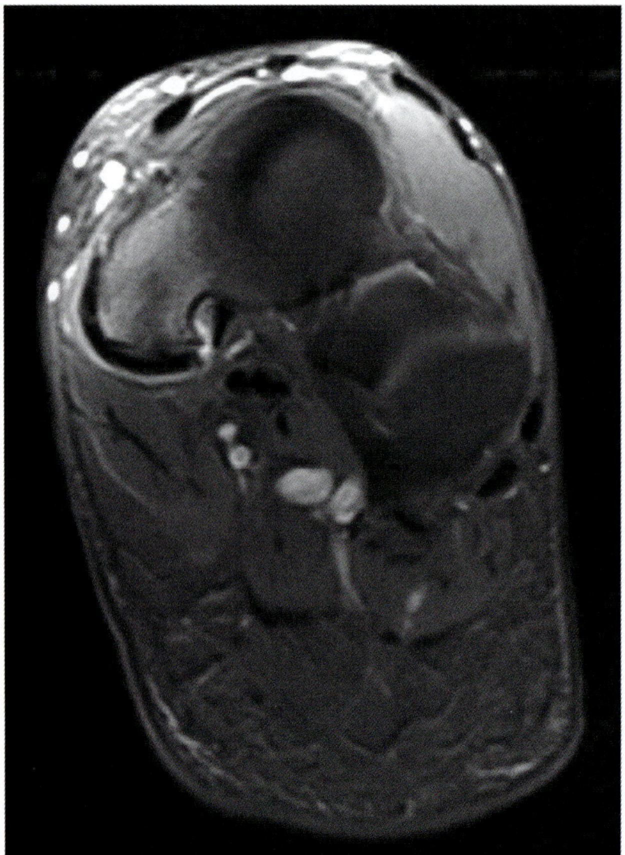

Fig. 3.100 Insertional tendinopathy at a variant posterior tibial tendon insertion site on the navicular in a 39-year-old woman with increasing shoe discomfort. Axial oblique T1-weighted fat-sat image after contrast administration shows a markedly hook-shaped configuration of the navicular with bone marrow edema, adjacent soft-tissue irritation, and peritendinitis at the fibro-osseous junction of the posterior tibial tendon.

the talonavicular joint, downward tilt of the longitudinal talar axis, abnormal spring ligament injury; bone marrow edema bordering on the tendon
- *Rare:* tendon subluxation due to rupture of the flexor retinaculum

Imaging Recommendation

Modalities of choice: ultrasound for evaluating morphology and determining tendon thickness; contrast-enhanced MRI for evaluating inflammatory response, detecting small partial tears, and especially for detecting secondary metatarsal degenerative changes.

> **! Note**
>
> Attention should be given to a possible accessory navicular bone, and to a possible lesion of the plantar calcaneonavicular ligament or sinus tarsi ligaments. Associated injuries are common. Most acute ruptures occur at the level of the medial malleolus.

Differential Diagnosis

- Differential diagnoses of planovalgus deformity (idiopathic, Charcot arthropathy, inflammatory cause)
- Activated osteoarthritis of the medial facet of the subtalar joint
- Tarsal tunnel syndrome
- Activated os tibiale externum

Treatment

- *Stage I:* usually treated conservatively with an orthotic insert with a hindfoot wedge, rest, nonsteroidal anti-inflammatory drugs, and physical therapy. Synovectomy is indicated for extensive tenosynovitis. Concomitant hindfoot deformity is corrected by a medial displacement calcaneal osteotomy.
- *Stage II:* augmentation of the posterior tibial tendon by a flexor digitorum longus tendon transfer. Hindfoot valgus is corrected by a medial displacement calcaneal osteotomy, and calcaneal lengthening (Evans osteotomy) may be added if forefoot abduction is present. Gastrocnemius tendon lengthening is appropriate if that muscle has become shortened. Rare cases may require a plantar-flexion osteotomy of the first metatarsal or cuneiform if forefoot supination is present.
- *Stage III:* conservative treatment may be tried with an ankle-foot orthotic or orthopedic shoe. Surgical treatment consists of corrective arthrodesis of the subtalar joint.
- *Stage IV:* Conservative: arthrodesis boot to stabilize the ankle and subtalar joints. Surgical: corrective arthrodesis of the ankle and subtalar joints.

Prognosis, Complications

Conservative and surgical treatment of stage I and II cases can yield a good functional result, although a 6–12-month rehabilitation period will be required. Cases at stage III or higher will have residual flexion deficits. Very long-standing deformity may lead to secondary degenerative changes in the midfoot and Chopart joint line.

Accessory Navicular

Definition

An accessory navicular is an accessory bone on the medial side of the foot, which arises from a separate ossification center that is not fused to the navicular bone. Synonyms are secondary navicular and os tibiale externum.

Symptoms

- Medial metatarsal pain at the level of the navicular
- Large bony protuberance (cornuate navicular) which is marked by local pain and irritation from footwear
- Complaints begin after ossification in adolescence; more common in girls

Predisposing Factors

The presence of this accessory bone is congenital, and complaints are often initiated by trauma or local pressure. Loosening of the fibrous attachment between the navicular and accessory navicular may lead to complaints. Fractures of the accessory bone may also occur.

Anatomy and Pathology

The accessory bone results from the congenital development of a separate ossification center that is not fused with the navicular but is attached to its medial aspect by fibrous tissue. After the os peroneum, the accessory navicular is the second most common accessory bone in the foot, being present in up to 20% of the population. The accessory navicular usually does not ossify until 9 or 10 years of age.

The three types of accessory navicular are described in ▶ Table 3.14. Types II and III together account for 70% of cases.

Imaging

Radiographs

The accessory bone is clearly visible in the DP view of the foot.

Ultrasound

Used only to narrow the differential diagnosis.

MRI

Interpretation Checklist

- Classify the accessory navicular by type
- Determine degree of activation: bone marrow edema, adjacent soft-tissue activation, status of the posterior tibial tendon, secondary changes

Examination Technique

- *Standard tendon protocol:* prone position, high-resolution multi-channel coil

Table 3.14 Classification of accessory navicular bones by types

Type	Description
I	This type is a small sesamoid bone embedded within the posterior tibial tendon. It is asymptomatic
II	Most of the posterior tibial tendon inserts on the accessory navicular. Chronic traction on the synchondrosis incites a soft-tissue or bony stress reaction, and complaints may be initiated by trauma
III	This type involves a partial bony coalition in which the accessory bone is fused to the navicular. The bony protuberance extends to the talar head at the medial navicular tuberosity, causing some of the tendon traction to be distributed to the parent navicular. The bony protuberance is a potential source of soft-tissue irritation

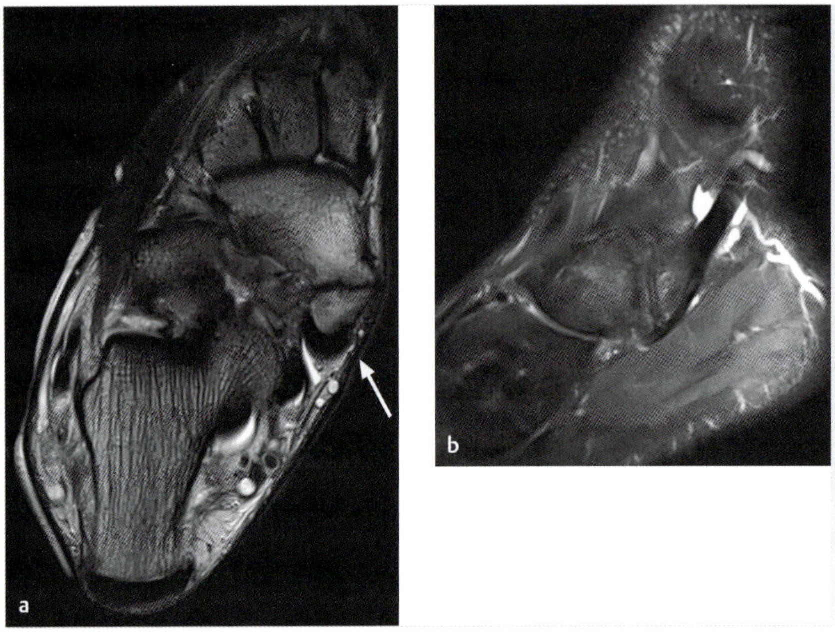

Fig. 3.101 a, b Type II accessory navicular.
a Axial oblique T1-weighted image shows a separate ossification center with fibrous attachment to the medial aspect of the navicular (arrow).
b Sagittal T1-weighted fat-sat image after contrast administration shows most of the posterior tibial tendon inserting on the accessory navicular, placing an increased traction stress on the syndesmosis.

- *Sequences:*
  - Sagittal and coronal PD-weighted fat-sat
  - Coronal T1-weighted
  - Axial T2-weighted (angled to joint plane)
  - T1-weighted fat-sat after contrast administration, axial oblique (angled to tendon plane) and sagittal

MRI Findings (▶ Fig. 3.101 and ▶ Fig. 3.102)

An ossicle within the posterior tibial tendon is identified by noting fatty marrow signal within the tendon (high T1-weighted signal intensity) approximately 5 mm proximal to the navicular. The possibility of a fracture or fragmentation should be considered in patients who have sustained trauma.

! Note

Trauma should particularly be considered in adolescents who participate in contact sports, even if a specific trauma history cannot be recalled.

Necrotic areas do not show fatty marrow signal or enhancement in T1-weighted sequences. MRI displays tendon degeneration in the form of peritendinitis with enhancement along the tendon sheath. More advanced degenerative changes are marked by intratendinous mucoid signals, partial tearing, adjacent soft-tissue activation, and fluid accumulation.

Imaging Recommendation

Modality of choice: MRI to evaluate bone activation and tendon quality.

Differential Diagnosis

- Metatarsal osteoarthritis
- Posterior tibial tendinosis
- Metatarsal fracture
- Arthritis

Treatment

- Orthotic
- Special padded shoe insert
- Orthopedic footwear
- Kidner operation (resection of the ossicle and reattachment of the posterior tibial tendon)
- Fusion to the navicular

Prognosis, Complications

Chronic activation may spread to the tendon, resulting in insufficiency and rupture. A pes planovalgus deformity may result.

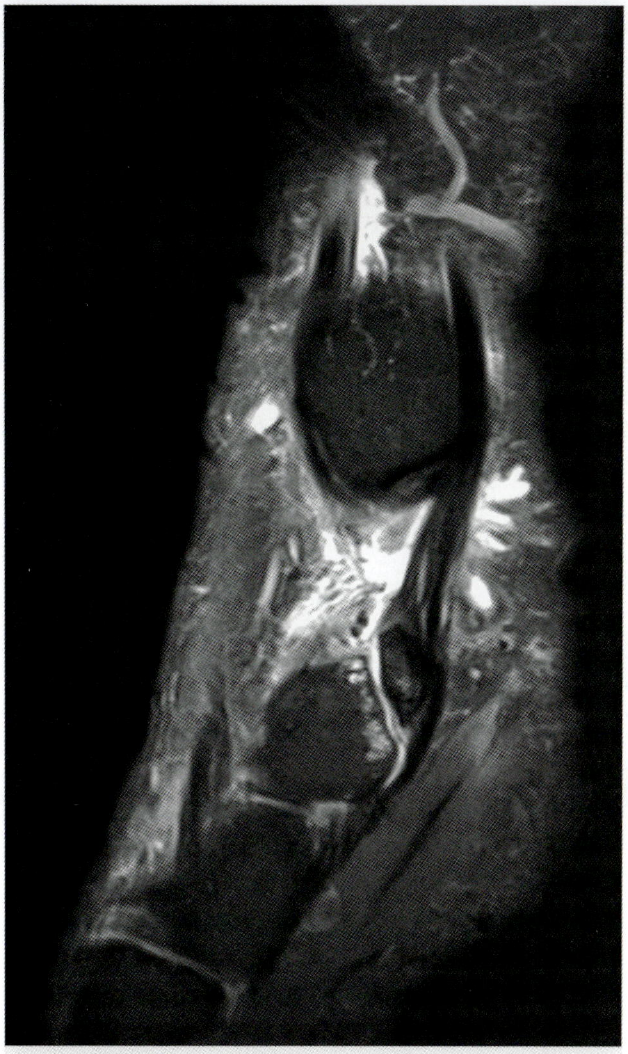

Fig. 3.102 Activated type II accessory navicular. Postcontrast sagittal T1-weighted fat-sat image shows activation of the fibro-osseous coalition of the accessory ossification center with contrast enhancement along the posterior tibial tendon sheath, within the synchondrosis, and in the navicular.

3.2.9 Anterior Tibial Tendon Pathology

U. Szeimies

Tendinosis, Insertional Tendinopathy

Definition

Insertional tendinopathy of the anterior tibial tendon is pathology involving the distal insertion of the tendon on the medial cuneiform bone and the base of the first metatarsal.

Symptoms

- Midfoot pain at the insertion of the anterior tibial tendon or in the course of the tendon
- Pain worsened by physical activity
- Pain may radiate to the anterior lower leg
- Possible palpable swelling over the distal part of the tendon

Predisposing Factors

- Overweight
- Older women predominantly affected
- More common in running athletes

Anatomy and Pathology

The anterior tibial tendon inserts on the medial side of the medial cuneiform bone and on the medial border of the first metatarsal. Distally the tendon traverses a tendon sheath approximately 7 cm in length on the dorsum of the foot and is spanned by the inferior extensor retinaculum. Its main action is dorsiflexion of the ankle joint. There are two factors that promote tendinosis: 1) blood flow is diminished on the dorsum of the foot beneath the retinaculum and 2) the extensor retinaculum compresses and kinks the tendon during dorsiflexion, causing an increased biomechanical stress. Insertional tendinopathy is a relatively rare form of tendinopathy.

Imaging

Radiographs

Radiographs usually show no abnormalities. In rare cases, soft-tissue calcifications may be found on the medial cuneiform and on the medial edge of the first metatarsal in patients with chronic insertional tendinopathy.

Ultrasound

- *Acute tendinopathy:* thickened tendon with uniformly decreased echogenicity, possible echo-free fluid in the tendon sheath (halo phenomenon)
- *Chronic tendinosis:* increasingly echogenic, inhomogeneous changes, caliber variations

MRI

Interpretation Checklist

- Extent of peritendinitis
- Evaluation for insertional tendinopathy, the quality of tendon and bone, osteophytes, partial tears

Examination Technique

- *Standard tendon protocol:* prone position, high-resolution multi-channel coil
- *Sequences:*
  - Sagittal and coronal PD-weighted fat-sat
  - Coronal T1-weighted
  - Axial T2-weighted (angled to joint plane)
  - T1-weighted fat-sat after contrast administration, axial oblique (angled to tendon plane) and sagittal

! Note

The tendon should be imaged over its entire length including the tarsal and metatarsal levels. If necessary, a sagittal T1-weighted sequence may be obtained to evaluate an osteophyte at the fibro-osseous junction of the insertion.

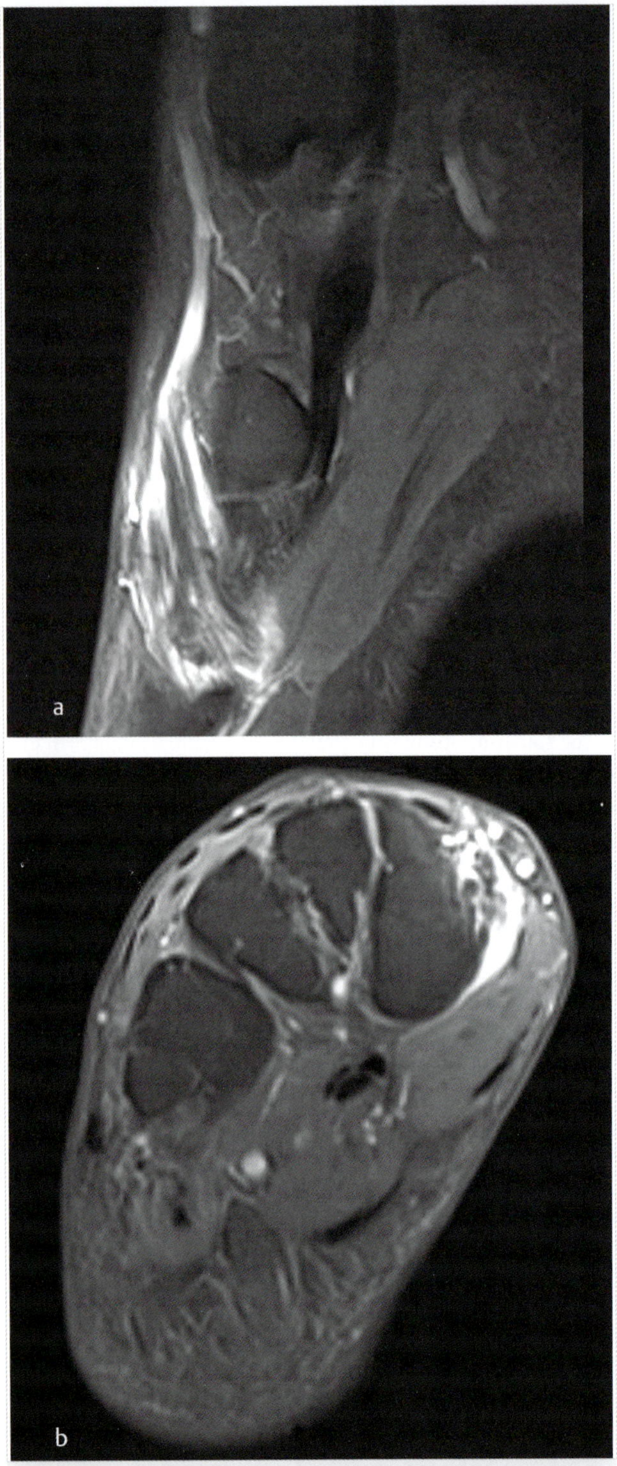

Fig. 3.103 a, b Insertional tendinopathy of the anterior tibial tendon in a 58-year-old woman with chronic medial midfoot pain.
a Sagittal T1-weighted fat-sat image after contrast administration shows markedly increased enhancement consistent with advanced distal tendinosis and insertional tendinopathy of the anterior tibial tendon.
b Axial oblique T1-weighted fat-sat image after contrast administration: tender soft-tissue swelling with increased enhancement at the fibro-osseous junction of the anterior tibial tendon on the medial cuneiform and the medial border of the first metatarsal.

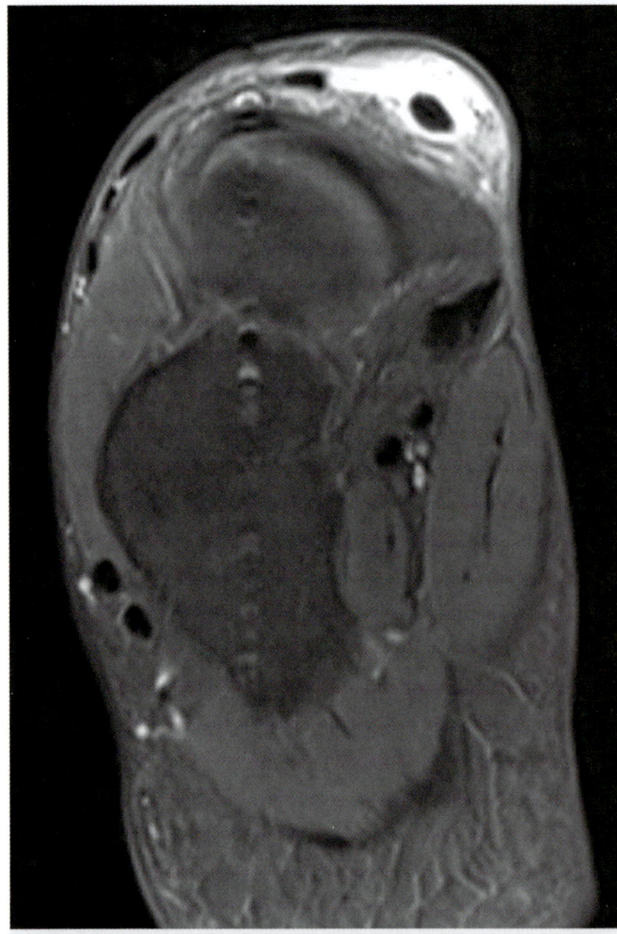

Fig. 3.104 Hyperacute anterior tibial tendonitis in a 41-year-old man with acute onset of soft-tissue swelling and tenderness on the medial midfoot after athletic activity. Axial oblique T1-weighted fat-sat image after contrast administration shows marked, florid peritendinitis of the right anterior tibial tendon extending from the ankle joint to the tendon insertion. The internal structure of the tendon appears intact.

MRI Findings (▶ Fig. 3.103 and ▶ Fig. 3.104)

- Contrast enhancement along the tendon sheath over the midfoot to the tendon insertion
- Enlarged transverse diameter
- Intratendinous hyperintensities due to internal degeneration
- Degenerative tendon vascularity with increased enhancement on postcontrast images
- Circumscribed longitudinal tear
- Bone marrow edema and increased enhancement at the bony insertion on the first metatarsal and medial cuneiform with possible enthesopathic spurs

Imaging Recommendation

Modality of choice: MRI.

Differential Diagnosis

- Tarsometatarsal osteoarthritis
- Bone overload (fatigue fracture)

Treatment

Conservative

- Nonsteroidal anti-inflammatory drugs
- Physical therapy (friction massage, ultrasound, eccentric stretching)
- Orthotics with a heel pad and longitudinal arch support
- Shockwave therapy
- Deep X-ray therapy
- Platelet-derived growth factor

Operative

- Debridement of the tendon insertion
- Tenosynovectomy and tendon reattachment with a bone anchor

Prognosis, Complications

Possible complications are a complete rupture and chronic tendinosis.

Rupture

Definition

A full-thickness tear of the anterior tibial tendon.

Symptoms

- Pain and loss of dorsiflexion in the ankle joint
- Rupture is often not perceived as such by the patient
- Possible chronic tendinopathy over a period of months with a gradual loss of tension
- Circumscribed defect in the course of the tendon, acute swelling
- Compensatory hyperextension of the big toe

Predisposing Factors

A complete spontaneous rupture is rare (< 1% of all muscle and tendon injuries). Underlying tendon degeneration, most common in patients over 50 years of age, leads to an increased risk in running sports, forced dorsiflexion from a plantar-flexed position (acute eccentric tendon load), especially in a setting of chronic inflammation, and in patients who have received corticosteroid injections. Spontaneous ruptures may occur in diabetes, gout, or rheumatoid arthritis. Proximal ruptures occur years after a tibial fracture with compartment syndrome.

Anatomy and Pathology

The anterior tibial tendon acts to dorsiflex the ankle joint and invert the foot at the subtalar joint. Most ruptures occur between the extensor retinaculum (cruciate crural ligament) and a point just above the actual tendon insertion on the medial cuneiform and the base of the first metatarsal.

Imaging

Radiographs

Radiographs generally show no abnormalities. Rarely, they can show soft-tissue calcifications in patients with a long history of tendinosis.

Ultrasound

An acute rupture or partial tear appears sonographically as a hypoechoic zone (hematoma) with echogenic torn edges. The peritendineum and tendon sheath may be partially preserved. With dynamic ultrasound, the examiner can visually assess reapproximation of the tendon ends on the monitor during maximum dorsiflexion and plantar flexion. Transverse scanning is important for assessing partial tears. A degenerative tear produces an "asparagus tip" sign.

MRI

Interpretation Checklist

- Localize the site of the tendon gap or dehiscence
- Evaluate the quality of the tendon ends
- Note degree of degeneration and mucoid swelling
- Note degree of inflammation in the tendon bed
- Evaluate the bony insertion on the medial cuneiform and first metatarsal
- Evaluate tendon quality for a possible extensor hallucis tendon transfer

Examination Technique

- *Standard tendon protocol:* prone position, high-resolution multi-channel coil
- *Sequences:*
  - Sagittal and coronal PD-weighted fat-sat
  - Coronal T1-weighted
  - Axial T2-weighted (angled to joint plane)
  - T1-weighted fat-sat after contrast administration, axial oblique (angled to tendon plane) and sagittal

MRI Findings (► Fig. 3.105)

The features of an anterior tibial tendon rupture are best appreciated in an axial oblique PD-weighted fat-sat sequence or T1-weighted fat-sat sequence after contrast administration.

- Empty tendon sheath with definable proximal and distal tendon ends
- Fluid detection and enhancement within the empty tendon sheath

Imaging Recommendation

Modalities of choice: ultrasound, MRI.

Differential Diagnosis

- Partial tear
- Tenosynovitis
- Synovitis in the anterior ankle joint

Treatment

Conservative

Splinting and rest for small partial tears and longitudinal tears and in older, sedentary patients.

Operative

- Reattachment with transosseous pull-through sutures or a bone anchor.

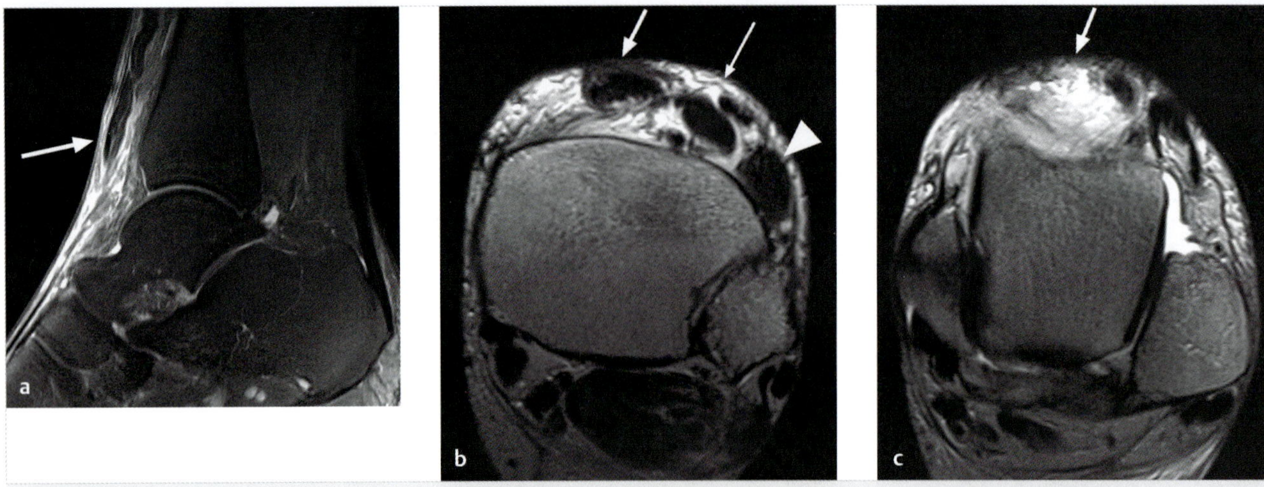

Fig. 3.105 a–c Complete rupture of the anterior tibial tendon in a 72-year-old man with acute dorsal foot trauma and pain.
a Sagittal PD-weighted fat-sat image shows a complete distal rupture of the left anterior tibial tendon with a retracted tendon stump at the level of the ankle joint.
b Axial T2-weighted slice proximal to the rupture displays the tibialis anterior (shorter arrow), extensor hallucis longus (longer arrow), and extensor digitorum (arrowhead).
c Axial T2-weighted slice at the level of the rupture shows absence of the anterior tibial tendon (arrow).

- End-to-end anastomosis of focal tears. Extensor hallucis transfer for motor replacement is appropriate in cases with large longitudinal tears or advanced degeneration or retraction of the tendon ends.

Prognosis, Complications

Progressive flattening of the pedal arch may occur and may be associated with Achilles tendon shortening in children.

3.2.10 Subtalar Joint: Sinus Tarsi Syndrome

U. Szeimies

Definition

Sinus tarsi syndrome is not a diagnosis, and further differentiation of the underlying pathogenic mechanism is advised. The pain syndrome often develops as a result of subtalar instability, injury to structures in the sinus tarsi, heavy scarring or impingement.

Symptoms

- Chronic hindfoot pain, more pronounced on the lateral side
- Feeling of subtalar instability
- Swelling in the acute stage
- Pain worsened by physical activity
- Pain relieved by infiltration with local anesthetic

Predisposing Factors

- Gout
- Rheumatoid arthritis
- Seronegative spondylarthropathy
- Sequel to a lateral ankle sprain or inversion trauma
- Pes planovalgus (impingement)

Anatomy and Pathology

The sinus tarsi contains the cervical ligament (restraint to inversion of the hindfoot; may be injured by inversion trauma) and the interosseous talocalcaneal ligament (restraint to eversion of the foot; injured by eversion trauma). The sinus tarsi is a laterally directed, funnel-shaped opening bounded posteriorly by the subtalar joint and anteriorly by the talonavicular joint. It is continuous medially with the tarsal canal. Its contents consist of fatty tissue, ligaments (interosseous ligament = talocalcaneal ligament, cervical ligament, inferior extensor retinaculum), blood vessels, and nerves.

The most important ligament is the interosseous ligament, located anterior to the cervical ligament and corresponding to the cruciate ligaments in the knee. The sinus tarsi ligaments stabilize the lateral side of the ankle joint and the hindfoot. They function as lateral stabilizers.

Imaging

Radiographs

Radiographs usually show no abnormalities and are used mainly to exclude osteoarthritis.

Ultrasound

Not indicated.

MRI

Interpretation Checklist

- Integrity of the sinus tarsi ligaments
- Contrast enhancement
- Degree of fibrosis

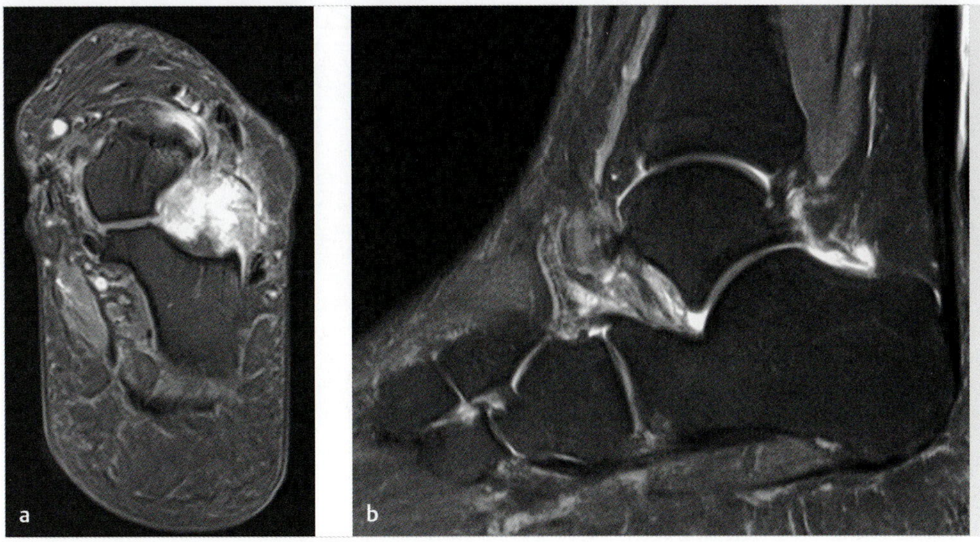

Fig. 3.106 a, b Chronic nonspecific pain in a 57-year-old woman with sinus tarsi syndrome.
a Axial T1-weighted fat-sat image after contrast administration shows intense enhancement in the sinus tarsi with elongated interosseous and cervical ligament fibers and massive fibrovascular reaction.
b Sagittal T1-weighted fat-sat image after contrast administration also shows signs of subtalar instability with synovitis in the posterior compartment of the subtalar joint.

- Signs of instability
- Evaluation of the subtalar joint
- Evaluation of the posterior tibial tendon

! Note

Always evaluate the interosseous ligament in patients with supination trauma.

Examination Technique

- *Standard tendon protocol:* prone position, high-resolution multi-channel coil
- *Sequences:*
  - Sagittal and coronal PD-weighted fat-sat
  - Coronal T1-weighted
  - Axial T2-weighted (angled to joint plane)
  - T1-weighted fat-sat after contrast administration, axial oblique (angled to tendon plane) and sagittal
  - True coronal slices through the ankle joint may be added, if required

MRI Findings (▶ Fig. 3.106)

- Obliteration of fatty tissue (chronic stage with fibrosis)
- Fat-suppressed, water-sensitive sequences in the acute stage show edema and enhancement
- Granulation tissue
- Fibrosis with synovial proliferation
- Contrast enhancement
- Fluid collection
- Thickening and poor delineation of the interosseous ligament

Imaging Recommendation

Modality of choice: contrast-enhanced MRI.

Differential Diagnosis

- Subtalar osteoarthritis
- Coalition
- Ganglion
- Other nerve compression syndromes
- Nonunion after a fracture of the talar lateral process or calcaneal anterior process
- Secondary osteoarthritis

Treatment

Conservative

- Nonsteroidal anti-inflammatory drugs
- Physical therapy
- Cortisone injections
- Rest

Operative

- Arthroscopic debridement
- Synovectomy
- Subtalar arthrodesis is indicated only if there is severe damage to the subtalar joint

Prognosis, Complications

The prognosis is favorable if treatment can address the underlying cause. If a morphologic substrate is not identified, there is a high likelihood of recurrence.

3.2.11 Differential Diagnosis of Chronic Hindfoot Pain

U. Szeimies

▶ Table 3.15 reviews the differential diagnosis of chronic pain at various locations in the hindfoot.

Table 3.15 Differential diagnosis of chronic hindfoot pain

Medial chronic hindfoot pain	Plantar chronic hindfoot pain	Lateral chronic hindfoot pain	Posterior chronic hindfoot pain	Diffuse chronic hindfoot pain
• Tendinosis and peritendinitis of the flexors (posterior tibial tendon disease: insufficiency, tendinosis, partial tear, insertion variants, accessory navicular) and the flexor hallucis longus tendon • Tarsal tunnel syndrome • Coalition of medial facet of subtalar joint • Plantar vein thrombosis • Os trigonum with irritation of the tarsal tunnel	• Disease of the plantar aponeurosis (plantar tendon fasciitis to partial tear, possibly with bursopathy, activated heel spur, Ledderhose disease) • Plantar chiasm syndrome (crossover effect involving the flexor hallucis longus and flexor digitorum longus tendons) • Baxter nerve entrapment • Medial plantar nerve compression syndrome (jogger's nerve)	• Peroneal tendon disease (peroneal split syndrome, tendinosis, peritendinitis, chronic subluxation, subdivided by location: tip of the fibula, os peroneum, peroneal tubercle, retinaculum, cuboid tunnel, insertion) • Sinus tarsi syndrome • Coalition in the hindfoot • Chronic syndesmosis injury, anterior syndesmosis insufficiency • Lateral instability (ankle joint, subtalar joint) • Nonunion of the calcaneal anterior process • Nonunion of the talar lateral process • Subtalar osteoarthritis • Pes planovalgus with subfibular impingement • Os trigonum	• Os trigonum • Calcaneal apophysitis • Achilles tendon disease (tendinosis, necrosis, xanthomatosis, Haglund exostosis) • Subachilles bursitis • Bony stress reaction, microfracture • Traction spur at the Achilles tendon insertion • Enthesopathy in ankylosing spondylitis	• Subtalar osteoarthritis, ankle instability • Coalition (fibrous, bony) • Bone marrow edema syndrome, algodystrophy • Bone marrow edema in children (tiger stripes) • Overuse edema, stress fracture • Ganglion cyst • Tarsal tunnel syndrome • Arthritis • Nerve compression syndromes

3.3 Bibliography

Capsule and Ligaments

Lateral Ligaments

Campbell SE, Warner M. MR imaging of ankle inversion injuries. Magn Reson Imaging Clin N Am 2008; 16: 1–18, v

Langner I, Frank M, Kuehn JP et al. Acute inversion injury of the ankle without radiological abnormalities: assessment with high-field MR imaging and correlation of findings with clinical outcome. Skeletal Radiol 2011; 40: 423–430

Saxena A, Luhadiya A, Ewen B, Goumas C. Magnetic resonance imaging and incidental findings of lateral ankle pathologic features with asymptomatic ankles. J Foot Ankle Surg 2011; 50: 413–415

Medial Ligaments

Chhabra A, Subhawong TK, Carrino JA. MR imaging of deltoid ligament pathologic findings and associated impingement syndromes. Radiographics 2010; 30: 751–761

Langner I, Frank M, Kuehn JP et al. Acute inversion injury of the ankle without radiological abnormalities: assessment with high-field MR imaging and correlation of findings with clinical outcome. Skeletal Radiol 2011; 40: 423–430

Syndesmosis

Bassett FH, Gates HS, Billys JB, Morris HB, Nikolaou PK. Talar impingement by the anteroinferior tibiofibular ligament. A cause of chronic pain in the ankle after inversion sprain. J Bone Joint Surg Am 1990; 72: 55–59

Cheung Y, Perrich KD, Gui J, Koval KJ, Goodwin DW. MRI of isolated distal fibular fractures with widened medial clear space on stressed radiographs: which ligaments are interrupted? AJR Am J Roentgenol 2009; 192: W7–12

Fischer W. MR-Skript. Skizzenbuch zur MRT des Bewegungsapparates. 4th ed. Self published; 2007

Hermans JJ, Beumer A, de Jong TA, Kleinrensink GJ. Anatomy of the distal tibiofibular syndesmosis in adults: a pictorial essay with a multimodality approach. J Anat 2010; 217: 633–645

Hermans JJ, Beumer A, Hop WC, Moonen AF, Ginai AZ. Tibiofibular syndesmosis in acute ankle fractures: additional value of an oblique MR image plane. Skeletal Radiol 2012; 41: 193–202

Langner I, Frank M, Kuehn JP et al. Acute inversion injury of the ankle without radiological abnormalities: assessment with high-field MR imaging and correlation of findings with clinical outcome. Skeletal Radiol 2011; 40: 423–430

Spring Ligament Injuries

Desai KR, Beltran LS, Bencardino JT, Rosenberg ZS, Petchprapa C, Steiner G. The spring ligament recess of the talocalcaneonavicular joint: depiction on MR images with cadaveric and histologic correlation. AJR Am J Roentgenol 2011; 196: 1145–1150

Harish S, Kumbhare D, O'Neill J, Popowich T. Comparison of sonography and magnetic resonance imaging for spring ligament abnormalities: preliminary study. J Ultrasound Med 2008; 27: 1145–1152

Kavanagh EC, Koulouris G, Gopez A, Zoga A, Raikin S, Morrison WB. MRI of rupture of the spring ligament complex with talo-cuboid impaction. Skeletal Radiol 2007; 36: 555–558

Mansour R, Teh J, Sharp RJ, Ostlere S. Ultrasound assessment of the spring ligament complex. Eur Radiol 2008; 18: 2670–2675

Mansour R, Jibri Z, Kamath S, Mukherjee K, Ostlere S. Persistent ankle pain following a sprain: a review of imaging. Emerg Radiol 2011; 18: 211–225

Melão L, Canella C, Weber M, Negrão P, Trudell D, Resnick D. Ligaments of the transverse tarsal joint complex: MRI-anatomic correlation in cadavers. AJR Am J Roentgenol 2009; 193: 662–671

Mengiardi B, Zanetti M, Schöttle PB et al. Spring ligament complex: MR imaging-anatomic correlation and findings in asymptomatic subjects. Radiology 2005; 237: 242–249

Toye LR, Helms CA, Hoffman BD, Easley M, Nunley JA. MRI of spring ligament tears. AJR Am J Roentgenol 2005; 184: 1475–1480

Williams BR, Ellis SJ, Deyer TW, Pavlov H, Deland JT. Reconstruction of the spring ligament using a peroneus longus autograft tendon transfer. Foot Ankle Int 2010; 31: 567–577

Bifurcated Ligament

Melão L, Canella C, Weber M, Negrão P, Trudell D, Resnick D. Ligaments of the transverse tarsal joint complex: MRI-anatomic correlation in cadavers. AJR Am J Roentgenol 2009; 193: 662–671

Calcaneocuboid Joint Injuries

Agnholt J, Nielsen S, Christensen H. Lesion of the ligamentum bifurcatum in ankle sprain. Arch Orthop Trauma Surg 1988; 107: 326–328

Andermahr J, Helling HJ, Maintz D, Mönig S, Koebke J, Rehm KE. The injury of the calcaneocuboid ligaments. Foot Ankle Int 2000; 21: 379–384

Dorn-Lange NV, Nauck T, Lohrer H, Arentz S, Konerding MA. Morphology of the dorsal and lateral calcaneocuboid ligaments. Foot Ankle Int 2008; 29: 942–949

Leland RH, Marymont JV, Trevino SG, Varner KE, Noble PC. Calcaneocuboid stability: a clinical and anatomic study. Foot Ankle Int 2001; 22: 880–884

Lohrer H, Arentz S. Calcaneocuboid joint instability: a novel operative technique for anatomic reconstruction. Foot Ankle Int 2004; 25: 349–356

Lohrer H, Nauck T, Arentz S, Vogl TJ. Dorsal calcaneocuboid ligament versus lateral ankle ligament repair: a case-control study. Br J Sports Med 2006; 40: 839–843

Lohrer H, Nauck T, Dorn-Lange NV, Arentz S, Konerding MA. Periosteal repair of the dorsal calcaneocuboid ligament: a comparative biomechanical study. Foot Ankle Int 2007; 28: 202–207

Patil V, Ebraheim N, Wagner R, Owens C. Morphometric dimensions of the dorsal calcaneocuboid ligament. Foot Ankle Int 2008; 29: 508–512

Valderrabano V, Engelhardt M, Küster H-H. Fuss und Sprunggelenk und Sport. Cologne: Deutscher Ärzteverlag; 2009

van Dorp KB, de Vries MR, van der Elst M, Schepers T. Chopart joint injury: a study of outcome and morbidity. J Foot Ankle Surg 2010; 49: 541–545

Ward KA, Soames RW. Morphology of the plantar calcaneocuboid ligaments. Foot Ankle Int 1997; 18: 649–653

Fractures

Ankle Fractures

Barbosa P, Bonnaire F, Kojima K. Malleoli. AO Foundation. Website: http://www.aofoundation.org; status: 26 Oct 2011

Cobb N. Oblique radiography in the diagnosis of ankle injuries. Proc R Soc Med 1965; 58: 334–336

Lauge N. Fractures of the ankle; analytic historic survey as the basis of new experimental, roentgenologic and clinical investigations. Arch Surg 1948; 56: 259–317

Lauge-Hansen N. Ligamentous ankle fractures; diagnosis and treatment. Acta Chir Scand 1949; 97: 544–550

Lauge-Hansen N. Fractures of the ankle. III. Genetic roentgenologic diagnosis of fractures of the ankle. Am J Roentgenol Radium Ther Nucl Med 1954; 71: 456–471

Vécsei V. Hajdu P. Operative Behandlung der Knöchelfrakturen des Erwachsenen. Vienna: Österreichische Gesellschaft für Unfallchirurgie. Website: http://www.unfallchirurgen.at/download/agenda/28_vecsei2.pdf; status: 26 Oct 2011

Weber BG. Die Verletzungen des oberen Sprunggelenks. Bern: Huber; 1966

Tibial Pilon Fractures

Feldman DS, Shin SS, Madan S, Koval KJ. Correction of tibial malunion and nonunion with six-axis analysis deformity correction using the Taylor Spatial Frame. J Orthop Trauma 2003; 17: 549–554

Griffiths GP, Thordarson DB. Tibial plafond fractures: limited internal fixation and a hybrid external fixator. Foot Ankle Int 1996; 17: 444–448

Hessmann M, Nork S, Sommer C, et al. Distal tibia. AO Foundation. Website: http://www.aofoundation.org; status: 26 Oct 2011

Kim HS, Jahng JS, Kim SS, Chun CH, Han HJ. Treatment of tibial pilon fractures using ring fixators and arthroscopy. Clin Orthop Relat Res 1997; 334: 244–250

Sanders R, Gorman RR, Ritter CA, et al. Replacement versus arthrodesis for post-traumatic ankle arthritis. Paper presented at the Annual Meeting of the Orthopedic Trauma Association; 2004

Thordarson DB. Complications after treatment of tibial pilon fractures: prevention and management strategies. J Am Acad Orthop Surg 2000; 8: 253–265

Topliss CJ, Jackson M, Atkins RM. Anatomy of pilon fractures of the distal tibia. J Bone Joint Surg Br 2005; 87: 692–697

Fracture of the Posterior Tibial Margin

Bartonícek J. Avulsed posterior edge of the tibia. Earle's or Volkmann's triangle? J Bone Joint Surg Br 2004; 86: 746–750

Earle H. Practical Observations in Surgery. London: Underwood; 1823

Magid D, Michelson JD, Ney DR, Fishman EK. Adult ankle fractures: comparison of plain films and interactive two- and three-dimensional CT scans. AJR Am J Roentgenol 1990; 154: 1017–1023

Mingo-Robinet J, López-Durán L, Galeote JE, Martinez-Cervell C. Ankle fractures with posterior malleolar fragment: management and results. J Foot Ankle Surg 2011; 50: 141–145

Niethard FU, Plaue R. The intra-articular fracture of the distal end of the tibia as a prognostic criterion [author's transl.]. Arch Orthop Unfallchir 1977; 87: 213–221

Volkmann R. Beiträge zur Chirurgie anschliessend an einen Bericht über die Thätigkeit der chirurgischen: Universitätsklinik zu Halle im Jahre 1873. Leipzig: Breitkopf und Härtel; 1875: 104–109

Volkmann R. Die Behandlung der complicierten Fracturen. In: Volkmann R, ed. Sammlung klinischer Vorträge in Verbindung mit deutschen Klinikern. Leipzig: Breitkopf und Härtel; 1875: 922–976

Maisonneuve Fracture

Imade S, Takao M, Miyamoto W, Nishi H, Uchio Y. Leg anterior compartment syndrome following ankle arthroscopy after Maisonneuve fracture. Arthroscopy 2009; 25: 215–218

Kalyani BS, Roberts CS, Giannoudis PV. The Maisonneuve injury: a comprehensive review. Orthopedics 2010; 33: 196–197

Millen JC, Lindberg D. Maisonneuve fracture. J Emerg Med 2011; 41: 77–78

Stufkens SA, van den Bekerom MP, Doornberg JN, van Dijk CN, Kloen P. Evidence-based treatment of maisonneuve fractures. J Foot Ankle Surg 2011; 50: 62–67

Tilleaux Fracture

Cone RO, Nguyen V, Flournoy JG, Guerra J. Triplane fracture of the distal tibial epiphysis: radiographic and CT studies. Radiology 1984; 153: 763–767

Cooperman DR, Spiegel PG, Laros GS. Tibial fractures involving the ankle in children. The so-called triplane epiphyseal fracture. J Bone Joint Surg Am 1978; 60: 1040–1046

Dailiana ZH, Malizos KN, Zacharis K, Mavrodontidis AN, Shiamishis GA, Soucacos PN. Distal tibial epiphyseal fractures in adolescents. Am J Orthop 1999; 28: 309–312

Dias LS, Giegerich CR. Fractures of the distal tibial epiphysis in adolescence. J Bone Joint Surg Am 1983; 65: 438–444

El-Karef E, Sadek HI, Nairn DS, Aldam CH, Allen PW. Triplane fracture of the distal tibia. Injury 2000; 31: 729–736

Feldman F, Singson RD, Rosenberg ZS, Berdon WE, Amodio J, Abramson SJ. Distal tibial triplane fractures: diagnosis with CT. Radiology 1987; 164: 429–435

Gourineni P, Gupta A. Medial joint space widening of the ankle in displaced Tillaux and Triplane fractures in children. J Orthop Trauma 2011; 25: 608–611

Kim JR, Song KH, Song KJ, Lee HS. Treatment outcomes of triplane and Tillaux fractures of the ankle in adolescence. Clin Orthop Surg 2010; 2: 34–38

Kleiger B, Mankin HJ. Fracture of the lateral portion of the distal tibial epiphysis. J Bone Joint Surg Am 1964; 46: 25–32

Lemburg SP, Lilienthal E, Heyer CM. Growth plate fractures of the distal tibia: is CT imaging necessary? Arch Orthop Trauma Surg 2010; 130: 1411–1417

Lynn MD. The triplane distal tibial epiphyseal fracture. Clin Orthop Relat Res 1972; 86: 187–190

Marmor L. An unusual fracture of the tibial epiphysis. Clin Orthop Relat Res 1970; 73: 132–135

Ogden JA, McCarthy SM. Radiology of postnatal skeletal development. VIII. Distal tibia and fibula. Skeletal Radiol 1983; 10: 209–220

Peiró A, Aracil J, Martos F, Mut T. Triplane distal tibial epiphyseal fracture. Clin Orthop Relat Res 1981: 196–200

von Laer L. Classification, diagnosis, and treatment of transitional fractures of the distal part of the tibia. J Bone Joint Surg Am 1985; 67: 687–698

Osteochondral Lesions of the Talus

Barnes CJ, Ferkel RD. Arthroscopic debridement and drilling of osteochondral lesions of the talus. Foot Ankle Clin 2003; 8: 243–257

Becher C, Thermann H. Results of microfracture in the treatment of articular cartilage defects of the talus. Foot Ankle Int 2005; 26: 583–589

Berndt AL, Harty M. Transchondral fractures (osteochondritis dissecans) of the talus. J Bone Joint Surg Am 1959; 41-A: 988–1020

Bosien WR, Staples OS, Russell SW. Residual disability following acute ankle sprains. J Bone Joint Surg Am 1955; 37-A: 1237–1243

Dipaola JD, Nelson DW, Colville MR. Characterizing osteochondral lesions by magnetic resonance imaging. Arthroscopy 1991; 7: 101–104

Elias I, Jung JW, Raikin SM, Schweitzer MW, Carrino JA, Morrison WB. Osteochondral lesions of the talus: change in MRI findings over time in talar lesions without operative intervention and implications for staging systems. Foot Ankle Int 2006; 27: 157–166

Giannini S, Buda R, Vannini F, Di Caprio F, Grigolo B. Arthroscopic autologous chondrocyte implantation in osteochondral lesions of the talus: surgical technique and results. Am J Sports Med 2008; 36: 873–880

Hangody L, Kish G, Módis L et al. Mosaicplasty for the treatment of osteochondritis dissecans of the talus: two to seven year results in 36 patients. Foot Ankle Int 2001; 22: 552–558

Hepple S, Winson IG, Glew D. Osteochondral lesions of the talus: a revised classification. Foot Ankle Int 1999; 20: 789–793

Loomer R, Fisher C, Lloyd-Smith R, Sisler J, Cooney T. Osteochondral lesions of the talus. Am J Sports Med 1993; 21: 13–19

Pritsch M, Horoshovski H, Farine I. Arthroscopic treatment of osteochondral lesions of the talus. J Bone Joint Surg Am 1986; 68: 862–865

Schenck RC, Goodnight JM. Osteochondritis dissecans. J Bone Joint Surg Am 1996; 78: 439–456

Schimmer RC, Dick W, Hintermann B. The role of ankle arthroscopy in the treatment strategies of osteochondritis dissecans lesions of the talus. Foot Ankle Int 2001; 22: 895–900

Taranow WS, Bisignani GA, Towers JD, Conti SF. Retrograde drilling of osteochondral lesions of the medial talar dome. Foot Ankle Int 1999; 20: 474–480

Verhagen RA, Maas M, Dijkgraaf MG, Tol JL, Krips R, van Dijk CN. Prospective study on diagnostic strategies in osteochondral lesions of the talus. Is MRI superior to helical CT? J Bone Joint Surg Br 2005; 87: 41–46

Fractures of the Talus

Brunner U, Schweiberer L. Injuries of the talus and calcaneus. [Article in German] Unfallchirurg 1996; 99: 136–151

Donnelly EF. The Hawkins sign. Radiology 1999; 210: 195–196

Early JS. Talus fracture management. Foot Ankle Clin 2008; 13: 635–657

Hawkins LG. Fractures of the neck of the talus. J Bone Joint Surg Am 1970; 52: 991–1002

Lutz M, Golser K, Sperner G, Gabl M, Wambacher M, Sailer R. Post-traumatic ischemia of the talus. Is talus necrosis unavoidable? [Article in German] Unfallchirurg 1998; 101: 461–467

Marti R. Talus- und Calcaneusfrakturen. In: Weber BG, Brunner C, Freuler F, eds. Die Frakturenbehandlung bei Kindern und Jugendlichen. Berlin: Springer; 1978

Metzger MJ, Levin JS, Clancy JT. Talar neck fractures and rates of avascular necrosis. J Foot Ankle Surg 1999; 38: 154–162

Prasarn ML, Miller AN, Dyke JP, Helfet DL, Lorich DG. Arterial anatomy of the talus: a cadaver and gadolinium-enhanced MRI study. Foot Ankle Int 2010; 31: 987–993

Schwarz N. Talusfraktur. Österreichische Gesellschaft für Unfallchirurgie 1–16. Website: http://www.unfallchirurgen.at/download/agenda/28_schwarz.pdf; status: 26 Oct 2011

Schwarz N, Eschberger J, Kramer J, Posch E. Radiologic and histologic observations in central talus fractures. [Article in German] Unfallchirurg 1997; 100: 449–456

Swanson TV, Bray TJ, Holmes GB. Fractures of the talar neck. A mechanical study of fixation. J Bone Joint Surg Am 1992; 74: 544–551

Calcaneal Fractures

Badillo K, Pacheco JA, Padua SO, Gomez AA, Colon E, Vidal JA. Multidetector CT evaluation of calcaneal fractures. Radiographics 2011; 31: 81–92

Brunner U, Kenn RW, Slawik J, Schweiberer L. Intra-articular calcaneus fracture. Classification in CT as a prerequisite for therapeutic decision and quantitative comparison. [Article in German] Unfallchirurg 1992; 95: 358–366

Buch BD, Myerson MS, Miller SD. Primary subtaler arthrodesis for the treatment of comminuted calcaneal fractures. Foot Ankle Int 1996; 17: 61–70

Daftary A, Haims AH, Baumgaertner MR. Fractures of the calcaneus: a review with emphasis on CT. Radiographics 2005; 25: 1215–1226

Eastwood DM, Gregg PJ, Atkins RM. Intra-articular fractures of the calcaneum. Part I: Pathological anatomy and classification. J Bone Joint Surg Br 1993; 75: 183–188

Essex-Lopresti P. The mechanism, reduction technique, and results in fractures of the os calcis. Br J Surg 1952; 39: 395–419

Howard JL, Buckley R, McCormack R et al. Complications following management of displaced intra-articular calcaneal fractures: a prospective randomized trial comparing open reduction internal fixation with nonoperative management. J Orthop Trauma 2003; 17: 241–249

Mutschler W. Fracture of the calcaneus—detailed diagnosis, classification and consequences for therapy. [Article in German] Unfallchirurg 1988; 91: 486–492

Myerson M, Manoli A. Compartment syndromes of the foot after calcaneal fractures. Clin Orthop Relat Res 1993: 142–150

Rammelt S, Gavlik JM, Zwipp H. Historical and current treatment of calcaneal fractures. J Bone Joint Surg Am 2001; 83-A: 1438–1440, author reply 1439–1440

Rammelt S, Amlang M, Barthel S, Zwipp H. Minimally-invasive treatment of calcaneal fractures. Injury 2004; 35 Suppl 2: SB55–SB63

Rubino R, Valderrabano V, Sutter PM, Regazzoni P. Prognostic value of four classifications of calcaneal fractures. Foot Ankle Int 2009; 30: 229–238

Sanders R. Intra-articular fractures of the calcaneus: present state of the art. J Orthop Trauma 1992; 6: 252–265

Thordarson DB, Krieger LE. Operative vs. nonoperative treatment of intra-articular fractures of the calcaneus: a prospective randomized trial. Foot Ankle Int 1996; 17: 2–9

Zwipp H, Tscherne H, Wülker N, Grote R. Intra-articular fracture of the calcaneus. Classification, assessment and surgical procedures. [Article in German] Unfallchirurg 1989; 92: 117–129

Pediatric Fractures

Petit P, Panuel M, Faure F et al. Acute fracture of the distal tibial physis: role of gradient-echo MR imaging versus plain film examination. AJR Am J Roentgenol 1996; 166: 1203–1206

Seifert J, Laun R, Paris S, Mutze S, Ekkernkamp A, Ostermann PA. Value of magnetic resonance tomography (MRI) in diagnosis of triplane fractures of the distal tibia. [Article in German] Unfallchirurg 2001; 104: 524–529

Vanhoenacker FM, Bernaerts A, Gielen J, Schepens E, De Schepper AM. Trauma of the pediatric ankle and foot. JBR-BTR 2002; 85: 212–218

Peritalar Dislocations

Buckingham WW, LeFlore I. Subtalar dislocation of the foot. J Trauma 1973; 13: 753–765

Forrester DM, Kerr R. Trauma to the foot. Radiol Clin North Am 1990; 28: 423–433

Heck BE, Ebraheim NA, Jackson WT. Anatomical considerations of irreducible medial subtalar dislocation. Foot Ankle Int 1996; 17: 103–106

Merianos P, Papagiannakos K, Hatzis A, Tsafantakis E. Peritalar dislocation: a follow-up report of 21 cases. Injury 1988; 19: 439–442

Milenkovic S, Radenkovic M, Mitkovic M. Open subtalar dislocation treated by distractional external fixation. J Orthop Trauma 2004; 18: 638–640

Perugia D, Basile A, Massoni C, Gumina S, Rossi F, Ferretti A. Conservative treatment of subtalar dislocations. Int Orthop 2002; 26: 56–60

Zimmer TJ, Johnson KA. Subtalar dislocations. Clin Orthop Relat Res 1989: 190–194

Midtarsal Joint Injuries

Jones FW. Structure and Function as Seen in the Foot. London: Balliere, Tindall & Cox; 1944: 246

Kenwright J, Taylor RG. Major injuries of the talus. J Bone Joint Surg Br 1970; 52: 36–48

Main BJ, Jowett RL. Injuries of the midtarsal joint. J Bone Joint Surg Br 1975; 57: 89–97

Richter M, Thermann H, Huefner T, Schmidt U, Goesling T, Krettek C. Chopart joint fracture-dislocation: initial open reduction provides better outcome than closed reduction. Foot Ankle Int 2004; 25: 340–348

Sangeorzan BJ, Hansen ST. Early and late posttraumatic foot reconstruction. Clin Orthop Relat Res 1989: 86–91

van Dorp KB, de Vries MR, van der Elst M, Schepers T. Chopart joint injury: a study of outcome and morbidity. J Foot Ankle Surg 2010; 49: 541–545

Axial Deformities of the Hindfoot

Osteoarthritis of the Ankle Joint with Varus or Valgus Deformity

Paley D. Principles of Deformity Correction. Berlin: Springer; 2003

Pes Planovalgus

Herzenberg JE, Goldner JL, Martinez S, Silverman PM. Computerized tomography of talocalcaneal tarsal coalition: a clinical and anatomic study. Foot Ankle 1986; 6: 273–288

Kulik SA, Clanton TO. Tarsal coalition. Foot Ankle Int 1996; 17: 286–296
Luhmann SJ, Schoenecker PL. Symptomatic talocalcaneal coalition resection: indications and results. J Pediatr Orthop 1998; 18: 748–754
Newman JS, Newberg AH. Congenital tarsal coalition: multimodality evaluation with emphasis on CT and MR imaging. Radiographics 2000; 20: 321–332, quiz 526–527, 532
Premkumar A, Perry MB, Dwyer AJ et al. Sonography and MR imaging of posterior tibial tendinopathy. AJR Am J Roentgenol 2002; 178: 223–232
Schweitzer ME, Karasick D. MR imaging of disorders of the posterior tibialis tendon. AJR Am J Roentgenol 2000; 175: 627–635
Staser J, Karmazyn B, Lubicky J. Radiographic diagnosis of posterior facet talocalcaneal coalition. Pediatr Radiol 2007; 37: 79–81

Pes Cavus

Aminian A, Sangeorzan BJ. The anatomy of cavus foot deformity. Foot Ankle Clin 2008; 13: 191–198, v
Charles YP, Louahem D, Diméglio A. Cavovarus foot deformity with multiple tarsal coalitions: functional and three-dimensional preoperative assessment. J Foot Ankle Surg 2006; 45: 118–126
Döderlein L, Wenz W, Schneider U. Der Hohlfuß. Berlin: Springer; 2000
Ippolito E, Fraracci L, Farsetti P, Di Mario M, Caterini R. The influence of treatment on the pathology of club foot. CT study at maturity. J Bone Joint Surg Br 2004; 86: 574–580
Niethard FU. Kinderorthopädie. 2nd ed. Chapter8. Stuttgart: Thieme; 2009: 160

Impingement

Anterolateral Impingement

Arnold H. Posttraumatic impingement syndrome of the ankle—indication and results of arthroscopic therapy. Foot Ankle Surg 2011; 17: 85–88
Cochet H, Pelé E, Amoretti N, Brunot S, Lafenêtre O, Hauger O. Anterolateral ankle impingement: diagnostic performance of MDCT arthrography and sonography. AJR Am J Roentgenol 2010; 194: 1575–1580
Donovan A, Rosenberg ZS. MRI of ankle and lateral hindfoot impingement syndromes. AJR Am J Roentgenol 2010; 195: 595–604
Edmonds EW, Chambers R, Kaufman E, Chambers HG. Anterolateral ankle impingement in adolescents: outcomes of nonoperative and operative treatment. J Pediatr Orthop 2010; 30: 186–191
Ferkel RD, Tyorkin M, Applegate GR, Heinen GT. MRI evaluation of anterolateral soft tissue impingement of the ankle. Foot Ankle Int 2010; 31: 655–661
Linklater J. MR imaging of ankle impingement lesions. Magn Reson Imaging Clin N Am 2009; 17: 775–800, vii–viii
Moustafa El-Sayed AM. Arthroscopic treatment of anterolateral impingement of the ankle. J Foot Ankle Surg 2010; 49: 219–223

Anteromedial and Anterior Impingement

Bauer T, Breda R, Hardy P. Anterior ankle bony impingement with joint motion loss: the arthroscopic resection option. Orthop Traumatol Surg Res 2010; 96: 462–468
Chhabra A, Subhawong TK, Carrino JA. MR imaging of deltoid ligament pathologic findings and associated impingement syndromes. Radiographics 2010; 30: 751–761
Donovan A, Rosenberg ZS. MRI of ankle and lateral hindfoot impingement syndromes. AJR Am J Roentgenol 2010; 195: 595–604
Hayeri MR, Trudell DJ, Resnick D. Anterior ankle impingement and talar bony outgrowths: osteophyte or enthesophyte? Paleopathologic and cadaveric study with imaging correlation. AJR Am J Roentgenol 2009; 193: W334-W338
Linklater J. MR imaging of ankle impingement lesions. Magn Reson Imaging Clin N Am 2009; 17: 775–800, vii–viii
Moon JS, Lee K, Lee HS, Lee WC. Cartilage lesions in anterior bony impingement of the ankle. Arthroscopy 2010; 26: 984–989
Murawski CD, Kennedy JG. Anteromedial impingement in the ankle joint: outcomes following arthroscopy. Am J Sports Med 2010; 38: 2017–2024
Scranton PE, McDermott JE, Rogers JV. The relationship between chronic ankle instability and variations in mortise anatomy and impingement spurs. Foot Ankle Int 2000; 21: 657–664
Tol JL, van Dijk CN. Etiology of the anterior ankle impingement syndrome: a descriptive anatomical study. Foot Ankle Int 2004; 25: 382–386

Posterior Impingement

Donovan A, Rosenberg ZS. MRI of ankle and lateral hindfoot impingement syndromes. AJR Am J Roentgenol 2010; 195: 595–604
Lee JC, Calder JD, Healy JC. Posterior impingement syndromes of the ankle. Semin Musculoskelet Radiol 2008; 12: 154–169
Linklater J. MR imaging of ankle impingement lesions. Magn Reson Imaging Clin N Am 2009; 17: 775–800, vii–viii
Peace KA, Hillier JC, Hulme A, Healy JC. MRI features of posterior ankle impingement syndrome in ballet dancers: a review of 25 cases. Clin Radiol 2004; 59: 1025–1033
Russell JA, Kruse DW, Koutedakis Y, McEwan IM, Wyon MA. Pathoanatomy of posterior ankle impingement in ballet dancers. Clin Anat 2010; 23: 613–621

Os Trigonum Syndrome

Abramowitz Y, Wollstein R, Barzilay Y et al. Outcome of resection of a symptomatic os trigonum. J Bone Joint Surg Am 2003; 85-A: 1051–1057
Mendez-Castillo A, Burd TA, Kenter K et al. Radiologic case study. Os trigonum syndrome. Orthopedics 1999; 22 (12): 1208, 1201–1202
Mouhsine E, Crevoisier X, Leyvraz PF, Akiki A, Dutoit M, Garofalo R. Post-traumatic overload or acute syndrome of the os trigonum: a possible cause of posterior ankle impingement. Knee Surg Sports Traumatol Arthrosc 2004; 12: 250–253
Russell JA, Kruse DW, Koutedakis Y, McEwan IM, Wyon MA. Pathoanatomy of posterior ankle impingement in ballet dancers. Clin Anat 2010; 23: 613–621
Zeichen J, Schratt E, Bosch U, Thermann H. Os trigonum syndrome. [Article in German] Unfallchirurg 1999; 102: 320–323

Instability

Syndesmosis

Grass R, Herzmann K, Biewener A, Zwipp H. Injuries of the inferior tibiofibular syndesmosis. [Article in German] Unfallchirurg 2000; 103: 520–532
Han SH, Lee JW, Kim S, Suh JS, Choi YR. Chronic tibiofibular syndesmosis injury: the diagnostic efficiency of magnetic resonance imaging and comparative analysis of operative treatment. Foot Ankle Int 2007; 28: 336–342
Hermans JJ, Beumer A, de Jong TA, Kleinrensink GJ. Anatomy of the distal tibiofibular syndesmosis in adults: a pictorial essay with a multimodality approach. J Anat 2010; 217: 633–645
Lin CF, Gross ML, Weinhold P. Ankle syndesmosis injuries: anatomy, biomechanics, mechanism of injury, and clinical guidelines for diagnosis and intervention. J Orthop Sports Phys Ther 2006; 36: 372–384
Miller AN, Paul O, Boraiah S, Parker RJ, Helfet DL, Lorich DG. Functional outcomes after syndesmotic screw fixation and removal. J Orthop Trauma 2010; 24: 12–16
Rammelt S, Zwipp H, Grass R. Injuries to the distal tibiofibular syndesmosis: an evidence-based approach to acute and chronic lesions. Foot Ankle Clin 2008; 13: 611–633, vii–viii
Schuberth JM, Jennings MM, Lau AC. Arthroscopy-assisted repair of latent syndesmotic instability of the ankle. Arthroscopy 2008; 24: 868–874
Stark E, Tornetta P, Creevy WR. Syndesmotic instability in Weber B ankle fractures: a clinical evaluation. J Orthop Trauma 2007; 21: 643–646
van den Bekerom MP, de Leeuw PA, van Dijk CN. Delayed operative treatment of syndesmotic instability. Current concepts review. Injury 2009; 40: 1137–1142
Zalavras C, Thordarson D. Ankle syndesmotic injury. J Am Acad Orthop Surg 2007; 15: 330–339
Zamzami MM, Zamzam MM. Chronic isolated distal tibiofibular syndesmotic disruption: diagnosis and management. Foot Ankle Surg 2009; 15: 14–19

Ankle Joint

Bonnel F, Toullec E, Mabit C, Tourné Y; Sofcot. Chronic ankle instability: biomechanics and pathomechanics of ligaments injury and associated lesions. Orthop Traumatol Surg Res 2010; 96: 424–432
Hubbard TJ, Cordova M. Effect of ankle taping on mechanical laxity in chronic ankle instability. Foot Ankle Int 2010; 31: 499–504
Joshy S, Abdulkadir U, Chaganti S, Sullivan B, Hariharan K. Accuracy of MRI scan in the diagnosis of ligamentous and chondral pathology in the ankle. Foot Ankle Surg 2010; 16: 78–80

Mabit C, Tourné Y, Besse JL et alSofcot (French Society of Orthopedic and Traumatologic Surgery). Chronic lateral ankle instability surgical repairs: the long term prospective. Orthop Traumatol Surg Res 2010; 96: 417–423

Martin B. Ankle sprain complications: MRI evaluation. Clin Podiatr Med Surg 2008; 25: 203–247, vi

Rein S, Fabian T, Zwipp H, Mittag-Bonsch M, Weindel S. Influence of age, body mass index and leg dominance on functional ankle stability. Foot Ankle Int 2010; 31: 423–432

Tourné Y, Besse JL, Mabit C; Sofcot. Chronic ankle instability. Which tests to assess the lesions? Which therapeutic options? Orthop Traumatol Surg Res 2010; 96: 433–446

Subtalar Joint

Bonnel F, Toullec E, Mabit C, Tourné Y; Sofcot. Chronic ankle instability: biomechanics and pathomechanics of ligaments injury and associated lesions. Orthop Traumatol Surg Res 2010; 96: 424–432

Budny A. Subtalar joint instability: current clinical concepts. Clin Podiatr Med Surg 2004; 21: 449–460, viii

Kamiya T, Kura H, Suzuki D, Uchiyama E, Fujimiya M, Yamashita T. Mechanical stability of the subtalar joint after lateral ligament sectioning and ankle brace application: a biomechanical experimental study. Am J Sports Med 2009; 37: 2451–2458

Langer P, Nickisch F, Spenciner D, Fleming B, DiGiovanni CW. In vitro evaluation of the effect lateral process talar excision on ankle and subtalar joint stability. Foot Ankle Int 2007; 28: 78–83

Lui TH. Arthroscopic-assisted lateral ligamentous reconstruction in combined ankle and subtalar instability. Arthroscopy 2007;23(5):554.e1–5

Mabit C, Tourné Y, Besse JL et alSofcot (French Society of Orthopedic and Traumatologic Surgery). Chronic lateral ankle instability surgical repairs: the long term prospective. Orthop Traumatol Surg Res 2010; 96: 417–423

Michelson J, Hamel A, Buczek F, Sharkey N. The effect of ankle injury on subtalar motion. Foot Ankle Int 2004; 25: 639–646

Pisani G, Pisani PC, Parino E. Sinus tarsi syndrome and subtalar joint instability. Clin Podiatr Med Surg 2005; 22: 63–77, vii

Ringleb SI, Udupa JK, Siegler S et al. The effect of ankle ligament damage and surgical reconstructions on the mechanics of the ankle and subtalar joints revealed by three-dimensional stress MRI. J Orthop Res 2005; 23: 743–749

Tochigi Y, Amendola A, Rudert MJ et al. The role of the interosseous talocalcaneal ligament in subtalar joint stability. Foot Ankle Int 2004; 25: 588–596

Tourné Y, Besse JL, Mabit C; Sofcot. Chronic ankle instability. Which tests to assess the lesions? Which therapeutic options? Orthop Traumatol Surg Res 2010; 96: 433–446

Weindel S, Schmidt R, Rammelt S, Claes L, v Campe A, Rein S. Subtalar instability: a biomechanical cadaver study. Arch Orthop Trauma Surg 2010; 130: 313–319

Chronic Disorders of Cartilage and Bone

Osteoarthritis of the Ankle and Subtalar Joint

AlOmran AS. Osteoarthritis of knee: correlation between radiographic and arthroscopic findings. Int Surg 2009; 94: 269–272

Bai LB, Lee KB, Song EK, Yoon TR, Seon JK. Total ankle arthroplasty outcome comparison for post-traumatic and primary osteoarthritis. Foot Ankle Int 2010; 31: 1048–1056

Dihlmann W, Stäbler A. Gelenke des Fußes einschließlich des oberen Sprunggelenks. In: Dihlmann W, Stäbler A, eds. Gelenke - Wirbelverbindungen. 4th ed. Stuttgart: Thieme; 2010: 692ff

Halstead J, Bergin D, Keenan AM, Madden J, McGonagle D. Ligament and bone pathologic abnormalities more frequent in neuropathic joint disease in comparison with degenerative arthritis of the foot and ankle: implications for understanding rapidly progressive joint degeneration. Arthritis Rheum 2010; 62: 2353–2358

Hayashi K, Tanaka Y, Kumai T, Sugimoto K, Takakura Y. Correlation of compensatory alignment of the subtalar joint to the progression of primary osteoarthritis of the ankle. Foot Ankle Int 2008; 29: 400–406

Kozanek M, Rubash HE, Li G, de Asla RJ. Effect of post-traumatic tibiotalar osteoarthritis on kinematics of the ankle joint complex. Foot Ankle Int 2009; 30: 734–740

Rodríguez-Merchán EC, Gómez-Cardero P. The outerbridge classification predicts the need for patellar resurfacing in TKA. Clin Orthop Relat Res 2010; 468: 1254–1257

von Knoch F, Reckord U, von Knoch M, Sommer C. Fracture of the lateral process of the talus in snowboarders. J Bone Joint Surg Br 2007; 89: 772–777

Witteveen AG, Sierevelt IN, Blankevoort L, Kerkhoffs GM, van Dijk CN. Intra-articular sodium hyaluronate injections in the osteoarthritic ankle joint: effects, safety and dose dependency. Foot Ankle Surg 2010; 16: 159–163

Chondromatosis, Multiple Intra-articular Loose Bodies

Breitenseher M. MR-Trainer obere Extremität. Stuttgart: Thieme; 2005

Dihlmann W, Stäbler A. Gelenke–Wirbelverbindungen. Chapter 14: Hüftgelenk; Chapter16: Gelenke des Fusses einschließlich des oberen Sprunggelenks. 4th ed. Stuttgart: Thieme; 2010: 593, 754

Galat DD, Ackerman DB, Spoon D, Turner NS, Shives TC. Synovial chondromatosis of the foot and ankle. Foot Ankle Int 2008; 29: 312–317

Gaulrapp H, Szeimies U. Diagnostik der Gelenke und Weichteile. Munich: Elsevier; 2008: 62

Kerimoglu S, Aynaci O, Saraçoglu M, Cobanoglu U. Synovial chondromatosis of the subtalar joint: a case report and review of the literature. J Am Podiatr Med Assoc 2008; 98: 318–321

Lee DK, Louk L, Bell BL. Synovial osteochondromatosis involvement in post-traumatic ankle injury. J Am Podiatr Med Assoc 2008; 98: 70–74

McKenzie G, Raby N, Ritchie D. A pictorial review of primary synovial osteochondromatosis. Eur Radiol 2008; 18: 2662–2669

Murphey MD, Vidal JA, Fanburg-Smith JC, Gajewski DA. Imaging of synovial chondromatosis with radiologic-pathologic correlation. Radiographics 2007; 27: 1465–1488

Oakley J, Yewlett A, Makwana N. Tenosynovial osteochondromatosis of the flexor hallucis longus tendon. Foot Ankle Surg 2010; 16: 148–150

Scholl DM, Taddie KL. Asymptomatic synovial chondromatosis of the ankle: an incidental finding. J Foot Ankle Surg 2010; 49: e13–e17

Sperling BL, Angel S, Stoneham G, Chow V, McFadden A, Chibbar R. Synovial chondromatosis and chondrosarcoma: a diagnostic dilemma. Sarcoma 2003; 7: 69–73

Testaverde L, Perrone A, Caporali L et al. CT and MR findings in synovial chondromatosis of the temporo-mandibular joint: our experience and review of literature. Eur J Radiol 2011; 78: 414–418

Osteochondral Lesions of the Talus

Arcq M. Fixation of osteochondrosis dissecans by bone-pins (author's transl). [Article in German] Arch Orthop Unfallchir 1974; 79: 297–312

Berndt AL, Harty M. Transchondral fractures (osteochondritis dissecans) of the talus. J Bone Joint Surg Am 1959; 41-A: 988–1020

Bohndorf K, Imhof H, Schibany N. Diagnostic imaging of acute and chronic osteochondral lesions of the talus. [Article in German] Orthopade 2001; 30: 12–19

Breitenseher M. MR-Trainer obere Extremität. Stuttgart: Thieme; 2005: 88

Cheng JC, Ferkel RD. The role of arthroscopy in ankle and subtalar degenerative joint disease. Clin Orthop Relat Res 1998: 65–72

Clinical Munchenwiler Evaluation Group. ICRS Cartilage Injury Evaluation Package. Edited April 2000. Website: http://www.cartilage.org; status: 26 Oct 2011

Dihlmann W, Stäbler A. Gelenke–Wirbelverbindungen. 4th ed. Stuttgart: Thieme; 2010: 735, 644

Elias I, Jung JW, Raikin SM, Schweitzer MW, Carrino JA, Morrison WB. Osteochondral lesions of the talus: change in MRI findings over time in talar lesions without operative intervention and implications for staging systems. Foot Ankle Int 2006; 27: 157–166

Ettl V, Kenn W, Radke S, Kirschner S, Goerttler-Krauspe I, Vispo-Seara JL. The role of MRI in therapy and follow-up after surgical treatment of osteochondrosis dissecans of the talus. [Article in German] Z Orthop Ihre Grenzgeb 2001; 139: 157–162

Furlong J, Morrison WB, Carrino JA. Imaging of the talus. Foot Ankle Clin 2004; 9: 685–701, v

Giannini S, Battaglia M, Buda R, Cavallo M, Ruffilli A, Vannini F. Surgical treatment of osteochondral lesions of the talus by open-field autologous chondrocyte implantation: a 10-year follow-up clinical and magnetic resonance imaging T2-mapping evaluation. Am J Sports Med 2009; 37 Suppl 1: 112S–118S

Han SH, Lee JW, Lee DY, Kang ES. Radiographic changes and clinical results of osteochondral defects of the talus with and without subchondral cysts. Foot Ankle Int 2006; 27: 1109–1114

Heywood CS, Benke MT, Brindle K, Fine KM. Correlation of magnetic resonance imaging to arthroscopic findings of stability in juvenile osteochondritis dissecans. Arthroscopy 2011; 27: 194–199

Kokkinakis M, Kafchitsas K, Rajeev A, Mortier J. Is MRI useful in the early follow-up after autologous osteochondral transplantation? Acta Orthop Belg 2008; 74: 636–642

Letts M, Davidson D, Ahmer A. Osteochondritis dissecans of the talus in children. J Pediatr Orthop 2003; 23: 617–625

Nelson DW, DiPaola J, Colville M, Schmidgall J. Osteochondritis dissecans of the talus and knee: prospective comparison of MR and arthroscopic classifications. J Comput Assist Tomogr 1990; 14: 804–808

O'Loughlin PF, Heyworth BE, Kennedy JG. Current concepts in the diagnosis and treatment of osteochondral lesions of the ankle. Am J Sports Med 2010; 38: 392–404

Outerbridge RE. The etiology of chondromalacia patellae. J Bone Joint Surg Br 1961; 43-B: 752–757

Schuman L, Struijs PA, van Dijk CN. Traumatic osteochondral lesions of the talar dome [Article in German] Orthopade 2001; 30: 66–72

Steinhagen J, Niggemeyer O, Bruns J. Etiology and pathogenesis of osteochondrosis dissecans tali. [Article in German] Orthopade 2001; 30: 20–27

Stroud CC, Marks RM. Imaging of osteochondral lesions of the talus. Foot Ankle Clin 2000; 5: 119–133

van Bergen CJ, de Leeuw PA, van Dijk CN. Treatment of osteochondral defects of the talus. Rev Chir Orthop Repar Appar Mot 2008; 94 Suppl: 398–408

Winalski CS, Alparslan L. Imaging of articular cartilage injuries of the lower extremity. Semin Musculoskelet Radiol 2008; 12: 283–301

Wirth S, Wieser A, Witt SN, Mutschler W, Reiser M. Visualization of radiographically occult osteochondrosis dissecans of the talus using MRI [Article in German] Unfallchirurg 2003; 106: 238–240

Avascular Necrosis of the Talus

Adelaar RS, Madrian JR. Avascular necrosis of the talus. Orthop Clin North Am 2004; 35: 383–395, xi

Babu N, Schuberth JM. Partial avascular necrosis after talar neck fracture. Foot Ankle Int 2010; 31: 777–780

Breitenseher M. MR-Trainer Untere Extremität. Stuttgart: Thieme; 2002: 94

Chiodo CP, Herbst SA. Osteonecrosis of the talus. Foot Ankle Clin 2004; 9: 745–755, vi

DiGiovanni CW, Patel A, Calfee R, Nickisch F. Osteonecrosis in the foot. J Am Acad Orthop Surg 2007; 15: 208–217

Dihlmann W, Stäbler A. Gelenke–Wirbelverbindungen. Chapter16: Gelenke des Fusses einschließlich des oberen Sprunggelenks. 4th ed. Stuttgart: Thieme; 2010: 777

Hawkins LG. Fractures of the neck of the talus. J Bone Joint Surg Am 1970; 52: 991–1002

Horst F, Gilbert BJ, Nunley JA. Avascular necrosis of the talus: current treatment options. Foot Ankle Clin 2004; 9: 757–773

Léduc S, Clare MP, Laflamme GY, Walling AK. Posttraumatic avascular necrosis of the talus. Foot Ankle Clin 2008; 13: 753–765

Pearce DH, Mongiardi CN, Fornasier VL, Daniels TR. Avascular necrosis of the talus: a pictorial essay. Radiographics 2005; 25: 399–410

Prasarn ML, Miller AN, Dyke JP, Helfet DL, Lorich DG. Arterial anatomy of the talus: a cadaver and gadolinium-enhanced MRI study. Foot Ankle Int 2010; 31: 987–993

Stoller DW, Tirman PFJ, Bredella MA. Diagnostic Imaging: Orthopaedics. Philadelphia: Elsevier; 2004: 6–90

Tehranzadeh J, Stuffman E, Ross SD. Partial Hawkins sign in fractures of the talus: a report of three cases. AJR Am J Roentgenol 2003; 181: 1559–1563

Avascular Necrosis of the Navicular

DiGiovanni CW. Fractures of the navicular. Foot Ankle Clin 2004; 9: 25–63

DiGiovanni CW, Patel A, Calfee R, Nickisch F. Osteonecrosis in the foot. J Am Acad Orthop Surg 2007; 15: 208–217

Dihlmann W, Stäbler A. Gelenke - Wirbelverbindungen. Chapter16: Gelenke des Fusses einschließlich des oberen Sprunggelenks. 4th ed. Stuttgart: Thieme; 2010: 732

Golano P, Fariñas O, Sáenz I. The anatomy of the navicular and periarticular structures. Foot Ankle Clin 2004; 9: 1–23

Sizensky JA, Marks RM. Imaging of the navicular. Foot Ankle Clin 2004; 9: 181–209

Calcaneal Apophysitis

Gaulrapp H, Szeimies U. Diagnostik der Gelenke und Weichteile. Chapter 9: Ferse. Munich: Elsevier; 2008: 207

James AM, Williams CM, Haines TP. Heel raises versus prefabricated orthoses in the treatment of posterior heel pain associated with calcaneal apophysitis (Sever's Disease): a randomised control trial. J Foot Ankle Res 2010; 3: 3

Kose O. Do we really need radiographic assessment for the diagnosis of non-specific heel pain (calcaneal apophysitis) in children? Skeletal Radiol 2010; 39: 359–361

Kose O, Celiktas M, Yigit S, Kisin B. Can we make a diagnosis with radiographic examination alone in calcaneal apophysitis (Sever's disease)? J Pediatr Orthop B 2010; 19: 396–398

Stein CJ, Micheli LJ. Overuse injuries in youth sports. Phys Sportsmed 2010; 38: 102–108

Volpon JB, de Carvalho Filho G. Calcaneal apophysitis: a quantitative radiographic evaluation of the secondary ossification center. Arch Orthop Trauma Surg 2002; 122: 338–341

Coalition

Bixby SD, Jarrett DY, Matheney T, Johnston P, Kasser J, Kleinman PK. Unilateral subtalar coalition: contralateral sustentaculum tali morphology. Radiology 2010; 257: 830–835

Bonasia DE, Phisitkul P, Saltzman CL, Barg A, Amendola A. Arthroscopic resection of talocalcaneal coalitions. Arthroscopy 2011; 27: 430–435

Cass AD, Camasta CA. A review of tarsal coalition and pes planovalgus: clinical examination, diagnostic imaging, and surgical planning. J Foot Ankle Surg 2010; 49: 274–293

Crim J. Imaging of tarsal coalition. Radiol Clin North Am 2008; 46: 1017–1026, vi

Dihlmann W, Stäbler A. Gelenke–Wirbelverbindungen. Chapter16: Gelenke des Fusses einschließlich des oberen Sprunggelenks. 4th ed. Stuttgart: Thieme; 2010

Guignand D, Journeau P, Mainard-Simard L, Popkov D, Haumont T, Lascombes P. Child calcaneonavicular coalitions: MRI diagnostic value in a 19-case series. Orthop Traumatol Surg Res 2011; 97: 67–72

Kernbach KJ. Tarsal coalitions: etiology, diagnosis, imaging, and stigmata. Clin Podiatr Med Surg 2010; 27: 105–117

Mubarak SJ, Patel PN, Upasani VV, Moor MA, Wenger DR. Calcaneonavicular coalition: treatment by excision and fat graft. J Pediatr Orthop 2009; 29: 418–426

Patel CV. The foot and ankle: MR imaging of uniquely pediatric disorders. Magn Reson Imaging Clin N Am 2009; 17: 539–547, vii

Philbin TM, Homan B, Hill K, Berlet G. Results of resection for middle facet tarsal coalitions in adults. Foot Ankle Spec 2008; 1: 344–349

Pouliquen JC, Duranthon LD, Glorion C, Kassis B, Langlais J. The too-long anterior process calcaneus: a report of 39 cases in 25 children and adolescents. J Pediatr Orthop 1998; 18: 333–336

Stoller DW, Tirman PFJ, Bredella MA. Diagnostic Imaging: Orthopaedics. Philadelphia: Elsevier; 2004: 6–102

Upasani VV, Chambers RC, Mubarak SJ. Analysis of calcaneonavicular coalitions using multi-planar three-dimensional computed tomography. J Child Orthop 2008; 2: 301–307

Zaw H, Calder JD. Tarsal coalitions. Foot Ankle Clin 2010; 15: 349–364

Achilles Tendon Pathology

Achillodynia

Calleja M, Connell DA. The Achilles tendon. Semin Musculoskelet Radiol 2010; 14: 307–322

Gaweda K, Tarczynska M, Krzyzanowski W. Treatment of Achilles tendinopathy with platelet-rich plasma. Int J Sports Med 2010; 31: 577–583

Hodgson RJ, Grainger AJ, O'Connor PJ et al. Imaging of the Achilles tendon in spondyloarthritis: a comparison of ultrasound and conventional, short and ultrashort echo time MRI with and without intravenous contrast. Eur Radiol 2011; 21: 1144–1152

Humphrey J, Chan O, Crisp T et al. The short-term effects of high volume image guided injections in resistant non-insertional Achilles tendinopathy. J Sci Med Sport 2010; 13: 295–298

Maffulli N, Testa V, Capasso G, Bifulco G, Binfield PM. Results of percutaneous longitudinal tenotomy for Achilles tendinopathy in middle- and long-distance runners. Am J Sports Med 1997; 25: 835–840

Maffulli N, Longo UG, Hüfner T, Denaro V. Surgical treatment for pain syndromes of the Achilles tendon [Article in German] Unfallchirurg 2010; 113: 721–725

Myerson MS, McGarvey W. Disorders of the Achilles tendon insertion and Achilles tendinitis. Instr Course Lect 1999; 48: 211–218

Peduto AJ, Read JW. Imaging of ankle tendinopathy and tears. Top Magn Reson Imaging 2010; 21: 25–36

Pierre-Jerome C, Moncayo V, Terk MR. MRI of the Achilles tendon: a comprehensive review of the anatomy, biomechanics, and imaging of overuse tendinopathies. Acta Radiol 2010; 51: 438–454

Porter DA, Schon LC. The Foot and Ankle in Sports. Philadelphia: Mosby; 2007

Reddy SS, Pedowitz DI, Parekh SG, Omar IM, Wapner KL. Surgical treatment for chronic disease and disorders of the achilles tendon. J Am Acad Orthop Surg 2009; 17: 3–14

Weber C, Wedegärtner U, Maas LC, Buchert R, Adam G, Maas R. MR imaging of the Achilles tendon: evaluation of criteria for the differentiation of asymptomatic and symptomatic tendons [Article in German] Rofo 2011; 183: 631–640

Wijesekera NT, Calder JD, Lee JC. Imaging in the assessment and management of Achilles tendinopathy and paratendinitis. Semin Musculoskelet Radiol 2011; 15: 89–100

Partial Tear

Irwin TA. Current concepts review: insertional achilles tendinopathy. Foot Ankle Int 2010; 31: 933–939

Maffulli N, Testa V, Capasso G, Bifulco G, Binfield PM. Results of percutaneous longitudinal tenotomy for Achilles tendinopathy in middle- and long-distance runners. Am J Sports Med 1997; 25: 835–840

Steenstra F, van Dijk CN. Achilles tendoscopy. Foot Ankle Clin 2006; 11: 429–438, VIII

Rupture

Amlang MH, Maffuli N, Longo UG, Stübig T, Imrecke J, Hüfner T. Surgical treatment of Achilles tendon rupture. [Article in German] Unfallchirurg 2010; 113: 712–720

Cottom JM, Hyer CF, Berlet GC, Lee TH. Flexor hallucis tendon transfer with an interference screw for chronic Achilles tendinosis: a report of 62 cases. Foot Ankle Spec 2008; 1: 280–287

Maffulli N, Tallon C, Wong J, Lim KP, Bleakney R. Early weightbearing and ankle mobilization after open repair of acute midsubstance tears of the achilles tendon. Am J Sports Med 2003; 31: 692–700

McGarvey WC, Singh D, Trevino SG. Partial Achilles tendon ruptures associated with fluoroquinolone antibiotics: a case report and literature review. Foot Ankle Int 1996; 17: 496–498

Myerson MS. Achilles tendon ruptures. Instr Course Lect 1999; 48: 219–230

Insertional Tendinopathy, Traction Spur

Den Hartog BD. Insertional Achilles tendinosis: pathogenesis and treatment. Foot Ankle Clin 2009; 14: 639–650

DeOrio MJ, Easley ME. Surgical strategies: insertional achilles tendinopathy. Foot Ankle Int 2008; 29: 542–550

Gaweda K, Tarczynska M, Krzyzanowski W. Treatment of Achilles tendinopathy with platelet-rich plasma. Int J Sports Med 2010; 31: 577–583

Kearney R, Costa ML. Insertional achilles tendinopathy management: a systematic review. Foot Ankle Int 2010; 31: 689–694

Rompe JD, Furia J, Maffulli N. Eccentric loading compared with shock wave treatment for chronic insertional achilles tendinopathy. A randomized, controlled trial. J Bone Joint Surg Am 2008; 90: 52–61

van Dijk CN, van Sterkenburg MN, Wiegerinck JI, Karlsson J, Maffulli N. Terminology for Achilles tendon related disorders. Knee Surg Sports Traumatol Arthrosc 2011; 19: 835–841

Haglund Exostosis

Irwin TA. Current concepts review: insertional achilles tendinopathy. Foot Ankle Int 2010; 31: 933–939

Jerosch J, Nasef NM. Endoscopic calcaneoplasty—rationale, surgical technique, and early results: a preliminary report. Knee Surg Sports Traumatol Arthrosc 2003; 11: 190–195

Lohrer H, Arentz S. Impingement lesion of the distal anterior Achilles tendon in sub-Achilles bursitis and Haglund-pseudoexostosis-a therapeutic challenge [Article in German] Sportverletz Sportschaden 2003; 17: 181–188

Lu CC, Cheng YM, Fu YC, Tien YC, Chen SK, Huang PJ. Angle analysis of Haglund syndrome and its relationship with osseous variations and Achilles tendon calcification. Foot Ankle Int 2007; 28: 181–185

Ortmann FW, McBryde AM. Endoscopic bony and soft-tissue decompression of the retrocalcaneal space for the treatment of Haglund deformity and retrocalcaneal bursitis. Foot Ankle Int 2007; 28: 149–153

Pavlov H, Heneghan MA, Hersh A, Goldman AB, Vigorita V. The Haglund syndrome: initial and differential diagnosis. Radiology 1982; 144: 83–88

Tennis Leg

Kwak HS, Lee KB, Han YM. Ruptures of the medial head of the gastrocnemius ("tennis leg"): clinical outcome and compression effect. Clin Imaging 2006; 30: 48–53

Kwak HS, Han YM, Lee SY, Kim KN, Chung GH. Diagnosis and follow-up US evaluation of ruptures of the medial head of the gastrocnemius ("tennis leg"). Korean J Radiol 2006; 7: 193–198

Abnormalities of the Flexor Hallucis Longus Tendon (Posterior Impingement, Os Trigonum Syndrome, Partial Tear)

Ogut T, Ayhan E. Hindfoot endoscopy for accessory flexor digitorum longus and flexor hallucis longus tenosynovitis. Foot Ankle Surg 2011; 17: e7–e9

Phisitkul P, Amendola A. False FHL: a normal variant posing risks in posterior hindfoot endoscopy. Arthroscopy 2010; 26: 714–718

Rodriguez D, Devos Bevernage B, Maldague P, Deleu PA, Leemrijse T. Tarsal tunnel syndrome and flexor hallucis longus tendon hypertrophy. Orthop Traumatol Surg Res 2010; 96: 829–831

Stoller DW, Tirman PFJ, Bredella MA. Diagnostic Imaging: Orthopaedics. Philadelphia: Elsevier; 2004: 6–14

Peroneal Tendon Pathology

Blitz NM, Nemes KK. Bilateral peroneus longus tendon rupture through a bipartite os peroneum. J Foot Ankle Surg 2007; 46: 270–277

Boya H, Pinar H. Stenosing tenosynovitis of the peroneus brevis tendon associated with hypertrophy of the peroneal tubercle. J Foot Ankle Surg 2010; 49: 188–190

Cerrato RA, Myerson MS. Peroneal tendon tears, surgical management and its complications. Foot Ankle Clin 2009; 14: 299–312

Chadwick C, Highland AM, Hughes DE, Davies MB. The importance of magnetic resonance imaging in a symptomatic "bipartite" os peroneum: a case report. J Foot Ankle Surg 2011; 50: 82–86

Cooper ME, Selesnick FH, Murphy BJ. Partial peroneus longus tendon rupture in professional basketball players: a report of 2 cases. Am J Orthop 2002; 31: 691–694

Dihlmann W, Stäbler A. Gelenke—Wirbelverbindungen. Chapter16: Gelenke des Fusses einschliesslich des oberen Sprunggelenks. 4th ed. Stuttgart: Thieme; 2010

Lanz J, Wachsmuth W. Praktische Anatomie. 2nd ed. Heidelberg: Springer; 2004: 314

Leonhardt H, Tillmann B, Töndury G, Zilles K, eds. Rauber/Kopsch: Lehrbuch und Atlas der Anatomie des Menschen in 4 Bänden. Band I: Bewegungsapparat. Stuttgart: Thieme; 1987: 583

Park HJ, Cha SD, Kim HS et al. Reliability of MRI findings of peroneal tendinopathy in patients with lateral chronic ankle instability. Clin Orthop Surg 2010; 2: 237–243

Patil V, Frisch NC, Ebraheim NA. Anatomical variations in the insertion of the peroneus (fibularis) longus tendon. Foot Ankle Int 2007; 28: 1179–1182

Rademaker J, Rosenberg ZS, Delfaut EM, Cheung YY, Schweitzer ME. Tear of the peroneus longus tendon: MR imaging features in nine patients. Radiology 2000; 214: 700–704

Rademaker J, Teichgräber UK, Schröder RJ, Oestmann JW, Felix R. MRI diagnosis of injuries and diseases of peroneal tendons [Article in German] Rontgenpraxis 2001; 53: 235–240

Saupe N, Mengiardi B, Pfirrmann CW, Vienne P, Seifert B, Zanetti M. Anatomic variants associated with peroneal tendon disorders: MR imaging findings in volunteers with asymptomatic ankles. Radiology 2007; 242: 509–517

Slater HK. Acute peroneal tendon tears. Foot Ankle Clin 2007; 12: 659–674, vii

Stäbler A, Freyschmidt J, eds. Handbuch diagnostische Radiologie, muskuloskelettales System 3. Chapter9.4: Reaktive und Stress bedingte Knochenerkrankungen, Belastung bedingte Erkrankungen der Sehnen und Sehnenansätze. Heidelberg: Springer; 2005: 62

Stoller DW, Tirman PFJ, Bredella MA. Diagnostic Imaging: orthopaedics. Philadelphia: Elsevier; 2004: 6–14

Taki K, Yamazaki S, Majima T, Ohura H, Minami A. Bilateral stenosing tenosynovitis of the peroneus longus tendon associated with hypertrophied peroneal tubercle in a junior soccer player: a case report. Foot Ankle Int 2007; 28: 129–132

Peroneal Tendon Subluxation and Dislocation

Dihlmann W, Stäbler A. Gelenke–Wirbelverbindungen. Chapter16: Gelenke des Fusses einschliesslich des oberen Sprunggelenks. 4th ed. Stuttgart: Thieme; 2010: 692

Jäger M, Wirth CJ, eds. Praxis der Orthopädie. 2nd ed. Stuttgart: Thieme; 1992

Neustadter J, Raikin SM, Nazarian LN. Dynamic sonographic evaluation of peroneal tendon subluxation. AJR Am J Roentgenol 2004; 183: 985–988

Raikin SM, Elias I, Nazarian LN. Intrasheath subluxation of the peroneal tendons. J Bone Joint Surg Am 2008; 90: 992–999

Saxena A, Ewen B. Peroneal subluxation: surgical results in 31 athletic patients. J Foot Ankle Surg 2010; 49: 238–241

Walther M, Morrison R, Mayer B. Retromalleolar groove impaction for the treatment of unstable peroneal tendons. Am J Sports Med 2009; 37: 191–194

Peroneal Split Syndrome

Dihlmann W, Stäbler A. Gelenke–Wirbelverbindungen. Chapter16: Gelenke des Fusses einschliesslich des oberen Sprunggelenks. 4th ed. Stuttgart: Thieme; 2010: 692

Freccero DM, Berkowitz MJ. The relationship between tears of the peroneus brevis tendon and the distal extent of its muscle belly: an MRI study. Foot Ankle Int 2006; 27: 236–239

Lamm BM, Myers DT, Dombek M, Mendicino RW, Catanzariti AR, Saltrick K. Magnetic resonance imaging and surgical correlation of peroneus brevis tears. J Foot Ankle Surg 2004; 43: 30–36

Stoller DW, Tirman PFJ, Bredella MA. Diagnostic Imaging: Orthopaedics. Philadelphia: Elsevier; 2004: 6–14

Zammit J, Singh D. The peroneus quartus muscle. Anatomy and clinical relevance. J Bone Joint Surg Br 2003; 85: 1134–1137

Posterior Tibial Tendon Pathology

Insufficiency, Tendinosis, Partial Tear, Complete Rupture

Bluman EM, Title CI, Myerson MS. Posterior tibial tendon rupture: a refined classification system. Foot Ankle Clin 2007; 12: 233–249, v

Gluck GS, Heckman DS, Parekh SG. Tendon disorders of the foot and ankle, part 3: the posterior tibial tendon. Am J Sports Med 2010; 38: 2133–2144

Hintermann B, Knupp M. Injuries and dysfunction of the posterior tibial tendon [Article in German] Orthopade 2010; 39: 1148–1157

Kohls-Gatzoulis J, Angel JC, Singh D, Haddad F, Livingstone J, Berry G. Tibialis posterior dysfunction: a common and treatable cause of adult acquired flatfoot. BMJ 2004; 329: 1328–1333

Kong A, Van Der Vliet A. Imaging of tibialis posterior dysfunction. Br J Radiol 2008; 81: 826–836

Perry MB, Premkumar A, Venzon DJ, Shawker TH, Gerber LH. Ultrasound, magnetic resonance imaging, and posterior tibialis dysfunction. Clin Orthop Relat Res 2003; 408: 225–231

Pufe T, Petersen WJ, Mentlein R, Tillmann BN. The role of vasculature and angiogenesis for the pathogenesis of degenerative tendons disease. Scand J Med Sci Sports 2005; 15: 211–222

Trnka HJ. Dysfunction of the tendon of tibialis posterior. J Bone Joint Surg Br 2004; 86: 939–946

Accessory Navicular

Choi YS, Lee KT, Kang HS, Kim EK. MR imaging findings of painful type II accessory navicular bone: correlation with surgical and pathologic studies. Korean J Radiol 2004; 5: 274–279

Dihlmann W, Stäbler A. Gelenke–Wirbelverbindungen. Chapter16: Gelenke des Fusses einschliesslich des oberen Sprunggelenks. 4th ed. Stuttgart: Thieme; 2010: 692

Leonard ZC, Fortin PT. Adolescent accessory navicular. Foot Ankle Clin 2010; 15: 337–347

Pastore D, Dirim B, Wangwinyuvirat M et al. Complex distal insertions of the tibialis posterior tendon: detailed anatomic and MR imaging investigation in cadavers. Skeletal Radiol 2008; 37: 849–855

Perdikakis E, Grigoraki E, Karantanas A. Os naviculare: the multi-ossicle configuration of a normal variant. Skeletal Radiol 2011; 40: 85–88

Pisani G. About the pathogenesis of the so-called adult acquired pes planus. Foot Ankle Surg 2010; 16: 1–2

Scott AT, Sabesan VJ, Saluta JR, Wilson MA, Easley ME. Fusion versus excision of the symptomatic Type II accessory navicular: a prospective study. Foot Ankle Int 2009; 30: 10–15

Stoller DW, Tirman PFJ, Bredella MA. Diagnostic Imaging: Orthopaedics. Philadelphia: Elsevier; 2004: 6–14

Anterior Tibial Tendon Pathology

Tendinosis, Insertional Tendinopathy

Beischer AD, Beamond BM, Jowett AJ, O'Sullivan R. Distal tendinosis of the tibialis anterior tendon. Foot Ankle Int 2009; 30: 1053–1059

Grundy JR, O'Sullivan RM, Beischer AD. Operative management of distal tibialis anterior tendinopathy. Foot Ankle Int 2010; 31: 212–219

Schneppendahl J, Gehrmann SV, Stosberg U, Regenbrecht B, Windolf J, Wild M. The operative treatment of the degenerative rupture of the anterior tibialis tendon [Article in German] Z Orthop Unfall 2010; 148: 343–347

Rupture

Ellington JK, McCormick J, Marion C et al. Surgical outcome following tibialis anterior tendon repair. Foot Ankle Int 2010; 31: 412–417

ElMaraghy A, Devereaux MW. Bone tunnel fixation for repair of tibialis anterior tendon rupture. Foot Ankle Surg 2010; 16: e47–e50

George AT, Babu A, Davis J. Traumatic rupture of the tibialis anterior tendon associated with chronic tibialis posterior dysfunction. Foot Ankle Surg 2009; 15: 46–52

Imhoff AB, Zollinger-Kies H. Fußchirurgie. Stuttgart: Thieme; 2004: 199

Khoury NJ, el-Khoury GY, Saltzman CL, Brandser EA. Rupture of the anterior tibial tendon: diagnosis by MR imaging. AJR Am J Roentgenol 1996; 167: 351–354

Rajagopalan S, Sangar A, Upadhyay V, Lloyd J, Taylor H. Bilateral atraumatic sequential rupture of tibialis anterior tendons. Foot Ankle Spec 2010; 3: 352–355

Sammarco VJ, Sammarco GJ, Henning C, Chaim S. Surgical repair of acute and chronic tibialis anterior tendon ruptures. J Bone Joint Surg Am 2009; 91: 325–332

Schneppendahl J, Gehrmann SV, Stosberg U, Regenbrecht B, Windolf J, Wild M. The operative treatment of the degenerative rupture of the anterior tibialis tendon [Article in German] Z Orthop Unfall 2010; 148: 343–347

Waizy H, Goede F, Plaass C, Stukenborg-Colsman C. Tendinopathy of the tibialis anterior tendon : surgical management [Article in German] Orthopade 2011; 40: 630–632, 634

Subtalar Joint: Sinus Tarsi Syndrome

Choudhary S, McNally E. Review of common and unusual causes of lateral ankle pain. Skeletal Radiol 2011; 40: 1399–1413

Helgeson K. Examination and intervention for sinus tarsi syndrome. N Am J Sports Phys Ther 2009; 4: 29–37

Herrmann M, Pieper KS. Sinus tarsi syndrome: what hurts? [Article in German] Unfallchirurg 2008; 111: 132–136

Lee KB, Bai LB, Park JG, Song EK, Lee JJ. Efficacy of MRI versus arthroscopy for evaluation of sinus tarsi syndrome. Foot Ankle Int 2008; 29: 1111–1116

Lee KB, Bai LB, Song EK, Jung ST, Kong IK. Subtalar arthroscopy for sinus Tarsi syndrome: arthroscopic findings and clinical outcomes of 33 consecutive cases. Arthroscopy 2008; 24: 1130–1134

Chapter 4

Midfoot

4 Midfoot

4.1 Trauma

R. Degwert and U. Szeimies

As described in the Integral Classification of Injuries (ICI), the midfoot consists of a proximal row of bones formed by the navicular and cuboid and a distal row formed by the medial, intermediate, and lateral cuneiforms. In the AO/ASIF (Arbeitsgemeinschaft für Osteosynthese / Association for the Study of Internal Fixation) system, the Chopart joint (also called the midtarsal or transverse tarsal joint) defines the boundary line between the midfoot and hindfoot, and injuries to that joint are classified as midfoot injuries. The Lisfranc joint marks the distal boundary of the midfoot, and injuries to that joint are assigned to the forefoot.

4.1.1 Fractures of the Tarsometatarsal Joint Line (Lisfranc Fractures)

Definition

A Lisfranc fracture is a fracture that involves the tarsometatarsal joint line, with or without articular dislocation. The joint was named after Jacques Lisfranc, who established the tarsometatarsal joint line as a level for foot amputations.

> **! Note**
>
> Lisfranc fractures are among the most commonly missed severe foot injuries. They may alter the biomechanics of the foot, leading to secondary degenerative changes and chronic pain.

Not infrequently, dislocations have already reduced spontaneously by the time the foot is examined, and the patient presents with a severe capsuloligamentous disruption. Superimposed or unperceived signs and symptoms from other injuries are common, as in the case of multiple trauma patients. Pain and swelling of the midfoot in a patient with no radiographic abnormalities should always prompt further investigation.

Symptoms

- Pain and swelling, predominantly affecting the medial column
- Inability to stand on the toes
- Limitation of motion
- Flattening of the pedal arches
- Shortening of the foot
- Possible compartment syndrome

Predisposing Factors

No specific predisposing factors are known. In principle, any laxity of the capsule and ligaments may increase susceptibility to a Lisfranc injury.

Anatomy and Pathology

Anatomy

► **Joints.** Key anatomic landmarks for the Lisfranc joint line are the tarsometatarsal joints between the cuneiforms, cuboid, and bases of the metatarsals, and the intermetatarsal joints between the trapezoid-shaped *bases* of the second through fourth metatarsals. Anatomically, these joints are amphiarthroses that allow for a small degree of springy motion. The base of the second metatarsal, which extends proximally into the cuneiform row, acts as a "keystone" to help stabilize the midfoot.

► **Ligaments.** The plantar metatarsal ligaments interconnect the second through fourth metatarsals; there is no comparable connection between the first and second metatarsals. The tough Lisfranc ligament connects the first ray to the second ray. This ligament is approximately 1.5 cm × 0.5 cm thick and consists of two bands—one longitudinal and one oblique, arranged in a Y-shaped configuration. The Lisfranc ligament extends from the medial cuneiform to the base of the first metatarsal and to the ligament at the base of the second metatarsal.

► **Pedal arches.** The longitudinal arch of the foot is supported by ligaments (plantar calcaneonavicular ligament, plantar ligament, plantar aponeurosis) and by the flexor muscles. The transverse arch derives its ligamentous support from the plantar calcaneonavicular ligament and deep transverse metatarsal ligament. It receives most of its muscular support from portions of the posterior tibial tendon and peroneus longus muscle ("stirrup" function) and from the intrinsic muscles and plantar fascia, all of which interact dynamically to maintain the integrity of the plantar vault.

► **Vessels and nerves.** The perforating branch of the dorsal pedal artery and the deep peroneal nerve run between the first and second metatarsals to the plantar arch and are highly susceptible to injuries.

Pathology

Lisfranc fractures are rare (0.2% of all fractures). They are caused mainly by high-impact trauma—in motor vehicle accidents, for example—but may also result from low-energy trauma due to a stumble or fall (axial compression trauma with the forefoot in a fixed position). Common associated injuries include lesions of the cuneiform bones and fractures of the calcaneocuboid joint, navicular, and metatarsal heads.

Mechanisms of Injury

- *Abduction injury:* This mechanism involves forceful abduction of the forefoot while the hindfoot is fixed in place, causing lateral displacement of the metatarsals with a fracture through the base of the second metatarsal (e.g., a fall from horseback with the foot fixed in the stirrup).
- *Plantar flexion injury:* This mechanism involves sudden, forceful plantar hyperflexion of the forefoot while the ankle joint is plantar-flexed and the hindfoot is in an equinus position,

Table 4.1 Quenu and Kuss classification of Lisfranc fracture-dislocations

Type	Description
A	Lateral dislocation of multiple rays
B	Partial dislocation with incomplete homolateral displacement
• B1	Isolated medial displacement of the first ray
• B2	Lateral displacement of the second through fifth metatarsals
C	Divergent dislocation in the Lisfranc joint line with medial displacement of the first metatarsal and lateral displacement of the other metatarsals

leading to dorsal dislocation of the proximal metatarsals. This may be caused, for example, by landing on tiptoes in ballet, falling backwards with the forefoot fixed, or sudden high-velocity compression in the longitudinal direction (most common form).

- *Dislocation injury:* homolateral dorsolateral dislocation of all five metatarsals.

Classification

The Quenu and Kuss system is most widely used for the classification of Lisfranc fracture-dislocations (▶ Table 4.1; ▶ Fig. 4.1 and ▶ Fig. 4.2).

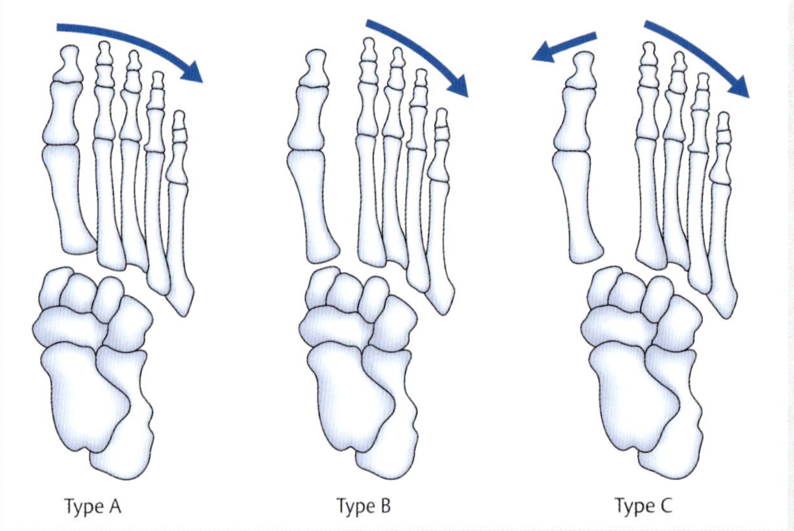

Fig. 4.1 Quenu and Kuss classification of Lisfranc fracture-dislocations.

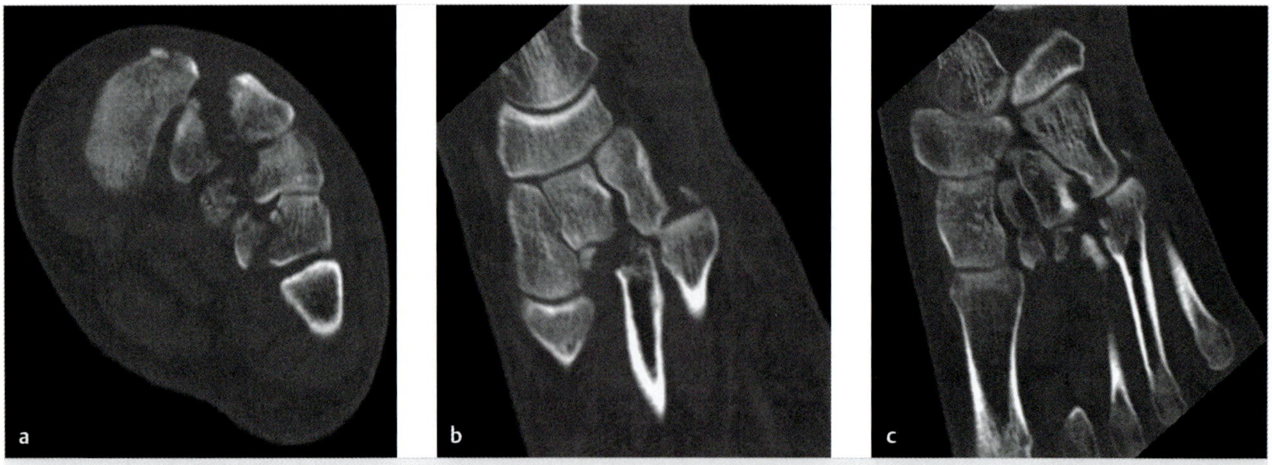

Fig. 4.2 a–c CT images of a Quenu and Kuss type B Lisfranc fracture-dislocation in a 36-year-old woman.
a Axial MPR with a 0.5-mm slice thickness and 0.3-mm interslice gap shows a fracture through the base of the second and third metatarsals with lateral displacement.
b Coronal reformatted image shows complete dorsolateral dislocation of the base of the second metatarsal accompanied by partial dorsolateral dislocation of the base of the third metatarsal.
c Coronal reformatted image shows fractures at the base of the fourth metatarsal and a bony capsular avulsion from the cuboid with lateral displacement. The first ray is intact and shows no evidence of a fracture.

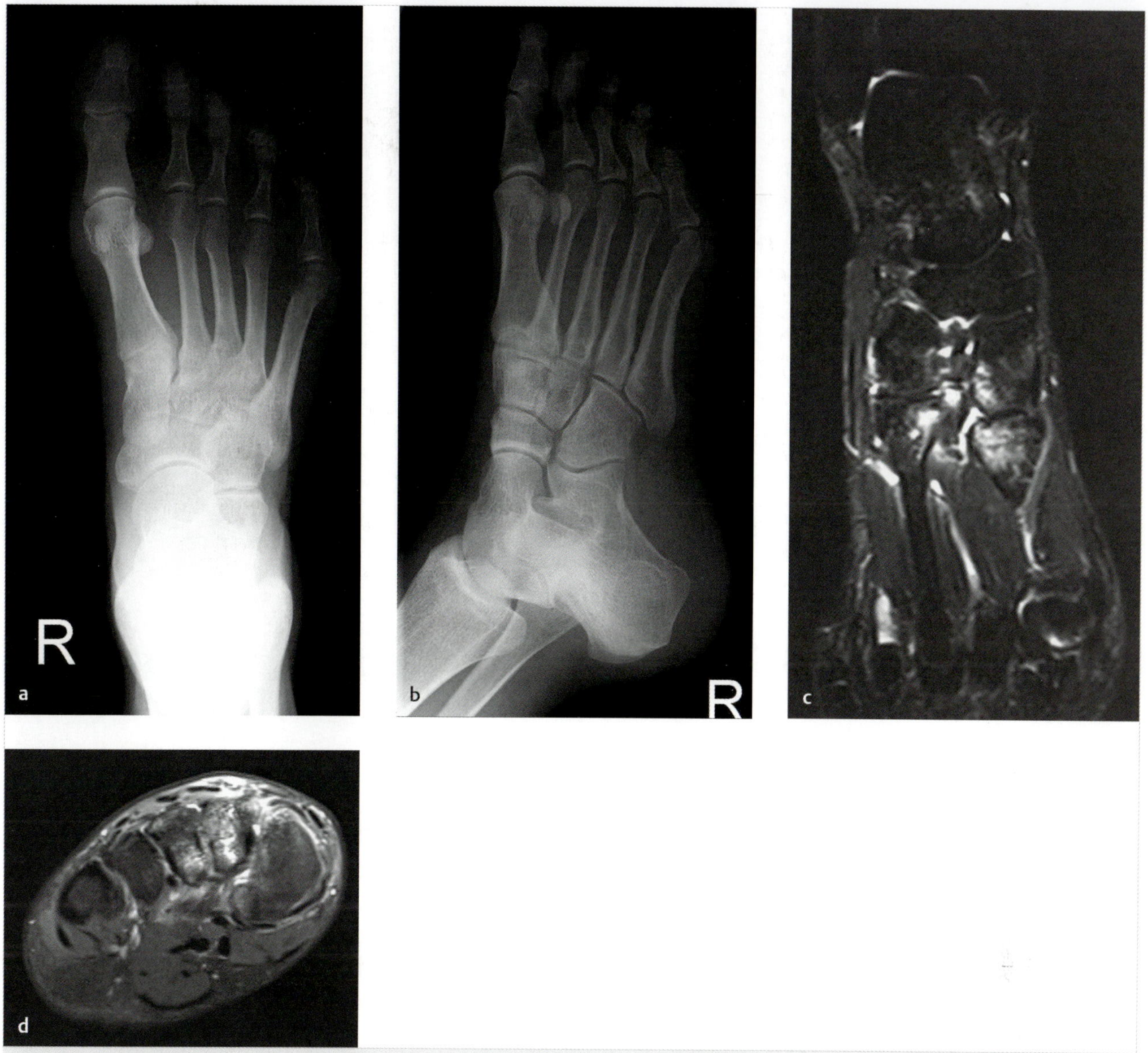

Fig. 4.3 a–d Lisfranc fracture. Four weeks earlier this female patient had suffered an ankle sprain followed by recurring pain in the midfoot, most pronounced between the bases of the first and second metatarsals. X-ray films taken elsewhere were reportedly negative.
a DP radiograph of the foot with the tube angled 20° from the vertical. The intertarsal joint line shows possible irregularities but is difficult to evaluate.
b Supine oblique radiograph of the foot reveals a fracture at the base of the second metatarsal, prompting further investigation by MRI.
c MRI: Coronal STIR sequence shows fracture edema along the Lisfranc joint line from the first to third metatarsals.
d Axial PD-weighted fat-sat image shows a basal fracture of the right second metatarsal, edema along the diaphysis of the second metatarsal, and marked contusional bone edema at the base of the first and third metatarsals.

Imaging (▶ Fig. 4.3 and ▶ Fig. 4.4)

Ultrasound

Ultrasound scans may show a plantar hematoma, a dislocation, or a surface discontinuity indicating the presence of a fracture. Ultrasound is useful only as an adjunct to other modalities.

Radiographs

- Dorsoplantar (DP) view of the foot with the tube angled 20° from the vertical
- Supine lateral view of the foot
- Special views: oblique midfoot, 45° lateromedial and 45° mediolateral
- If necessary, the study may include static or dynamic stress radiographs. Anesthesia may be given to evaluate forefoot abduction relative to the stabilized hindfoot and midfoot or relative to the opposite side.

! Note

Abnormalities are often difficult to appreciate on X-ray films due to superimposed structures. Approximately 20% of all injuries are missed on AP and oblique radiographs.

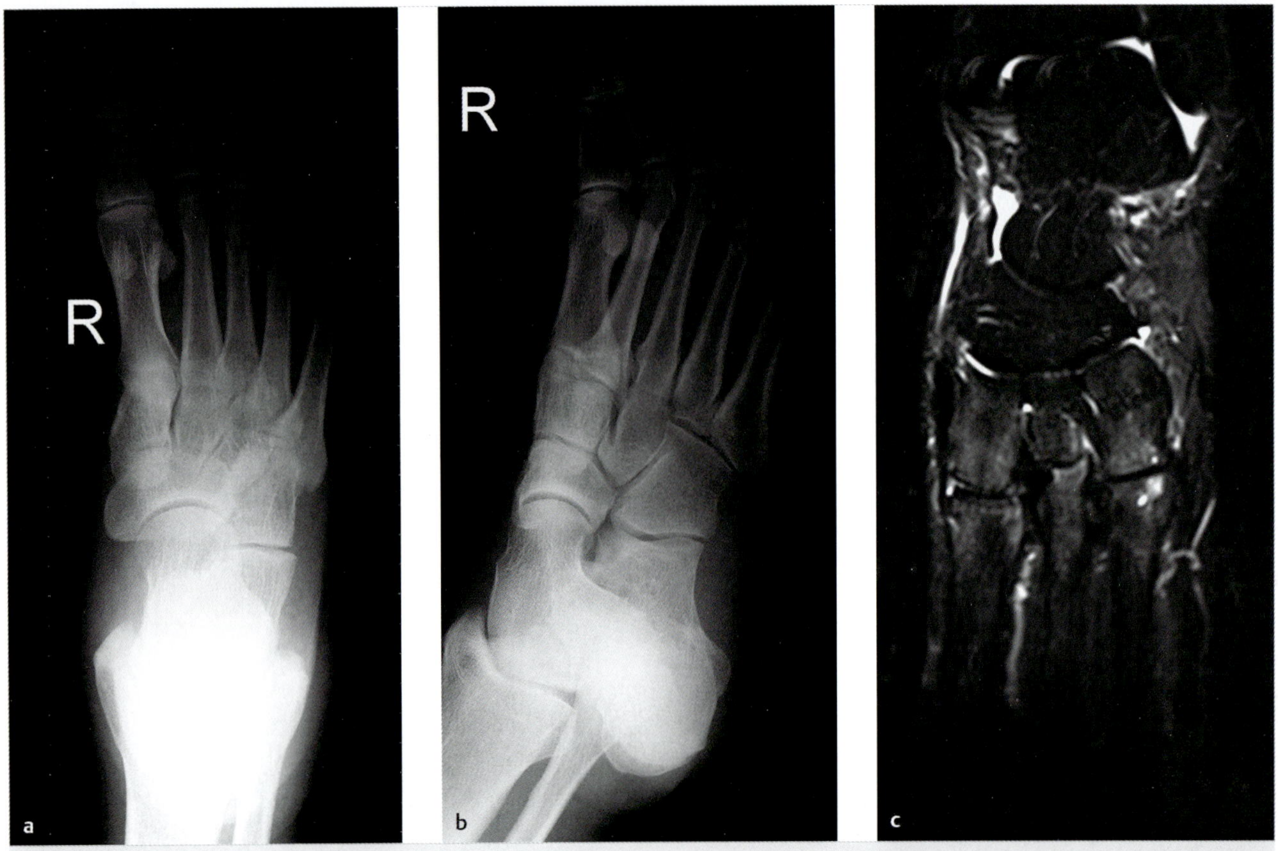

Fig. 4.4 a–c Fractures of the tarsometatarsal joint line (Lisfranc fracture) caused by direct impact trauma. X-ray films taken on site were declared to be negative, but the patient continued to have pain. Only sectional imaging can define the full extent of the injury and direct surgical planning.
a DP radiograph of the foot shows intermetatarsal unsharpness between the first and second metatarsals with a normal distance between the medial cuneiform and base of the second metatarsal.
b Supine oblique radiograph of the foot shows a questionable fracture at the base of the second metatarsal.
c MRI: Coronal STIR sequence shows contusional edema along the tarsometatarsal joint line from the first to third metatarsals.

Important signs:

- Distance between the medial cuneiform and second metatarsal > 2.5 mm: injury to the Lisfranc ligament
- Disruption of the normally straight line along the medial border of the second metatarsal and the intermediate cuneiform on a DP radiograph

CT

Accurate evaluation requires high-resolution midfoot CT with isotropic voxels (ca. 0.5-mm slice thickness) and multiplanar reformatting (MPR) views. Three-dimensional (3D) rendering is helpful in patients with complex fracture-dislocations and may include bone segmentation to improve visualization of the fractured joint lines and aid preoperative planning (ideally the radiologist and foot surgeon can work together on interactive displays at the CT workstation).

MRI

MRI is excellent for visualizing a traumatic injury to the Lisfranc ligament.

Interpretation Checklist

- Evaluate the alignment of the Lisfranc joint line
- Evaluate articular step-offs and degree of disintegration
- Describe axial malalignment
- Accurately describe the capsuloligamentous structures, even in the absence of gross incongruity
- Specifically address the integrity of the Lisfranc ligament
- Check for associated injuries

! Note

Clinical and radiologic findings may suggest the possibility of an impending compartment syndrome. Sometimes this can be difficult to recognize. Suggestive signs are marked soft-tissue swelling and possible denervation edema of muscles on MRI.

Examination Technique

- *Standard protocol:* prone position, high-resolution multichannel coil

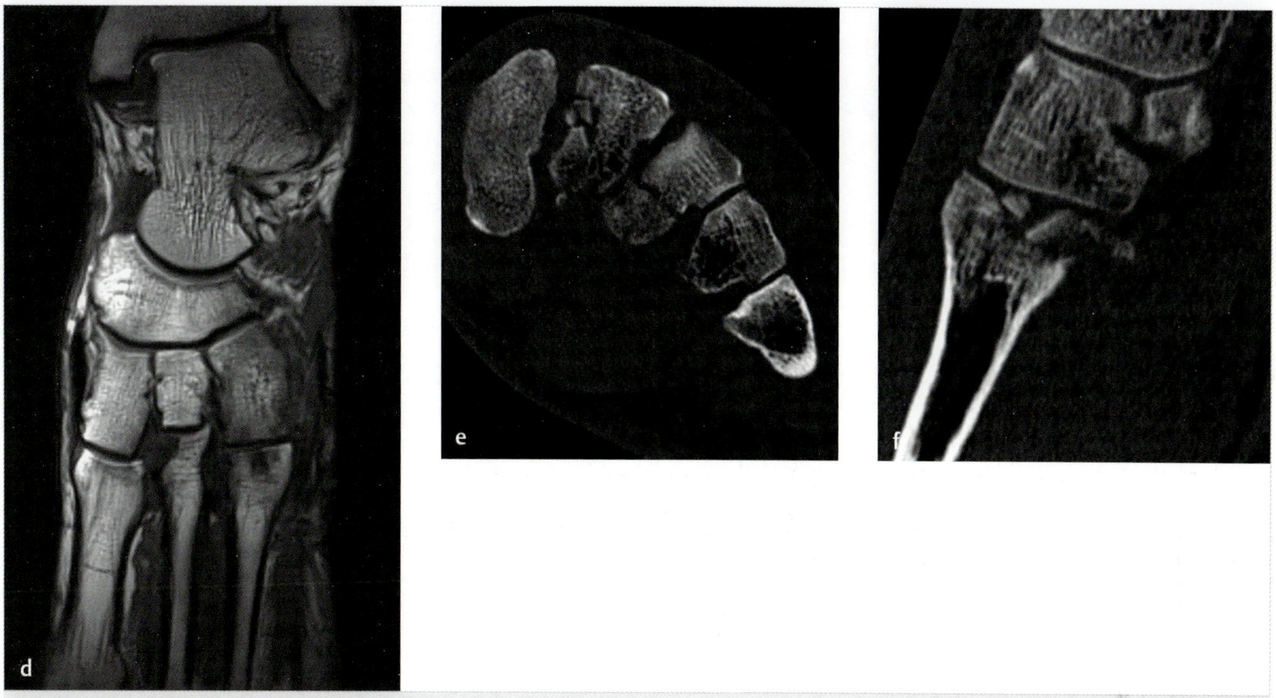

Fig. 4.4 d–f Fractures of the tarsometatarsal joint line (Lisfranc fracture) caused by direct impact trauma. X-ray films taken on site were declared to be negative, but the patient continued to have pain. Only sectional imaging can define the full extent of the injury and direct surgical planning.
d Coronal T1-weighted image shows a bony avulsion with bleeding and tearing of the Lisfranc ligament at the base of the second metatarsal, accompanied by intracapsular hemorrhage of the Lisfranc joint at the level of the third metatarsal.
e Axial CT shows a multipart fracture of the base of the second metatarsal with bony avulsion of the Lisfranc ligament and a nondisplaced fracture of the third metatarsal base.
f Sagittal CT shows disintegration of the tarsometatarsal articular surface of the second metatarsal.

- *Sequences:*
  - Coronal double-oblique STIR (short-tau inversion recovery) and T1-weighted
  - Sagittal PD (proton density)-weighted fat-sat (aligned on the metatarsal showing greatest clinical abnormality; use different sagittal planes for the first and fifth metatarsals)
  - Axial T2-weighted
  - Contrast administration is not required
  - Fat-suppressed water-sensitive sequences (STIR is best for fracture detection, while PD-weighted fat-sat gives better anatomical detail)
  - Always image the Lisfranc joint line in three planes

MRI Findings

- Areas of hemorrhage and edema in the soft tissues of the midfoot
- Marked bone marrow edema caused by fractures and contusions or cancellous bone fractures at the bases of the metatarsals, the cuneiforms, and the cuboid

! Note

Joints should be carefully surveyed in all planes to confirm normal articulation

Imaging Recommendation

Modalities of choice: In clinically suspicious cases and especially in cases with abnormal X-ray findings, sectional imaging studies should be initiated without delay. Start with high-resolution MRI of the midfoot, giving attention to possible ligamentous and bony injuries. Fracture-dislocations with multiple fragments are more anatomically complex and should be evaluated further by CT with MPRs and 3D rendering.

Differential Diagnosis

- Cuneiform dislocation
- Lateral sprain injury (e.g., bifurcate ligament, anterior talofibular ligament, calcaneofibular ligament)
- Jones fracture of the fifth metatarsal base
- Navicular fracture
- Subtalar sprain

Treatment

Conservative

- Rarely indicated
- Appropriate for grade I 4.1.2 Lisfranc Ligament Injury (p. 136)
- For dislocations of the Lisfranc joint line with no apparent tendency to redislocate: non–weight bearing in a short leg cast for 4 to 6 weeks, followed by progression to full weight-bearing in a walker boot
- Further rehabilitation may include sensorimotor training (e.g., the Janda program), training therapy, tailored gait and coordination exercises, and orthotic care

- Mobilization may be supported by injection or infiltration therapy, chiropractic therapy, osteopathy, and orthovolt therapy
- The patient should not return to sports participation for 4 to 6 months

Operative

Surgical treatment is indicated in patients with > 2 mm of displacement and in patients with unstable injuries.

- *Complete dislocation:* emergency reductions can be done in nonfasted patients (closed technique may be used) and then stabilized surgically with a Kirschner wire, screw arthrodesis, or an external fixation device. Reductions should be centered on the second metatarsal (the "key fragment"), followed by reduction and stabilization of the first metatarsal and then the third through fifth metatarsals.
- *Fracture with a subluxated position:* Surgical planning is based on CT scans and, if necessary, MRI. Reduction begins with the second ray, then proceeds to the first ray and the lateral rays. The tarsometatarsal joints can be transfixed with screws or stabilized by dorsal plating. Kirschner wires should be used in patients with critical soft tissues. The only indication for primary arthrodesis is the complete destruction of the first through third tarsometatarsal joints. Transfixation should be in line with the Lisfranc ligament for grade II and III ligament injuries.
- *Postoperative care:* non-weight bearing in a walker boot for 6 to 8 weeks. A foot that is stable for exercise can be mobilized without weight bearing. Progression to full weight bearing may be started when radiographs confirm fracture healing and transfixation screws have been removed. Screws placed across articular surfaces are removed at 6 to 8 weeks.

Prognosis, Complications

Possible complications:

- Compartment syndrome: requires emergency incision of the four plantar compartments and the dorsal compartment. Compartmental pressures should be measured, if possible, but decompression incisions should be made, even if doubt exists
- Injury to the dorsal pedal artery
- Persistent or chronic instability, deformity, displacement, posttraumatic osteoarthritis, chronic pain, and loss of foot mechanics
- Rare: avascular necrosis of the cuneiforms, complex regional pain syndrome (CRPS)

4.1.2 Lisfranc Ligament Injury

Definition

A Lisfranc ligament injury is an injury of the ligament that connects the medial cuneiform to the second metatarsal.

Symptoms

The clinical picture is highly variable, ranging from nonspecific local pain on pressure and weight bearing to deformity with diastasis between the first and second rays.

- Pain in the first tarsometatarsal joint
- Swelling of the midfoot region
- Inability to bear weight on the affected foot
- Pain on palpation along the tarsometatarsal joints and in response to a pronation or abduction stress
- It often takes several days for plantar hematoma to appear
- Inability to stand on the toes (always compare both sides)

Predisposing Factors

None.

Anatomy and Pathology

See also 4.1.1 Fractures of the Tarsometatarsal Joint Line (Lisfranc Fractures) (p. 131)

Anatomy

Injury to the Lisfranc ligament is discussed as a separate entity because of its major functional importance. The weak point in the six articulations comprising the Lisfranc joint line is the absence of a direct intermetatarsal connection between the bases of the first and second metatarsals. The first ray is connected to the second ray only by the cuneometatarsal ligament (Lisfranc ligament, ▶ Fig. 4.5). Unlike the four lateral metatarsals, whose bases are interconnected by stable ligament bands,

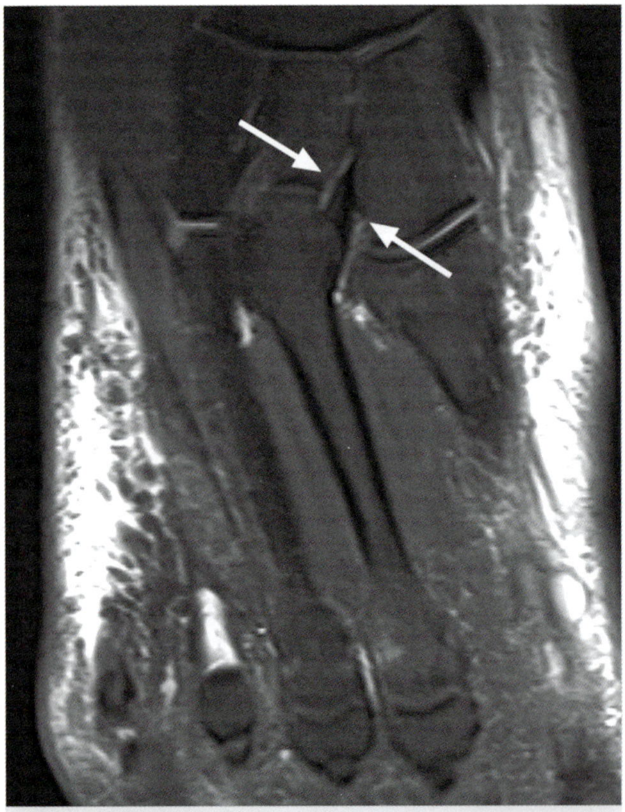

Fig. 4.5 Normal MRI appearance of the Lisfranc ligament. Coronal PD-weighted fat-sat image shows a hypointense interosseous ligament running obliquely from the medial cuneiform to the base of the second metatarsal (arrows).

no transverse ligament exists between the first and second metatarsal bases. The strongest ligament within the Lisfranc ligament complex is the interosseous ligament; the plantar and dorsal elements are weaker. These anatomic factors account for the high relevance of injuries to the Lisfranc ligament.

Pathology

Mechanism of Injury

A rupture of the Lisfranc ligament leads to significant instability. The injury is often missed or misinterpreted on initial examination, resulting in significant, persistent complaints. Most injuries occur when the midfoot is twisted while the forefoot is fixed to the ground (e.g., by a cleated shoe). This force causes dorsal displacement of the second metatarsal base with associated diastasis between the bases of the first and second metatarsals.

Classification

- Classification by the width of the diastasis (can provide a rough guide):
  - Stage I: < 2 mm diastasis
  - Stage II: > 2 mm diastasis
- Nunley and Vertullo classification (a more precise classification); ▶ Table 4.2

Imaging

Ultrasound

Ultrasound has only a minor role in the routine work-up of these injuries. Increased distance between the medial cuneiform and second metatarsal base, or diastasis increasing to more than 2.5 mm on the weight-bearing radiograph, provide indirect signs of a ruptured Lisfranc ligament. Plantar hematoma may be noted in recent injuries.

Radiographs

- *Radiographs of the foot in three planes.* Caution: non–weight-bearing radiographs often show no abnormalities!
- *Dorsoplantar (DP) and lateral weight-bearing radiographs with side-to-side comparison.* The following are indirect signs of a Lisfranc ligament rupture:
  - DP: difference in the gap between the base of the first and second cuneiforms is > 2.5 mm
  - Lateral: depressed position of the first metatarsal relative to the fifth metatarsal (measured from the plantar cortex of the first metatarsal at the level of the base to the plantar cortex of the fifth metatarsal)
- *Alternative stress radiographs:* abduction and adduction stress can be applied under fluoroscopic control according to the mechanism of injury (may require anesthesia). Stress radiographs can yield more qualitative information than weight-bearing views.

CT

CT is used only to exclude a fracture in cases where MRI findings are equivocal and have therapeutic implications.

MRI

Interpretation Checklist

- Continuity of the Lisfranc ligament
- Location of the tear
- Bony avulsion
- Complete fiber disintegration in all portions of the ligament
- Evaluate alignment
- Alignment and congruity of the first and second Lisfranc joints and of the remaining tarsometatarsal articulations
- Exclude associated injuries

Examination Technique

- *Standard protocol:* Prone position, high-resolution multichannel coil; contrast administration is not required.
- *Sequences:*
  - Double-oblique coronal PD-weighted fat-sat and T1-weighted images of the midfoot
  - Sagittal PD-weighted fat-sat (aligned on the first or second metatarsal)
  - Axial PD-weighted fat-sat
  - Axial T2-weighted
  - Coronal STIR sequence may be added to check for any associated bone contusions or fractures

MRI Findings (▶ Fig. 4.6 and ▶ Fig. 4.7)

Often the Lisfranc ligament is not completely torn from its attachment, and fat-suppressed images show hyperintense bleeding in and along the ligament with very poor delineation of individual fiber structures. These findings suggest a sprain of the Lisfranc ligament, which may also cause significant instability. There may be associated bleeding into the joint capsule and soft tissues as well as focal bone contusion edema or malalignment of the first and second metatarsals.

Imaging Recommendation

The modality of choice is MRI. In recent years MRI has replaced weight-bearing and stress radiographs in clinically suspicious

Table 4.2 Nunley and Vertullo classification of Lisfranc ligament injuries

Grade	Description
I	Sprain of the Lisfranc ligament. Weight-bearing radiographs show no abnormalities. MRI may show signal change in the Lisfranc ligament complex but does not show a discontinuity
II	2–5 mm diastasis on weight-bearing radiographs. Lateral radiographs show no difference between the affected and unaffected foot. MRI may reveal a partial tear of the ligaments
III	Extensive disruption of the dorsal and plantar elements with pronounced instability of the first ray; diastasis between the first and second metatarsals; decreased medial arch height on weight-bearing radiograph (plantar cortex of the first metatarsal is lower than that of the fifth metatarsal)

cases with no radiographic abnormalities. MRI is well tolerated even by patients in pain and is sensitive enough to visualize the ligament injury. It can also detect other injuries that may be missed on radiographs.

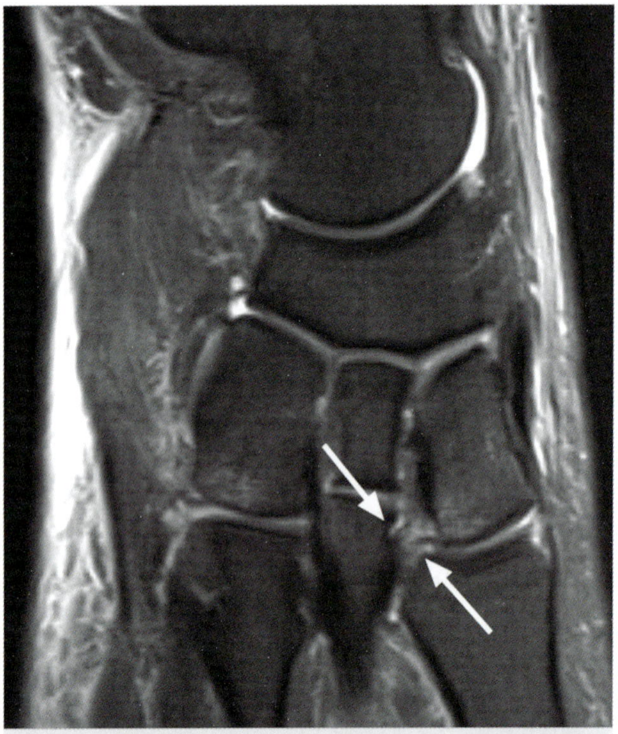

Fig. 4.6 Rupture of the Lisfranc ligament in a 19-year-old woman with persistent midfoot pain following a stumble. The ligament (arrows) has low signal intensity in the coronal PD-weighted fat-sat image. The interosseous fibers are elongated, edematous, and show continuity disruption. A faint, focal area of bone contusion is visible at its attachment to the distal medial cuneiform. Injury to the capsule and ligaments of the third tarsometatarsal joint is also noted.

Differential Diagnosis

- Injury to the calcaneocuboid joint
- Proximal metatarsal fractures
- Cuneiform fractures

Treatment

Conservative

- Nunley and Vertullo grade I injuries with less than 2 mm of diastasis can be treated conservatively in a walker boot or non–weight-bearing short leg cast for 4 to 6 weeks.
- Progress to weight bearing supported by an orthotic insert.
- Sports participation may be resumed at 4 to 6 months.
- With chronic instability, consider secondary surgical treatment by arthrodesis.

Operative

- *Fresh injury of grade II or higher (> 2 mm diastasis):* closed reduction and screw fixation of the ruptured ligament. If other instabilities are also present, additional fixation screws can be placed between the first and second metatarsals and through the first tarsometatarsal joint. The screws are removed at 8 weeks, followed by progression to full weight bearing aided by orthotics.
- *Chronic instability with intact joints:* ligament reconstruction with plantaris longus tendon is an option. Fixation screws are placed for 8 weeks as in a fresh injury.
- *Chronic instability with significant degenerative changes in the first tarsometatarsal joint or with an established secondary fixed deformity:* arthrodesis of the first tarsometatarsal joint is combined with correction of the deformity.

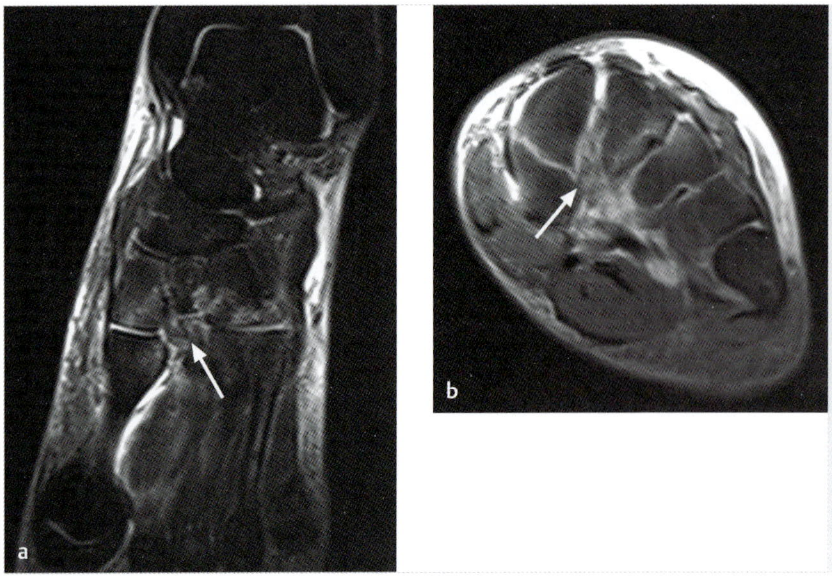

Fig. 4.7 a, b Severe Lisfranc joint injury with an extensive rupture of the Lisfranc ligament.
a Coronal STIR sequence shows bone contusions and fracture edema along the Lisfranc joint line with distal avulsion and bleeding of the Lisfranc ligament (arrow).
b Axial PD-weighted fat-sat image shows fractures of the medial cuneiform and second metatarsal base with advanced traumatic disintegration of the Lisfranc ligament (arrow). Fractures of the third and fourth metatarsal bases are also visible.

Prognosis, Complications

Prognosis

! Note

A good outcome requires prompt treatment that is tailored to the stage of the injury.

Most patients can return to their original performance level after appropriate treatment. The prognosis is significantly poorer if treatment is delayed.

Possible Complications

- Lisfranc fractures are often combined with ligamentous injuries
- Underestimating or missing the injury (sometimes due to spontaneous reduction)
- Compartment syndrome
- Chronic joint instability with chronic pain, painful posttraumatic (midfoot) osteoarthritis

4.1.3 Navicular Fracture

Definition

Fracture of the boat-shaped bone located between the talus and cuneiforms.

Symptoms

- Pain
- Hematoma
- Malalignment or deformity
- Decreased forefoot mobility and weight-bearing ability
- Forefoot malalignment (medial angulation of the forefoot due to dislocation of the talar head)
- Stress fracture: load-dependent complaints

Predisposing Factors

- Tarsal coalition
- Hindfoot arthrodesis
- Vascular insufficiency predisposing to stress fractures

Anatomy and Pathology

Anatomy

The navicular bone is the keystone of the medial longitudinal arch or medial column of the foot. It is a bony slab with surfaces that articulate with the talar head (spheroidal type of joint motion) and with the medial, intermediate, and lateral cuneiforms. The talonavicular joint is the central joint for all complex movements of the foot. The navicular is at risk for posttraumatic osteonecrosis due to the relatively poor blood supply to its central third.

The navicular bone consists of three segments:

- Proximal segment: talar facet
- Middle segment: body, tuberosity, and cuboid facet
- Distal segment: distal facet and adjacent bone

Pathology

Mechanism of Injury

Navicular fractures comprise 37% of all fractures of the foot. Associated injuries are common. The complex motions of the bone give rise to various potential mechanisms of navicular fractures: forced plantar flexion and inversion, forced eversion, and direct or indirect trauma. A stress fracture is the result of excessive pronation of the foot, which may occur in running athletes, for example. Several morphologic types of navicular fracture are distinguished:

- *Avulsion fractures* (bony avulsions of the dorsal capsule): These fractures are caused by forced plantar flexion and inversion that is sufficient to avulse the insertion of the talonavicular ligament.
- *Tuberosity fractures* (insertion of the posterior tibial tendon, anterior deltoid ligament, and spring ligament): Avulsion fractures of the navicular tuberosity result from forced eversion of the foot causing a bony avulsion of the medial stabilizing structures (insertion of the posterior tibial tendon, anterior deltoid ligament, and spring ligament).
- *Navicular body fractures:* Fractures of the navicular body result from direct or indirect trauma caused by a fall and plantar flexion, or by plantar flexion and abduction of the metatarsal joint.
- *Stress fractures:* A stress fracture results from excessive pronation, which may occur in running athletes, for example. Chopart fracture-dislocations account for 15% of all talar injuries and 1% of all dislocations. Approximately 80% of patients have a chain of injuries in the affected limb. A "nutcracker" fracture of the navicular is caused by forcible adduction, which is usually combined with an axial force (also tearing the bifurcate ligament).

! Note

Because high-impact trauma is common, the patterns of injury are often complex. It is important, therefore, to evaluate the entire Chopart (midtarsal) joint. Dislocations without bony involvement are extremely rare, because considerable force is needed to dislocate the joint due to the strong ligament restraints. Dislocations are usually one component of a complex foot injury.

Classifications

- *AO/ASIF and OTA* (Orthopaedic Trauma Association) classifications:
  - 83A: simple
  - 83B: comminuted
- *Classification of Sangeorzan et al:* ▸ Table 4.3
- *Special fracture types*:
  - Avulsion fracture: dorsal cortical avulsion at the insertion of the dorsal talonavicular ligament
  - Fracture of the navicular tuberosity: bony avulsion of the posterior tibial tendon insertion
  - Stress fracture: most commonly affects the central (hypovascular) third

Table 4.3 Sangeorzan classification of navicular fractures

Type	Description
1	Transverse fracture with bony avulsion of the anterior tibial tendon
2	Transverse fracture with a nondisplaced lateral fragment and displaced medial fragment (most common type)
3	Comminuted fracture with central or lateral fragmentation (comminution) plus injury to the calcaneocuboid joint and hindfoot varus deformity

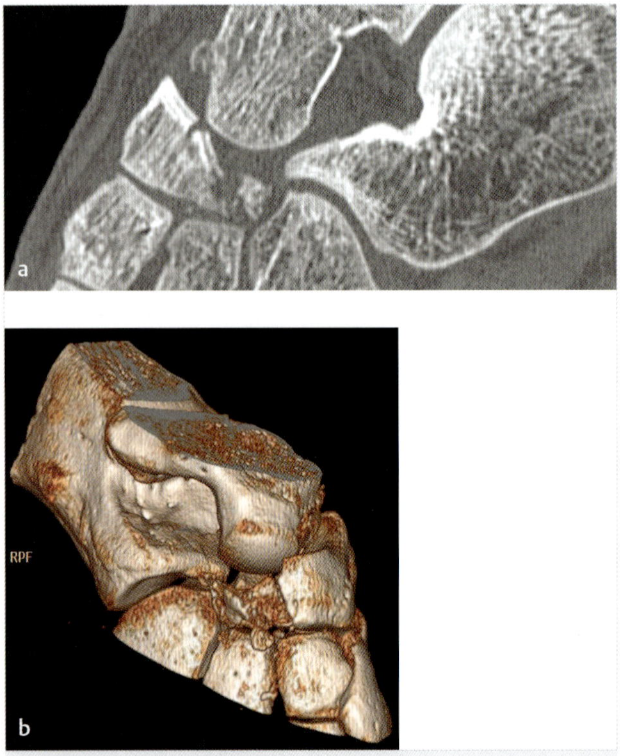

Fig. 4.8 a, b CT for planning the operative treatment of a lateral comminuted navicular fracture.
a Sagittal reformatted image (data set with 0.5-mm slice thickness, 0.3-mm interslice gap, 120 kV, 80 mA) of the navicular fracture shows impaction of the articular surface in the talonavicular joint.
b A 3D VR (virtual reality) image provides a more detailed view of the articular surfaces.

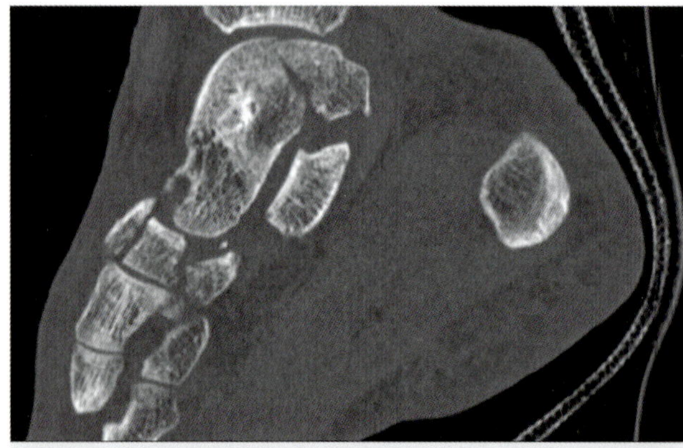

Fig. 4.9 CT following a severe compression injury. Sagittal reformatted CT image of a complex hindfoot and midfoot fracture displays multiple navicular fragments with detachment of the posterior talar dome.

Imaging

Radiographs

The initial imaging study of choice is plain radiography in four planes. If a fracture is not found, it may be necessary to obtain stress radiographs with a forefoot adduction or abduction stress as well as AP or posteroanterior (PA) (i.e., dorsoplantar or plantodorsal) and lateral weight-bearing views of the foot. Comparative views of the opposite foot may also be obtained if necessary.

The best landmark for radiographic orientation is the Cyma line, which is an S-shaped line formed by the talonavicular and calcaneocuboid joints on the lateral radiograph. Any break or incongruity in the S-shaped curve is suggestive of a fracture.

Navicular stress fractures are detected in only 33% of initial plain radiographs. It takes 3 to 10 days for bone resorption to appear at the fracture site. If a stress fracture is suspected, MRI should be instituted without delay.

Ultrasound

Ultrasound can demonstrate (plantar) hematoma, displacement, and a visible step-off or fracture. It is used only as an adjunct to radiographs and CT.

CT (▶ Fig. 4.8 and ▶ Fig. 4.9)

CT is used for fracture classification and preoperative planning.

- High-resolution (isotropic voxel) imaging of the navicular
- MPRs with submillimeter reconstruction for the complete visualization of adjacent articulating bones and joint lines, and (segmented) 3D volume-rendered imaging to evaluate complex fragments and fractured articular surfaces

MRI

MRI would not be indicated for an isolated navicular fracture. It may be used for the further evaluation of capsuloligamentous structures in dislocation injuries. MRI is appropriate in patients with a suspected stress fracture or suspected posttraumatic osteonecrosis.

Interpretation Checklist

- *Stress fracture:*
  - See also the section on Calcaneal Fractures (p. 53) in Chapter 3 and Navicular Fractures (p. 139) in Chapter 4
  - Determine extent of the stress fracture or area of bone marrow edema
  - Evaluate the bony overload reaction or fracture

- Evaluate the subchondral articular surface, surface impactions, and morphologic abnormalities
- Narrow the differential diagnosis (transient bone marrow edema syndrome, activated osteoarthritis)
- *Osteonecrosis:*
  - Extent of osteonecrosis, articular surface collapse, joint line involvement, and morphologic abnormalities
  - Initial degenerative changes in adjacent joints

Examination Technique

Contrast administration is not necessary for the evaluation of a stress fracture. It is sometimes helpful in the evaluation of osteonecrosis.

- *Standard protocol:* prone position, high-resolution multichannel coil
- *Sequences:*
  - Double-oblique coronal STIR and T1-weighted images
  - Sagittal PD-weighted fat-sat (aligned on the ankle joint)
  - Coronal PD-weighted fat-sat if required
  - Osteonecrosis additionally requires sagittal and coronal T1-weighted fat-sat imaging after contrast administration

MRI Findings

- *Stress fracture*: intense focal bone marrow edema, usually running horizontal to the talonavicular articular surface. T1-weighted imaging in advanced cases shows linear hypointensities, followed later by decreased height and flattening of the navicular with subchondral sclerosis
- *Osteonecrosis:* edema formation in the STIR sequence, usually covering a larger area with central intensity. T1-weighted imaging shows circumscribed complete loss of fatty marrow signal and absence of enhancement, sometimes with peripheral hyperperfusion

Imaging Recommendation

Modalities of choice: CT for traumatic navicular fractures, MRI for stress fractures and for evaluating osteonecrosis.

Differential Diagnosis

- Injury to the bifurcate ligament (Chopart ligament) or calcaneocuboid ligament
- Bipartite navicular
- Os tibiale externum
- Cuboid fracture
- Deltoid ligament injury
- Rupture of the posterior tibial tendon

Treatment

The basic goal is to restore the anatomy (length and stability) of the medial column of the foot.

Conservative

- Conservative treatment is an option for nondisplaced fractures or dislocations, well-positioned fractures and dislocations after reduction, ligamentous injuries after reduction, and fatigue fractures with a favorable healing tendency.
- Nondisplaced fractures: non–weight-bearing short leg cast for 8 to 10 weeks, then gradual progression to full weight bearing.
- Stress fractures: non–weight bearing for 6 to 10 weeks. Increasingly, percutaneous screw fixation is used due to the high risk of fracture nonunion.

Operative

- Goal: anatomical restoration of congruent joint lines, ligamentous stability, and especially the stability of the medial column
- Indication for surgical treatment: all fractures with shortening of one of the two foot columns, and depressed articular fractures with a step-off > 2 mm
- The exact procedure depends on the pattern of injury, since most patients will have a combination of different midfoot fractures and/or dislocations. Injuries will often require cancellous bone grafting or the use of synthetic bone substitutes. Temporary Kirschner-wire fixation may be necessary when dealing with small fragments, an injury prone to redislocation, or to secure the reconstructed capsule and ligaments. The K-wires are removed at approximately 6 weeks.

! Note

Open fractures and fracture-dislocations in the Chopart joint line are emergency indications for surgical treatment. If a compartment syndrome is suspected, immediate incision is required. If radiographs cannot positively confirm bony consolidation, high-resolution (submillimeter) CT with MPRs can often add significant information. Metal artifacts will generally pose no problems in scanners with isotropic voxel resolution.

The treatment of posttraumatic osteoarthritis includes arthrodesis of the talonavicular joint. Preoperative planning should employ MRI to evaluate for activated osteoarthritis in neighboring joints. If degenerative changes are found in adjacent joints, a double arthrodesis (which includes the subtalar joint) or triple arthrodesis (which also includes the calcaneocuboid joint) can be performed.

Prognosis, Complications

Possible acute complications after navicular injuries:

- Compartment syndrome
- Redislocation
- Defects in the soft-tissue envelope, infection
- Algodystrophy, decreased blood flow or avascular necrosis (can occur even with closed fracture-dislocations, slightly more common in the talus than the navicular)

Possible long-term sequelae of a navicular fracture:

- Posttraumatic osteoarthritis, chronic pain (common)
- Nonunion
- Deformity, joint instability
- Change in the bony architecture of the foot (shortening of the medial column), adversely affecting foot biomechanics

4.1.4 Cuboid Fracture

Definition

Fracture of the cube-shaped bone on the lateral side of the foot.

Symptoms

- Difficulty bearing weight on the affected foot
- Pain and swelling on the lateral side of the foot

! Note

Cuboid injury may be misdiagnosed as a simple lateral ankle sprain.

Predisposing Factors

It has been suggested that a talonavicular or talocalcaneal coalition may predispose to cuboid fractures.

Anatomy and Pathology

Anatomy

The cuboid bone is an important structural component of the lateral column of the foot. It articulates proximally with the calcaneus, medially with the navicular and lateral cuneiform, and distally with the fourth and fifth metatarsals. Its undersurface bears a groove, the peroneal sulcus, in which the long peroneal tendon runs beneath the transverse arch of the foot.
The cuboid consists of three segments:

- *Proximal segment:* calcaneal facet and adjacent bone
- *Middle segment:* body and tuberosity
- *Distal segment:* metatarsal facets with adjacent bone, including the peroneal sulcus

Pathology

Mechanism of Injury

Fractures of the cuboid are rare, and most occur through indirect mechanisms. Avulsion fractures (bony capsule and ligament avulsion in a midfoot sprain, ▶ Fig. 4.10) are distinguished from compression fractures, which are usually concomitant with other fractures. Other possible mechanisms of injury are forcible abduction of the forefoot or a lateral force applied directly to the side of the foot while the forefoot is in a fixed position.

A special type of cuboid injury is the “nutcracker” fracture, in which the cuboid is compressed between the calcaneus and base of the fourth and fifth metatarsals due to forced abduction combined with an axial stress in the midtarsal joint.

Cuboid fractures are important because they affect the lateral column of the foot and thus may lead to instability or valgus displacement of the forefoot.

Classification

AO/ASIF and OTA classifications:

- 84A: Simple
- 84B: Comminuted

Imaging

Ultrasound

Ultrasound may show bony flake fragments resulting from an avulsion fracture or dislocation as well as larger fragments or step-offs caused by the fracture. The adjacent ligaments (calcaneocuboid or bifurcate ligament) cannot be accurately evaluated with ultrasound. Ultrasound can detect a hematoma, if present.

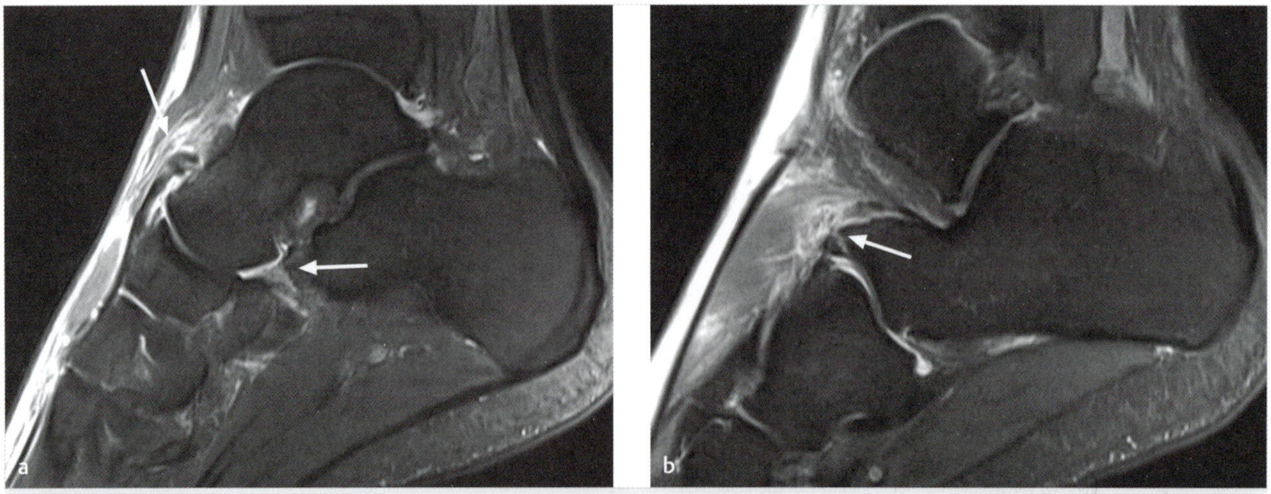

Fig. 4.10 a, b MRI of a fresh capsuloligamentous injury in the Chopart joint (talonavicular and calcaneocuboid joints) following supination trauma in a 44-year-old man. Isolated cuboid fractures are rare. Most occur as an avulsion injury of the Chopart joint with a bony avulsion of the capsule and ligaments due to a midfoot sprain.
a Sagittal PD-weighted fat-sat image shows a talar-side rupture of the talonavicular and calcaneocuboid joint capsule with injury to the bifurcate ligament (arrows).
b Sagittal PD-weighted fat-sat image shows a bony avulsion of the calcaneocuboid joint capsule with an avulsion fracture of the dorsal tip of the anterior calcaneal process, altering the alignment of the calcaneocuboid joint (arrow).

Radiographs

Radiographs of the foot in two planes and with 45° of inversion are useful for detecting abnormalities of joint position and alignment. Avulsion fractures of the calcaneocuboid ligament are usually seen most clearly on the AP radiograph. The 45° oblique inversion view shows the dorsal portions of the calcaneocuboid joint, including the anterior process of the calcaneus and the articular facets for the fourth and fifth metatarsals.

The lateral view is useful for evaluating the plantar peroneal sulcus.

CT

High-resolution thin-slice CT employs isotropic voxels and a submillimeter slice thickness so that optimum MPRs can be generated in all planes. Also 3D views can be rendered for evaluation of complex fracture types and multiple fragments. The volume segmentation of adjacent tarsal bones can be done to generate clearer views of a fractured articular surface.

MRI

Interpretation Checklist

When applied to complex fractures, MRI can be used to evaluate alignment in the Chopart joint, adjacent ligamentous structures, articular step-offs, and the position and integrity of the peroneal tendons.

Examination Technique

- *Standard protocol:* prone position, high-resolution multichannel coil
- *Sequences:*
  - Double-oblique coronal STIR and T1-weighted images
  - Sagittal PD-weighted fat-sat
  - Axial T2-weighted
  - If necessary: axial oblique PD-weighted fat-sat (angled to the tendon plane)

MRI Findings

- Bone contusion edema
- Detached bone fragments
- Significant bleeding into adjacent joint spaces and soft tissues
- Fluid or hematoma detection around the peroneal tendons, possibly displaced by a fragment
- With dislocation injuries: abnormal alignment in the Chopart joint

Imaging Recommendation

Modalities of choice: radiographs for small bony avulsion fractures, CT for fractures with articular involvement to accurately assess the step-off. In the case of more complex fractures (nutcracker) with dislocations, MRI is useful for evaluating the capsules and ligaments all along the Chopart joint line and midfoot. MRI is also useful for evaluating the peroneal tendons. MRI is the modality of choice for imaging suspected stress fractures.

Treatment

Conservative

Isolated, nondisplaced fractures can be immobilized in a plaster cast or splint for 6 to 10 weeks.

Operative

Displaced fractures are an indication for operative treatment with the goal of reconstructing the articular surfaces and the lateral column of the foot. With compression fractures of the cuboid, the use of a distractor may be the only way to restore the length of the lateral column. Defects are repaired with a corticocancellous bone graft or bone substitute. Larger fragments with articular involvement are stabilized by screw fixation, smaller fragments with Kirschner wires. Bone length can be maintained with a heavy-duty H-plate, taking care to place the screws in the stable subcortical cancellous bone of the articular surfaces. Very unstable fractures may require temporary plating or external fixation across joints to obtain adequate stabilization. Complete destruction of the calcaneocuboid joint may warrant primary arthrodesis.

Differential Diagnosis

- Midfoot sprain
- Os peroneum fracture
- Rupture of the peroneal tendon

Prognosis, Complications

Possible complications are as follows:

- Compartment syndrome
- Posttraumatic osteoarthritis
- Nonunions
- Limited motion in the midfoot
- Impingement of the long peroneal tendon in the peroneal sulcus (if lateral contour is not restored)
- Loss of lateral column length with secondary pes planovalgus
- Rare secondary tearing of the posterior tibial tendon due to improper treatment of a nutcracker fracture

4.1.5 Cuneiform Fractures

Definition

These fractures involve any of the three small bones of the tarsus: the medial, intermediate, and lateral cuneiforms.

Symptoms

- Edema
- Hematoma
- Tenderness to pressure
- Tenderness to compression
- Crepitation
- Possible generalized midfoot pain, depending on associated injuries, or a single painful focus in the medial midfoot
- Inability to bear weight on the affected foot

Predisposing Factors

No significant factors are known.

Anatomy and Pathology

Anatomy

The medial, intermediate, and lateral cuneiforms articulate distally with the first, second, and third metatarsals to form the medial part of the Lisfranc joint. The lateral cuneiform has a lateral facet that articulates with the cuboid and the base of the fourth metatarsal. Viewed in frontal section, the intermediate and lateral cuneiforms have a wedge shape that tapers toward the plantar side, thus forming the transverse arch of the foot. Each of the cuneiforms articulates with four other bones.

The cuneiforms can be divided into three segments:

- *Proximal segment:* articular surfaces for the navicular and cuboid, and proximal intercuneiform facets
- *Middle segment:* bodies and distal intercuneiform facets
- *Distal segment:* has articular surfaces for the metatarsals and adjacent bones

Pathology

Mechanism of Injury

The three cuneiforms and their joints in the foot are small and relatively well protected from injuries. Fractures may occur through a direct or indirect mechanism. Isolated fractures, especially of the lateral cuneiform, are very rare and usually result from indirect trauma. Most cuneiform fractures result from direct trauma or occur as part of a complex foot injury (e.g., Lisfranc fracture/dislocation) caused by forcible abduction or adduction of the forefoot.

Classification

The AO/ASIF classification distinguishes between simple and complex fractures but is rarely used in everyday practice:

- **A** Simple cuneiform fracture
  - **A1** Medial cuneiform
  - **A2** Intermediate cuneiform
  - **A3** Lateral cuneiform
- **B** Complex cuneiform fracture
  - **B1** Medial cuneiform
  - **B2** Intermediate cuneiform
  - **B3** Lateral cuneiform

For routine reporting, cuneiform fractures are usually characterized descriptively rather than with an alphanumeric system.

Imaging

Ultrasound

Cuneiform injuries are difficult to detect sonographically. At most, scans may contribute information by showing cortical surface irregularities (displacement, step-offs, fragments) or detecting a possible hematoma. Given their frequency, attention should always be given to possible associated injuries (e.g., vascular injuries due to direct trauma or tendon ruptures).

Radiographs

Radiographs of the foot are obtained in two planes, and oblique views are taken in 45° of eversion and 45° of inversion. Changes in bone alignment are most clearly appreciated in the DP view. Lines drawn along the medial and lateral borders of the metatarsals should run straight to the corresponding cuneiform with no offset. Lesions in the dorsal cortex are clearly visible in the lateral view. The 45° inversion view displays the first tarsometatarsal joint and plantar cortex. If doubt exists, a view of the opposite foot may be taken for comparison.

CT (▶ Fig. 4.11)

CT examination is indicated in patients with severe midfoot injuries and equivocal findings on plain radiographs. Even if radiographs have detected fractures, CT can be used for further classification and for detecting other fractures that were occult on plain films. It is common to detect cortical avulsion fractures on the plantar side of multiple cuneiforms that do not show obvious displacement or articular step-offs. In addition 3D reconstructions are helpful in evaluating complex fractures.

MRI

MRI is particularly recommended in patients with suspected ligamentous or other associated injuries. Because the signs and symptoms are often diffuse and are rarely sufficient to support the diagnosis of an isolated cuneiform fracture, MRI is preferred over CT.

Interpretation Checklist

- Accurately describe alignment in three planes
- Describe the capsuloligamentous structures, especially the Lisfranc ligament
- Exclude other injuries

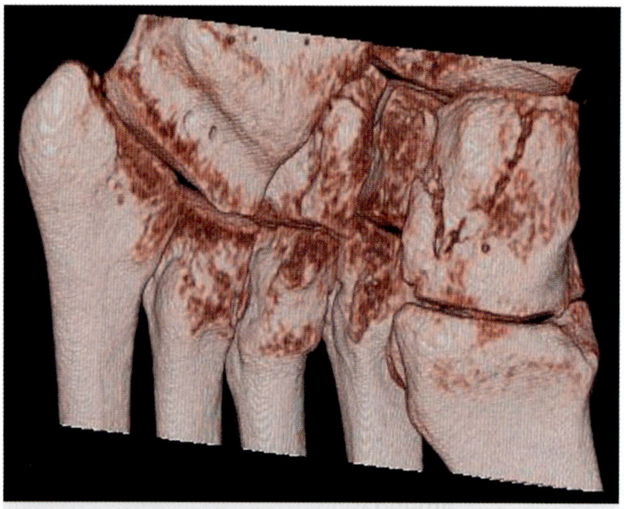

Fig. 4.11 Sprain injury in a 45-year-old man. CT displays a fresh fracture of the medial cuneiform. A 3D VR (virtual reality) image from the plantar aspect demonstrates the fracture in the medial cuneiform. MRI also showed a significant capsuloligamentous injury along the Lisfranc joint line. The fracture was treated surgically.

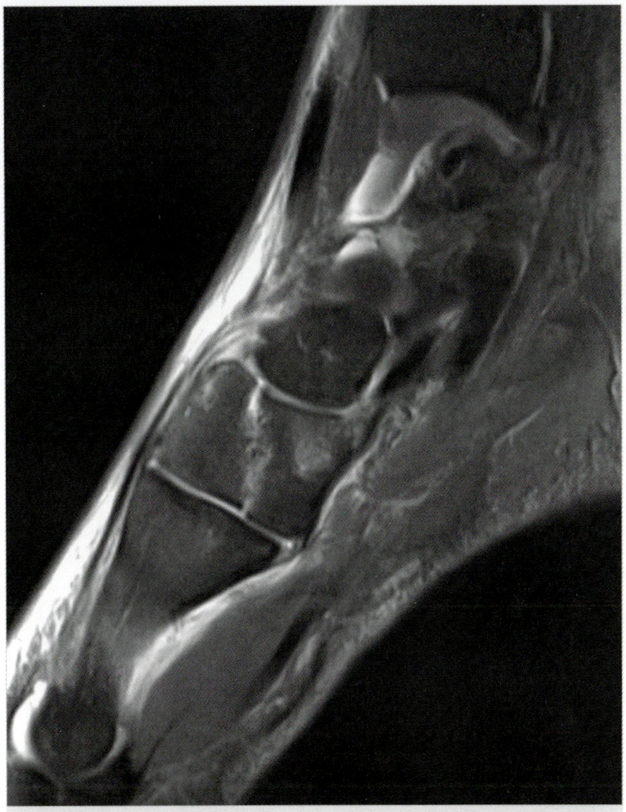

Fig. 4.12 MRI of a fresh fracture of the medial cuneiform following a severe midfoot sprain. Sagittal PD-weighted fat-sat image shows an oblique fracture line through the medial cuneiform. Severe capsuloligamentous injuries were also present, necessitating surgical treatment.

Examination Technique

- *Standard protocol:* prone position, high-resolution multichannel coil
- *Sequences:*
  - Double-oblique coronal STIR and T1-weighted images
  - Sagittal PD-weighted fat-sat (aligned on the cuneiform showing greatest clinical abnormality)
  - Axial T2-weighted
  - Axial PD-weighted fat-sat

MRI Findings (▶ Fig. 4.12)

- Bone contusion edema
- Small cortical avulsion fractures
- Hemorrhagic areas, especially in the plantar soft tissues
- Joint effusion
- Bleeding into capsuloligamentous structures
- Possible abnormal alignment (somewhat unusual)

Imaging Recommendation

Modalities of choice: Radiographs are taken for initial evaluation. CT is indicated for persistent suspicion or severe trauma and to evaluate fragments or articular step-offs. MRI may be used to evaluate capsuloligamentous tears with altered alignment, stress edema, and stress fractures.

Differential Diagnosis

- Other midfoot or hindfoot injuries
- Normal variants (bipartite medial cuneiform)
- Rubinstein–Tabyi syndrome (congenital "fourth" cuneiform located between the medial and intermediate cuneiforms)

Treatment

Conservative

Nondisplaced fractures with no associated midfoot injuries can be treated conservatively with a short leg cast or walker boot. Progression to exercise and weight bearing depends on the severity of the instability.

Operative

The goal is to restore the anatomy of the medial and lateral columns. Thus, displaced fractures and comminuted fractures are an indication for surgical treatment. Surgery is followed by 6 to 8 weeks of non–weight bearing in a short leg cast or walker boot.

Prognosis, Complications

Possible complications are as follows:

- Risk of compartment syndrome in patients with high-impact trauma and pronounced swelling
- With direct trauma: risk of neurovascular and tendon injury with a corresponding functional deficit
- Frequent persistent limited motion and risk of posttraumatic osteoarthritis

4.2 Chronic, Posttraumatic, and Degenerative Changes

U. Szeimies

4.2.1 Osteoarthritis

Talonavicular, Naviculocuneiform, and Calcaneocuboid Joints

Definition

Degenerative changes in the bones articulating with the navicular (talus and cuneiforms) and between the calcaneal anterior process and the cuboid (calcaneocuboid joint).

Symptoms

- Joint pain
- Feeling of stiffness
- Recurrent swelling
- Warm-up pain and pain during exercise
- Later on, pain at night
- Difficulty walking
- Effusion
- Decreased walking distance
- Limited motion or loss of function

- Crepitation
- Muscle splinting
- Muscular atrophy
- Increasing deformity or axial malalignment
- Instability
- Coarse joint contours
- Palpable osteophytes

Predisposing Factors

- Primary osteoarthritis: idiopathic
- Secondary osteoarthritis: posttraumatic (following a fracture or dislocation)
- Inflammatory causes (chronic rheumatoid arthritis, other arthritis, previous bacterial infection)
- Congenital deformities
- Metabolic disorders
- Age
- Sex (predilection for females)
- Overweight
- Genetic factors
- Köhler disease I (navicular ischemia and deformity)

Anatomy and Pathology

The talonavicular joint is most commonly affected. Rheumatoid arthritis should always be considered in the differential diagnosis of talonavicular joint pain. Following initial cartilage damage due to exogenous or endogenous causes, the destruction of chondrocytes leads to a decrease in the synthesis of proteoglycan and collagen. A mismatch develops between the stresses imposed on the cartilage and its ability to withstand them, leading both primarily and secondarily to generalized cartilage wear. The initial cartilage damage incites a reactive synovitis. Osteoarthritis usually runs a progressive course that includes periods of activation.

The naviculocuneiform joint is an amphiarthrosis that permits very little motion. The strong pull of the posterior tibial tendon transmits tension to the plantar vault through its attachments to the navicular, cuneiform, and cuboid bones. Additional attachments extend this functional unit to the second, third, and fourth metatarsals.

Imaging

Radiographs

Weight-bearing radiographs of the foot in three planes will show classic signs of osteoarthritis such as joint space narrowing, subchondral sclerosis, subchondral cysts, and osteophytes. Deviations of bone alignment may be noted in patients with chronic instability.

Ultrasound

Not indicated.

MRI

Interpretation Checklist

- Degree of activation of the degenerative process
- Cartilage quality
- Degree of cartilage loss as an aid to treatment planning (conservative or operative)
- Alignment in the Chopart joint line
- Signs of instability
- Monoarticular findings
- Differentiation from rheumatoid arthritis

Examination Technique

- *Standard protocol:* prone position, high-resolution multichannel coil
- *Sequences:*
  - Sagittal and coronal PD-weighted fat-sat
  - Coronal T1-weighted
  - Axial T2-weighted (angled to the plane of the ankle joint)
  - Axial oblique T1-weighted fat-sat after contrast administration (angled to the tendon plane of the talonavicular joint) and sagittal

MRI Findings (▶ Fig. 4.13 and ▶ Fig. 4.14)

- Joint space narrowing with cartilage defects
- Subchondral bony activation edema or areas of bone marrow edema
- Effusion
- Reactive synovitis

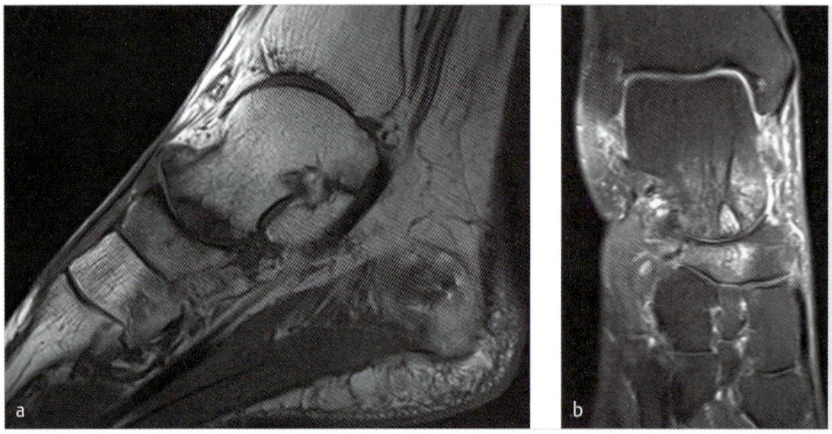

Fig. 4.13 a, b Activated talonavicular osteoarthritis in a 73-year-old woman with pain refractory to treatment.
a Sagittal T1-weighted image shows a completely obliterated joint space with an area of exposed bone in the talonavicular joint. Other findings: osteophytes along the joint capsule, an area of subchondral bone softening in the talar head, and initial deformity of the navicular.
b Coronal PD-weighted fat-sat image shows areas of bone marrow edema in the talar neck and navicular, subchondral cysts in the articulating bone ends, especially the talus, and adjacent soft-tissue edema.

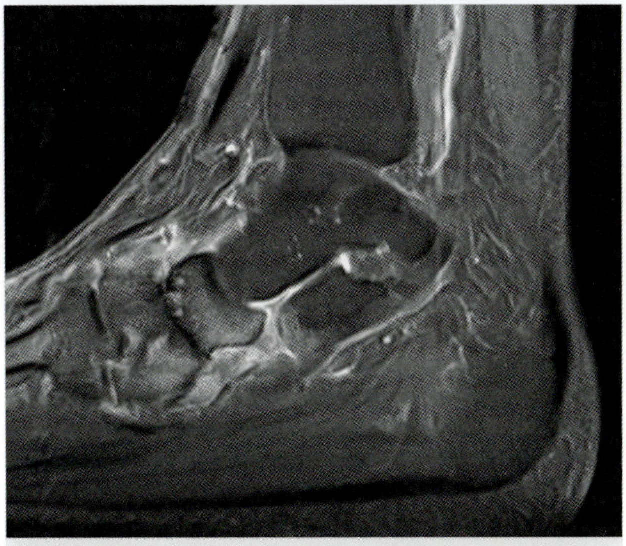

Fig. 4.14 Activated osteoarthritis in the naviculocuneiform joint. Sagittal T1-weighted fat-sat image after contrast administration shows advanced, destructive osteoarthritic changes between the navicular and the medial, intermediate and lateral cuneiforms with joint space obliteration, subchondral cysts, and marked edema of surrounding bone and soft tissues.

- Edematous joint capsule showing increased contrast enhancement
- Adjacent fluid collection and enhancement in subcutaneous fat
- Altered alignment along the Chopart joint line
- Activated osteophytes
- Subchondral cysts
- Cortical collapse in the articulating bone ends
- Remodeling of the articular surfaces
- Advanced destructive changes with adjacent joint involvement, also signs of hindfoot and midfoot tendon overload

Imaging Recommendation

Modalities of choice: radiographs for initial evaluation; MRI for further investigation of equivocal X-ray findings and to assess activation.

Differential Diagnosis

- Os tibiale externum
- Os supranaviculare
- Köhler disease I
- Stress fracture of the navicular
- Rheumatoid or bacterial arthritis
- Tumors

Treatment

Conservative

- Orthotic inserts with a heel pad and support for the sustentaculum tali
- Midfoot rocker, which may be combined with a stiff sole if necessary
- Physical therapy
- Oral or local treatment with nonsteroidal anti-inflammatory drugs to reduce swelling, relieve inflammation, and control pain
- Intra-articular hyaluronic acid or steroids

Operative

The joint spaces are too small for effective arthroscopic debridement and synovectomy. Surgical treatment is basically limited to arthrodesis of the affected joints.

Prognosis, Complications

Arthrodesis can preserve bone lengths and positions, although fusion of the talonavicular or calcaneocuboid joint will render the midfoot largely immobile. This contrasts with fusion of the naviculocuneiform joint, which has fewer functional effects.

Progressive osteoarthritis with secondary foot deformity may develop.

First and Second Tarsometatarsal Joints, Lisfranc Joint Line

Definition

Degenerative changes in the tarsometatarsal joints of the midfoot.

Symptoms

- Midfoot pain on weight bearing
- Local tenderness
- Warm-up pain
- Pain at rest
- Swelling
- Instability
- Chronic midfoot pain with functional impairment
- Flattening of the plantar arch
- Lack of stress transfer from hindfoot to forefoot

Predisposing Factors

Osteoarthritis of the Lisfranc joint line is an overuse condition. Heavy pressure loads with increased flattening of the plantar arch lead to wear and tear of the articular cartilage and may occur in a setting of age-related degeneration, overweight, arthritis, congenital and acquired deformities of the first ray, abnormal curvature of the metatarsals, or pes equinus. Secondary osteoarthritis is relatively common after sports-related injuries of the midfoot (American football, windsurfing, foot caught in a stirrup, motor vehicle accidents, crush injuries, direct impact trauma) and in patients with missed or improperly treated Lisfranc injuries. Other risk factors are a shortened gastrocnemius and a generally high ligamentous laxity.

Anatomy and Pathology

The tarsometatarsal joints along the Lisfranc joint line are rigid joints (amphiarthroses) with strong ligamentous attachments that stabilize the plantar vault. The most important of these attachments is the Lisfranc ligament, which connects the second metatarsal to the medial cuneiform. It has dorsal, plantar, and interosseous components. The dorsal ligament of the Lisfranc complex is the weakest ligament. The plantar part of the Lisfranc ligament is twice as thick as the dorsal part. The interosseous part is the strongest and most important component (see ▶ Fig. 4.5).

Imaging

Radiographs

The midfoot is X-rayed in three planes to evaluate the joint line. Standing DP and lateral radiographs are very useful for detecting any instability.

Ultrasound

Not indicated.

MRI

Interpretation Checklist

- Evaluate the Lisfranc ligament (continuity, activation, signs of instability)
- Evaluate the articular cartilage in the tarsometatarsal joints
- Effusion
- Synovitis
- Bone marrow edema
- Alignment
- Stress fractures

Examination Technique

- *Standard midfoot protocol:* prone position, high-resolution multi-channel coil
- *Sequences:*
  - Sagittal and coronal PD-weighted fat-sat
  - Coronal T1-weighted
  - Axial T2-weighted
  - Coronal STIR sequence, if required
  - T1-weighted fat-sat after contrast administration, axial to the midfoot and coronal to the midfoot

MRI Findings (▶ Fig. 4.15)

- Activated osteoarthritis of the tarsometatarsal joints
- Edema of the articulating bone ends
- Synovitis
- Subchondral sclerosis and cysts
- Adjacent edema
- Contrast enhancement in the soft tissues, especially on the dorsum of the foot
- Enhancement, thickening, and poor delineation of the Lisfranc ligament in the first and second tarsometatarsal joints
- Malalignment with slightly increased offset in the joints, followed later by subluxation
- Rare: bony avulsion of the Lisfranc ligament

Imaging Recommendation

Modalities of choice: radiographs for initial evaluation, MRI to evaluate instability and after trauma.

Differential Diagnosis

- Bone overload
- Stress fracture
- Anterior tibial tendinopathy
- Arthritis
- Charcot arthropathy
- Silfverskiöld disease (dorsal hump between the medial cuneiform and first metatarsal, exostosis, local tenderness, shoe irritation, adjacent peritendinitis of the extensor tendons)

Treatment

- Shoe inserts
- Braces
- Percutaneous screw arthrodesis

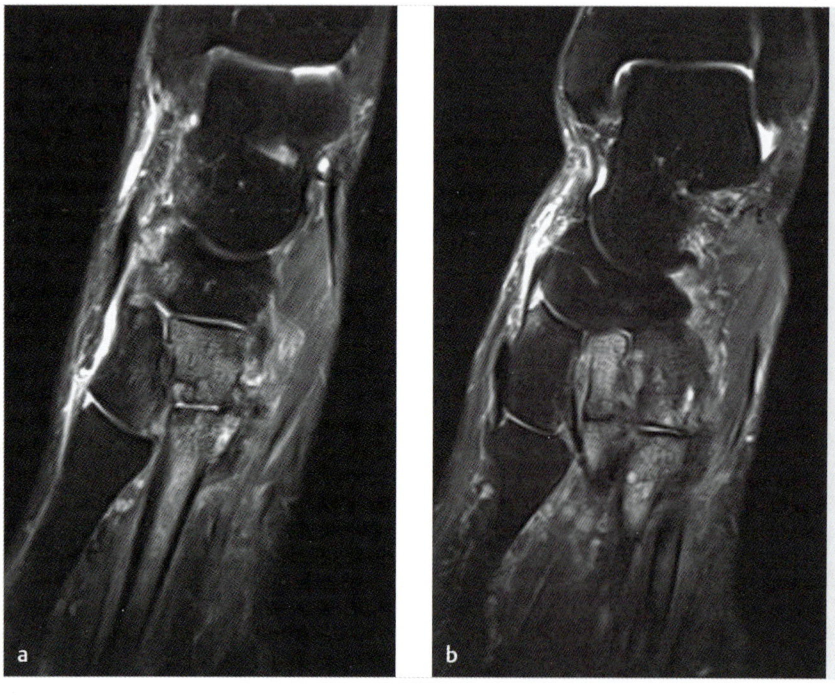

Fig. 4.15 a, b Activated osteoarthritis of the tarsometatarsal joints (Lisfranc osteoarthritis) in a patient with chronic refractory midfoot pain.
a Coronal PD-weighted fat-sat image shows advanced Lisfranc osteoarthritis with multiple subchondral cysts and a massive activation reaction.
b Coronal PD-weighted fat-sat image. The Lisfranc joint space is completely obliterated at this level. There are multiple subchondral cysts, areas of bone edema, and edema of adjacent soft tissues.

Prognosis, Complications

Posttraumatic instabilities often lead quickly to osteoarthritis, which can be managed only by surgical fusion of the tarsometatarsal joints.

4.2.2 Instability

Calcaneocuboid Joint

Definition

The calcaneocuboid joint may become unstable following injury to the joint capsule and calcaneocuboid ligaments.

Symptoms

- Lateral foot pain in response to rapid direction changes or walking on uneven ground
- Focal tenderness over the calcaneocuboid joint
- Feeling of instability

Predisposing Factors

Prior unhealed injury of the calcaneocuboid joint capsule and ligaments.

Anatomy and Pathology

Elongation of the calcaneocuboid ligaments and/or joint capsule may lead to increased joint play with associated pain.

Imaging (▶ Fig. 4.16)

Radiographs

DP stress radiograph of the foot shows increased joint-space opening (> 5°) in the calcaneocuboid joint.

Ultrasound

Not indicated.

MRI

MRI is useful for the evaluation of osteoarthritis.

Interpretation Checklist

- Evaluate cartilage quality in the calcaneocuboid and adjacent joints
- Joint activation (effusion, synovitis, bone marrow edema)
- Continuity of the adjacent ligaments
- Evaluate the joint capsule
- Scar tissue

! Note

Take care to evaluate all the ligaments of the hindfoot and midfoot (especially in the sinus tarsi) as well as the individual tendons.

Examination Technique

- *Standard protocol:* prone position, high-resolution multichannel coil
- *Sequences:*
  - Sagittal and coronal PD-weighted fat-sat
  - Coronal T1-weighted
  - Axial T2-weighted (angled to the plane of the ankle joint)
  - Axial oblique T1-weighted fat-sat after contrast administration (angled to the tendon plane of the talonavicular joint) and sagittal

MRI Findings

MRI findings are often subtle. Even if stress radiographs show increased opening of the calcaneocuboid joint space, MRI may show no abnormalities in the early stage, especially if the patient has been resting the foot or taking anti-inflammatory pain relievers. In most cases the ligaments of the calcaneocuboid joint show no discontinuities, and obvious ligament laxity is noted only in severe cases (thickened with ill-defined margins).

Otherwise MRI may show activation of the capsule and ligaments manifested by a thickened joint capsule, mild irritative synovitis, reactive effusion, and thinned articular cartilage. Abnormal alignment may be found in advanced stages.

Imaging Recommendation

Modality of choice: radiography.

Differential Diagnosis

- Sinus tarsi syndrome
- Peroneal tendon injuries
- Fracture of the calcaneal anterior process

Treatment

- Stabilizing the foot by physical therapy, bracing and taping
- Infiltration of the calcaneocuboid joint
- If complaints persist: reconstruction of the lateral ligaments with the plantaris longus tendon

Prognosis, Complications

The prognosis is good if mechanical stabilization of the calcaneocuboid joint can be achieved, especially in patients with intact articular cartilage.

Medial Column (First Tarsometatarsal, Talonavicular, and Naviculocuneiform Joints)

Definition

Posttraumatic or degenerative instability of the joints in the medial column of the foot.

Symptoms

- Pain in the affected joint
- Flattened longitudinal arch
- Forefoot abduction

Predisposing Factors

Pes planovalgus deformity.

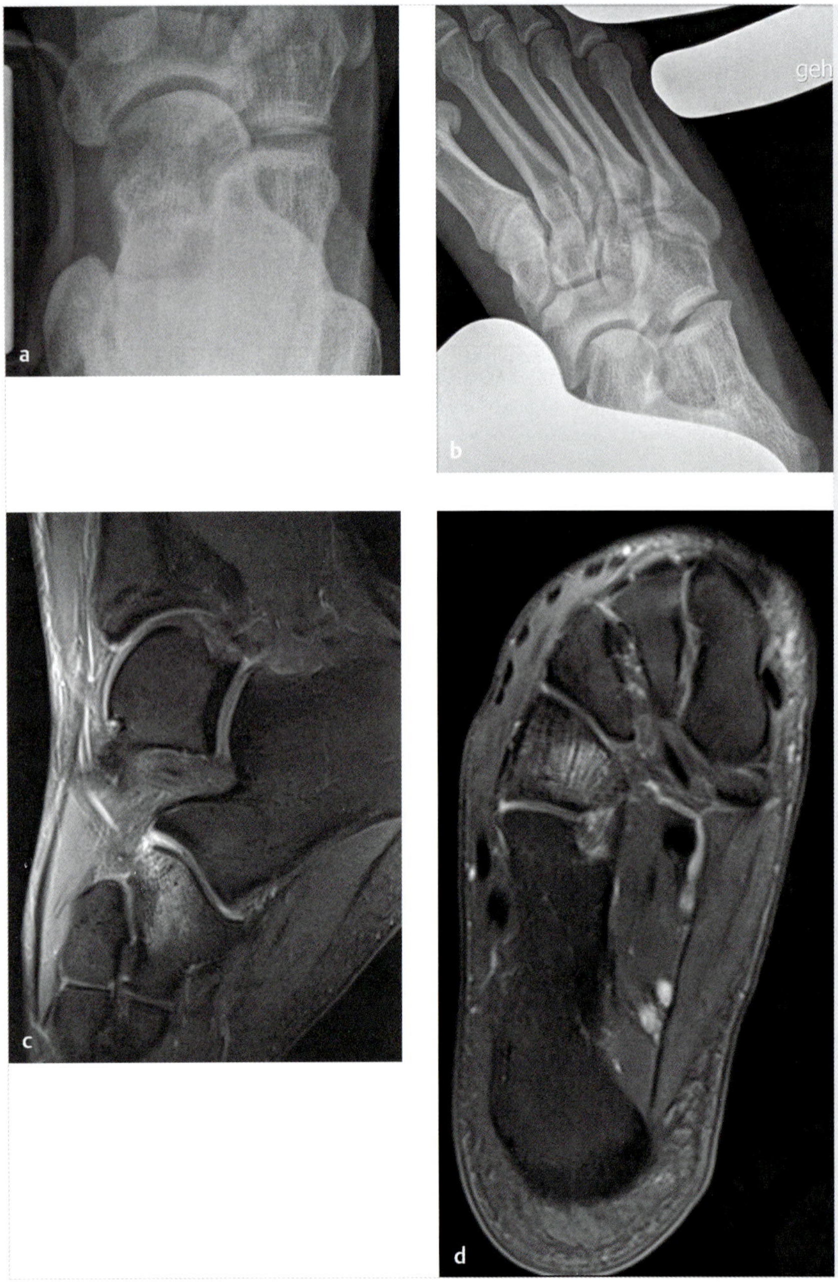

Fig. 4.16 a–d Instability of the calcaneocuboid joint. A 23-year-old male with persistent pain on the lateral side of the midfoot at 1 year after a supination-type injury of the ankle and midfoot.
a DP radiograph of the midfoot.
b Stress radiograph shows slightly increased lateral opening of the calcaneocuboid joint space.
c Sagittal T1-weighted fat-sat MRI after contrast administration shows activation in the dorsal plantar portion of the right cuboid and in the plantar calcaneocuboid ligament.
d Axial oblique T1-weighted fat-sat image after contrast administration shows enhancement along the plantar calcaneocuboid ligament with no apparent disruption of continuity.

Anatomy and Pathology

The medial column is stabilized by the interaction of the posterior tibial tendon, peroneus longus tendon (inserts on the plantar side of the first metatarsal base), and anterior tibial tendon. In addition, the first tarsometatarsal joint is stabilized by the Lisfranc ligament complex. Instabilities of the medial column result from damage to one or more of these anatomic structures.

Imaging

Radiographs

Weight-bearing radiographs of the foot are obtained in three planes, and the sides are compared. The principal findings are flattening of the longitudinal arch, an increased distance between the base of the second metatarsal and the medial cuneiform, plantar gapping of the affected joint, and skewing of the bone axes relative to one another.

Ultrasound

Not indicated.

MRI

MRI is most commonly used to identify the cause and direct preoperative planning.

Interpretation Checklist

- Evaluate the joints (effusion and synovitis are early signs of instability), cartilage quality, activated osteoarthritis, bone marrow edema, and the capsuloligamentous

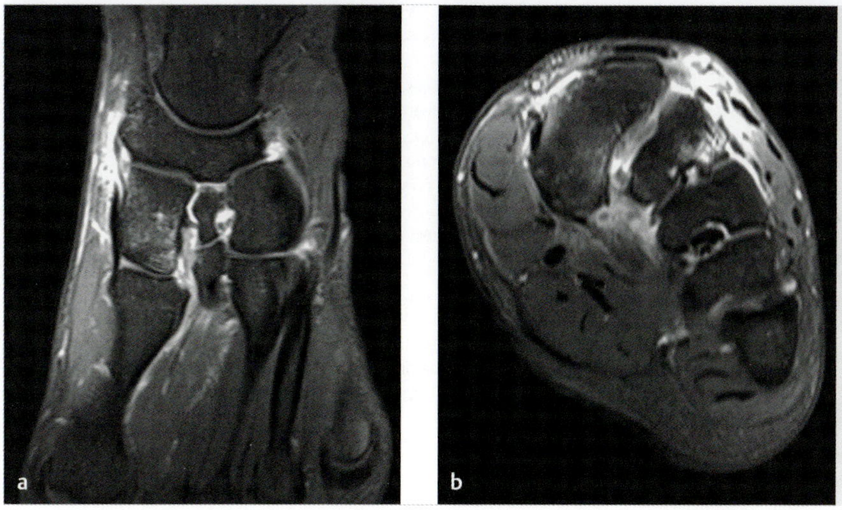

Fig. 4.17 **a, b Posttraumatic instability of the first tarsometatarsal joint** following an old midfoot injury with an undiagnosed sprain of the Lisfranc ligament. The patient complained of medial column pain on weight bearing.
a Coronal T1-weighted fat-sat image after contrast administration shows an intense activation reaction along the Lisfranc ligament with activation of the capsule and ligaments in the first tarsometatarsal joint and between the navicular and medial cuneiform.
b Axial T1-weighted fat-sat image after contrast administration shows enhancement of adjacent soft tissues and thickening of the Lisfranc ligament.

structures and tendons of the hindfoot and midfoot (tendinosis, peritendinitis)
- Look for other systemic diseases (rheumatoid arthritis, Charcot arthropathy)

Examination Technique

- *Standard protocol:* prone position, high-resolution multichannel coil
- *Sequences:*
  - Sagittal and coronal PD-weighted fat-sat
  - Coronal T1-weighted
  - Axial T2-weighted (angled to the midfoot joint plane)
  - Axial oblique T1-weighted fat-sat after contrast administration (angled to the tendon plane of the talonavicular joint) and sagittal

MRI Findings (▶ Fig. 4.17)

- Activation process along the medial column with edema and slight thickening of the capsuloligamentous structures
- Reactive effusion and moderate synovitic enhancement in the joints
- Possible early signs of osteoarthritis with thinning of the articular cartilage
- Altered alignment with decreased coverage of the talar head by the navicular articular surface
- Bone activation edema
- With tendon insufficiency (usually posterior tibial tendon insufficiency), corresponding signs that include tendinosis and peritendinitis

Imaging Recommendation

Modality of choice: radiography. MRI may be used for further investigation.

Differential Diagnosis

- Insertional tendinopathy of the anterior tibial tendon
- Navicular stress fracture
- Charcot neuroarthropathy
- Rupture of the Lisfranc ligament

Treatment

- Treatment of the underlying disease
- Shoe orthosis with a heel pad and medial arch support for symptom relief
- If degenerative changes are present: arthrodesis of the affected joint

Prognosis, Complications

The prognosis depends on the underlying disease.

4.3 Bibliography

Trauma

Lisfranc Fracture, Lisfranc Ligament Injury

Anderson RB, Hunt KJ, McCormick JJ. Management of common sports-related injuries about the foot and ankle. J Am Acad Orthop Surg 2010; 18: 546–556

Aronow MS. Treatment of the missed Lisfranc injury. Foot Ankle Clin 2006; 11: 127–142, ix

Baierlein SA. Frakturklassifikationen. Stuttgart: Thieme; 2011

Bulut G, Yasmin D, Heybeli N, Erken HY, Yildiz M. A complex variant of Lisfranc joint complex injury. J Am Podiatr Med Assoc 2009; 99: 359–363

Castro M, Melão L, Canella C et al. Lisfranc joint ligamentous complex: MRI with anatomic correlation in cadavers. AJR Am J Roentgenol 2010; 195: W447-W455

Chaney DM. The Lisfranc joint. Clin Podiatr Med Surg 2010; 27: 547–560

Coetzee JC. Making sense of lisfranc injuries. Foot Ankle Clin 2008; 13: 695–704, ix

Crim J. MR imaging evaluation of subtle Lisfranc injuries: the midfoot sprain. Magn Reson Imaging Clin N Am 2008; 16: 19–27, v

Della Rocca GJ, Sangeorzan BJ. Navicular and midfoot injuries. In: DiGiovanni C, Greisberg J, eds. Core knowledge in orthopaedics: foot and ankle. Philadelphia: Elsevier; 2007: 297–309

DeOrio M, Erickson M, Usuelli FG, Easley M. Lisfranc injuries in sport. Foot Ankle Clin 2009; 14: 169–186

de Palma L, Santucci A, Sabetta SP, Rapali S. Anatomy of the Lisfranc joint complex. Foot Ankle Int 1997; 18: 356–364

Granata JD, Philbin TM. The midfoot sprain: a review of Lisfranc ligament injuries. Phys Sportsmed 2010; 38: 119–126

Grivas TB, Vasiliadis ED, Koufopoulos G, Polyzois VD, Polyzois DG. Midfoot fractures. Clin Podiatr Med Surg 2006; 23: 323–341, vi

Gupta RT, Wadhwa RP, Learch TJ, Herwick SM. Lisfranc injury: imaging findings for this important but often-missed diagnosis. Curr Probl Diagn Radiol 2008; 37: 115–126

Haapamaki V, Kiuru M, Koskinen S. Lisfranc fracture-dislocation in patients with multiple trauma: diagnosis with multidetector computed tomography. Foot Ankle Int 2004; 25: 614–619

Hatem SF. Imaging of lisfranc injury and midfoot sprain. Radiol Clin North Am 2008; 46: 1045–1060, vi

Heckmann JD, Rockwood CA Jr, Green DP. Fractures and dislocations of the foot. Fractures in Adults. 2nd ed. Philadelphia: Lippincott; 1984: 1703–1832

Johnson A, Hill K, Ward J, Ficke J. Anatomy of the lisfranc ligament. Foot Ankle Spec 2008; 1: 19–23

Kalia V, Fishman EK, Carrino JA, Fayad LM. Epidemiology, imaging, and treatment of Lisfranc fracture-dislocations revisited. Skeletal Radiol 2012; 41: 129–136

Kummer B. Biomechanik. Form und Funktion des Bewegungsapparates. Cologne: Deutscher Ärzte Verlag; 2005

Lattermann C, Goldstein JL, Wukich DK, Lee S, Bach BR. Practical management of Lisfranc injuries in athletes. Clin J Sport Med 2007; 17: 311–315

Macmahon PJ, Dheer S, Raikin SM et al. MRI of injuries to the first interosseous cuneometatarsal (Lisfranc) ligament. Skeletal Radiol 2009; 38: 255–260

Mantas JP, Burks RT. Lisfranc injuries in the athlete. Clin Sports Med 1994; 13: 719–730

Müller-Mai CM, Ekkernkamp A. Frakturen. Klassifikation und Behandlungsoptionen. Heidelberg: Springer; 2010

Nunley JA, Vertullo CJ. Classification, investigation, and management of midfoot sprains: Lisfranc injuries in the athlete. Am J Sports Med 2002; 30: 871–878

Raikin SM, Elias I, Dheer S, Besser MP, Morrison WB, Zoga AC. Prediction of midfoot instability in the subtle Lisfranc injury. Comparison of magnetic resonance imaging with intraoperative findings. J Bone Joint Surg Am 2009; 91: 892–899

Rhim B, Hunt JC. Lisfranc injury and Jones fracture in sports. Clin Podiatr Med Surg 2011; 28: 69–86

Stoller DW, Tirman PFJ, Bredella MA. Diagnostic Imaging: orthopedics. Salt Lake City, Utah: Amirsys; 2004

Turco VJ. Injuries to the Foot and Ankle. In: Nicholas JA, Hershmann EB. The lower extremity and spine in sports medicine. St. Louis: Mosby; 1995: 1229–1250

Valderrabano V, Engelhardt M, Küster H-H, eds. Fuß und Sprunggelenk und Sport. Empfehlungen von Sportarten aus orthopädischer und sportmedzinischer Sicht. Cologne: Deutscher Ärzte Verlag; 2009

Watson TS, Shurnas PS, Denker J. Treatment of Lisfranc joint injury: current concepts. J Am Acad Orthop Surg 2010; 18: 718–728

Woodward S, Jacobson JA, Femino JE, Morag Y, Fessell DP, Dong Q. Sonographic evaluation of Lisfranc ligament injuries. J Ultrasound Med 2009; 28: 351–357

Wülker N, Stephens MM, Cracchiolo A, eds. Operationsatlas Fuß und Sprunggelenk. 2nded. Stuttgart: Thieme; 2007: 129–135

Navicular Fracture

Andermahr J, Jubel A, Rehm KE, Koebke J. Erkrankungen und Verletzungen des Rückfußes. Cologne: Deutscher Ärzte Verlag; 2011

Baierlein SA. Frakturklassifikationen. Stuttgart: Thieme; 2011

Brockwell J, Yeung Y, Griffith JF. Stress fractures of the foot and ankle. Sports Med Arthrosc 2009; 17: 149–159

Della Rocca GJ, Sangeorzan BJ. Navicular and midfoot injuries. In: DiGiovanni C, Greisberg J, eds. Core knowledge in orthopaedics: foot and ankle. Philadelphia: Elsevier; 2007: 297–309

DiGiovanni CW. Fractures of the navicular. Foot Ankle Clin 2004; 9: 25–63

Goulart M, O'Malley MJ, Hodgkins CW, Charlton TP. Foot and ankle fractures in dancers. Clin Sports Med 2008; 27: 295–304

Heckmann JD, Rockwood CA Jr, Green DP. Fractures and dislocations of the foot. Fractures in Adults. 2nd ed. Philadelphia: Lippincott; 1984: 1703–1832

Kummer B. Biomechanik. Form und Funktion des Bewegungsapparates. Cologne: Deutscher Ärzte Verlag; 2005

McCormick JJ, Bray CC, Davis WH, Cohen BE, Jones CP, Anderson RB. Clinical and computed tomography evaluation of surgical outcomes in tarsal navicular stress fractures. Am J Sports Med 2011; 39: 1741–1748

Miller T, Kaeding CC, Flanigan D. The classification systems of stress fractures: a systematic review. Phys Sportsmed 2011; 39: 93–100

Müller-Mai CM, Ekkernkamp A. Frakturen. Klassifikation und Behandlungsoptionen. Heidelberg: Springer; 2010

Nyska M, Margulies JY, Barbarawi M, Mutchler W, Dekel S, Segal D. Fractures of the body of the tarsal navicular bone: case reports and literature review. J Trauma 1989; 29: 1448–1451

Rammelt S, Biewener A, Grass R, Zwipp H. Foot injuries in the polytraumatized patient. [Article in German] Unfallchirurg 2005; 108: 858–865

Stoller DW, Tirman PFJ, Bredella MA. Diagnostic Imaging: orthopedics. Salt Lake City, Utah: Amirsys; 2004

Torg JS, Moyer J, Gaughan JP, Boden BP. Management of tarsal navicular stress fractures: conservative versus surgical treatment: a meta-analysis. Am J Sports Med 2010; 38: 1048–1053

Turco VJ. Injuries to the Foot and Ankle. In: Nicholas JA, Hershmann EB. The lower extremity and spine in sports medicine. St. Louis: Mosby; 1995: 1229–1250

Valderrabano V, Engelhardt M, Küster H-H, eds. Fuß & Sprunggelenk und Sport. Empfehlungen von Sportarten aus orthopädischer und sportmedzinischer Sicht. Cologne: Deutscher Ärzte Verlag; 2009

Wülker N, Stephens MM, Cracchiolo A, eds. Operationsatlas Fuß und Sprunggelenk. 2nd ed Stuttgart: Thieme; 2007: 129–135

Cuboid Fracture

Andermahr J, Jubel A, Rehm KE, Koebke J. Erkrankungen und Verletzungen des Rückfußes. Cologne: Deutscher Ärzte Verlag; 2011

Baierlein SA. Frakturklassifikationen. Stuttgart: Thieme; 2011

Della Rocca GJ, Sangeorzan BJ. Navicular and midfoot injuries. In: DiGiovanni C, Greisberg J, eds. Core knowledge in orthopaedics: foot and ankle. Philadelphia: Elsevier; 2007: 297–309

Dodson NB, Dodson EE, Shromoff PJ. Imaging strategies for diagnosing calcaneal and cuboid stress fractures. Clin Podiatr Med Surg 2008; 25: 183–201, vi

Heckmann JD, Rockwood CA Jr, Green DP. Fractures and dislocations of the foot. Fractures in Adults. 2nd ed. Philadelphia: Lippincott; 1984: 1703 – 1832

Hunter JC, Sangeorzan BJ. A nutcracker fracture: cuboid fracture with an associated avulsion fracture of the tarsal navicular. AJR Am J Roentgenol 1996; 166: 888

Kummer B. Biomechanik. Form und Funktion des Bewegungsapparates. Cologne: Deutscher Ärzte Verlag; 2005

Mihalich RM, Early JS. Management of cuboid crush injuries. Foot Ankle Clin 2006; 11: 121–126, ix

Müller-Mai CM, Ekkernkamp A. Frakturen. Klassifikation und Behandlungsoptionen. Heidelberg: Springer; 2010

Rammelt S, Grass R, Zwipp H. Nutcracker fractures of the navicular and cuboid. [Article in German] Ther Umsch 2004; 61: 451–457

Ruffing T, Muhm M, Winkler H. Nutcracker fracture of the cuboid in children. [Article in German] Unfallchirurg 2010; 113: 495–500

Wülker N, Stephens MM, Cracchiolo A, eds. Operationsatlas Fuß und Sprunggelenk. 2nded. Stuttgart: Thieme; 2007: 129–135

Cuneiform Fractures

Baierlein SA. Frakturklassifikationen. Stuttgart: Thieme; 2011

Della Rocca GJ, Sangeorzan BJ. Navicular and midfoot injuries. In: DiGiovanni C, Greisberg J, eds. Core knowledge in orthopaedics: foot and ankle. Philadelphia: Elsevier; 2007: 297–309

Heckmann JD, Rockwood CA Jr, Green DP. Fractures and dislocations of the foot. Fractures in Adults. 2nd ed. Philadelphia: Lippincott; 1984: 1703–1832

Miersch D, Wild M, Jungbluth P, Betsch M, Windolf J, Hakimi M. A transcuneiform fracture-dislocation of the midfoot. Foot (Edinb) 2011; 21: 45–47

Müller-Mai CM, Ekkernkamp A. Frakturen. Klassifikation und Behandlungsoptionen. Heidelberg: Springer; 2010

Olson RC, Mendicino SS, Rockett MS. Isolated medial cuneiform fracture: review of the literature and report of two cases. Foot Ankle Int 2000; 21: 150–153

Sener RN. Bilateral extra tarsal bones in Rubinstein-Taybi syndrome: the fourth cuneiform bones. Eur Radiol 1999; 9: 483–484

Shah K, Odgaard A. Fracture of the lateral cuneiform only: a rare foot injury. J Am Podiatr Med Assoc 2007; 97: 483–485

Taylor SF, Heidenreich D. Isolated medial cuneiform fracture: a special forces soldier with a rare injury. South Med J 2008; 101: 848–849

Wülker N, Stephens MM, Cracchiolo A, eds. Operationsatlas Fuß und Sprunggelenk. 2nded. Stuttgart: Thieme; 2007: 129–135

Osteoarthritis

Talonavicular, Naviculocuneiform and Calcaneocuboid Joints

Fessell DP, Jacobson JA. Ultrasound of the hindfoot and midfoot. Radiol Clin North Am 2008; 46: 1027–1043, vi

Mittlmeier T, Beck M. Injuries of the midfoot [Article in German] Chirurg 2011; 82: 169–186, quiz 187–188

Randt T, Dahlen C, Schikore H, Zwipp H. Dislocation fractures in the area of the middle foot–injuries of the Chopart and Lisfranc joint [Article in German] Zentralbl Chir 1998; 123: 1257–1266

Richter M, Wippermann B, Krettek C, Schratt HE, Hufner T, Therman H. Fractures and fracture dislocations of the midfoot: occurrence, causes and long-term results. Foot Ankle Int 2001; 22: 392–398

Swords MP, Schramski M, Switzer K, Nemec S. Chopart fractures and dislocations. Foot Ankle Clin 2008; 13: 679–693, viii

van Dorp KB, de Vries MR, van der Elst M, Schepers T. Chopart joint injury: a study of outcome and morbidity. J Foot Ankle Surg 2010; 49: 541–545

First and Second Tarsometatarsal Joints, Lisfranc Joint Line

Castro M, Melão L, Canella C et al. Lisfranc joint ligamentous complex: MRI with anatomic correlation in cadavers. AJR Am J Roentgenol 2010; 195: W447-W455

Chaney DM. The Lisfranc joint. Clin Podiatr Med Surg 2010; 27: 547–560

Coetzee JC. Making sense of lisfranc injuries. Foot Ankle Clin 2008; 13: 695–704, ix

Crim J. MR imaging evaluation of subtle Lisfranc injuries: the midfoot sprain. Magn Reson Imaging Clin N Am 2008; 16: 19–27, v

Dihlmann W, Stäbler A. Gelenke–Wirbelverbindungen. Kap.16: Gelenke des Fußes einschließlich des oberen Sprunggelenks. 4thed. Stuttgart: Thieme; 2010: 729

Fessell DP, Jacobson JA. Ultrasound of the hindfoot and midfoot. Radiol Clin North Am 2008; 46: 1027–1043, vi

Granata JD, Philbin TM. The midfoot sprain: a review of Lisfranc ligament injuries. Phys Sportsmed 2010; 38: 119–126

Gupta RT, Wadhwa RP, Learch TJ, Herwick SM. Lisfranc injury: imaging findings for this important but often-missed diagnosis. Curr Probl Diagn Radiol 2008; 37: 115–126

Johnson A, Hill K, Ward J, Ficke J. Anatomy of the lisfranc ligament. Foot Ankle Spec 2008; 1: 19–23

Hatem SF. Imaging of lisfranc injury and midfoot sprain. Radiol Clin North Am 2008; 46: 1045–1060, vi

Kaar S, Femino J, Morag Y. Lisfranc joint displacement following sequential ligament sectioning. J Bone Joint Surg Am 2007; 89: 2225–2232

Macmahon PJ, Dheer S, Raikin SM et al. MRI of injuries to the first interosseous cuneometatarsal (Lisfranc) ligament. Skeletal Radiol 2009; 38: 255–260

Menz HB, Munteanu SE, Zammit GV, Landorf KB. Foot structure and function in older people with radiographic osteoarthritis of the medial midfoot. Osteoarthritis Cartilage 2010; 18: 317–322

Patel A, Rao S, Nawoczenski D, Flemister AS, DiGiovanni B, Baumhauer JF. Midfoot arthritis. J Am Acad Orthop Surg 2010; 18: 417–425

Raikin SM, Elias I, Dheer S, Besser MP, Morrison WB, Zoga AC. Prediction of midfoot instability in the subtle Lisfranc injury. Comparison of magnetic resonance imaging with intraoperative findings. J Bone Joint Surg Am 2009; 91: 892–899

Rao S, Baumhauer JF, Becica L, Nawoczenski DA. Shoe inserts alter plantar loading and function in patients with midfoot arthritis. J Orthop Sports Phys Ther 2009; 39: 522–531

Watson TS, Shurnas PS, Denker J. Treatment of Lisfranc joint injury: current concepts. J Am Acad Orthop Surg 2010; 18: 718–728

Woodward S, Jacobson JA, Femino JE, Morag Y, Fessell DP, Dong Q. Sonographic evaluation of Lisfranc ligament injuries. J Ultrasound Med 2009; 28: 351–357

Wülker N, Stephens MM, Cracchiolo A, eds. Operationsatlas Fuß und Sprunggelenk. 2nded. Stuttgart: Thieme; 2007: 136

Instability

Calcaneocuboid Joint

van Dorp KB, de Vries MR, van der Elst M, Schepers T. Chopart joint injury: a study of outcome and morbidity. J Foot Ankle Surg 2010; 49: 541–545

Medial column (First Tarsometatarsal, Talonavicular and Naviculocuneiform Joints

Granata JD, Philbin TM. The midfoot sprain: a review of Lisfranc ligament injuries. Phys Sportsmed 2010; 38: 119–126

King DM, Toolan BC. Associated deformities and hypermobility in hallux valgus: an investigation with weightbearing radiographs. Foot Ankle Int 2004; 25: 251–255

Myerson MS, Cerrato R. Current management of tarsometatarsal injuries in the athlete. Instr Course Lect 2009; 58: 583–594

Patel A, Rao S, Nawoczenski D, Flemister AS, DiGiovanni B, Baumhauer JF. Midfoot arthritis. J Am Acad Orthop Surg 2010; 18: 417–425

Raikin SM, Elias I, Dheer S, Besser MP, Morrison WB, Zoga AC. Prediction of midfoot instability in the subtle Lisfranc injury. Comparison of magnetic resonance imaging with intraoperative findings. J Bone Joint Surg Am 2009; 91: 892–899

Chapter 5

Forefoot

5 Forefoot

5.1 Trauma

R. Degwert, U. Szeimies, and M. Walther

Metatarsal Fractures

Definition

Fractures of the first through fifth metatarsals are caused by direct or indirect trauma or by a disproportion between recurrent loads and bony stress tolerance (stress fracture; see also Calcaneal Fractures (p. 53) in Chapter 3 and 4.1.3 Navicular Fractures (p. 139) in Chapter 4).

Symptoms

- Swelling and hematoma on the dorsum of the foot
- Deformities: shortening, axial deviation, rotational malalignment (rarely visible on radiographs, detected more easily by physical examination)
- Load-dependent pain at the fracture site or in the sole of the foot, occasionally localized to one point
- Diffuse pain over the top of the forefoot (especially on weight bearing)
- Occasional crepitation
- Tender to axial pressure
- Tenderness to percussion
- With stress fractures: increasing pain on weight bearing

Predisposing Factors

- *Fitness level:*
  - Stress fractures in young runners, dancers, musicians
  - Stress fractures of the fifth metatarsal, usually in young professional soccer players after intensive training
  - "March fracture," that is, a fatigue fracture in response to unaccustomed walking or running; common in soldiers or long-distance runners who suddenly increase their level of training
- *Pre-existing foot deformities*, especially hindfoot varus or forefoot adduction, high vertical loading rate
- *Non–custom-made shoe inserts:* Support to the medial longitudinal arch can increase plantar forces and place more pressure on the fifth metatarsal, increasing the fracture risk to that bone.
- *Steroid therapy*
- *Long-term steroid therapy for rheumatoid arthritis:* spontaneous serial fractures of metatarsal bones

Anatomy and Pathology

Anatomy

The midfoot is formed by five metatarsal bones. Each consists of a broad proximal base (which includes the metaphysis), a diaphysis (shaft), and a round distal head. The strong plantar ligaments (longitudinal plantar ligament) are attached to the bases of the metatarsals. The diaphysis gives attachment to the intrinsic muscles of the foot, and the necks of the metatarsals are interconnected by the intermetatarsal ligaments. The metatarsal heads are weight bearing. A physiologic load distribution on the heads depends on an anatomically correct position and alignment of the bones. Even slight deviations in the sagittal or frontal plane may cause painful and persistent metatarsalgia.

The bases of the metatarsals are stabilized by their firm attachments to the cuneiform and cuboid bones (amphiarthroses). The first and fifth metatarsals are tethered less firmly, making them slightly more mobile and allowing small movements in flexion and extension. In this way they can contribute to pronation and supination of the foot, making it easier to walk on uneven ground. The second metatarsal fits snugly between the medial and lateral cuneiforms, giving it the most stable basal attachment. The second metatarsal is the longest of the metatarsals and also the most prominent on the dorsum of the foot.

The growth zone with the epiphyseal plate is located at the proximal end of the first metatarsal. The growth zones of the second through fourth metatarsals are located at the distal ends.

The first metatarsal is considerably thicker than the other metatarsals. The inferior surface of its head bears two depressions for the sesamoid bones. The first metatarsal and both sesamoids bear approximately one-half of the body weight. The sesamoids are embedded in the tendons of the abductor hallucis (medial) and flexor hallucis brevis (lateral). The base of the first metatarsal gives attachment to the peroneus longus (plantar flexion and pronation) and tibialis anterior (supination).

The fifth metatarsal extends farther proximally than the other metatarsals. The tuberosity on the lateral side of its base gives attachment to the peroneus brevis tendon and slips of the plantar aponeurosis.

In normal walking the vertical load on the foot is approximately equal to the body weight. Running increases the vertical load to approximately 2.5 times the body weight. The vertical load is accompanied by a significant mediolateral load and by shear loads acting in a "forward–backward" direction.

Pathology

Mechanisms of metatarsal injury

Metatarsal fractures account for 5 to 6% of all fractures and approximately 50% of fractures in the foot. In soccer players, 78% of lower limb fractures involve the fifth metatarsal alone. These injuries may be caused by direct or indirect trauma. Stress fractures of the foot most commonly affect the metatarsals (in professional soccer players: 0.04 injuries per 1,000 hours played). The frequency distribution of metatarsal fractures is as follows: fifth metatarsal > third metatarsal > second metatarsal > first metatarsal > fourth metatarsal. Concomitant fractures of multiple bones are common.

Metatarsal fractures can have various pathogenic mechanisms:

- Twisting or rotation of the body with the toes planted: fractures of the metatarsal shaft (spiral fractures) and central metatarsals

- Direct impact or crush injury or an indirect (axial) traumatizing force
- Stress fracture: overuse injury resulting from excessive stress on a bone (running or dancing) or decreased bone density

! Note

Proximal fractures of the first through fourth metatarsals, though rare, require special attention because they are often associated with injuries of the Lisfranc ligament or tarsometatarsal joints.

Fracture mechanisms in specific metatarsals:

- *First metatarsal:* Hyperextension, hyperflexion or abduction may cause a fracture involving the metatarsophalangeal joint of the big toe. Dancers are more likely to sustain lateral avulsion fractures of the proximal or distal first metatarsal, which are often associated with a capsular tear. First metatarsal fractures may be markedly displaced by the pull of the attached tibialis anterior and peroneus longus tendons.
- *Second through fourth metatarsals:* The interosseous ligaments and interosseous muscles prevent the gross displacement of shaft fractures in the second through fourth metatarsals. Stress fractures are common in the proximal portions of the second and third metatarsals. With fractures of the metatarsal head, the head fragment tends to undergo plantar displacement due to the greater pull of the superficial flexor tendons relative to the extensor tendons.
- *Fifth metatarsal:* Fractures of the fifth metatarsal are assigned to three different zones. The joint between the bases of the fourth and fifth metatarsals is the landmark for defining the zones.
  - Zone I: The tuberosity of the fifth metatarsal is subject to avulsion injuries (most common injury of the fifth ray) caused by inversion and plantar flexion at the ankle joint. The cause is less the pull of the peroneus brevis than the slips of the plantar aponeurosis that are attached there.
  - Zone II: The "Jones fracture" is a transverse fracture distal to the tuberosity but proximal to the metaphysis. It results from a vertical or mediolateral force acting on the base of the fifth metatarsal while the body weight is over the lateral portion of the plantar-flexed foot (e.g., during a sudden direction change without heel contact).
  - Zone III: The proximal diaphysis is subject to fractures with intra-articular involvement of the cuboid-fifth metatarsal joint. Zone III fractures are the most difficult fractures from an anatomical and mechanical standpoint because the base of the fifth metatarsal receives its blood supply from the proximal side. As a result, conservatively treated fractures may take 2 to 21 months to heal and are at high risk for nonunion. These fractures often occur as stress injuries in athletes, and it is within this context that the decision between operative or conservative treatment must be made.

Classification

- *AO/ASIF classification of metatarsal fractures* (▸ Fig. 5.1 and ▸ Table 5.1). This classification includes special designations:

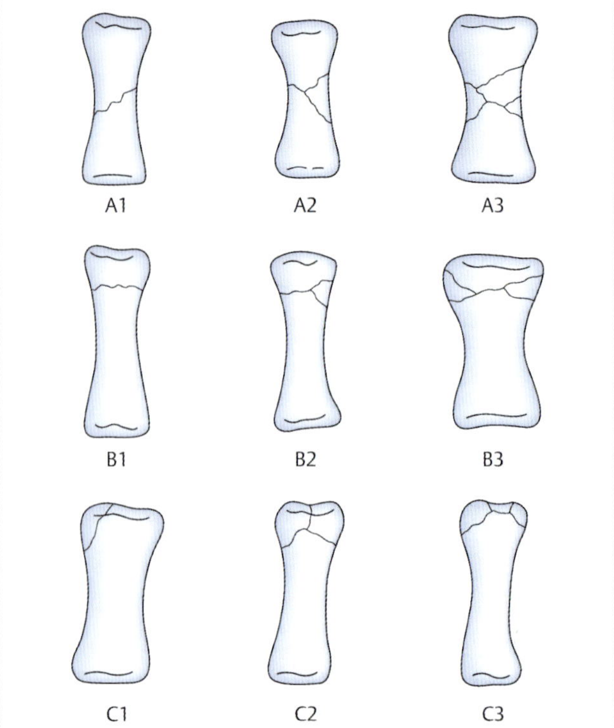

Fig. 5.1 Current AO/ASIF classification of metatarsal fractures. A final version of the classification is in progress (see http://www.aofoundation.org).

Table 5.1 AO/ASIF classification of metatarsal fractures

Type	Description
A	Proximal and distal extra-articular, simple diaphyseal fracture
B	Proximal and distal with partial articular involvement, diaphyseal wedge fracture
C	Proximal and distal with articular involvement, multipart diaphyseal fracture

the Jones fracture and pseudo-Jones fracture (tuberosity avulsion fracture of the fifth metatarsal).

- *Fractures of the fifth metatarsal:* Jones fracture (named after Sir Robert Jones 1902; ▸ Fig. 5.2), as described above.
- *Other classification:* the Dameron and Quill classification of proximal fifth metatarsal fractures (▸ Table 5.2) is widely used but requires an accurate description of fracture location.

Imaging

Ultrasound

Ultrasound can demonstrate associated soft-tissue injuries, hematoma, and vascular injuries. A dynamic ultrasound examination can assess the stability of the Lisfranc joint line. Step-offs in the cortex of the metatarsals are consistently visualized owing to the superficial location of the bones.

Radiography

Radiographs of the foot are taken in three planes with the foot resting on the film cassette. A 45° inversion view may be added if necessary.

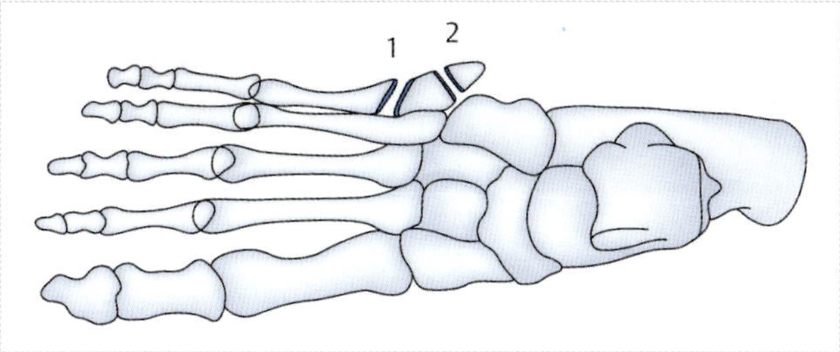

Fig. 5.2 Jones fracture. A true Jones fracture at the base of the fifth metatarsal (1) differs from a pseudo-Jones fracture (2), which is a more proximal avulsion fracture at lower risk for nonunion.

The following points should be noted during interpretation of the films:

- *Metatarsal head:* axial or rotational malalignment
- *Neck:* plantar or lateral displacement
- *Midshaft:* oblique, transverse, spiral, or comminuted fracture
- *Base* (▶ Fig. 5.3): Lisfranc fractures are often difficult to evaluate on radiographs due to superimposed structures. Generally these cases are investigated further by CT.

Table 5.2 Dameron and Quill classification of proximal fifth metatarsal fractures

Type	Description
1	Avulsion fracture of the tuberosity
2	Fracture at the metaphyseal–diaphyseal junction
3	Stress fracture of the proximal shaft
4	Distal shaft fractures including the head and neck

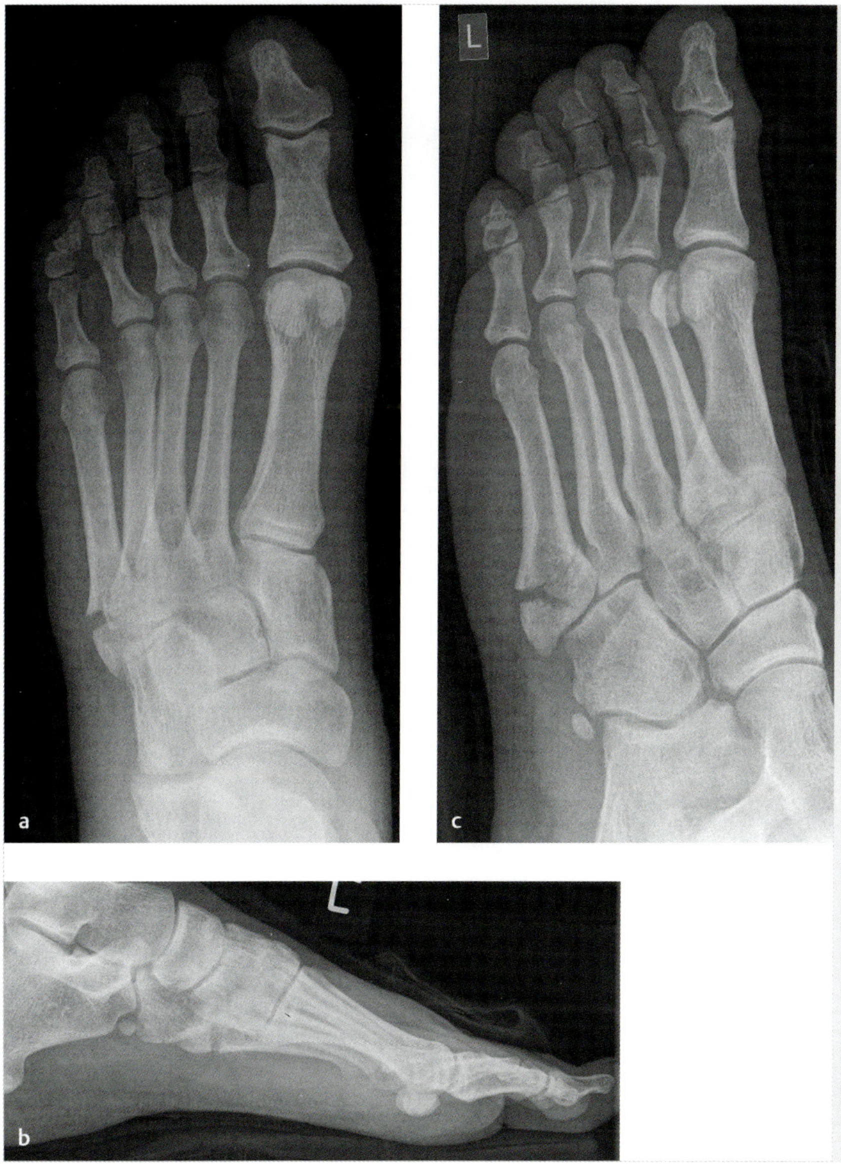

Fig. 5.3 a–c Radiographs in three planes of a basal fracture of the fifth metatarsal. The films demonstrate the fractured metatarsal base with articular involvement.
a DP projection.
b Lateral projection.
c Oblique view.

> **! Note**
>
> Multiple fractures may be present.

If a stress fracture is suspected, radiographic abnormalities often do not appear until pain has persisted for 2 to 6 weeks. In this case repeat radiographs or MR images may have to be obtained 10 to 14 days later. Stress fractures will usually present as a transverse line and may show angulation and periosteal reaction or marked callus formation. Sites of heavy callus ossification may resemble a malignant tumor on radiographs, and these changes were sometimes biopsied in years past. Equivocal cases should be investigated by MRI.

MRI

Interpretation Checklist

- Alignment of the joint lines
- Involvement of articular surfaces
- Dimensions of articular step-offs
- Displacement and fragmentation
- Evaluation of flexor and extensor tendons
- Exclusion of associated disorders

Examination Technique

- *Standard protocol:* prone position, high-resolution multichannel coil
- *Sequences:*
  - STIR and T1-weighted coronal oblique (double-angled)
  - PD-weighted fat-sat sagittal (centered on metatarsal with dominant clinical signs—different sagittal sections for first and fifth metatarsals)
  - T2-weighted axial
  - All scans without contrast

MRI Findings

Fractures and bone contusions or cancellous fractures cause areas of bone edema that are defined with high sensitivity by STIR sequences. This allows for an accurate description of all posttraumatic bone edema and fractures. A true fracture appears as a hypointense line and/or as a cortical discontinuity or step-off. MRI also permits a detailed description of all ligamentous structures, most notably the Lisfranc ligament and capsular ligaments along the Lisfranc joint line, and an accurate evaluation of the metatarsophalangeal joints.

CT (▶ Fig. 5.4)

Basal fractures of the metatarsals are investigated by CT to exclude a Lisfranc fracture-dislocation. CT is also used for fracture classification and in cases with equivocal radiographic findings.

Scintigraphy

Scintigraphy can be used to image stress fractures, but this modality has been almost completely replaced by MRI, which provides higher specificity without radiation exposure.

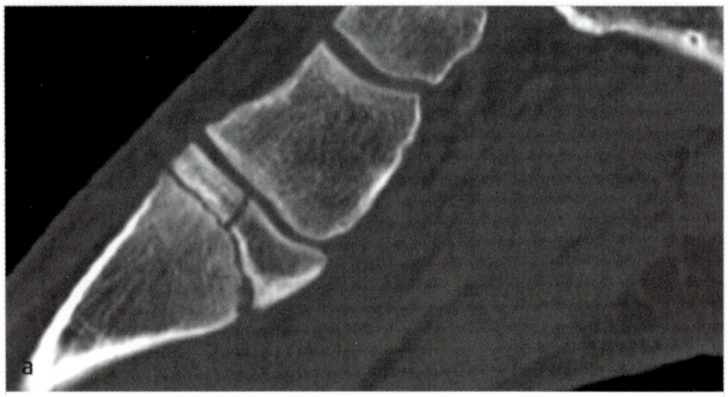

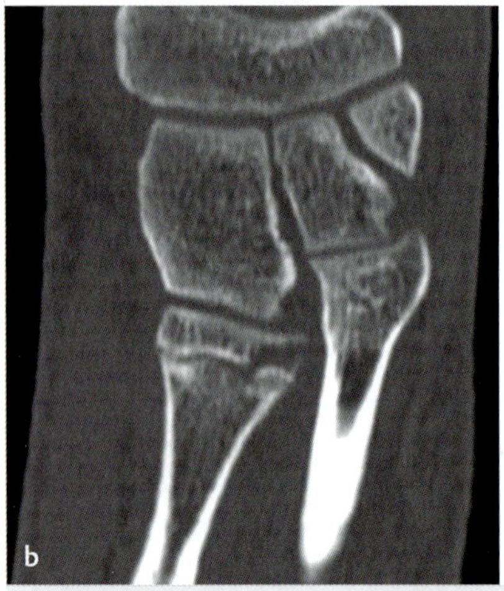

Fig. 5.4 a, b Soccer injury in a 15-year-old boy. CT demonstrates a fracture of the first metatarsal (Salter–Harris type III).
a Sagittal MPR does not show a significant step in the articular surface.
b Coronal MPR (slice thickness 0.5 mm, interslice gap 0.3 mm, 50 mA, 120 kV) shows a transverse epiphyseal fracture of the left first metatarsal with plantar-side involvement of the epiphyseal plate and no significant displacement.

Imaging Recommendation

Modality of choice: MRI for the exclusion of a Lisfranc ligament injury and other soft-tissue injuries. Stress fractures can also be seen and diagnosed at an early stage on MRI. The presence of a hypointense fracture line distinguishes that injury from a stress reaction without a fracture.

Differential Diagnosis

- Lisfranc fracture
- Navicular fracture
- Cuboid or cuneiform fracture, occasionally associated with tarsometatarsal dislocation
- Cuboid fracture with associated fractures of the calcaneus, fifth metatarsal or navicular
- Navicular avulsion fracture
- Rare joint injuries accompanying a cuboid fracture
- Turf toe
- Accessory tarsal bones (os peroneum in the peroneus longus tendon, os vesalianum in the peroneus brevis tendon)
- Köhler disease type II
- Morton neuroma

- Joplin neuroma
- Metatarsalgia

Treatment

The goal of treatment is an anatomic reconstruction, especially of articular surfaces and bone length. Axial malalignment consistently gives rise to secondary complaints based on an abnormal plantar pressure distribution. The risk of a compartment syndrome is particularly high after direct trauma.
Indications for immediate operative treatment:

- Associated neurologic deficit
- Compartment syndrome (5–9 compartments)
- Open fractures
- Devitalization of the skin
- Vascular compression

> **! Note**
>
> The first and fifth metatarsals are treated differently from the second through fourth metatarsals because of their specific anatomy. Metatarsals II–IV have little risk of secondary displacement because they are stabilized by the intermetatarsal ligaments. Fractures managed conservatively require close-interval radiographic follow-ups to ensure that any secondary displacement is not missed.

Conservative

- First metatarsal fractures, being located in a major weight-bearing zone, require a short leg cast for 6 weeks with partial weight bearing.
- Fractures of a single metatarsal shaft with lateral or medial displacement or < 2 mm of shortening will normally heal with 3 weeks of non–weight bearing and immobilization in a plaster splint.
- For a nondisplaced metatarsal shaft fracture: shoe with a stiff sole and full weight bearing according to pain tolerance, plus a schedule of regular radiographic follow-ups
- Fractures of the metatarsal base: cast immobilization and non-weight bearing for 6 to 8 weeks
- All incomplete or minimally displaced fifth metatarsal fractures, stress fractures, and nondisplaced avulsion fractures of the fifth metatarsal base:
  - Conservative treatment in a plaster splint and non-weight bearing for 6 to 8 weeks
  - More than 2 mm of secondary displacement is an indication for operative treatment
  - With stress fractures of the fifth metatarsal: cast immobilization for 6 to 20 weeks. (These fractures have a high risk of nonunion and displacement and require prolonged rehabilitation, so most are treated operatively today.)
- In children with open growth plates and with no rotational malalignment, no axial deviation in the frontal plane, and no more than 20° of anterior or posterior angulation: cast immobilization for 2 to 3 weeks for metaphyseal fractures and 3 to 5 weeks for diaphyseal fractures

Operative

- *Criteria for operative treatment:*
  - Shortening of the affected ray
  - Proximal and distal articular surface involvement (especially when incongruity is present)
  - Lateral displacement of ≥ 3 mm or axial deviation > 10°
  - Subcapital and capital fractures
  - Displaced intra-articular fractures of the metatarsal heads
  - Neurovascular impairment
  - Open fractures
  - Fractures of multiple metatarsals
  - Displaced complex and comminuted fractures
  - Displacement, even by a small degree, of the first and fifth metatarsals
  - Avulsion fractures of the fifth metatarsal base with > 2 mm displacement and > 30% articular surface involvement
  - Unsatisfactory outcome of conservative treatment (secondary displacement)
- *Main goal of operative treatment:* minimal malalignment in the sagittal plane and reconstruction of the load-bearing columns or restoration of bone length and axial alignment
- *First metatarsal:* Plate and screw fixation of shaft fractures, temporary or permanent arthrodesis for basal or Lisfranc fractures, screw or K-wire fixation of head fractures
- *Second through fourth metatarsals:* K-wire, plate and screw fixation of shaft fractures, temporary or permanent arthrodesis for basal or Lisfranc fractures, screw or K-wire fixation for head fractures
- *Fifth metatarsal* (▸ Fig. 5.5): cerclage wiring for displaced avulsion fractures or screw fixation of fractures with a large fragment; intramedullary screw or plating and bone grafting for metaphyseal and diaphyseal fractures

Prognosis and Complications

Prognosis

The prognosis is generally good.

Possible Complications

- Secondary soft-tissue necrosis and compartment syndrome in patients with complex injuries
- Osteomyelitis in open fractures
- Plantar displacement of head fragment due to dominant flexor tension causing an abnormal plantar pressure distribution and metatarsalgia
- Delayed healing and nonunion are common in fractures of the fifth metatarsal and basal fractures of the second metatarsal
- Posttraumatic splayfoot and flatfoot
- Neurovascular injuries
- Reflex sympathetic dystrophy (complex regional pain syndrome, CRPS)
- Rare: entrapment of a sural nerve branch with positive Tinel sign and resulting digital dysesthesias in displaced avulsion fractures of the fifth metatarsal base

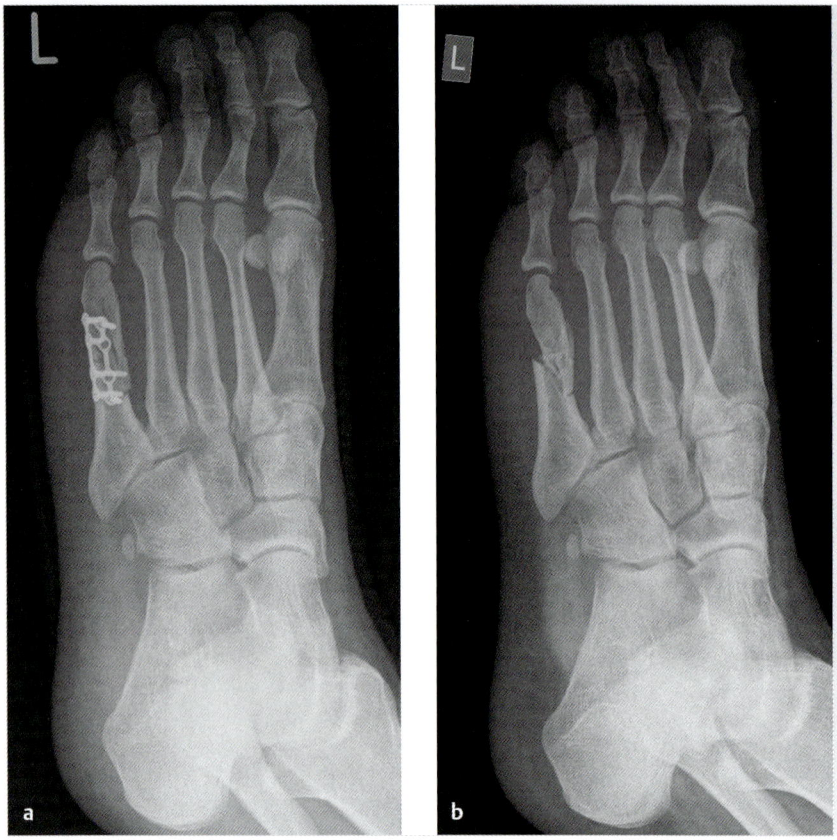

Fig. 5.5 a, b Fracture of the fifth metatarsal, pre- and postoperative views.
a Oblique view of a multipart fracture of the fifth metatarsal shaft with no articular involvement (A3 in AO/ASIF classification).
b Appearance after rigid internal fixation.

Capsuloligamentous Injuries of the First Metatarsophalangeal Joint (Turf Toe, Sand Toe), Plantar Plate Tear

Definition

Hyperextension of the first metatarsophalangeal joint may cause injury to the plantar plate. The spectrum of severity is very broad and ranges from stretching of the capsule to a complete tear, rupture of the flexor hallucis brevis tendon, and associated injuries of the sesamoid bones. The direction of the traumatizing force determines whether the brunt of the damage occurs to plantar structures (turf toe with hyperextension of the first metatarsophalangeal joint) or to dorsal structures (sand toe with hyper-plantar flexion).

Symptoms

- Pain aggravated by weight bearing
- Swelling
- Hematoma
- Limited motion
- Plantar tenderness
- Pain on dorsiflexion
- Weakened flexion against a resistance
- Metatarsalgiform pain

Predisposing Factors

- Flexible athletic shoes that permit a large range of hallux dorsiflexion
- Artificial turf (harder than natural grass)
- Dorsiflexion of the toes with a high axial compression load on the big toe. (Note that the big toe normally bears twice the weight of the lesser toes; the maximum force acting on the first metatarsophalangeal joint is approximately 40–60% of the body weight)
- Decreased range of motion of the first metatarsophalangeal joint
- Prior injuries

Anatomy and Pathology

Anatomy

The plantar plate of the metatarsophalangeal joints is a separate structure that helps support the body weight. Like the menisci, it has a fibrocartilagelike composition that enables it to withstand compressive loads. It is the principal stabilizer of the first metatarsophalangeal joint and is centered by the medial and lateral metatarsosesamoid ligaments. The collateral ligaments function as secondary stabilizers along with the abductor hallucis, adductor hallucis, and flexor hallucis brevis muscles. The flexor hallucis brevis divides into medial and lateral tendons at the level of the first metatarsophalangeal joint, and the two sesamoids are embedded within the lateral and medial heads.

Pathology

Mechanisms of Injury

- Bowers and Martin coined the term "turf toe" in 1976 to describe a hyperextension injury of the first metatarsophalan-

Table 5.3 Classification of capsuloligamentous injuries of the first metatarsophalangeal (MP) joint

Grade	Injury	Signs and symptoms
1	Stretching or small partial tear of the capsuloligamentous complex of the first MP joint	• Localized plantar or medial tenderness • Minimal swelling and no hematoma • Slight limitation of motion • Most patients can bear full weight with mild symptoms (common with chronic injury)
2	Partial tear of the capsuloligamentous complex of the first MP joint	• Increased tenderness, which may be diffuse • Moderate swelling and hematoma • Mild-to-moderate limitation of motion • Moderate pain and slight limp on weight bearing • Symptoms worsen within 24 hours
3	(Nearly) complete tear of the capsuloligamentous complex and a plantar plate tear at its origin on the head and neck of the first metatarsal (hyperextension mechanism) with impaction of the proximal phalanx into the dorsal metatarsal head; possible fracture of the medial sesamoid or diastasis of a bipartite sesamoid; rarely, distal rupture of the capsuloligamentous complex with proximal displacement of the sesamoid	• Marked pain and tenderness on both the plantar and dorsal sides of the first metatarsophalangeal joint • Marked swelling and obvious hematoma • Significant limitation of motion • Inability to bear weight

geal joint sustained by football players on artificial turf. This type of injury is most common in American football, soccer, and dancing; 83% are caused by playing sports on an artificial surface, and 45% of national football league players experience this injury at some time during their career.

- Traumatic tears of the plantar plate of the second through fourth metatarsals are very rare and may result in dorsal subluxation of the proximal phalanx.
- A common mechanism of injury is forcible bending of the first metatarsophalangeal joint past its physiologic range of motion. A variety of structures may be injured, depending on the direction of the traumatizing force.
- Sand toe: dorsal capsuloligamentous injury of the first metatarsophalangeal joint caused by plantar hyperflexion; relatively common in professional beach volleyball players. Injuries that do not heal completely often cause significant functional disability.

Classification

The classification of capsuloligamentous injuries of the first metatarsophalangeal joint is shown in ▶ Table 5.3.

Imaging

Radiography

- *Big toe, DP view:* position of the sesamoids
- *Big toe, lateral view (or lateral dorsiflexion view):* evaluates sesamoid position or sesamoid fractures
- *Forefoot, axial view:* demonstrates the sesamoids (according to pain tolerance)

Ultrasound

Ultrasound can demonstrate a hematoma or possible tendon rupture.

CT

Not indicated.

MRI

Interpretation Checklist

- Alignment of the first metatarsophalangeal joint in the sagittal plane
- Evaluation of the sesamoids (edema or necrosis, bipartite sesamoid, fragmentation, degeneration)

Examination Technique

- *Standard examination:* prone position, high-resolution multichannel coil
- *Sequences:*
  - PD-weighted fat-sat and T1-weighted coronal oblique
  - PD-weighted fat-sat sagittal (2- to 2.5-mm slice thickness, centered on first metatarsal)
  - T2-weighted axial
  - Contrast administration is useful for evaluating chronic injuries; T1-weighted fat-sat with IV contrast, coronal and sagittal

! Note

Match the examination technique to the structures of interest by using thin slices (2–2.5 mm), a small field of view, and multichannel technology. Only high-resolution imaging permits an accurate assessment of these fine anatomic structures.

MRI Findings (▶ Fig. 5.6 and ▶ Fig. 5.7)

- Joint position (plantar plate tears allow dorsal or extensor-side subluxation of the first metatarsophalangeal joint)
- Capsular injuries on the extensor side, which are best displayed on sagittal images; collateral ligament injuries on coronal images
- With a capsuloligamentous injury or tear, bleeding within the injured structures causes increased signal intensity on fluid-sensitive sequences
- Discontinuity in the plantar plate

Imaging Recommendation

Modality of choice: MRI for evaluating the plantar plate, sesamoids, and collateral ligaments.

Differential Diagnosis

- Tendon injuries
- Fractures
- Freiberg–Köhler disease (stress fracture of the metatarsal head)
- Metatarsalgia
- Sesamoid injuries
- Bipartite sesamoid

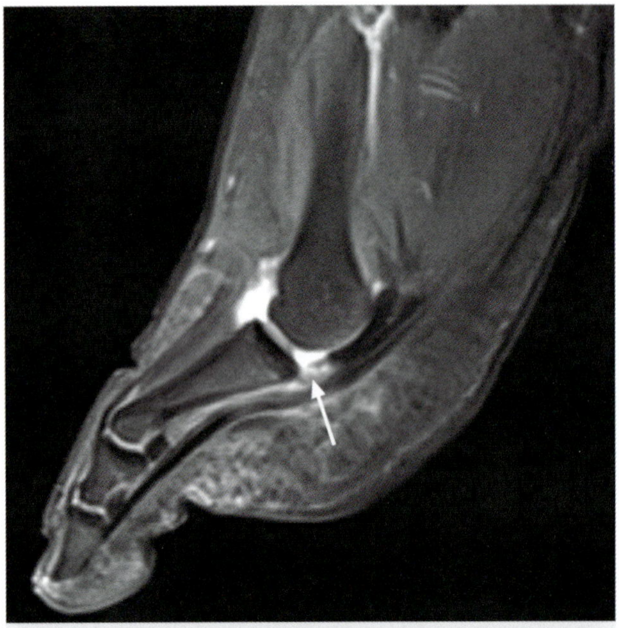

Fig. 5.6 Plantar plate tear in a 31-year-old woman. Sagittal fat-saturated PD-weighted image shows a central plantar plate tear at the level of the left second metatarsophalangeal joint (arrow). Effusion is noted in the adjacent metatarsophalangeal joint.

Treatment

Conservative

The extent of soft-tissue injuries determines the treatment strategy and affects the prognosis:

- *Grade 1:* tape and stiff soles; sports participation may be continued
- *Grade 2:* tape and stiff soles; 3 to 14 days' rest before returning to sports
- *Grade 3:* restricted weight bearing for 1 to 3 days on two forearm crutches, then a walking cast or walker for 1 week; approximately 6 weeks' rest before return to sports

Operative

- Indications for operative treatment:
  - Large capsular avulsion with an unstable joint
  - Diastasis of a bipartite sesamoid
  - Displaced sesamoid fracture
  - Retraction of the sesamoids (indicates avulsion of flexor hallucis brevis)
  - Traumatic hallux valgus deformity
  - Vertical instability (positive Lachman test)
  - Intra-articular loose body
  - Chondral injury
  - Persistent instability after conservative therapy
- Repair of the joint capsule and ruptured tendons
- Removal of small fragments, internal fixation of larger bone fragments, internal fixation of a fractured sesamoid

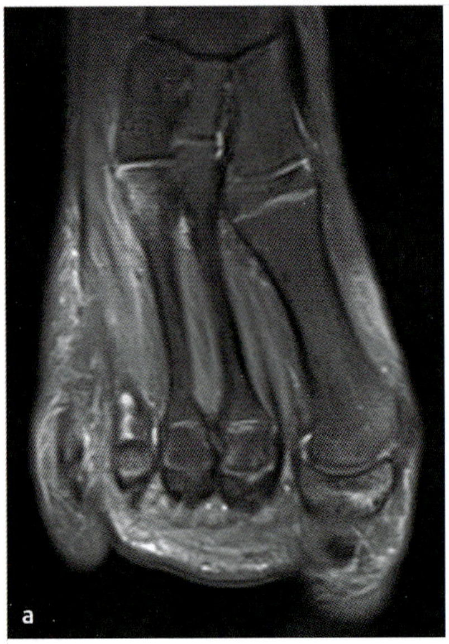

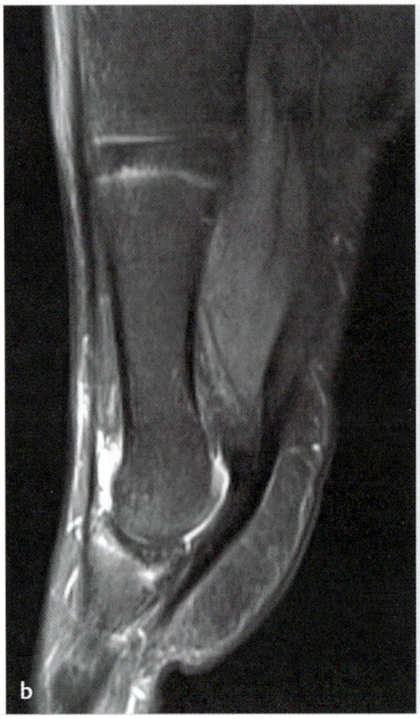

Fig. 5.7 a, b MRI in a 14-year-old girl with a recent sprain of the big toe.
a Coronal fat-saturated PD-weighted image shows subluxation of the first metatarsophalangeal joint with lateral deviation of the proximal phalanx, rupture of the medial capsule and ligaments, and cancellous bone edema in the proximal phalanx on the articular side.
b Sagittal fat-saturated PD-weighted image shows an intact plantar plate at the first metatarsophalangeal joint with intact flexor tendons. Contusional edema is noted in the proximal phalanx along with small hemorrhagic areas that include the proximal epiphyseal plate of the first metatarsal.

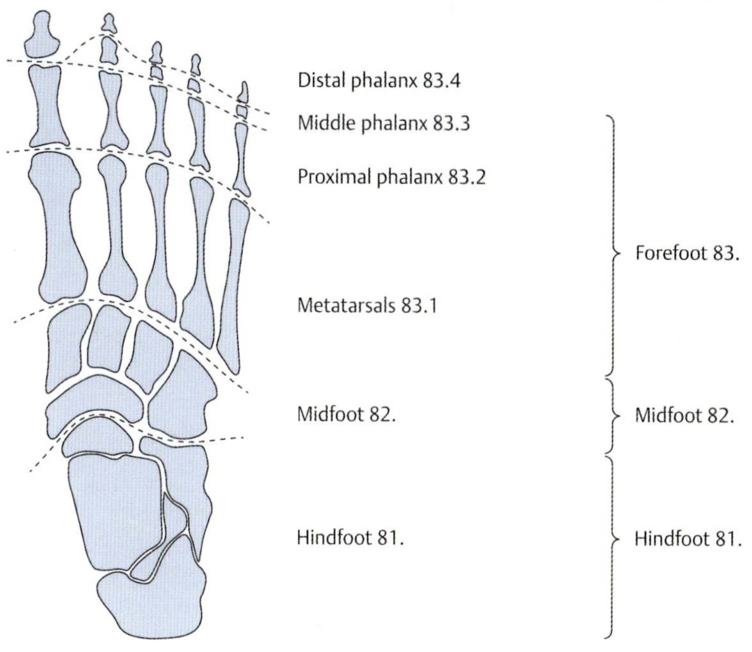

Fig. 5.8 ICI classification of toe fractures.

Possible Complications

- Persistent instability
- Functional weakening of flexor hallucis brevis with weakened push-off during running and jumping
- Metatarsalgia
- Posttraumatic osteoarthritis
- Possible mallet toe development after plantar plate injuries below the lesser metatarsals

Phalangeal Fractures

Definition

Fractures involving one or more digits (phalanges) of the first through fifth toe.

Symptoms

- Painful limitation of motion, especially during push-off
- Swelling
- Hematoma
- Displaced fracture with malalignment
- Tenderness to pressure

Predisposing Factors

There are no true predisposing factors, although the risk of phalangeal fractures is increased by certain athletic activities (such as contact sports or football, soccer, rugby) or sports in which the toes are subject to high stresses (e.g., sprinting, dancing, skimboarding: deceleration trauma caused by sudden stopping of the skimboard at the shoreline or by a fall into shallow water).

The phalanges are a site of predilection for bone tumors, especially enchondromas, which may lead to pathologic fractures.

Anatomy and Pathology

Anatomy

The second through fifth toes are each comprised of a proximal, middle, and distal phalanx. The middle phalanx is absent in the big toe. The proximal end of each phalanx, called the base, bears a concave articular surface, while the distal end is rounded to form a convex head. Between the proximal and distal ends is the shaft (diaphysis). The metatarsophalangeal and interphalangeal joints are connected by collateral ligaments and by a plantar fibrous thickening of the joint capsule (plantar ligaments).

Pathology

Mechanism of Injury

Toe fractures are a common injury. Most are caused by direct trauma to the big or small toe (entrapment, crushing, severe impact, stubbing). The majority of these injuries are nondisplaced fractures (< 2 mm) without articular involvement. Severe toe fractures or even amputations may occur in small children who ride on an escalator while wearing flip-flops (soft, open-back rubber sandals).

Classification (▶ Fig. 5.8)

The ICI classification describes the location of an injury by enumerating all 28 bones of the foot in relation to the three main anatomical regions from proximal to distal: hindfoot (81), midfoot (82), and forefoot (83). The letter A stands for extra-articular, B for intra-articular, and C for fracture-dislocation.

Imaging

Radiography (▶ Fig. 5.9)

- *Radiographs of the forefoot in two planes*
- *Big toe, DP view:* position of the sesamoids

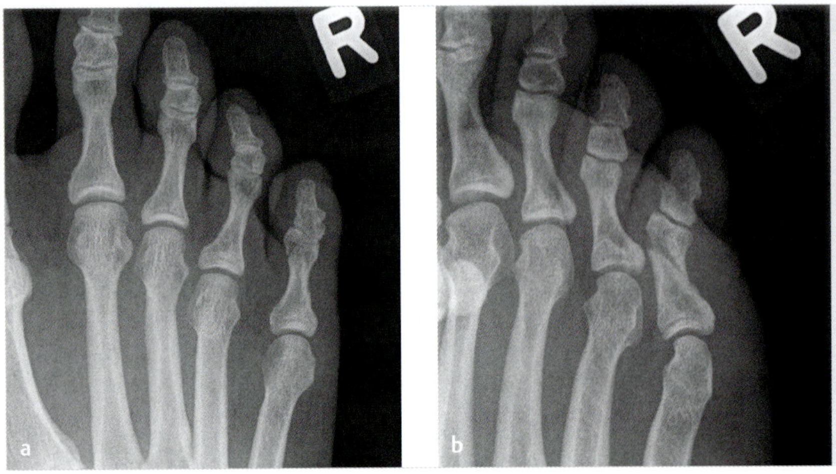

Fig. 5.9 a, b Distal oblique shaft fracture of the proximal phalanx of the small toe, stabilized by taping.
a DP radiograph.
b Oblique radiograph.

- *Big toe, lateral view (or lateral dorsiflexion view):* evaluate sesamoid position, sesamoid fractures
- *Sesamoid view:* displays the sesamoids and their joint spaces (according to pain tolerance). A bipartite sesamoid usually presents rounded edges that are unlike the sharp corners and margins of a sesamoid fracture.

Ultrasound

Not indicated.

CT

There is no primary indication for CT, though it is sometimes used for preoperative planning in complex comminuted fractures of the first metatarsophalangeal joint.

MRI

MRI is used to investigate suspected sesamoid necrosis and to help distinguish a bipartite sesamoid from a sesamoid fracture.

Differential Diagnosis

- Sesamoid necrosis in the fragmentation stage
- Bipartite sesamoid
- Accessory sesamoids at the second through fifth metatarsophalangeal joints

Treatment

Conservative

A proven treatment is to tape the fractured toe to an adjacent toe with a small gauze pad placed between the taped toes.

A forefoot offloading shoe is usually sufficient to relieve pressure on the forefoot.

Operative

! Note

Displaced fractures can be reduced under local anesthesia. Care must be taken to position the fragments in correct rotational alignment.

Unstable displaced fractures and fractures with articular involvement can be stabilized with a K-wire or immobilized with miniscrews or plates. This particularly applies to fractures of the big toe. Bony avulsions of the collateral ligaments can also be reduced and fixed with screws or a K-wire. Open fractures of the first metatarsophalangeal joint can be immobilized with a mini-external fixation device.

Sesamoid fractures showing 3 mm or more of dehiscence are currently treated more aggressively by internal fixation with a double-threaded screw. Minimally displaced sesamoid fractures can be managed conservatively.

Prognosis and Complications

There is little risk of fracture nonunion in the toes. Fractures involving the lesser toe joints consistently lead to a permanent limitation of motion. Sesamoid fractures have a high risk of nonunion.

5.2 Chronic, Posttraumatic, and Degenerative Changes

M. Walther and U. Szeimies

Hallux valgus

Definition

Hallux valgus is the term applied to a static subluxation of the first metatarsophalangeal joint combined with lateral deviation of the big toe and medial deviation of the first metatarsal. Other components may be a pronated position of the big toe, lateral tilt of the articular surface of the first metatarsal, and lateral subluxation of the sesamoids.

Symptoms

Symptoms range from an absence of complaints to chronic inflammation over the pseudoexostosis. Secondary mechanical sequelae include transfer metatarsalgia caused by reduced stress transfer across the big toe.

Predisposing Factors

- Positive family history
- Connective tissue diseases
- Gender (90% of patients are female)
- Pes planovalgus
- Inflammatory joint diseases

Anatomy and Pathology

- Lateral deviation of the big toe combined with medialization of the first metatarsal
- Lateral decentering of the sesamoids, ranging to complete dislocation
- Varying degrees of pseudoexostosis
- Hallux pronation deformity or even intraduction (partial overlap of the first and second toes)

Imaging

Radiography

Stress radiographs of the foot are taken in three planes. The following parameters are determined:

- Hallux valgus angle (normal: < 15°)
- Intermetatarsal angle (normal: < 9°)
- Position of the sesamoids (partial or complete dislocation)
- Position of the articular surface
- First metatarsal: distal metatarsal articular angle (DMAA; normal: < 6°)
- Proximal phalanx: proximal articular set angle (PASA; normal: < 15°)
- Hallux interphalangeal angle (angle between the axis of the first metatarsal and proximal phalanx; normal: < 5°)
- Pseudoexostosis
- Hallux valgus interphalangeal angle (normal: < 10°)
- Length of the metatarsals
- Shape of the metatarsophalangeal joint
- Congruity
- First talometatarsal joint and joint with medial cuneiform: shape of articular surface, os intermetatarseum

Ultrasound

Not indicated.

CT, MRI (▶ Fig. 5.10)

There is no indication for sectional imaging.

Imaging Recommendation

Modality of choice: radiography. Stress radiographs of the foot in three planes.

Differential Diagnosis

- Hallux rigidus
- Gout
- Pseudogout
- Turf toe

Treatment

Conservative

The symptoms of hallux valgus can be reduced by conservative measures such as physical therapy, exercise therapy, bracing, shoe inserts, and a wide toebox.

Operative

The only way to correct the deformity is by surgery. More than 150 surgical procedures have been published. The most widely used techniques are the chevron, scarf, basal osteotomy, and corrective fusion of the first tarsometatarsal joint. The greater the deformity, the more proximal the level of the corrective osteotomy.

Prognosis and Complications

The prognosis is good following successful surgical realignment of the first ray. Several factors may compromise the functional outcome:

- Pre-existing cartilage lesions
- Limited motion in the first metatarsophalangeal joint
- Crystal arthropathy, rheumatoid disease

Possible complications include recurrent deformity, hallux varus, progressive osteoarthritis of the first metatarsophalangeal joint, and osteonecrosis of the first metatarsal head.

Hallux rigidus

Definition

Hallux rigidus is defined as a painful, degenerative limitation of motion in the first metatarsophalangeal joint combined with dorsal osteophyte formation.

Symptoms

- Painful limitation of motion
- Synovitis and swelling
- Osteophytes on the dorsal aspect of the proximal phalanx and first metatarsal
- Bilateral in 80% of cases
- Not typically associated with hallux valgus

Predisposing Factors

- Trauma (turf toe injury)
- Flattened metatarsal head
- Elevated first ray
- Positive family history

Anatomy and Pathology

Trauma or incongruity in the first metatarsophalangeal joint gives rise to progressive degenerative changes with joint space narrowing, osteophyte formation, and limited motion.

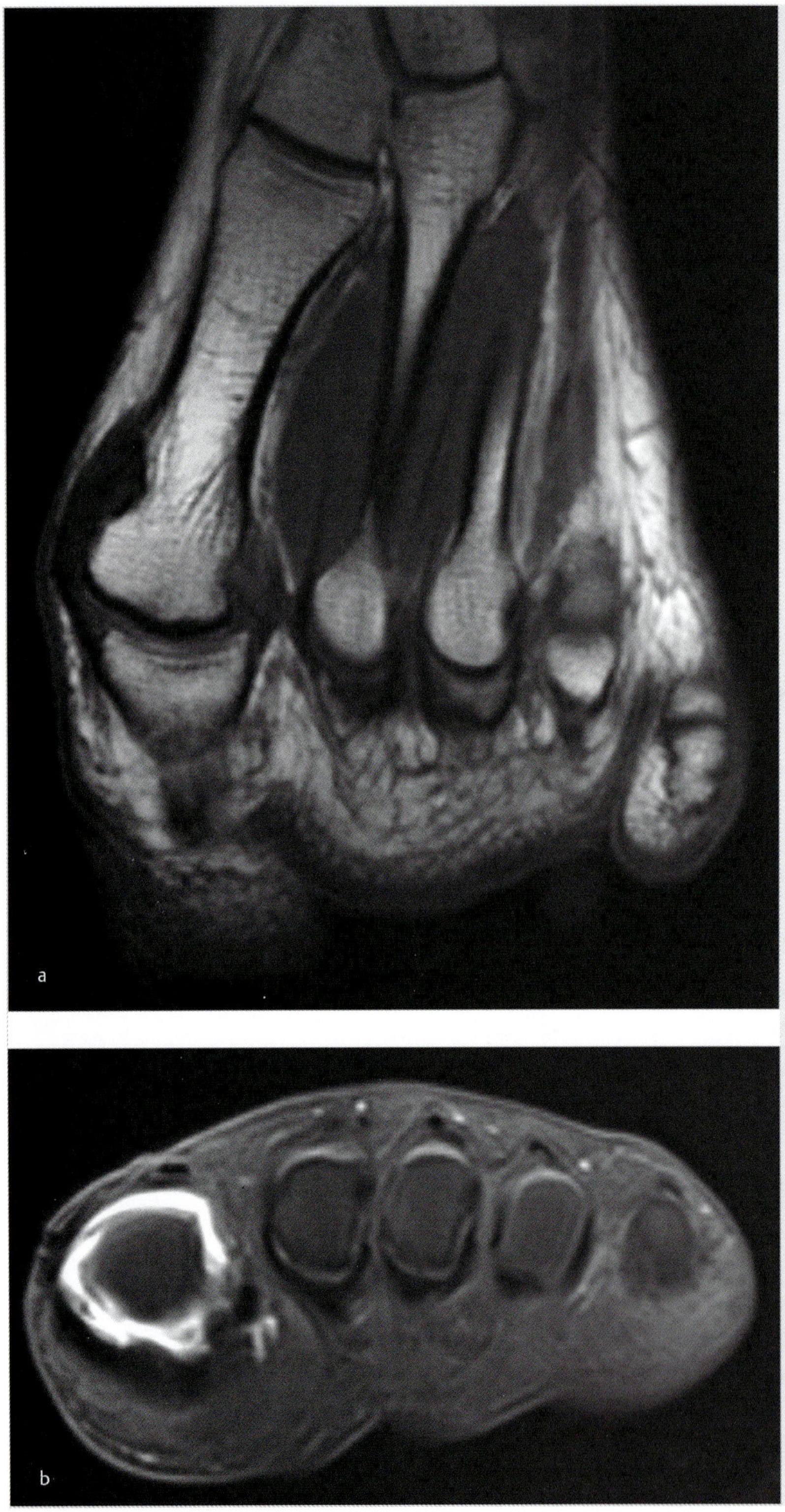

Fig. 5.10 a, b Activated hallux valgus in a 27-year-old woman. The foot was imaged to exclude other pathology. The diagnosis of hallux valgus is not a primary indication for MRI.
a Coronal T1-weighted image shows lateral deviation of the big toe with medialization of the first metatarsal and subluxation of the first metatarsophalangeal joint.
b Axial fat-saturated T1-weighted image after contrast administration shows intense synovial enhancement consistent with chronic activation of hallux valgus.

Imaging

Radiography

The clinical and radiographic stages of hallux rigidus are outlined in ▶ Table 5.4.

Ultrasound

A longitudinal scan over the first metatarsophalangeal joint shows projecting, echogenic bony lines (osteophytes), often with bizarre shapes, a hypoechoic joint effusion, and possible echogenic thickening of the synovial membrane (Doppler-positive).

Table 5.4 Grading of hallux rigidus based on clinical and radiographic findings

Grade	Description
0	Dorsiflexion 40–60°, normal radiograph, no clinical abnormalities
1	Dorsiflexion 30–40°, possible dorsal osteophyte with minimal joint space narrowing; subjective feeling of joint stiffness and pain on passive dorsiflexion
2	Dorsiflexion 10–30°, circumferential osteophytes with flattening of the first metatarsal head
3	Dorsiflexion 10° or less, radiographic cyst formation with little or no residual joint space; constant pain with significant metatarsophalangeal joint stiffness
4	Dorsiflexion 10° or less, further progress of radiographically visible joint space narrowing, degenerative changes in the sesamoid joints and cyst formation

CT, MRI

Not indicated.

Imaging Recommendation

Modality of choice: radiographs of the affected foot in three planes.

Differential Diagnosis

- Intra-articular loose body
- Arthrofibrosis
- Osteochondritis dissecans
- Rheumatoid arthritis
- Sesamoid necrosis
- Uric arthritis

Treatment

Conservative

- Orthotics with a steel spring under the first ray (“rigidus spring”)
- Physical therapy with mobilization and traction
- Nonsteroidal anti-inflammatory drugs (NSAIDs), local or systemic, as needed
- Steroid injection into the joint
- Hyaluronic acid

Operative

- *Grades 1 and 2 (and 3):* removal of bone spurs (cheilectomy); plantar-flexion osteotomy if necessary
- *Grade (3 and) 4:* arthrodesis of the first metatarsophalangeal joint, replacement arthroplasty, resection arthroplasty

Prognosis and Complications

Approximately 75% of patients benefit from treatment with an improved range of motion. Pain symptoms are improved in 90% of cases.

Hammer, Claw and Mallet Toes, Chronic Plantar Plate Tear

Definition

Toe deformity:

- *Hammer toe:* dorsiflexion of the metatarsophalangeal joint combined with flexion of the proximal interphalangeal joint and a neutral or hyperextended distal interphalangeal joint
- *Mallet toe:* flexion contracture of the distal interphalangeal joint
- *Claw toe:* dorsiflexion of the metatarsophalangeal joint combined with flexion contracture of the proximal and distal interphalangeal joints

Symptoms

- Second toe most commonly affected
- Corn over the dorsal side of the proximal interphalangeal joint
- Metatarsalgia
- Initially flexible deformity
- Advanced stage marked by increasing contracture with subluxation or dislocation of the metatarsophalangeal joint
- With mallet toe: painful hyperkeratosis beneath the toenail

Predisposing Factors

- Long second toe
- Hallux valgus
- Diabetes mellitus
- Frequent wearing of tight shoes
- Neuromuscular diseases
- Trauma (rare)
- Inflammatory joint diseases

Anatomy and Pathology

Anatomy

The long extensor tendon inserts on the distal phalanx of the toe but functions as an extensor of the proximal and distal interphalangeal joints only when the metatarsophalangeal joint is in a neutral or flexed position. The extensor brevis inserts on the middle phalanx as does the short flexor, while the long flexor inserts on the distal phalanx. No muscles insert on the proximal phalanx itself. The intrinsic muscles of the foot (lumbricals and interossei) act as stabilizers. The function of the intrinsic muscles depends on the position of the toe at the metatarsophalangeal joint. When the joint is flexed, they act as extensors of the proximal interphalangeal joint; when the joint is extended, they act as flexors of the proximal interphalangeal joint.

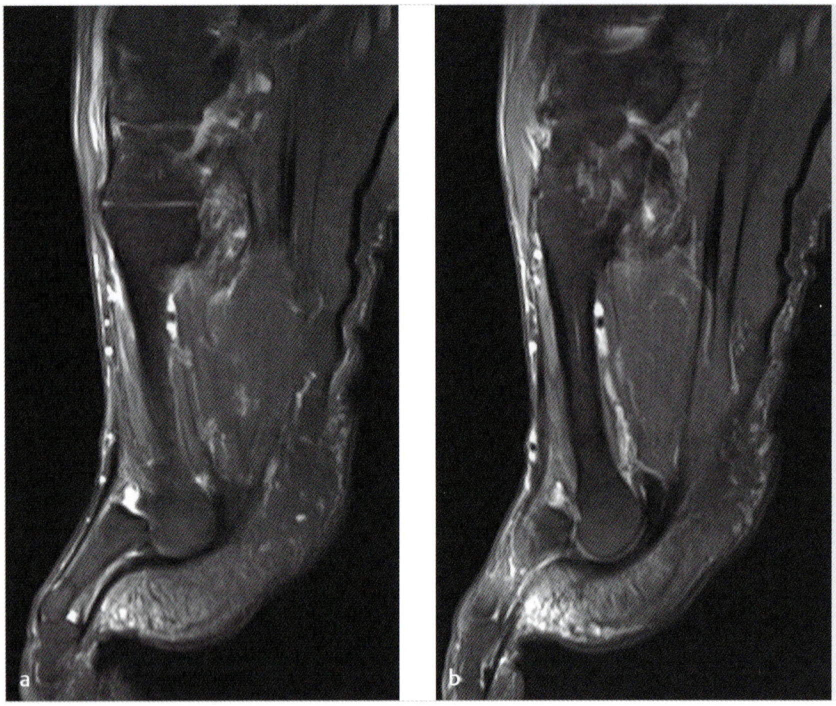

Fig. 5.11 a, b Dislocated second metatarsophalangeal joint in a 50-year-old woman. MRI was performed to exclude a Morton neuroma.
a Sagittal fat-saturated PD-weighted image shows significant dislocation of the second metatarsophalangeal joint without significant activation.
b Sagittal fat-saturated PD-weighted image. Chronic forefoot pain is best evaluated by acquiring thin sagittal slices and scrolling through them to examine all the metatarsophalangeal joints. Dislocation or subluxation associated with hammer toes is difficult to appreciate in axial and coronal sections.

The position of the metatarsophalangeal joint is a key factor, therefore. The extrinsic muscles of the foot always generate more force than the intrinsic muscles.

A central stabilizing element of the toe is the plantar plate, which is formed by expansions of the plantar aponeurosis and plantar joint capsule. The static stabilizing effect of the plantar plate, combined with the dynamic action of the intrinsic foot muscles, acts to restore the proximal phalanx to a neutral position after the push-off phase of gait.

Pathology

Both walking and footwear tend to force the proximal phalanx of the toe into a dorsiflexed position. Meanwhile the muscles exert only a weak plantar-flexing force on the proximal phalanx, while the long and short flexors can only flex the proximal and distal interphalangeal joints. All of these factors contribute to the development of hammer toe, which is the most common toe deformity. Clawing of the toes is most often encountered in neuromuscular diseases.

Imaging (▶ Fig. 5.11, ▶ Fig. 5.12, ▶ Fig. 5.13)

Radiography

Radiographs of the forefoot in two planes show the following:
- Axial deformity of the toes, most clearly appreciated in the oblique view
- Possible dislocation of the toe at the metatarsophalangeal joint with an associated plantar plate tear
- Degenerative changes in the affected joints

Ultrasound

Defects in the plantar plate can be detected by longitudinal scanning with a high-frequency transducer (> 13 MHz).

CT, MRI

Hammer toe, claw toe, and mallet toe are not indications for sectional imaging in themselves. MRI is rarely used for toe deformities. It may be used in patients with coexisting, unexplained midfoot or forefoot pain, or an exacerbation of pain in order to exclude other causes (metatarsal fatigue fracture, Morton neuroma, osteonecrosis, Köhler disease, etc.). MRI can be a useful adjunct for the precise differentiation of metatarsalgia, especially involving the second ray, in evaluations of the plantar plate.

Interpretation Checklist

- Quality of the plantar plate
- Complete rupture
- Congruity of the second metatarsophalangeal joint
- Quality of the cartilage
- Synovitis
- Joint effusion
- Keratosis
- Bone marrow signal in the midfoot and forefoot
- Evaluation of flexor and extensor tendons
- Exclusion of associated pathology

Examination Technique

- *Standard examination:* prone position, high-resolution multichannel coil
- *Sequences:*
  - PD-weighted fat-sat coronal and sagittal (high resolution over the second metatarsophalangeal joint)
  - T1-weighted coronal
  - T1-weighted axial
  - T1-weighted fat-sat after contrast administration, coronal and sagittal

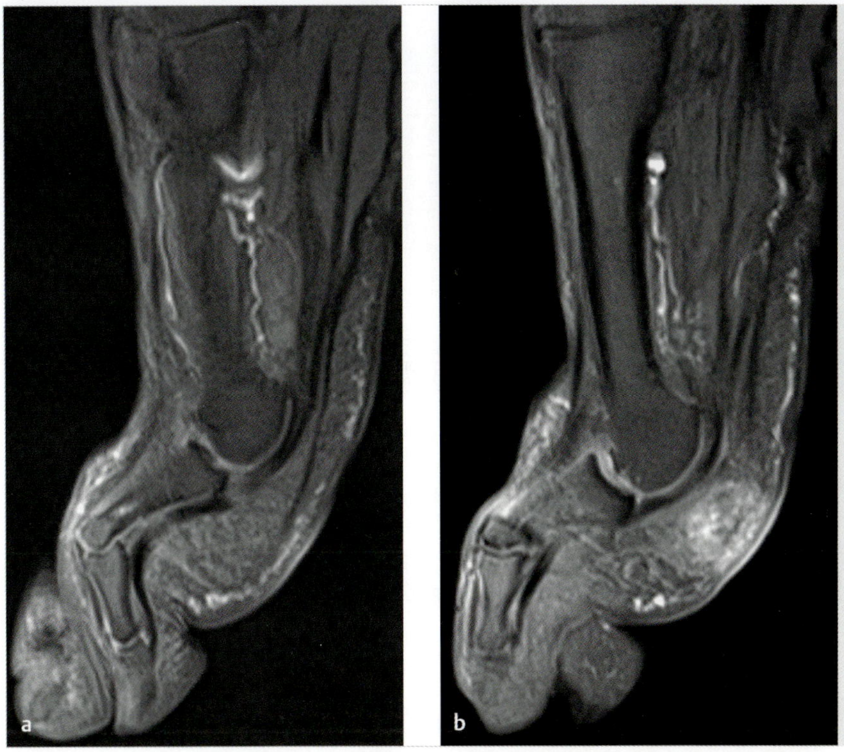

Fig. 5.12 a, b Hammer toe with plantar keratosis. The presence of a hammer toe is not an indication for MRI, which is usually carried out to exclude associated pathology such as a Morton neuroma or fatigue fracture.
a Sagittal fat-saturated T1-weighted image after contrast administration shows hammer toe deformity with extension of the metatarsophalangeal joint and flexion of the proximal interphalangeal joint.
b Sagittal fat-saturated T1-weighted image after contrast administration shows plantar keratosis under the second metatarsal head from repetitive unphysiologic loads.

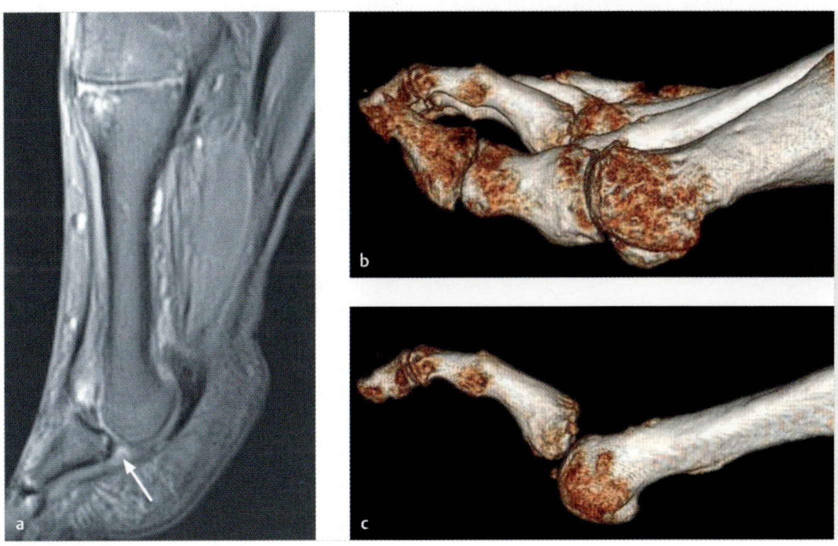

Fig. 5.13 a–c Plantar plate tear with subluxation of the second metatarsophalangeal joint in a 70-year-old woman.
a Sagittal fat-saturated T1-weighted image after contrast administration shows complete avulsion of the plantar plate (arrow) from the base of the right second proximal phalanx with proximal subluxation of the volar plate and activated osteoarthritic changes in the second metatarsophalangeal joint.
b Sagittal 3D CT reconstruction for bony evaluation of the second metatarsophalangeal joint. The first ray overlaps the affected joint.
c Sagittal segmented 3D CT reconstruction. The other metatarsals and phalanges were removed by automated segmentation to aid evaluation of the sagittal joint position.

MRI Findings

The plantar plate at the second metatarsophalangeal joint is a hypointense fibrous thickening of the plantar joint capsule between the metatarsal head and the base of the proximal phalanx. Tears or degenerative changes are relatively common in the distal joint capsule at the level of the proximal phalanx. The plantar plate is best depicted in fat-sat PD-weighted sequences with a slice thickness of 2 to 3 mm. Imaging after contrast administration or chronic degeneration sometimes shows focally increased enhancement relating to degenerative vascularization. Chronic insufficiency of the plantar plate causes increased enhancement of the capsule and ligaments of the second metatarsophalangeal joint. Other possible findings:

- Synovitis
- Joint effusion
- Malalignment
- Subluxation
- Occasional bone overload with marrow edema in the articulating bone ends
- Initial cartilage lesions
- Plantar keratosis under the second metatarsal head
- Possible keratosis under the fifth metatarsal head due to compensatory weight transfer to the lateral side of the foot

Imaging Recommendation

Modality of choice: radiography.

Table 5.5 Bragard classification of osteonecrosis

Stage	Description
I	Flattening of the metatarsal head and decreased subchondral bone density
II	Sclerosis and fragmentation, deformation of the metatarsal head, thickening of the cortex
III	Metatarsophalangeal osteoarthritis with intra-articular loose bodies, most common in women 20–30 years of age. Second metatarsal is most commonly affected, third metatarsal is occasionally affected

Differential Diagnosis

- Morton neuroma
- Arthritis
- Köhler disease
- Stress fracture

Treatment

Conservative

- Cushioning inserts
- Toe pads
- Physical therapy
- Shoes with a toebox and soft top
- Steroid injections into a painful metatarsophalangeal joint

Operative

Surgical correction is geared toward the extent of the deformity, the number of joints affected, and the degree of rigidity. Combinations of different techniques are most commonly used:

- *Metatarsophalangeal joint:* lengthening the extensor tendons, arthrolysis, Weil osteotomy, plantar plate repair
- *Proximal interphalangeal joint:* transfer of flexor digitorum longus to the proximal phalanx to stabilize the metatarsophalangeal joint, resection arthroplasty, arthrodesis
- *Distal interphalangeal joint:* long flexor tendon release, dermatotenodesis with or without resection of the joint

Prognosis and Complications

The goal of conservative treatment is to reduce local pressure-related complaints and prevent progression. As a rule, existing deformities are not reversible. The goal of operative treatment is to improve the position of the toes; a normal range of motion cannot be achieved.

! Note

Patients should be informed they will still have functional limitations after surgery.

Osteonecrosis, Köhler Disease Type II

Definition

Osteonecrosis is an aseptic necrosis that generally affects the second metatarsal head and may rarely affect the third or fourth metatarsal. Köhler disease type II is also known as Köhler–Freiberg disease.

Symptoms

- Pain and swelling
- Later, enlargement of the joint with locking and limited motion
- Osteonecrosis: disease of adolescence (peak incidence: 11–17 years of age)
- Late sequelae with symptomatic osteoarthritis often delayed until adulthood

Predisposing Factors

- Long second metatarsal
- Prior history of trauma (repetitive microtrauma or a single event)
- Wearing high heels

Anatomy and Pathology

A long second metatarsal is subject to increased stresses. Repeated microtrauma leads to trabecular fractures, occluded blood vessels, and local necrosis. Revascularization occurs from the periosteum and metaphysis.

Imaging

Radiography

The Bragard staging classification is based on radiographs of the forefoot in two planes (▶ Table 5.5).

Ultrasound

Ultrasound does not have a role in routine examinations. Scans of osteonecrosis may show the following:

- Cartilage irregularities
- Dorsal flattening of the metatarsal head
- Joint effusion
- Intra-articular loose bodies
- Synovitis
- Longitudinal scan over the second (or third) metatarsophalangeal joint in the acute stage shows hypoechoic joint effusion and a rough, echogenic bony surface of the metatarsal head, increased when destructive changes are present

CT, MRI

Generally there is no need for sectional imaging tests when the diagnosis is known. MRI may be used to investigate unexplained metatarsalgia in patients with no radiographic abnormalities, and the imaging pattern of osteonecrosis should be known.

Interpretation Checklist

- Evaluate the quality of the subchondral bone
- Extent of osteonecrosis
- Degree of activation in the metatarsophalangeal joint
- Signs of early osteoarthritis

Examination Technique

- *Standard examination:* prone position, high-resolution multichannel coil
- *Sequences:*
  - PD-weighted fat-sat coronal and sagittal (high resolution over the second metatarsophalangeal joint)
  - T1-weighted coronal
  - T1-weighted axial
  - T1-weighted fat-sat after contrast administration, coronal and sagittal

MRI Findings (▶ Fig. 5.14 and ▶ Fig. 5.15)

- The findings are like those in any osteonecrosis with initial bone marrow edema (difficult to distinguish from bone stress reaction; bone overload may occasionally affect the third metatarsal and is sometimes associated with plantar keratosis)
- Effusion in the metatarsophalangeal joint
- Synovitis

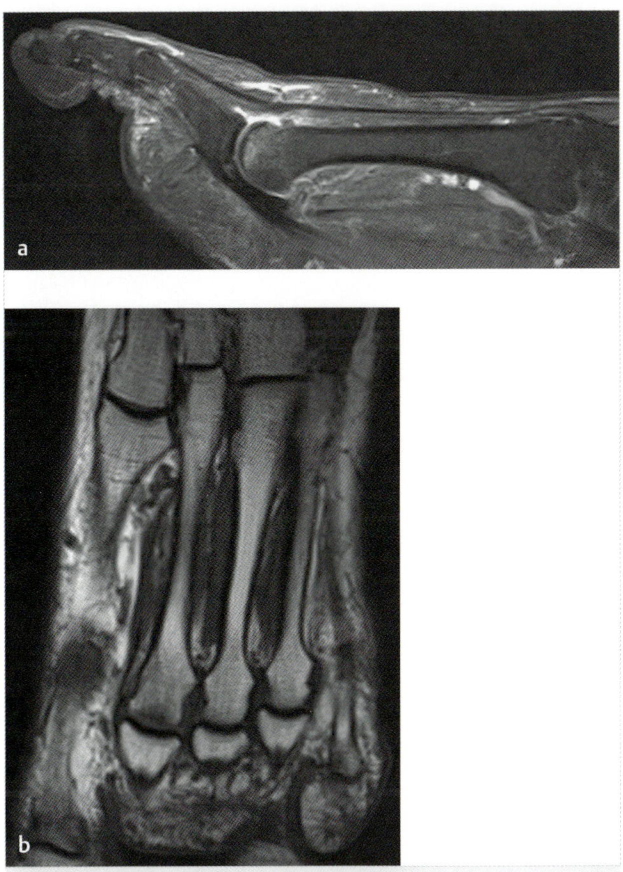

Fig. 5.14 a, b Florid Köhler disease type II involving the head of the second metatarsal.
a Sagittal fat-saturated PD-weighted image shows focal bone marrow edema in the head of the second metatarsal with mild reactive effusion in the metatarsophalangeal joint.
b Coronal T1-weighted image shows flattening and cortical infraction of the metatarsal head in Köhler disease type II.

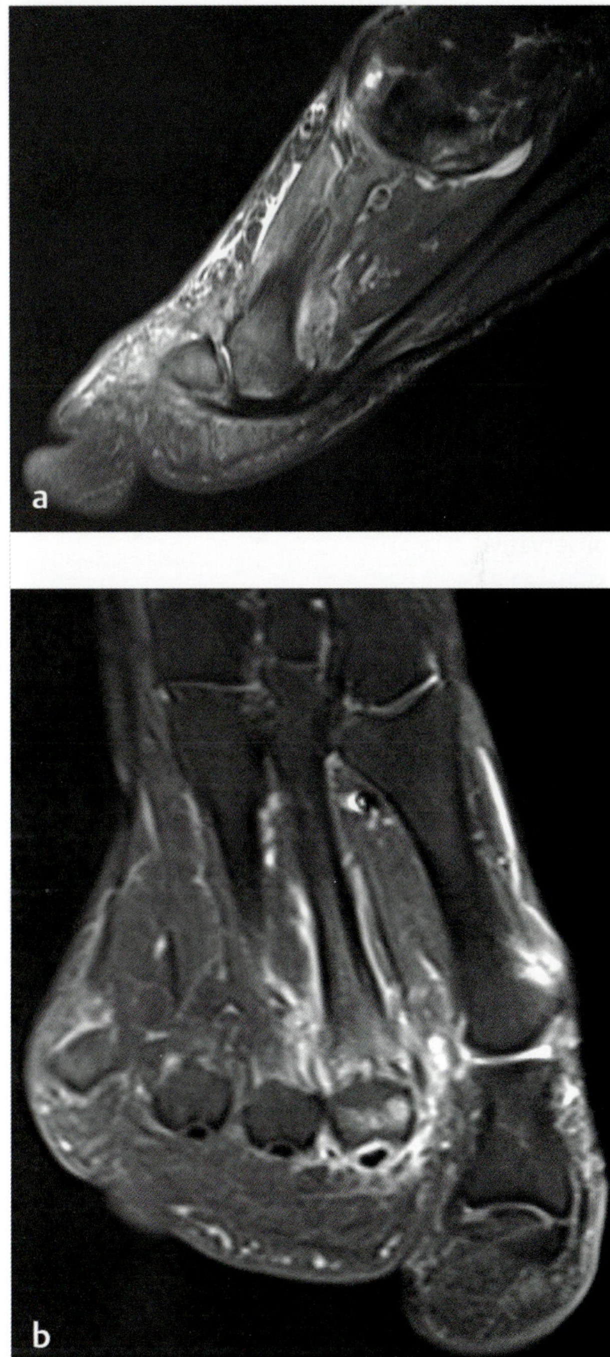

Fig. 5.15 a, b Advanced Köhler disease type II in a 59-year-old woman with severe forefoot pain.
a Sagittal fat-saturated T1-weighted image after contrast administration shows patchy bone marrow edema and enhancement in the second metatarsal head with subchondral infraction, deformation, and loss of metatarsophalangeal joint congruity.
b Coronal fat-saturated T1-weighted image after contrast administration shows an extensive irritative reaction in the metatarsophalangeal joint with synovitis and in adjacent soft tissues.

- With advanced osteonecrosis: cortical infraction in the metatarsal head with flattening, loss of joint congruity, and loss of T1-weighted signal in the subchondral region
- Later: advanced deformation of the metatarsal head with sclerosis (signal void in all pulse sequences)
- Dominant findings may be secondary degenerative changes with possible activated osteoarthritis

Imaging Recommendation

Modality of choice: radiography. MRI is used in equivocal cases.

Differential Diagnosis

- Stress fracture
- Arthritis
- Plantar plate tear
- Morton neuroma
- Gout
- Neuroarthropathy
- Osteoarthritis

Treatment

Conservative

- Stress reduction
- Steroid injections
- Cushioning inserts
- Shoe with wide toebox

Operative

- Removal of intra-articular loose bodies and synovectomy
- Cheilectomy
- Corrective osteotomy
- Resection arthroplasty (Stainsby operation)

Prognosis and Complications

The functional results of joint resections are poor. Every effort should be made, therefore, to preserve the joint whenever possible. Functional deficits usually persist in the metatarsophalangeal joint.

Sesamoid Pathology

Definition

This category includes numerous sesamoid disorders such as fractures, turf toe injuries, a mobile bipartite sesamoid, osteochondrosis, degenerative changes in the subsesamoid joint space, osteonecrosis, and insertional tendinopathy of flexor hallucis longus, all of which present with largely identical symptoms.

Symptoms

- Plantar pain under the first metatarsal head
- Pain on dorsiflexion of the first metatarsophalangeal joint
- With turf toe injury: possible complete rupture of the plantar structures with a palpable defect

Predisposing Factors

- Depression of the first metatarsal (pes cavus)
- Hyperactivity of the peroneus longus
- Atrophy of the plantar fat pad
- Bipartite sesamoid
- Trauma
- Turf toe injury

Anatomy and Pathology

Anatomy

The sesamoid bones and collateral ligaments stabilize the metatarsophalangeal joint of the big toe on the plantar side. The dorsal surface of the sesamoids articulates with the plantar surface of the first metatarsal head.

Pathology

- *Bipartite sesamoid:* a medial and/or lateral sesamoid bone comprising two separate pieces—a congenital condition having no pathologic significance. Trauma or chronic overload may cause the fibrous attachment between the ossification centers to loosen, resulting in clinical complaints.
- *Sesamoid fracture:* usually a transverse fracture following hyperextension trauma or a direct blow to the foot.
- *Turf toe:* usually a hyperextension injury, rarely a flexion injury, with capsular lesions that range from minor to a complete tear. Concomitant injury to the collateral ligaments may be present.
- *Osteochondrosis:* defect in the sesamoid cartilage.
- *Sesamoid osteoarthritis:* degenerative changes in the subsesamoid joint space, usually occurring in association with hallux valgus, hallux rigidus, osteonecrosis, or after a sesamoid fracture with a step in the articular surface. Characterized by an increasing loss of substance in the cartilage, metatarsal head, and sesamoid.
- *Osteonecrosis:* aseptic necrosis of the sesamoid bone. Repetitive microtrauma has been postulated as a cause.
- *Flexor hallucis brevis insertional tendinopathy:* tendinopathy of the short hallux flexor at its insertion on the sesamoid bone.

Imaging

Radiography (▶ Fig. 5.16)

Axial sesamoid view and a lateral view of the first metatarsophalangeal joint:
- Dehiscence due to fracture or a mobile bipartite sesamoid
- Joint space narrowing in osteoarthritis

Ultrasound

Ultrasound does not have a role in routine examinations.

CT

CT may be indicated when radiographs are suspicious for a fracture or to evaluate the fragments in osteonecrosis with fragmentation. Scans should be high-resolution with a 0.5-mm slice thickness, and multiplanar reformatting (MPR) should be performed.

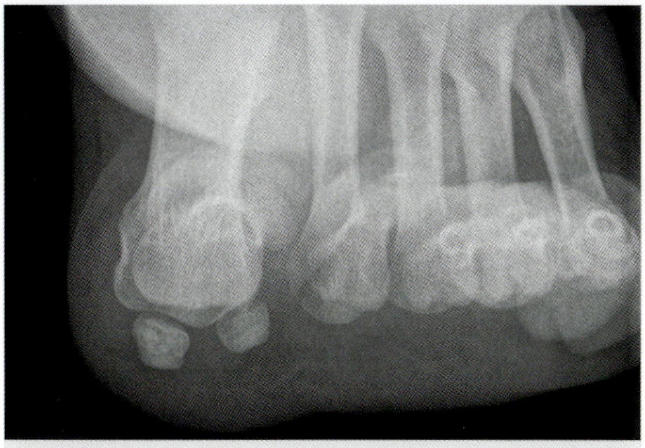

Fig. 5.16 Special radiographic view of the sesamoids shows no abnormalities.

MRI

Sesamoiditis is not a diagnosis in the true sense but describes only a nonspecific state of sesamoid irritation, which may have various causes. Many cases involve a bony overload that can eventually lead to osteonecrosis with subsequent fragmentation and involvement of the flexor hallucis brevis tendon and first metatarsophalangeal joint.

Interpretation Checklist

- Degree of sesamoid activation
- Bone marrow edema
- Contrast enhancement
- Exclusion or confirmation of osteonecrosis
- Shape of sesamoids
- Position
- Bipartite sesamoid
- Evaluation of the subsesamoid joint space
- Osteoarthritis
- Evaluation of flexor hallucis longus and brevis tendons
- Insertional tendinopathy
- Tendinosis
- Peritendinitis
- Evaluation of the plantar plate
- Capsule and ligaments of the first metatarsophalangeal joint

Examination Technique

- *Standard examination:* prone position, high-resolution multichannel coil
- *Sequences:*
  - PD-weighted fat-sat coronal and sagittal
  - T1-weighted coronal
  - T2-weighted axial
  - T1-weighted fat-sat after contrast administration, coronal and sagittal

MRI Findings (▶ Fig. 5.17, ▶ Fig. 5.18, ▶ Fig. 5.19)

- Bone marrow edema in medial or lateral sesamoid with increased enhancement
- With osteonecrosis: noncontrast T1-weighted sequence shows low signal intensity with absence of fatty marrow

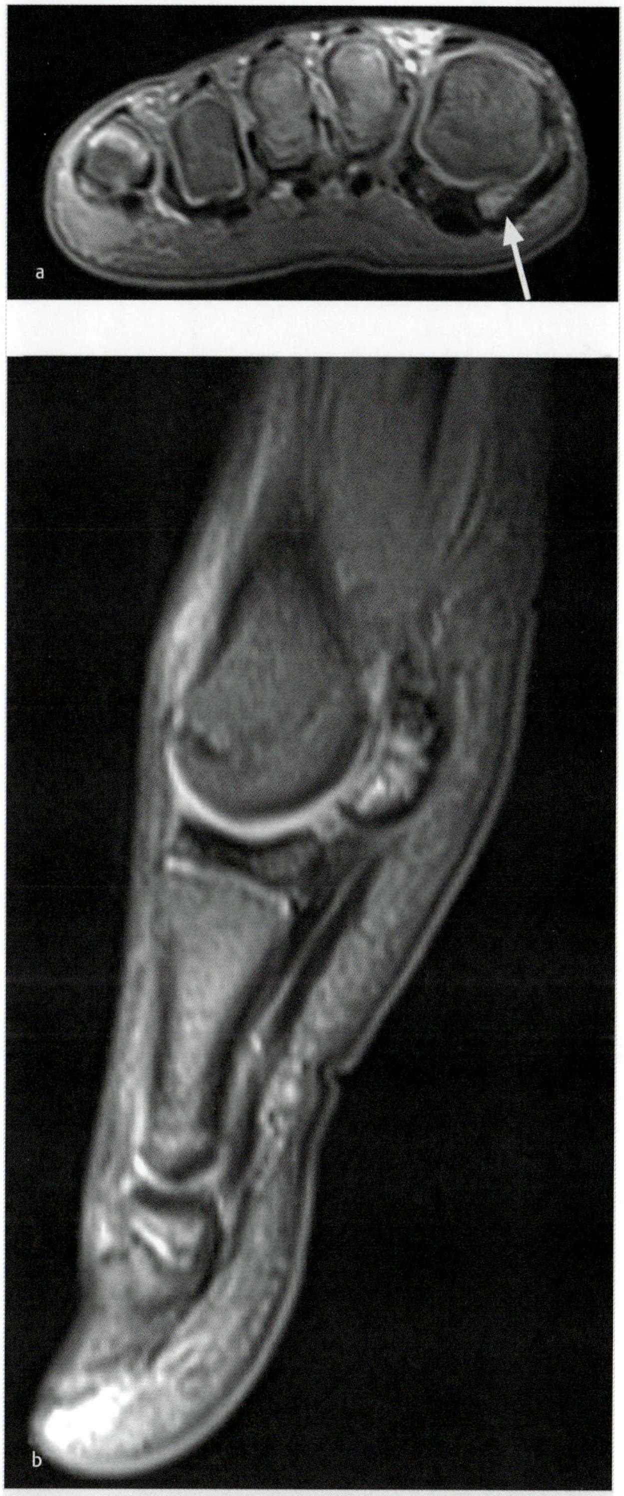

Fig. 5.17 a, b Activated medial sesamoid in a 14-year-old boy.
a Axial fat-saturated T1-weighted image after contrast administration shows homogeneous enhancement of the medial sesamoid (arrow) and plantar keratosis under the fifth metatarsal head due to unphysiologic weight bearing caused by pain under the first metatarsophalangeal joint.
b Sagittal fat-saturated T1-weighted image after contrast administration excludes sesamoid necrosis and fragmentation. Findings are consistent with chronic irritation of the sesamoid.

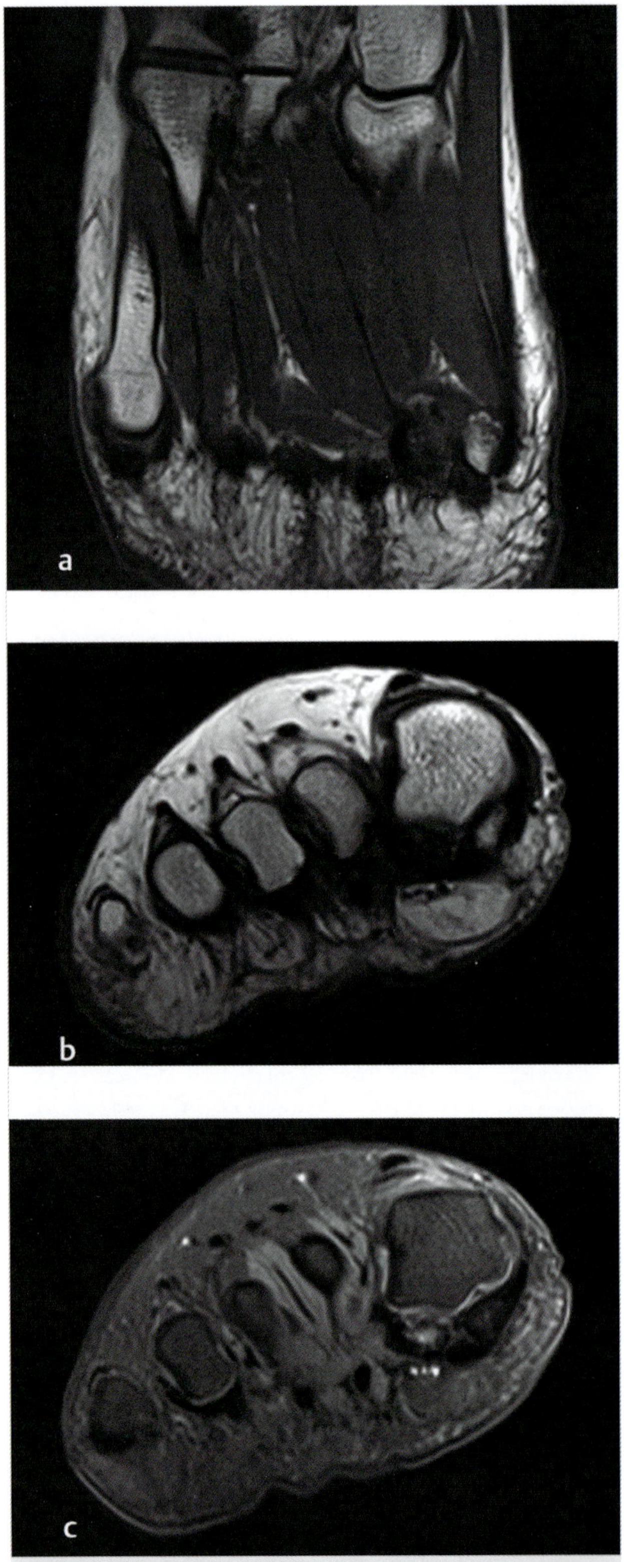

Fig. 5.18 a–c Sesamoid necrosis.
a Coronal T1-weighted image shows absence of fatty marrow signal in the lateral sesamoid compared with the other bony structures.
b Axial T1-weighted image. Absence of fatty marrow signal in the lateral sesamoid is consistent with complete necrosis.
c Axial fat-saturated T1-weighted image after contrast administration. Despite focal enhancement, the complete absence of fatty marrow signal indicates osteonecrosis.

- Altered shape
- Decreased height
- Fragmentation with possible adjacent activation and enhancement
- Osteophytes with activated osteoarthritis in the subsesamoid joint space
- Increased enhancement along the flexor tendon sheath with bone marrow edema and enhancement at the fibro-osseous junction of the flexor hallucis brevis tendon; possible abnormal tendon position
- Lateral plantar keratosis under the fourth and fifth metatarsal heads due to compensatory or abnormal loading

Imaging Recommendation

Modality of choice: radiography. MRI is used in equivocal cases.

Differential Diagnosis

- Metatarsal stress fracture
- Synovitis
- Plantar fascial fibromatosis (Ledderhose disease)
- Morton neuroma (medial side of first metatarsal head: Joplin neuroma)
- Hallux rigidus

Treatment

Conservative

- *Fracture without dehiscence:* short leg cast with sole extended at the front
- *Osteonecrosis:* relieve pressure, prescribe NSAIDs
- *Turf toe:* depends on severity; tape, stiff insert, short leg cast with extended sole
- *Osteoarthritis, bipartite sesamoid:* soft cushioning insert, steroid injection, NSAIDs

Operative

- *Fracture:* fresh gaping fracture can be treated by internal fixation (interference screws, cancellous bone grafting if needed); simultaneous correction of axial malalignment if present
- *Older fracture, bipartite sesamoid:* resection of the smaller bone fragment
- *Osteonecrosis at the fragmentation stage, osteoarthritis of the subsesamoid joint space:* resection of the painful sesamoid bone

Prognosis and Complications

Conservative treatment can often improve symptoms in sesamoid disorders. If pain persists resection of the sesamoids can be considered. Pain is relieved in about 90% of patients. However, residual complaints can persist, as well as a moderate weakness in plantar flexion of the big toe.

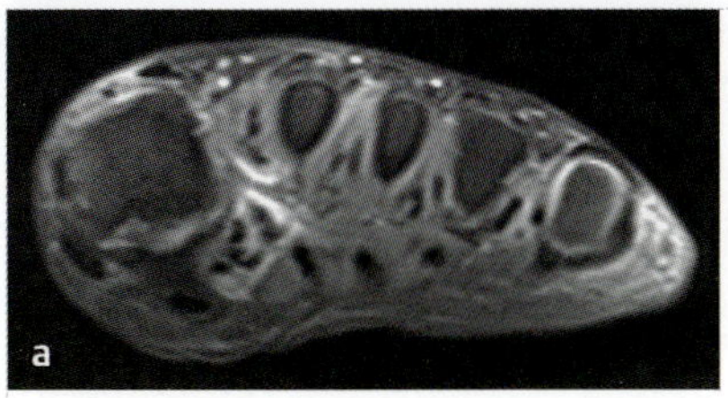

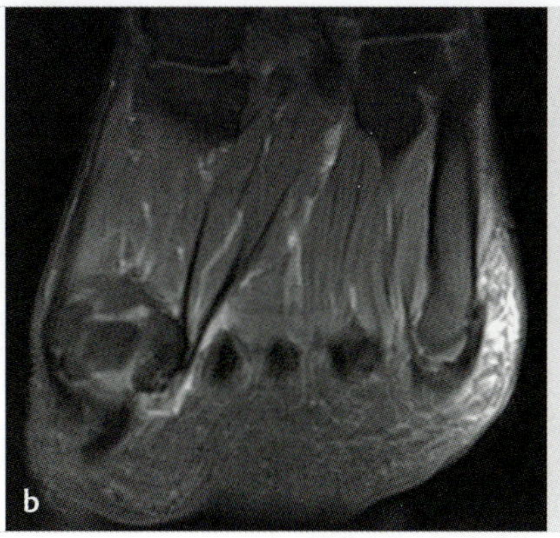

Fig. 5.19 a, b A 40-year-old man with chronic pain on the medial side of the first metatarsophalangeal joint during push-off. Insertional tendinopathy on the sesamoid bone.
a Axial fat-saturated T1-weighted image after contrast administration shows florid insertional tendinopathy with enhancement in the distal tendon of the lateral head of the flexor hallucis brevis.
b Coronal fat-saturated T1-weighted image after contrast administration shows enhancing fibrovascular granulation tissue at the fibro-osseous tendon junction on the lateral sesamoid.

5.3 Bibliography

Metatarsal Fractures

Baierlein SA. Frakturklassifikationen. Stuttgart: Thieme; 2011

Beck M, Mittlmeier T. Metatarsal fractures. [Article in German] Unfallchirurg 2008; 111: 829–839, quiz 840

Buddecke DE, Polk MA, Barp EA. Metatarsal fractures. Clin Podiatr Med Surg 2010; 27: 601–624

Cakir H, Van Vliet-Koppert ST, Van Lieshout EM, De Vries MR, Van Der Elst M, Schepers T. Demographics and outcome of metatarsal fractures. Arch Orthop Trauma Surg 2011; 131: 241–245

Dameron TB. Fractures and anatomical variations of the proximal portion of the fifth metatarsal. J Bone Joint Surg Am 1975; 57: 788–792

Dameron TB. Fractures of the proximal fifth metatarsal: selecting the best treatment option. J Am Acad Orthop Surg 1995; 3: 110–114

Goulart M, O'Malley MJ, Hodgkins CW, Charlton TP. Foot and ankle fractures in dancers. Clin Sports Med 2008; 27: 295–304

Hatch RL, Alsobrook JA, Clugston JR. Diagnosis and management of metatarsal fractures. Am Fam Physician 2007; 76: 817–826

Heckmann JD, Rockwood CA Jr, Green DP. Fractures and Dislocations of the Foot. Fractures in Adults. 2nd ed. Philadelphia: Lippincott; 1984: 1703–1832

Jones R. Fracture of the base of the fifth metatarsal bone by indirect violence. Ann Surg 1902; 35: 697–700, 2

Lehman RC, Torg JS, Pavlov H, DeLee JC. Fractures of the base of the fifth metatarsal distal to the tuberosity: a review. Foot Ankle 1987; 7: 245–252

Meurman KO. Less common stress fractures in the foot. Br J Radiol 1981; 54: 1–7

Müller-Mai CM, Ekkernkamp A. Frakturen. Klassifikation und Behandlungsoptionen. Heidelberg: Springer; 2010

Quill GE. Fractures of the proximal fifth metatarsal. Orthop Clin North Am 1995; 26: 353–361

Rhim B, Hunt JC. Lisfranc injury and Jones fracture in sports. Clin Podiatr Med Surg 2011; 28: 69–86

Schünke M, Schulte E, Schumacher U. Allgemeine Anatomie und Bewegungssystem. Prometheus LernAtlas der Anatomie. Stuttgart: Thieme; 2005

Shrivastava N, Greisberg C, DiGiovanni W, Greisberg J. Metatarsal and Phalangeal Fractures. Foot and Ankle: Core Knowledge in Orthopaedics. Philadelphia: Elsevier; 2007: 310–320

Stewart IM. Jones's fracture: fracture of base of fifth metatarsal. Clin Orthop 1960; 16: 190–198

Torg JS, Balduini FC, Zelko RR, Pavlov H, Peff TC, Das M. Fractures of the base of the fifth metatarsal distal to the tuberosity. Classification and guidelines for non-surgical and surgical management. J Bone Joint Surg Am 1984; 66: 209–214

Turco VJ. Injuries to the foot and ankle. In: Nicholas JA, Hershmann EB. The Lower Extremity and Spine in Sports Medicine. St. Louis: Mosby; 1995: 1229–1250

Van Laer L, Kraus R, Linhart WE. Frakturen der Metatarsalia. In: Van Laer L, ed. Frakturen und Luxationen im Wachstumsalter. Stuttgart: Thieme; 2007: 411–414

Vorlat P, Achtergael W, Haentjens P. Predictors of outcome of non-displaced fractures of the base of the fifth metatarsal. Int Orthop 2007; 31: 5–10

Capsuloligamentous Injuries of the First Metatarsophalangeal Joint (Turf Toe, Sand Toe), Plantar Plate Tear

Ashman CJ, Klecker RJ, Yu JS. Forefoot pain involving the metatarsal region: differential diagnosis with MR imaging. Radiographics 2001; 21: 1425–1440

Bowers KD, Martin RB. Turf-toe: a shoe-surface related football injury. Med Sci Sports 1976; 8: 81–83

Brophy RH, Gamradt SC, Ellis SJ et al. Effect of turf toe on foot contact pressures in professional American football players. Foot Ankle Int 2009; 30: 405–409

Clanton TO, Ford JJ. Turf toe injury. Clin Sports Med 1994; 13: 731–741

Coker TP, Arnold JA, Weber DL. Traumatic lesions of the metatarsophalangeal joint of the great toe in athletes. Am J Sports Med 1978; 6: 326–334

Coughlin MJ, Kemp TJ, Hirose CB. Turf toe: soft tissue and osteocartilaginous injury to the first metatarsophalangeal joint. Phys Sportsmed 2010; 38: 91–100

Crain JM, Phancao JP, Stidham K. MR imaging of turf toe. Magn Reson Imaging Clin N Am 2008; 16: 93–103, vi

Donnelly LF, Betts JB, Fricke BL. Skimboarder's toe: findings on high-field MRI. AJR Am J Roentgenol 2005; 184: 1481–1485

Frey C, Andersen GD, Feder KS. Plantarflexion injury to the metatarsophalangeal joint ("sand toe"). Foot Ankle Int 1996; 17: 576–581

Heckmann JD, Rockwood CA Jr, Green DP. Fractures and Dislocations of the Foot. Fractures in Adults. 2nd ed. Philadelphia: Lippincott; 1984: 1703–1832

McCormick JJ, Anderson RB. The great toe: failed turf toe, chronic turf toe, and complicated sesamoid injuries. Foot Ankle Clin 2009; 14: 135–150

McCormick JJ, Anderson RB. Rehabilitation following turf toe injury and plantar plate repair. Clin Sports Med 2010; 29: 313–323, ix

Rao JP, Banzon MT. Irreducible dislocation of the metatarsophalangeal joints of the foot. Clin Orthop Relat Res 1979: 224–226

Rodeo SA, O'Brien S, Warren RF, Barnes R, Wickiewicz TL, Dillingham MF. Turf-toe: an analysis of metatarsophalangeal joint sprains in professional football players. Am J Sports Med 1990; 18: 280–285

Schünke M, Schulte E, Schumacher U. Allgemeine Anatomie und Bewegungssystem. Prometheus LernAtlas der Anatomie. Stuttgart: Thieme; 2005

Shrivastava N, Greisberg C, DiGiovanni W, Greisberg J. Metatarsal and Phalangeal Fractures. Foot and Ankle: Core Knowledge in Orthopaedics. Philadelphia: Elsevier; 2007: 310–320

Valderrabano V, Engelhardt M, Küster H-H. Fuß und Sprunggelenk und Sport. Cologne: Deutscher Ärzteverlag; 2009

Wilson L, Dimeff R, Miniaci A, Sundaram M. Radiologic case study. First metarsophalangeal plantar plate injury (turf toe). Orthopedics 2005; 28: 344–, 417–419

Yao L, Do HM, Cracchiolo A, Farahani K. Plantar plate of the foot: findings on conventional arthrography and MR imaging. AJR Am J Roentgenol 1994; 163: 641–644

Phalangeal Fractures

Dauber W. Feneis Bildlexikon der Anatomie. 10thed. Stuttgart: Thieme; 2008

Lim KB, Tey IK, Lokino ES, Yap RT, Tawng DK. Escalators, rubber clogs, and severe foot injuries in children. J Pediatr Orthop 2010; 30: 414–419

Merriman D, Carmichael K, Battle SC. Skimboard injuries. J Trauma 2008; 65: 487–490

Nihal A, Trepman E, Nag D. First ray disorders in athletes. Sports Med Arthrosc 2009; 17: 160–166

Pagenstert GI, Valderrabano V, Hintermann B. Medial sesamoid nonunion combined with hallux valgus in athletes: a report of two cases. Foot Ankle Int 2006; 27: 135–140

Van Vliet-Koppert ST, Cakir H, Van Lieshout EM, De Vries MR, Van Der Elst M, Schepers T. Demographics and functional outcome of toe fractures. J Foot Ankle Surg 2011; 50: 307–310

Wolansky R. Krankheitsbilder in der Podologie. Stuttgart: Hippokrates; 2006

Zwipp H, Baumgart F, Cronier P et al. Integral classification of injuries (ICI) to the bones, joints, and ligaments—application to injuries of the foot. Injury 2004; 35 Suppl 2: SB3–SB9

Hallux Valgus

Cong Y, Cheung JT, Leung AK, Zhang M. Effect of heel height on in-shoe localized triaxial stresses. J Biomech 2011; 44: 2267–2272

Huang PJ, Lin YC, Fu YC, et al. Radiographic evaluation of minimally invasive distal metatarsal osteotomy for hallux valgus. Foot Ankle Int 2011;32(5): S503–S507

Kennedy JG, Collumbier JA. Bunions in dancers. Clin Sports Med 2008; 27: 321–328

Shannak O, Sehat K, Dhar S. Analysis of the proximal phalanx size as a guide for an Akin closing wedge osteotomy. Foot Ankle Int 2011; 32: 419–421

Shirzad K, Kiesau CD, DeOrio JK, Parekh SG. Lesser toe deformities. J Am Acad Orthop Surg 2011; 19: 505–514

Trnka HJ, Zembsch A, Easley ME, Salzer M, Ritschl P, Myerson MS. The chevron osteotomy for correction of hallux valgus. Comparison of findings after two and five years of follow-up. J Bone Joint Surg Am 2000; 82-A: 1373–1378

Hallux Rigidus

Botek G, Anderson MA. Etiology, pathophysiology, and staging of hallux rigidus. Clin Podiatr Med Surg 2011; 28: 229–243, vii

DeCarbo WT, Lupica J, Hyer CF. Modern techniques in hallux rigidus surgery. Clin Podiatr Med Surg 2011; 28: 361–383, ix

Fuhrmann RA. First metatarsophalangeal arthrodesis for hallux rigidus. Foot Ankle Clin 2011; 16: 1–12

Galli MM, Hyer CF. Hallux rigidus: what lies beyond fusion, resectional arthroplasty, and implants. Clin Podiatr Med Surg 2011; 28: 385–403, ix

Sanhudo JA, Gomes JE, Rodrigo MK. Surgical treatment of advanced hallux rigidus by interpositional arthroplasty. Foot Ankle Int 2011; 32: 400–406

Hammer, Claw, and Mallet Toes, Chronic Plantar Plate Tear

Ashman CJ, Klecker RJ, Yu JS. Forefoot pain involving the metatarsal region: differential diagnosis with MR imaging. Radiographics 2001; 21: 1425–1440

Baravarian B, Thompson J, Nazarian D. Plantar plate tears: a review of the modified flexor tendon transfer repair for stabilization. Clin Podiatr Med Surg 2011; 28: 57–68

Cong Y, Cheung JT, Leung AK, Zhang M. Effect of heel height on in-shoe localized triaxial stresses. J Biomech 2011; 44: 2267–2272

Lui TH, Chan LK, Chan KB. Modified plantar plate tenodesis for correction of claw toe deformity. Foot Ankle Int 2010; 31: 584–591

Lui TH. Correction of crossover deformity of second toe by combined plantar plate tenodesis and extensor digitorum brevis transfer: a minimally invasive approach. Arch Orthop Trauma Surg 2011; 131: 1247–1252[E-pub ahead of print]

Shirzad K, Kiesau CD, DeOrio JK, Parekh SG. Lesser toe deformities. J Am Acad Orthop Surg 2011; 19: 505–514

Walther M, Simons P, Nass K, Röser A. Fusion of the first tarsometatarsal joint using a plantar tension band osteosynthesis [Article in German] Oper Orthop Traumatol 2011; 23: 52–59

Weil L, Sung W, Weil LS, Malinoski K. Anatomic plantar plate repair using the Weil metatarsal osteotomy approach. Foot Ankle Spec 2011; 4: 145–150

Osteonecrosis, Köhler Disease Type II

Ashman CJ, Klecker RJ, Yu JS. Forefoot pain involving the metatarsal region: differential diagnosis with MR imaging. Radiographics 2001; 21: 1425–1440

Blitz NM, Yu JH. Freiberg's infraction in identical twins: a case report. J Foot Ankle Surg 2005; 44: 218–221

Gregg JM, Schneider T, Marks P. MR imaging and ultrasound of metatarsalgia—the lesser metatarsals. Radiol Clin North Am 2008; 46: 1061–1078, vi–vii

Sesamoid Pathology

Ashman CJ, Klecker RJ, Yu JS. Forefoot pain involving the metatarsal region: differential diagnosis with MR imaging. Radiographics 2001; 21: 1425–1440

Boike A, Schnirring-Judge M, McMillin S. Sesamoid disorders of the first metatarsophalangeal joint. Clin Podiatr Med Surg 2011; 28: 269–285, vii

Chou LB. Disorders of the first metatarsophalangeal joint: diagnosis of great-toe pain. Phys Sportsmed 2000; 28: 32–45

Cohen BE. Hallux sesamoid disorders. Foot Ankle Clin 2009; 14: 91–104

Kanatli U, Ozturk AM, Ercan NG, Ozalay M, Daglar B, Yetkin H. Absence of the medial sesamoid bone associated with metatarsophalangeal pain. Clin Anat 2006; 19: 634–639

Lee S, James WC, Cohen BE, Davis WH, Anderson RB. Evaluation of hallux alignment and functional outcome after isolated tibial sesamoidectomy. Foot Ankle Int 2005; 26: 803–809

Chapter 6

Abnormalities of the Plantar Soft Tissues

6 Abnormalities of the Plantar Soft Tissues

A. Roeser and U. Szeimies

6.1 Plantar Fasciitis, Rupture of the Plantar Fascia

Definition

Plantar fasciitis is caused by excessive loads at the origin of the plantar fascia on the calcaneal tuberosity. It is associated with inflammatory and degenerative changes in the plantar fascia and calcaneal fat pad. Partial tearing may occur with advanced degenerative changes, and trauma to the fascia may cause partial or complete ruptures.

Symptoms

- Weight-bearing pain on the bottom of the heel
- Pain worse with initial steps in the morning
- Pain may radiate laterally around the posterior calcaneal tuberosity due to irritation of the first branch of the lateral plantar nerve (Baxter nerve)
- Point of maximum tenderness is usually anteromedial to the main weight-bearing zone below the heel
- With rupture: plantar hematoma with tenderness

Predisposing Factors

- Overweight
- Repetitive strains (running, jumping, ball sports)

Anatomy and Pathology

The plantar fascia is a thick, multilayered aponeurosis that spans the sole of the foot in three directions and chiefly supports the longitudinal arch with its five longitudinal slips that insert on the corresponding proximal phalanges. Transverse fibers give distal support to the longitudinal slips. Vertical fibers extend around the short toe flexors, dividing the sole of the foot into three well-known compartments (large toe, small toe, and central compartment) while other fibers run through the fat pad to the skin. The loculation of the fat pad limits its mobility relative to the skin.

The plantar fascia originates from a broad area on the anterior and medial calcaneal tuberosity. Distally it splits into digital slips that insert on the proximal phalanges of all the toes.

Imaging

Radiographs

- *Lateral view of the calcaneus:* bony plantar heel spur, possible intramuscular calcifications in the flexor digitorum brevis
- *Weight-bearing views of the foot in three planes:* to exclude hindfoot deformity

Ultrasound

- Longitudinal plantar ultrasound scan shows hypoechoic thickening of the plantar fascia (thickening to > 6 mm is definitely pathologic).
- Plantar heel spur appears as an echogenic exostosis beneath the plantar fascia, and bursopathy appears as a hypoechoic zone.
- Progression to chronic stage is marked by increasing inhomogeneous disintegration of the fascia, with partial tears causing loss of clear delineation. Involvement of the flexor digitorum brevis muscle bellies may be associated with hypoechoic hemorrhage and tearing of the perimysium.

MRI

Interpretation Checklist

- Extent of inflammation
- Accurate localization
- Describe longitudinal extent
- Involvement of fibro-osseous junction
- Fibro-osteitis
- Local zones of softening in the aponeurosis
- Risk of rupture
- Partial tearing
- Extent of inflammation in adjacent soft tissue of the heel
- Associated findings (other tendons in the hindfoot, degenerative joint changes, bone edema)

Examination Technique

Except in the case of a recent acute rupture, IV contrast administration is recommended for better visualization of the acute and chronic inflammatory component with tendon vascularization, peritendinitis, and fibro-osteitis.

- *Standard protocol:* prone position, high-resolution multichannel coil
- *Sequences:*
  - Sagittal T1-weighted and PD-weighted fat-sat
  - Axial T2-weighted and PD-weighted fat-sat
  - Sagittal and coronal T1-weighted fat-sat after contrast administration

MRI Findings (▶ Fig. 6.1, ▶ Fig. 6.2, ▶ Fig. 6.3)

- Edema and contrast uptake in the proximal plantar tendon, usually more pronounced on the medial side, with enhancement in the adjacent soft tissues of the heel
- Zones of mucoid degeneration within the tendon
- Partial tear appears hyperintense in the PD-weighted fat-saturated (fat-sat) sequence
- Degenerative tendon vascularity with increased enhancement

! Note

Even subtle findings may often cause significant complaints. The extent of activation does not always correlate with the symptomatic picture.

Imaging Recommendation

Modality of choice: ultrasonography. MRI may be used as needed.

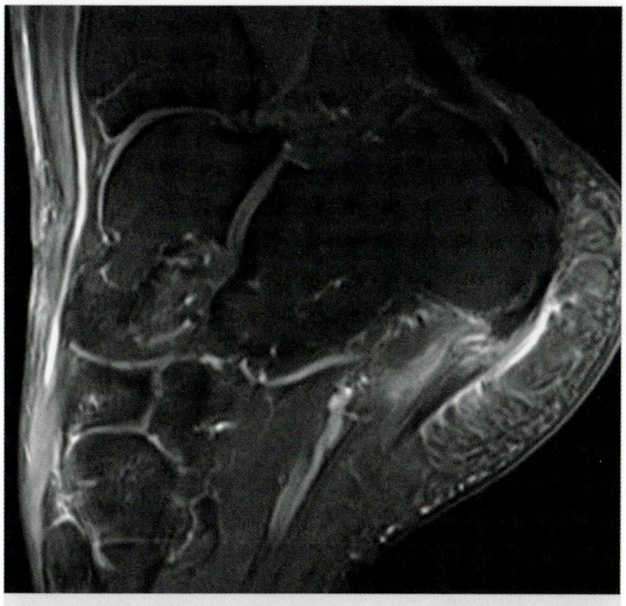

Fig. 6.1 Plantar fasciitis in a 39-year-old woman with increasing chronic heel pain. The patient had an occupation that required prolonged standing. Sagittal T1-weighted fat-sat image after contrast administration shows definite signs of activated insertional tendinopathy of the plantar fascia (plantar fasciitis) with thickening of the plantar aponeurosis at the fibro-osseous junction, initial degenerative vascularization, and increased enhancement in the adjacent soft tissues, especially the fatty tissue of the heel.

Differential Diagnosis

- Calcaneal stress fracture
- Tumors
- Infection
- Fat pad atrophy
- Fibromatosis of the plantar fascia
- Flexor hallucis longus tendinitis
- Compression of the tibial nerve or lateral plantar nerve (Baxter nerve)
- Radiculopathy at the S1 level
- Diseases with a chronic inflammatory or rheumatoid etiology: seronegative spondylarthropathy (human leukocyte antigen [HLA]-B27), psoriatic arthritis, reactive arthritis (titer assay); heel pain is usually bilateral

Treatment

Conservative

Conservative treatment is the preferred initial course of action for plantar fasciitis:

- Orthotic inserts that support or align the medial longitudinal arch while removing all weight from the fascial bundle
- Eccentric stretching exercises for the calf and plantar muscles (at-home program of exercises done 2 or 3 times daily)
- Nocturnal splints that position the ankle joint in dorsiflexion, especially recommended for pain during initial steps in the morning
- Oral NSAIDs / Cox-2 inhibitors
- Ultrasonic therapy, transverse friction massage
- Injection therapy (local anesthetics, steroids, platelet rich plasma [PRP], botulinum toxin)
- Local anesthetic, 2 to 3 x steroids, platelet-derived growth factor
- Orthovoltage therapy
- Shockwave therapy
- For acute rupture or partial tear: rest from sports participation, ice, NSAIDs, orthotics, ultrasound

Operative

If all conservative options have been exhausted and have been unsuccessful for 6 months, surgical intervention is available as a last recourse:

- Surgical decompression and neurolysis of the first branch of the lateral plantar nerve (Baxter nerve; preoperative work-up includes neurologic tests, measurement of nerve conduction velocity)
- Half-thickness notching of the medial part of the plantar fascia at its origin with resection of the bony heel spur (the plantar fascia is not completely divided)
- Endoscopic plantar fascial release

Prognosis, Complications

Prognosis

The disease runs a self-limiting but protracted course in approximately 80% of cases.

Surgical Complications

- Persistent pain
- Superficial or deep infection
- Scar pain
- Deep venous thrombosis
- Translocation of pain to the midfoot after complete division of the plantar fascia due to altered tension on the longitudinal arch

6.2 Plantar Heel Spur

Definition

A plantar heel spur is a bony excrescence on the inferomedial aspect of the calcaneal tuberosity.

Symptoms

The clinical presentation of heel pain is like that previously described for plantar fasciitis. The presence of a plantar heel spur does cause the heel pain; the underlying cause is the degenerative changes in the plantar fascia and fat pad that were described above. A fracture of the heel spur may cause the pain to intensify.

Predisposing Factors

See section 6.1 Plantar Fasciitis, Rupture of the Plantar Fascia (p. 178).

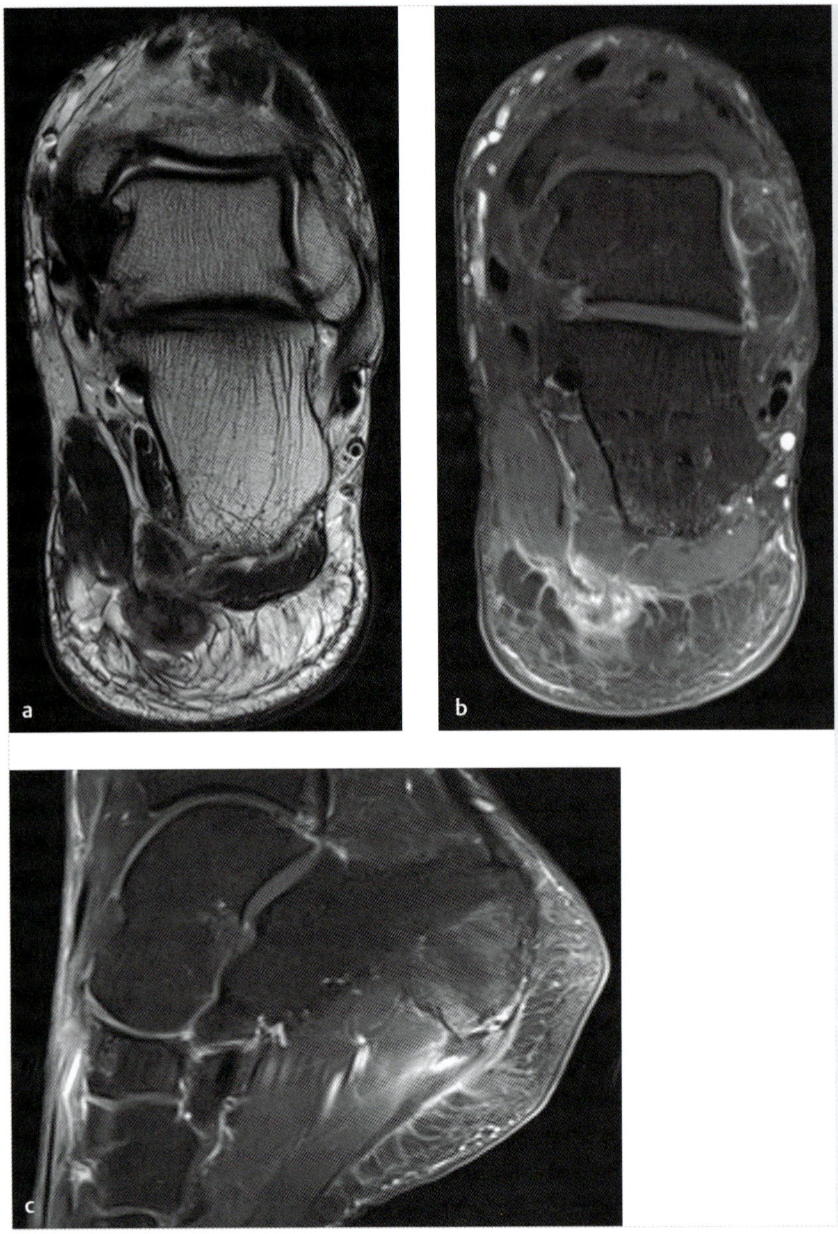

Fig. 6.2 a–c Plantar fasciitis.
a Coronal T2-weighted image shows marked thickening of the plantar aponeurosis on the medial side.
b T1-weighted fat-sat image after contrast administration shows intense enhancement within the tendon and in adjacent soft tissues including the muscles and calcaneal fat pad.
c Sagittal T1-weighted fat-sat image after contrast administration shows definite features of plantar fasciitis with intratendinous enhancement at the fibro-osseous junction.

Anatomy and Pathology

A heel spur is an intramuscular calcification in the flexor digitorum brevis located close to its origin on the plantar calcaneal tuberosity. The combined presence of a plantar and posterior heel spur may reflect a systemic insertional tendinopathy.

Imaging

Radiographs (▶ Fig. 6.4)

- The spur usually points forward, reflecting an adaptation to unphysiologic pressure loads.
- Bony plantar spur may be on the calcaneus or broken from it.
- Stress radiographs of the foot are obtained in three planes to exclude a hindfoot deformity.

Ultrasound

Longitudinal plantar scan shows a protrusion on the echogenic bony undersurface of the calcaneus beneath the plantar fascia, pointing away from the surface. Hypoechoic bursopathy may be evident between the spur and fascia.

MRI

Interpretation Checklist

- Assessment of the activation of the heel spur
- Extent of bone marrow edema
- Involvement of the plantar tendon
- Inflammation in the soft tissues of the heel

Examination Technique

- *Standard protocol:* prone position, high-resolution multichannel coil

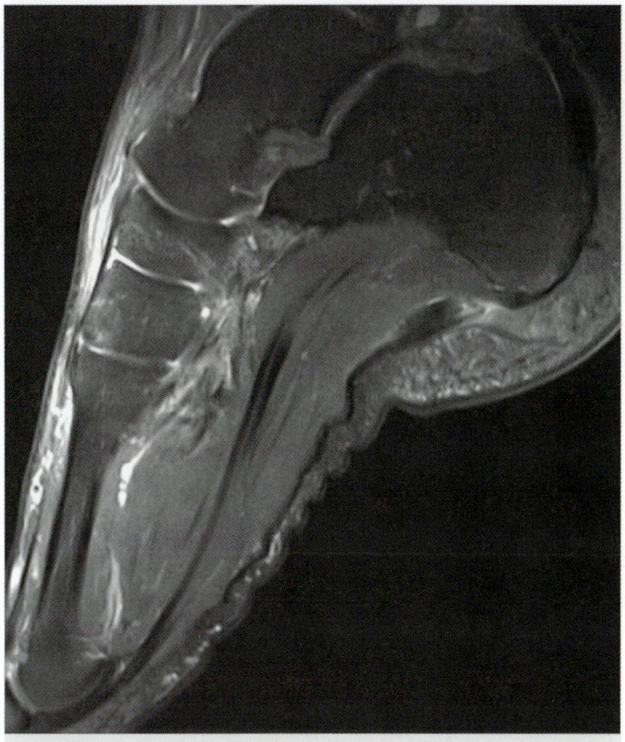

Fig. 6.3 **A 55-year-old man with acute stabbing pain due to a complete rupture of the plantar fascia.** The patient gave no history of trauma. Sagittal PD-weighted fat-sat image shows a complete rupture of the plantar fascia near its insertion with slight retraction of the tendon end.

- *Sequences:*
  - Sagittal T1-weighted and PD-weighted fat-sat
  - Axial T2-weighted and PD-weighted fat-sat
  - Sagittal and coronal T1-weighted fat-sat after contrast administration

MRI Findings

- Heel spur is clearly visible in the T1-weighted sagittal sequence
- Possible activation of the spur with bone-marrow edema and contrast enhancement at the fibro-osseous junction
- Edema in the plantar fat pad below the heel spur

Imaging Recommendation

Modalities of choice: radiography; contrast-enhanced MRI to assess activation of the heel spur and the integrity of the plantar aponeurosis.

Differential Diagnosis

- Plantar fasciitis
- Bursopathy
- Calcaneal stress fracture
- Tumor
- Infection
- Compression of the tibial nerve or lateral plantar nerve (Baxter nerve)
- S1 radiculopathy

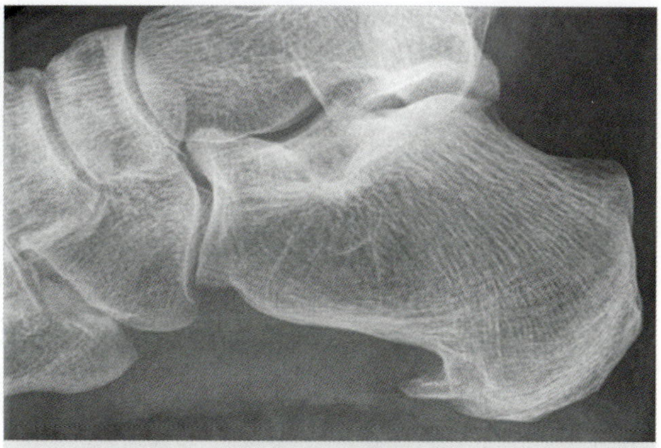

Fig. 6.4 **Plantar heel spur.** Lateral radiograph of the calcaneus.

- Diseases with a chronic inflammatory or rheumatoid etiology: seronegative spondylarthropathy (HLA-B27), psoriatic arthritis, reactive arthritis (titer assay); heel pain is usually bilateral
- Plantar vein thrombosis

Treatment

Conservative

! Note

When planning treatment, note that a plantar heel spur is usually the result of plantar fasciitis; it rarely occurs as a separate entity.

The initial course of action for a plantar heel spur is conservative treatment. Shockwave therapy is becoming increasingly important.

Operative

An acutely fractured heel spur can be managed by removing the spur and notching the plantar fascia, but only after conservative options have been tried.

Prognosis, Complications

See section 6.1 Plantar Fasciitis, Rupture of the Plantar Fascia (p. 178).

6.3 Ledderhose Disease

Definition

Ledderhose disease is defined as the presence of benign, firm, fibrous nodules in the sole of the foot, often located along the medial border of the plantar fascia.

Symptoms

- Complaints relating to footwear pressure on the nodules
- Load-dependent pain in the sole of the foot

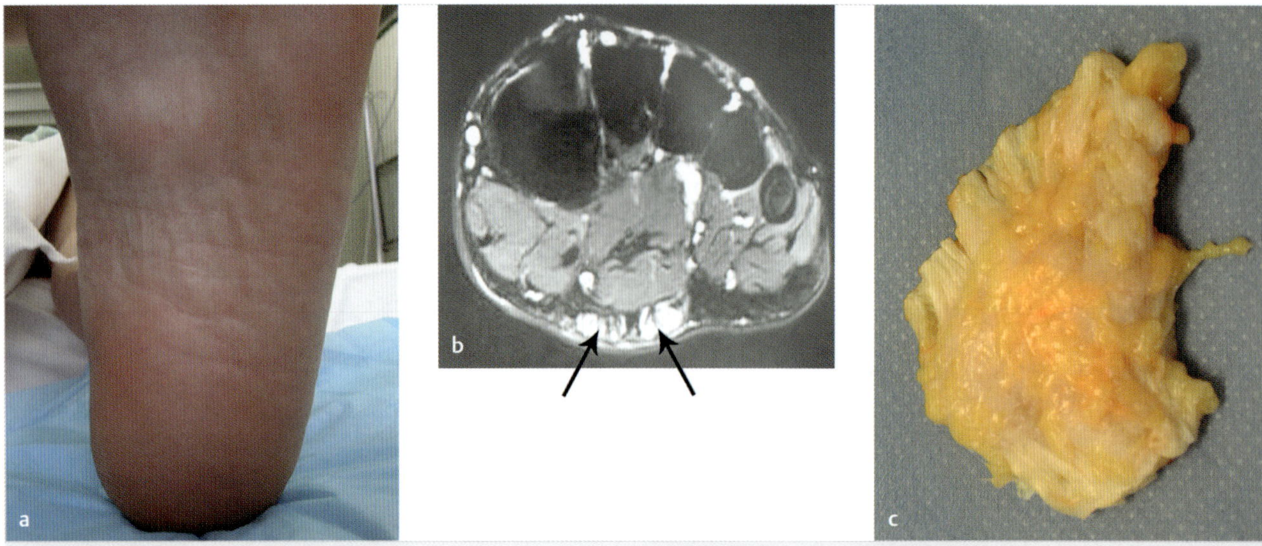

Fig. 6.5 a–c Plantar fibromatosis affecting the medial middle third of the plantar fascia.
a Clinical appearance.
b MRI appearance.
c Surgically resected area of plantar fibromatosis.

Predisposing Factors

- Etiology unclear
- Males predominantly affected
- Correlation with Dupuytren disease
- Association with diabetes mellitus
- Increased alcohol consumption has been cited as a predisposing factor

Anatomy and Pathology (▶ Fig. 6.5)

The medial border of the plantar fascia is most commonly affected. Formation of the nodules proceeds in various phases (proliferative, maturation phase). Well-differentiated fibroblasts develop which invade the deep soft-tissue structures of the plantar fascia or superficially infiltrate the skin. The slight contractile activity of the myofibroblasts leads to shortening and contracture of the plantar fascia.

Imaging

Radiographs

Radiographs do not advance the diagnosis of the soft-tissue masses. Weight-bearing radiographs can be taken after surgical removal of the plantar fascia to evaluate the secondary change in the medial longitudinal arch.

Ultrasound

Longitudinal and transverse plantar scans demonstrate individual or multiple, superficial, hypoechoic nodules in the plantar fascia.

MRI

Interpretation Checklist

- Confirm the presumptive diagnosis
- Preoperative planning
- Note number, size, and exact location of the nodules
- Assess the integrity of the plantar fascia

Examination Technique

- *Standard protocol:* prone position, high-resolution multichannel coil
- *Sequences:*
- Sagittal T1-weighted and PD-weighted fat-sat
- Axial T2-weighted and PD-weighted fat-sat
- Sagittal and axial T1-weighted fat-sat after contrast administration

MRI Findings (▶ Fig. 6.6)

The single or multiple nodular thickenings along the middle third of the plantar fascia are usually difficult to identify because their high cellularity and very low water content cause them to appear isointense in most sequences. They have scant vascularity and are often poorly visualized after contrast administration. They are most clearly depicted in the PD-weighted fat-sat sequence and unenhanced T2-weighted sequence.

The plantar fascia should be fully surveyed over its entire length. If necessary, a skin marker capsule can be placed to identify the area of maximum localized pain.

! Note

Even tiny nodules with an unimpressive MRI appearance may be very painful and should be identified

Imaging Recommendation

Modality of choice: MRI.

Differential Diagnosis

Fibrosarcoma.

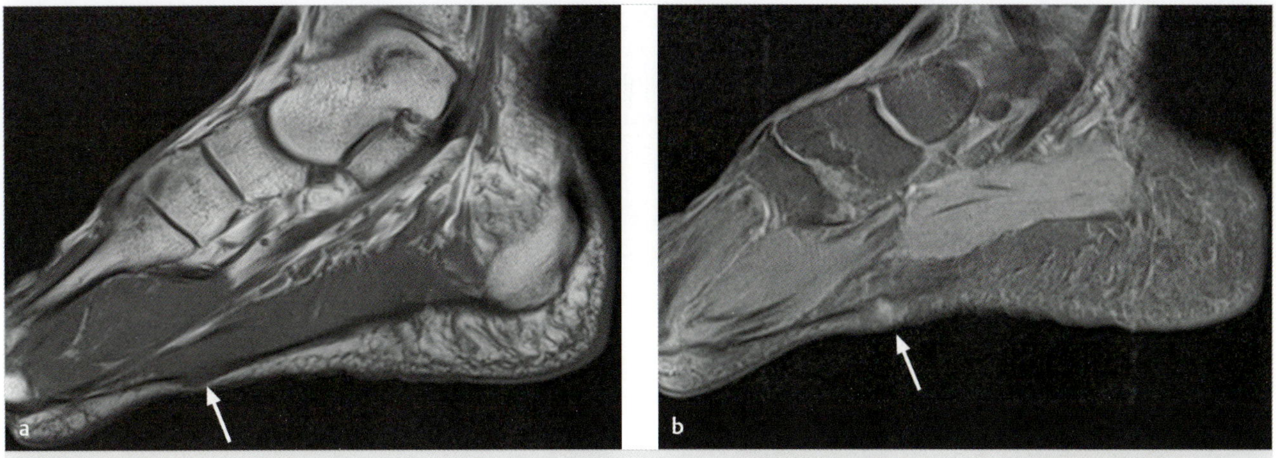

Fig. 6.6 a, b Ledderhose disease (plantar fibromatosis) in a patient with painful nodular thickening below the pedal arch along the plantar tendon.
a Sagittal T1-weighted image shows fusiform nodular thickening within the plantar tendon (arrow).
b Sagittal T1-weighted fat-sat image after contrast administration shows somewhat unusual enhancement of the very cellular fibrotic nodule in Ledderhose disease. Ordinarily the nodular thickenings show little or no increased enhancement (arrow).

Treatment

Conservative

- Orthotic shoe inserts that relieve pressure on the nodules
- NSAIDs

Operative

- Complete or partial resection of the plantar fascia in patients with increasing pressure-related complaints after an unsuccessful trial of shoe inserts
- Prophylactic surgical removal is not indicated

Prognosis, Complications

Possible complications are as follows:
- High recurrence rate after local removal of nodules
- Scar pain
- Plantar nerve injury with dys- or hypoesthesia, neuroma formation

6.4 Atrophy of the Plantar Fat Pad

Definition

Degenerative changes in the plantar calcaneal fat pad or the fat pad at the level of the metatarsal heads can decrease the resilience and water content of the fat pad, compromising its function as a shock absorber.

Symptoms

- Load-dependent heel pain or metatarsalgia
- Secondary deformity of the small toe

Predisposing Factors

- Splayfoot deformity
- Pes planovalgus
- Overweight
- Diabetes mellitus

Anatomy and Pathology

Anatomy

The plantar fat pad has an important role in cushioning the impact forces on the heel during walking. The fat pad can cushion and diffuse the massive heel-strike forces by virtue of its anatomic design: a honeycomb arrangement of fibroelastic fibers with septa anchored to both skin and bone arranged in a U-shaped pattern around the calcaneal tuberosity.

Pathology (▶ Fig. 6.7)

Degenerative changes in the fat pad, characterized by a loss of resilience and water content, compromise its shock-absorbing function and increase the loads on the calcaneal tuberosity. In addition, degenerative changes in the distal portion of the plantar aponeurosis near its insertion may lead to changes in the fat pad and plantar plate at the level of the metatarsal heads. Secondary degenerative changes in the metatarsophalangeal joints with associated secondary deformities of the small toe may result.

Imaging

Radiographs

Weight-bearing radiographs of the foot in three planes:
- Evaluation of the longitudinal arch
- Presence of splayfoot deformity
- Metatarsal alignment
- Exclude a deformity of the small toe

Ultrasound

Longitudinal and transverse plantar scans show thinning of the echogenic plantar fat pad.

MRI

Fat pad atrophy is usually a clinical diagnosis and there is no need for MRI. But MRI can be used to narrow the differential

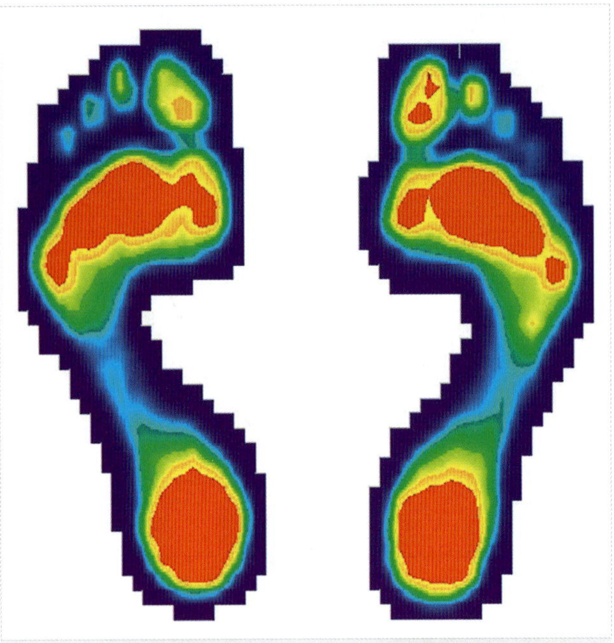

Fig. 6.7 Abnormal pressure distribution analysis in a 55-year-old female endurance athlete with atrophy of the plantar fat pad. The pressure distribution map shows pressure peaks (red) concentrated in areas below the metatarsal heads and calcaneal tuberosity. The arch is very pronounced and is occupied by scant fatty tissue.

diagnosis (plantar fasciitis, activated heel spur, bone overload, or fatigue fracture of the calcaneus).

Interpretation Checklist

- Evaluate the plantar fat pad
- Determine extent of edema and contrast enhancement
- Determine extent of fibrosis and chronicity of the inflammatory condition
- Detect or exclude bone marrow edema in the calcaneus

Examination Technique

- *Standard protocol:* prone position, high-resolution multichannel coil
- *Sequences:*
  - Sagittal T1-weighted and PD-weighted fat-sat
  - Axial T2-weighted and PD-weighted fat-sat
  - Sagittal and coronal T1-weighted fat-sat after contrast administration

MRI Findings

- Patchy, sometimes irregular areas of edema in a visibly thinned plantar fat pad
- Unenhanced T1-weighted sequence may show hypointense fibrotic areas in chronic cases
- Thickening of the skin

Imaging Recommendation

Most cases are diagnosed clinically, but MRI is useful for interpreting equivocal symptoms and excluding other possible diagnoses.

Differential Diagnosis

- Plantar fasciitis
- Stress fractures of the calcaneus or metatarsals
- Morton neuroma
- Peripheral polyneuropathy
- Tarsal tunnel syndrome with atrophy of the intrinsic muscles
- Chronic inflammatory joint disease

Treatment

Conservative

Orthotic inserts that relieve pressure on the metatarsal heads and cushion the heel.

Operative

- Lengthening the Achilles tendon in patients with splayfoot deformity
- With massive fat pad atrophy at the level of the metatarsal heads with pronounced metatarsalgia and plantar prominence of the metatarsal heads: an elevating distal osteotomy of the metatarsals or condylectomy may be performed
- Cushioning shoe inserts are usually essential after surgery

Prognosis, Complications

Prognosis

The disease runs a chronic course and is generally managed by shoe inserts and surgical treatment.

Possible Complications

- Persistence of metatarsalgia
- Limited motion in the operated metatarsophalangeal joints
- Development of secondary toe deformities
- Formation of plantar ulcers in patients with coexisting polyneuropathy

6.5 Plantar Vein Thrombosis

Definition

Plantar vein thrombosis refers to the occlusion of the plantar venous plexus by a thrombus.

Symptoms

- Plantar foot pain
- Plantar swelling of the foot

Predisposing Factors

- Foot trauma with soft-tissue swelling
- Previous surgery
- Varicosity with chronic venous insufficiency
- Coagulation disorders
- Neoplasms
- Anticardiolipin antibody syndrome
- Estrogen use

Anatomy and Pathology

Anatomy

The plantar venous plexus is located between the tarsal bones and the flexor digitorum brevis muscle.

Pathology

Immobilization and an incompetent calf muscle pump lead to decreased venous and lymphatic drainage with an alteration of blood flow. Blood viscosity changes and endothelial cell alterations have been cited as additional factors in the pathogenesis of plantar vein thrombosis.

Imaging

Radiographs

Radiographs are unrewarding. The principal imaging tools for plantar vein thrombosis are ultrasound and MRI.

Ultrasound

Doppler sonography can detect abnormal flow signals in the plantar veins of the foot. The thrombi prevent compression of the veins by the ultrasound probe.

MRI

> **! Note**
>
> The examiner should consider this diagnosis during MRI and keep the typical imaging features in mind. Imaging of the hindfoot and midfoot should always include an evaluation of the soft-tissue structures (vessels, nerves, muscles).

A diagnosis of plantar vein thrombosis should be considered in patients with unexplained diffuse hindfoot and midfoot pain predominantly affecting the sole of the foot.

Interpretation Checklist

- Narrow the differential diagnosis
- Extent of thrombosis
- Assessment of clot organization
- Fresh or older?
- Extent of recanalization

Examination Technique

- *Standard protocol:* prone position, high-resolution multichannel coil
- *Sequences:*
  - Sagittal T1-weighted and PD-weighted fat-sat
  - Axial T2-weighted and PD-weighted fat-sat
  - Sagittal and axial T1-weighted fat-sat after contrast administration

MRI Findings (▶ Fig. 6.8)

- Hypointense thrombotic material in the deep plantar veins
- Absent or abnormal flow signal in unenhanced sequences
- Normal vein has high signal intensity in the T2-weighted sequence, while a thrombus is hypointense or dark
- Enlarged veins
- Filling defect after contrast administration with hypointense thrombus and increased enhancement of the vein wall

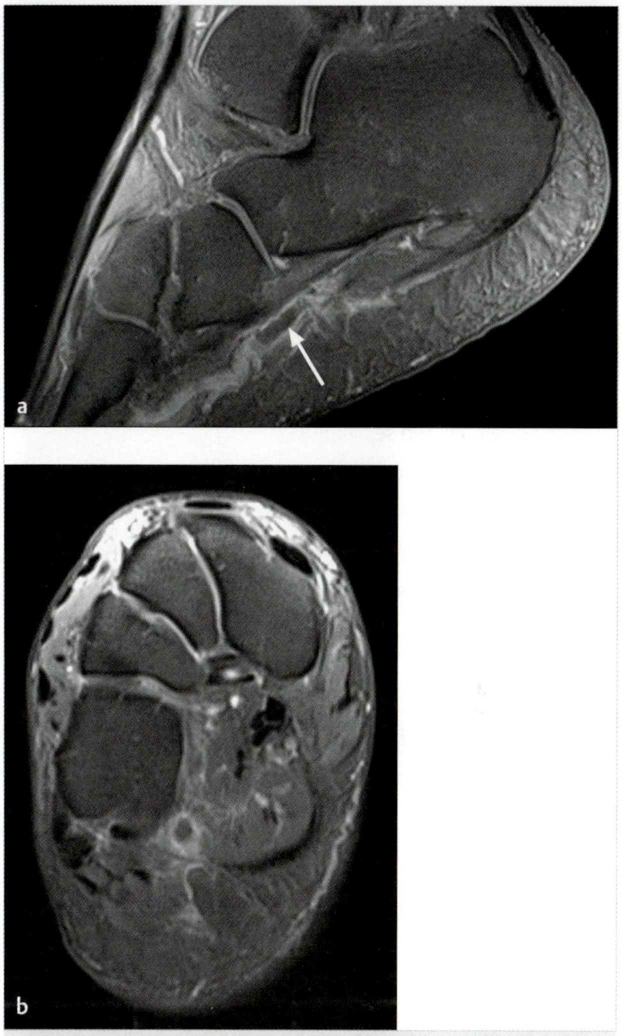

Fig. 6.8 a, b Subacute plantar vein thrombosis in a 68-year-old man with nonspecific midfoot pain.
a Sagittal T1-weighted fat-sat image after contrast administration demonstrates the thrombus (arrow) in an enlarged, contrast-filled plantar vein and shows incipient peripheral recanalization.
b Axial T1-weighted fat-sat image after contrast administration shows a hypointense central thrombus faintly outlined by intraluminal contrast medium. Increased enhancement of the vein wall and surroundings is noted as evidence of inflammatory change.

> **! Note**
>
> Often the thrombosis is limited to just one vein, which is responsible for the patient's complaints.

Imaging Recommendation

Modality of choice: duplex sonography.

Differential Diagnosis

- Hematoma or abscess
- Plantar compartment syndrome
- Tumors

Treatment

Conservative options:
- Activation of the foot and calf muscle pump
- Compression stocking
- Pharmacologic treatment of thrombosis

Prognosis, Complications

- Course is benign and self-limiting
- Complication: chronic venous insufficiency

6.6 Hallucis longus and Digitorum longus Intersection Syndrome

Definition

This syndrome involves an irritation of the flexor hallucis longus tendon or less commonly the flexor digitorum longus tendon at the plantar intersection of those tendons. Pathologic changes may range from degenerative tendon changes to rupture (degenerative or traumatic).

Symptoms

- Flexor tendon rupture distal to the intersection: painful weakness of active plantar flexion of the distal phalanx of the big or small toe
- Flexor tendon rupture proximal to the intersection: swelling and tenderness at the level of the rupture site due to retraction of the proximal tendon end
- Even with a rupture, the distal phalanx of the big or small toe still has some active residual plantar flexion due to intertendinous cross-connections at the level of the intersection
- Weakness on pressing the big toe down into the ground
- With an old rupture: increasing hyperextension deformity at the interphalangeal joint of the big toe with shoe interference

Predisposing Factors

- Degenerative tendon changes (high-risk activities: dancing, running, jumping sports)
- Rare traumatic rupture caused by a penetrating stab wound or laceration in the sole of the foot
- Rheumatoid arthritis, chronic inflammatory diseases

Anatomy and Pathology

Irritation of the flexor hallucis longus tendon at the level of the sustentaculum tali has clinical features analogous to a flexion contracture of the thumb. There are three main segments in the course of the flexor hallucis longus tendon where irritation or other tendon pathology are most likely to occur:
- at the level of the sustentaculum tali (flexor hallucis longus tendon runs in a fibro-osseous tunnel);
- between the sesamoids and tendon intersection;
- irritation distal to the sesamoids near the tendon insertion.

As a result of intertendinous cross-connections that exist at the level of the flexor tendon intersection (the "knot of Henry"), both tendons can contribute to active flexion of the distal phalanges of the toes distal to their intersection. With a tendon rupture at that level, the cross-connections will prevent significant retraction of the tendon ends. With a rupture proximal to the intersection, the proximal tendon end may undergo considerable retraction.

Imaging

Radiographs

- *Radiographs of the foot in three planes:* to exclude fractures, instabilities, and sesamoid pathology
- *Radiographs of the ankle joint in two planes:* to exclude bony impingement on the posteromedial hindfoot at the level of the subtalar joint and ankle joint (os trigonum, intra-articular loose bodies, periarticular calcifications, soft-tissue calcifications)

Ultrasound

Ultrasound scans show a normal hypoechoic ring around the flexor hallucis longus tendon in cross-section and a fluid line in longitudinal section. Ultrasound can define the stump of a ruptured tendon, which is usually surrounded by fluid. The distal stump moves with passive plantar flexion and dorsiflexion of the toes.

MRI

MRI is diagnostic by showing tenosynovitis of the flexor hallucis longus tendon at the level of the irritation or rupture:
- Sustentaculum tali
- Between the sesamoids and knot of Henry (tendon intersection)
- Distal to the sesamoids

! Note

A fluid collection around the flexor hallucis longus tendon between the sustentaculum and tendon intersection is a very common incidental finding on MRI. It has no pathologic significance and does not require treatment.

Interpretation Checklist

- Location and extent of tenosynovitis for preoperative planning
- Assessment of tendon quality
- Partial tear
- Dehiscence

Examination Technique

- *Standard protocol:* prone position, high-resolution multi-channel coil

- *Sequences:*
  - Sagittal and coronal PD-weighted fat-sat
  - Coronal T1-weighted
  - Axial T2-weighted
  - T1-weighted fat-sat after IV contrast administration, axial oblique (angled to the tendon plane) and sagittal

MRI Findings

The findings are most clearly displayed in the axial oblique T1-weighted fat-sat sequence after contrast administration. The tendon appears flattened and has an irregular surface. The typical enhancement pattern with peritendinitis is much less pronounced due to absence of the protective paratenon and should not be misinterpreted. The irregular tendon surface with flattening and thinning is much more characteristic of the tendon pathology in an intersection syndrome than the extent of peritendinitis.

Imaging Recommendation

Modality of choice: MRI.

Differential Diagnosis

Differentiation is required from proximal irritation of the flexor hallucis longus tendon or tenosynovitis at the level of the sustentaculum due to tendon thickening, a low-lying muscle belly, or os trigonum.

Treatment

Conservative

Cross-connections between the flexor hallucis longus and flexor digitorum longus tendons may provide for good residual function of the toes, in which case no further treatment is required.

Operative

The most common interventions are decompression of the tendon by incision of the fibrous canal and tenosynovectomy. The following options may be considered for traumatic ruptures due to stabs or cuts and in young, athletically active patients:

- End-to-end repair of a fresh rupture
- Proximal rupture: transposition of the flexor hallucis longus tendon stump to the flexor digitorum longus
- Tendon reconstruction with an interposed graft (fascia lata or similar material, flexor digitorum longus from a lesser toe, flexor digitorum longus of the second toe)

Prognosis, Complications

Possible complications:

- High risk of tenodesis with limited motion and weakness of the interphalangeal joint
- A hyperextension deformity of the interphalangeal joint with shoe interference can be managed by interphalangeal joint arthrodesis, combined if necessary with proximal advancement of the flexor hallucis longus tendon to the first metatarsal.

6.7 Metatarsalgia

Definition

Metatarsalgia is defined as pain at the midfoot level that is aggravated by walking or running. Metatarsalgia is not a disease in the strict sense but a symptom of overuse injury to the midfoot. The cause is multifactorial and requires further investigation (forefoot and hindfoot deformities).

Symptoms

- Corns and hyperkeratotic areas on plantar sites exposed to increased mechanical stresses
- Midfoot pain worse with prolonged walking or standing, improves with rest

Predisposing Factors

The most common predisposing factor is splayfoot, but other forefoot and hindfoot deformities are also significant:

- Overweight
- Tight-fitting shoes (narrow toebox)
- Shoes with high heels
- Connective tissue weakness

Anatomy and Pathology

A splayfoot deformity develops due to weakness or insufficiency of the intrinsic muscles of the foot. Excessive loading and degeneration of the intermetatarsal ligaments leads to depression of the metatarsal heads, which in turn causes a greater pressure concentration on the metatarsal heads and painful plantar hyperkeratosis. The dropped position of the metatarsal heads causes excessive loading and stretching of the plantar plate at the level of the metatarsophalangeal joints. This results in subluxations or dislocations of the metatarsophalangeal joints (DP or mediolateral displacement) with the development of fixed toe deformities and corns over the proximal and distal interphalangeal joints. Effusion and synovitic swelling develop in the metatarsophalangeal joints, often combined with bursae and exostoses on the medial and lateral sides of the foot (hallux valgus, tailor's bunion).

Imaging

Radiographs (▶ Fig. 6.9)

Weight-bearing radiographs of the foot are obtained in three planes to exclude possible mechanical causes of metatarsalgia. All the pathologies mentioned below can be identified on the X-rays:

- Relative overlength of individual metatarsals
- Instability of the first tarsometatarsal joint
- Prominent plantar condyles of the metatarsal heads
- Splayfoot deformity
- Hallux valgus
- Varus fifth toe
- Splayfoot, pes cavus, or pes planovalgus deformity
- Valgus or varus angulation of the calcaneus

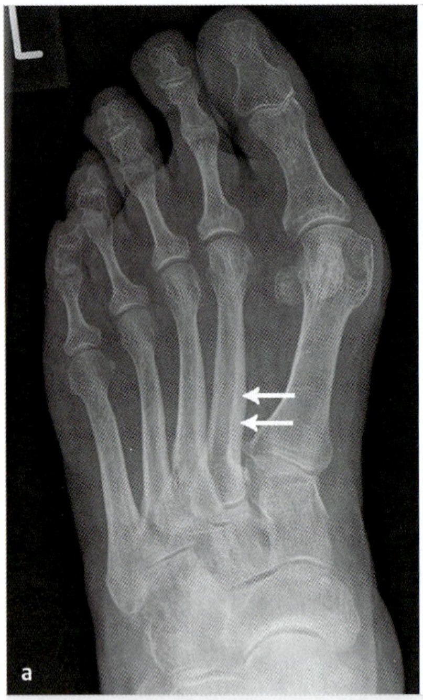

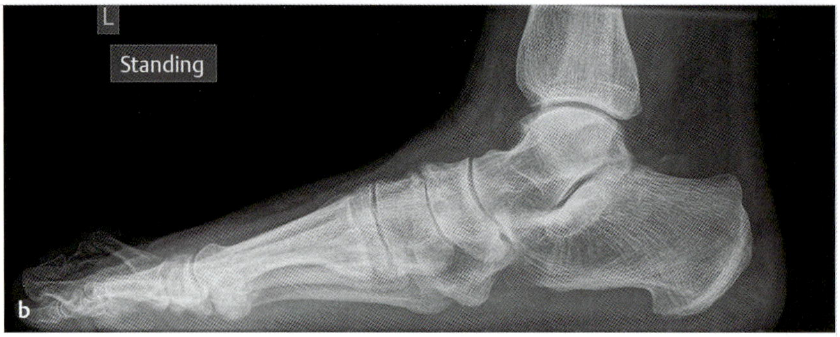

Fig. 6.9 a, b Cortical thickening of the second metatarsal in a patient with clinical metatarsalgia and a fixed hammer toe deformity of the second digit.
a DP radiograph of the left foot.
b Standing lateral radiograph.

Ultrasound

Ultrasound can help narrow the differential diagnosis: joint effusion, change in plantar fascia, Morton neuroma, etc.

MRI

Metatarsalgia is not a primary indication for MRI. The main application of MRI in this setting is to investigate the precipitating cause.

Interpretation Checklist

MRI is used to investigate the cause, for example:

- Indirect signs of instability in the Lisfranc joint line
- Instability or osteoarthritis of the metatarsophalangeal or interphalangeal joints
- Instability or rupture of the plantar plate
- Excessive loads on the metatarsals and especially the metatarsal heads

Plantar keratosis is often noted as a result of altered stress distribution on the ball of the foot, for example:

- Activated osteoarthritis of the first metatarsophalangeal joint
- Morton neuroma
- Insufficiency of the plantar plate at D II leading to plantar keratosis below the fifth metatarsal head

Examination Technique

- *Standard protocol:* prone position, high-resolution multichannel coil centered on the forefoot
- *Sequences:*
  - Axial and coronal T1-weighted
  - Coronal PD-weighted fat-sat (or STIR)
  - Sagittal PD-weighted fat-sat (with high resolution over the second tarsometatarsal joint)
  - Axial and coronal T1-weighted fat-sat after contrast administration

MRI Findings (▶ Fig. 6.10 and ▶ Fig. 6.11)

MRI can define the actual cause of the metatarsalgia (e.g., Morton neuroma, stress fracture, joint instability, or activated osteoarthritis). When imaged in the T1-weighted sequence, plantar keratosis appears as a hypointense tissue density with indistinct margins within the hyperintense fatty tissue. It often shows intense enhancement after contrast administration.

Imaging Recommendation

The diagnosis relies mainly on clinical findings.

Differential Diagnosis

- Prominent plantar condyles of the metatarsal heads
- Overlong second or third metatarsal
- Metatarsal stress fractures
- Posttraumatic metatarsal deformity
- Morton neuroma
- Rheumatoid deformity of the forefoot
- Osteonecrosis of the metatarsal heads
- Instability of the Lisfranc joint line or first tarsometatarsal joint
- Gouty arthritis
- Plantar warts
- Metatarsophalangeal joint deformities
- Varus or valgus position of the hindfoot
- Pes equinovarus, pes cavus, or pes planus deformity

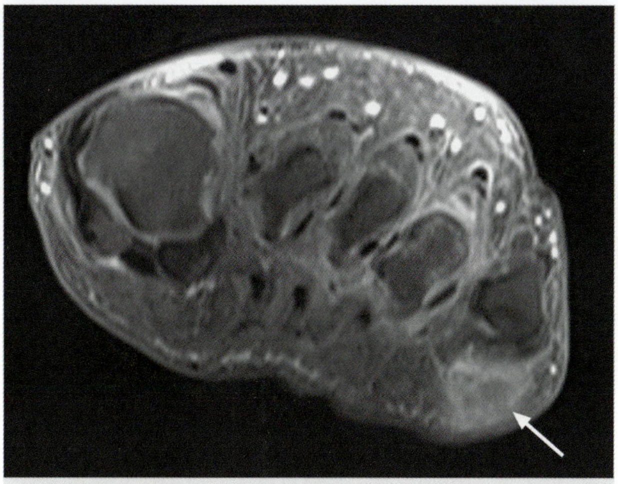

Fig. 6.10 Chronic metatarsalgia of the fourth toe with increasing pain on the lateral border of the foot. Axial T1-weighted fat-sat image after contrast administration shows signs of activation with contrast enhancement in the fourth metatarsophalangeal joint. To reduce pain, the patient has shifted the body weight to the outside of the foot during gait, leading to the development of enhancing lateral plantar keratosis (arrow).

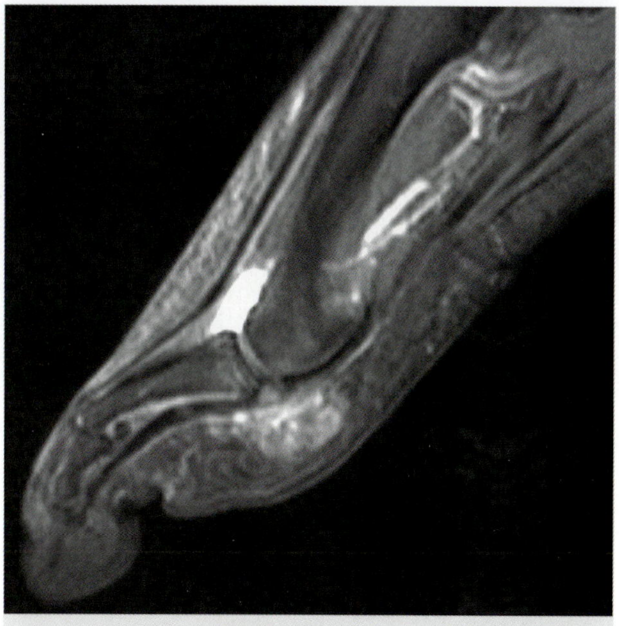

Fig. 6.11 Keratosis in metatarsalgia. A 67-year-old woman complained of pain under the ball of her foot when walking. Sagittal T1-weighted fat-sat image after contrast administration shows activation of the third metatarsophalangeal joint with synovitis and marked overloading of the plantar soft tissues in the ball of the foot.

- Transfer metatarsalgia after the correction of hallux valgus or after a resection arthroplasty of the first metatarsophalangeal joint

Treatment

! Note

Accurate localization of the mechanical overload based on a detailed examination of the foot is essential for successful treatment.

Conservative

Most patients will show good response to conservative treatment:

- Pressure-relieving, cushioning orthotic inserts with retro capital support, a rocker sole with cutout ("butterfly rocker") to relieve pressure on the second and third metatarsal heads
- Optimization of footwear
- Infiltration of the metatarsophalangeal joints with a local anesthetic containing cortisone
- Tangential removal or trimming of calluses (plane, scalpel blade); medical foot care for patients with known diabetes mellitus or diabetic foot syndrome
- Strengthening the intrinsic foot muscles with sensomotoric inserts and physiotherapy
- NSAIDs

! Note

Repeated steroid injections into the plantar fat pad should be avoided due to the risk of atrophy!

Operative

- DuVries or Coughlin condylectomy: for local pressure relief of specific metatarsal condyles
- Distal, proximal, or diaphyseal metatarsal osteotomies to elevate the metatarsal heads
- Girdlestone flexor digitorum longus transfer to correct additional toe deformities and stabilize the metatarsophalangeal joints
- Resection arthroplasty (resection of the second through fifth metatarsal heads), especially in rheumatoid arthritis with destroyed cartilage surface
- Stainsby procedure with reconstruction of the plantar tie bar in inflammatory joint disease with extended rupture of the plantar plate

Prognosis, Complications

Prognosis

The prognosis is good if the mechanical cause can be eliminated by conservative or operative means. Plantar fat pad atrophy and calf muscle shortening are always limiting factors in the treatment of plantar pressure complaints.

Surgical Complications

- Nonunion
- Limitation of motion in the metatarsophalangeal joints
- Transfer metatarsalgia with pressure loads shifted to an adjacent metatarsal
- Overcorrection
- Avascular necrosis of the metatarsal head

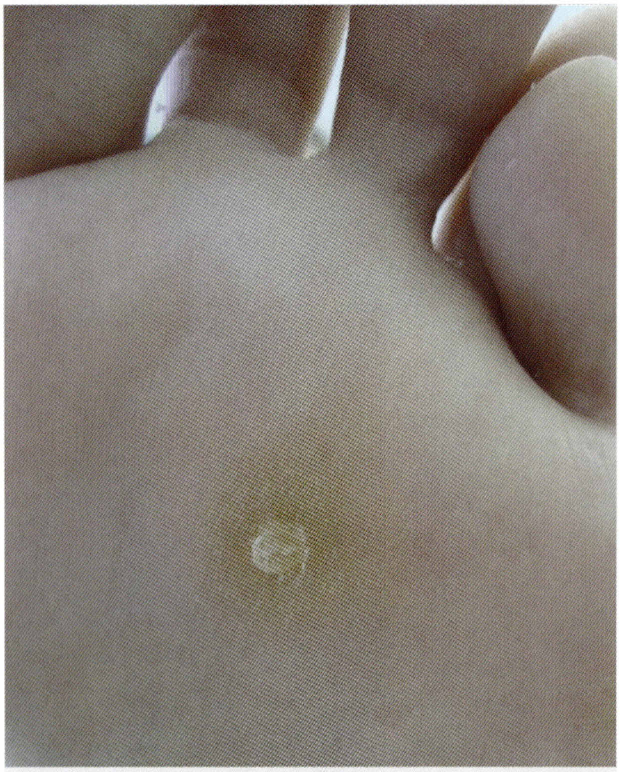

Fig. 6.12 Clinical appearance of a plantar wart.

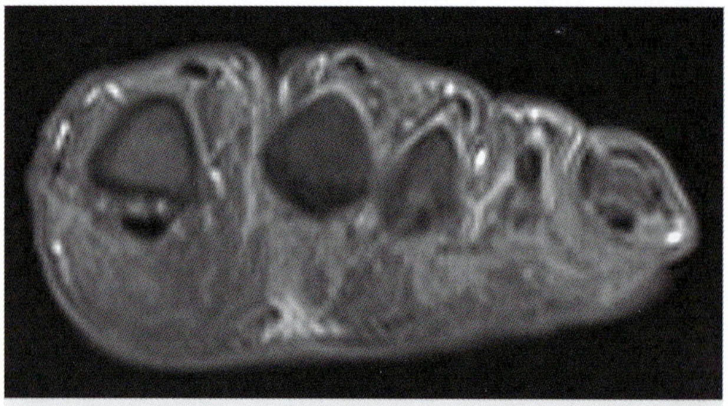

Fig. 6.13 MRI appearance of a plantar wart. Axial T1-weighted fat-sat image after contrast administration displays the wart as a deep, subcutaneous, localized enhancing area in the plantar soft tissues. The evaluation of a plantar wart is not ordinarily an indication for MRI, but it was performed in this case to exclude metatarsalgia as the patient had significant pain on weight bearing.

6.8 Plantar Warts

Definition

Plantar warts are painful, deeply penetrating zones of epithelial hyperplasia with vascular inclusions. They are benign lesions caused by infection with the human papillomavirus.

Symptoms

- Painful, hyperkeratotic area on the sole of the foot
- Presence of a central pore

Predisposing Factors

Viral infection through a macerated skin site.

Anatomy and Pathology (▶ Fig. 6.12)

A hyperkeratotic area with a central pore may occur at various sites on the sole of the foot. Removal of the surface exposes black dots that represent thrombosed capillaries. Plantar warts disrupt the normal contour of the skin. They may be solitary or may form a mosaic cluster. Their growth is exophytic at non-weight-bearing sites but endophytic on the weight-bearing sole of the foot.

Imaging

Ultrasound

Not required.

MRI (▶ Fig. 6.13)

Not required.

Imaging Recommendation

Clinical findings are diagnostic.

Differential Diagnosis

A plantar wart is distinguished from a corn, which can arise by various mechanisms in connection with foot deformities and overuse. See section 6.7 Metatarsalgia (p. 187). A corn does not have vascular inclusions, however, and does not disrupt the contour of the skin.

Treatment

Treatment depends on the age of the patient, the location of the plantar wart, clinical complaints, and the number and size of the warts:
- Keratolysis (salicylic acid)
- Pressure-relieving and cushioning insoles, custom-fitted shoe
- Tangential removal or trimming of calluses (plane, scalpel blade); contraindicated in patients with known diabetes mellitus or diabetic foot syndrome
- Virostatic agent (5-fluorouracil)
- Excision
- Laser vaporization, cryotherapy

Prognosis, Complications

- Spontaneous resolution is common in children
- Risk of recurrence

6.9 Compartment Syndrome of the Interosseous Muscles

Definition

A compartment syndrome develops as a result of complex midfoot and hindfoot injuries that cause a pressure build-up in the compartments of the foot muscles.

Symptoms

- Midfoot swelling
- Plantar hematoma
- Deformity, shortening, or widening of the foot
- Intracutaneous hemorrhage
- Painful passive dorsiflexion of the metatarsophalangeal joints

! Note

Severe foot pain that is not relieved by opioid analgesics is always suspicious for a compartment syndrome. Unlike a compartment syndrome in the lower leg, the neurologic deficits in the foot are difficult to assess by physical examination. Therefore a compartment pressure measurement should be performed whenever a compartment syndrome is suspected. If doubt exists, proceed with surgical decompression!

Predisposing Factors

- Severe, complex midfoot and hindfoot injuries or fractures
- Comatose patient, multiple injuries, decreased vigilance

Anatomy and Pathology

Anatomy

There are five named compartments in the foot:

- *Forefoot compartment:* four interosseous muscles, adductor hallucis
- *Medial compartment:* abductor hallucis, flexor hallucis brevis
- *Lateral compartment:* flexor digiti minimi, abductor digiti quinti
- *Superficial compartment:* flexor digitorum brevis, lumbricals
- *Calcaneal compartment:* quadratus plantae

Pathology

A communication exists between the deep posterior tibial compartment and the superficial and calcaneal compartments in the foot. This means that even in patients with complex hindfoot injuries, the foot is at risk for the development of a compartment syndrome.

Increased tissue pressure in a compartment due to fluid collections or muscular edema may compromise blood flow to the muscles and neurovascular structures, resulting in ischemic injury. Because the muscle fasciae are noncompliant, they cannot readily expand to compensate for the elevated pressure within the compartment. Myoglobinemia and impaired renal function are two signs that may indicate the destruction of muscle cells.

Imaging

Radiographs

- Radiographs of the ankle joint in two planes
- Radiographs of the foot in three planes
- Broden views may be obtained to exclude a fracture

Ultrasound

Not indicated.

MRI

MRI is unrewarding, and the diagnosis is made clinically. It is unwise to order time-consuming tests that would delay intervention.

Imaging Recommendation

Diagnosis relies on clinical findings and tissue pressure measurements. Pressures higher than 30 mmHg or more than 10 to 30 mmHg below the diastolic blood pressure are abnormal (normal = 8 mmHg).

Differential Diagnosis

- Acute arterial occlusion
- Plantar vein thrombosis
- Peripheral nerve lesion (peroneal nerve, tibial nerve, plantar nerve)

Treatment

! Note

A prompt diagnosis is important to prevent serious tissue injury and late sequelae in the form of foot or toe deformities.

Two dorsal approaches are available for decompressing the forefoot compartment: between the first and second metatarsals and between the third and fourth metatarsals. A medial incision is used for decompression of the medial, lateral and superficial compartments.

Prognosis, Complications

Prognosis

The prognosis is good following a prompt diagnosis and incision. Pressure elevations lasting more than 6 hours will cause irreversible muscle and nerve damage.

Possible Complications

- Hammer toe deformity and impaired function in the metatarsophalangeal joints due to contractures
- Rarely, amputation is necessary due to severe ischemia and necrosis
- Ulcers and sensory disturbances
- Tenodesis or lysis of adhesions after split-thickness skin grafting of the primary skin incisions

6.10 Bibliography

Plantar Fasciitis, Rupture of the Plantar Fascia

Chimutengwende-Gordon M, O'Donnell P, Singh D. Magnetic resonance imaging in plantar heel pain. Foot Ankle Int 2010; 31: 865–870

Drake M, Bittenbender C, Boyles RE. The short-term effects of treating plantar fasciitis with a temporary custom foot orthosis and stretching. J Orthop Sports Phys Ther 2011; 41: 221–231

Fabrikant JM, Park TS. Plantar fasciitis (fasciosis) treatment outcome study: plantar fascia thickness measured by ultrasound and correlated with patient self-reported improvement. Foot (Edinb) 2011; 21: 79–83

Gerdesmeyer L, Frey C, Vester J et al. Radial extracorporeal shock wave therapy is safe and effective in the treatment of chronic recalcitrant plantar fasciitis: results of a confirmatory randomized placebo-controlled multicenter study. Am J Sports Med 2008; 36: 2100–2109

Hafner S, Han N, Pressman MM, Wallace C. Proximal plantar fibroma as an etiology of recalcitrant plantar heel pain. J Foot Ankle Surg 2011; 50: 153–157

Ibrahim MI, Donatelli RA, Schmitz C, Hellman MA, Buxbaum F. Chronic plantar fasciitis treated with two sessions of radial extracorporeal shock wave therapy. Foot Ankle Int 2010; 31: 391–397

Jeswani T, Morlese J, McNally EG. Getting to the heel of the problem: plantar fascia lesions. Clin Radiol 2009; 64: 931–939

League AC. Current concepts review: plantar fasciitis. Foot Ankle Int 2008; 29: 358–366

Louwers MJ, Sabb B, Pangilinan PH. Ultrasound evaluation of a spontaneous plantar fascia rupture. Am J Phys Med Rehabil 2010; 89: 941–944

McNally EG, Shetty S. Plantar fascia: imaging diagnosis and guided treatment. Semin Musculoskelet Radiol 2010; 14: 334–343

Metzner G, Dohnalek C, Aigner E. High-energy Extracorporeal Shock-Wave Therapy (ESWT) for the treatment of chronic plantar fasciitis. Foot Ankle Int 2010; 31: 790–796

Patel A, DiGiovanni B. Association between plantar fasciitis and isolated contracture of the gastrocnemius. Foot Ankle Int 2011; 32: 5–8

Soomekh DJ. Current concepts for the use of platelet-rich plasma in the foot and ankle. Clin Podiatr Med Surg 2011; 28: 155–170

Stoita R, Walsh M. Operative treatment of plantar fasciitis preserving the function of the plantar fascia: technique tip. Foot Ankle Int 2009; 30: 1022–1025

Walther M, Radke S, Kirschner S, Ettl V, Gohlke F. Power Doppler findings in plantar fasciitis. Ultrasound Med Biol 2004; 30: 435–440

Watson TS, Anderson RB, Davis WH, Kiebzak GM. Distal tarsal tunnel release with partial plantar fasciotomy for chronic heel pain: an outcome analysis. Foot Ankle Int 2002; 23: 530–537

Plantar Heel Spur

Gerdesmeyer L, Frey C, Vester J et al. Radial extracorporeal shock wave therapy is safe and effective in the treatment of chronic recalcitrant plantar fasciitis: results of a confirmatory randomized placebo-controlled multicenter study. Am J Sports Med 2008; 36: 2100–2109

Ibrahim MI, Donatelli RA, Schmitz C, Hellman MA, Buxbaum F. Chronic plantar fasciitis treated with two sessions of radial extracorporeal shock wave therapy. Foot Ankle Int 2010; 31: 391–397

Lohrer H, Nauck T, Dorn-Lange NV, Schöll J, Vester JC. Comparison of radial versus focused extracorporeal shock waves in plantar fasciitis using functional measures. Foot Ankle Int 2010; 31: 1–9

Ledderhose Disease

Bancroft LW, Peterson JJ, Kransdorf MJ. Imaging of soft tissue lesions of the foot and ankle. Radiol Clin North Am 2008; 46: 1093–1103, vii

de Palma L, Santucci A, Gigante A, Di Giulio A, Carloni S. Plantar fibromatosis: an immunohistochemical and ultrastructural study. Foot Ankle Int 1999; 20: 253–257

Dürr HR, Krödel A, Trouillier H, Lienemann A, Refior HJ. Fibromatosis of the plantar fascia: diagnosis and indications for surgical treatment. Foot Ankle Int 1999; 20: 13–17

Heyd R, Dorn AP, Herkströter M, Rödel C, Müller-Schimpfle M, Fraunholz I. Radiation therapy for early stages of morbus Ledderhose. Strahlenther Onkol 2010; 186: 24–29

Jeswani T, Morlese J, McNally EG. Getting to the heel of the problem: plantar fascia lesions. Clin Radiol 2009; 64: 931–939

McNally EG, Shetty S. Plantar fascia: imaging diagnosis and guided treatment. Semin Musculoskelet Radiol 2010; 14: 334–343

Murphey MD, Ruble CM, Tyszko SM, Zbojniewicz AM, Potter BK, Miettinen M. From the archives of the AFIP: musculoskeletal fibromatoses: radiologic-pathologic correlation. Radiographics 2009; 29: 2143–2173

Sammarco GJ, Mangone PG. Classification and treatment of plantar fibromatosis. Foot Ankle Int 2000; 21: 563–569

Atrophy of the Plantar Fat Pad

Cichowitz A, Pan WR, Ashton M. The heel: anatomy, blood supply, and the pathophysiology of pressure ulcers. Ann Plast Surg 2009; 62: 423–429

Coughlin MJ, Mann R, Saltzman C. Surgery of the Foot and Ankle. Vol. I. 8thed. Philadelphia: Mosby / Elsevier; 2007

Miller-Young JE, Duncan NA, Baroud G. Material properties of the human calcaneal fat pad in compression: experiment and theory. J Biomech 2002; 35: 1523–1531

Snow SW, Bohne WH. Observations on the fibrous retinacula of the heel pad. Foot Ankle Int 2006; 27: 632–635

Waldecker U, Lehr HA. Is there histomorphological evidence of plantar metatarsal fat pad atrophy in patients with diabetes? J Foot Ankle Surg 2009; 48: 648–652

Wearing SC, Smeathers JE, Urry SR, Sullivan PM, Yates B, Dubois P. Plantar enthesopathy: thickening of the enthesis is correlated with energy dissipation of the plantar fat pad during walking. Am J Sports Med 2010; 38: 2522–2527

Plantar Vein Thrombosis

Barros MV, Labropoulos N. Plantar vein thrombosis—evaluation by ultrasound and clinical outcome. Angiology 2010; 61: 82–85

Bernathova M, Bein E, Bendix N, Bodner G. Sonographic diagnosis of plantar vein thrombosis: report of 3 cases. J Ultrasound Med 2005; 24: 101–103

Elsner A, Schiffer G, Jubel A, Koebke J, Andermahr J. The venous pump of the first metatarsophalangeal joint: clinical implications. Foot Ankle Int 2007; 28: 902–909

Geiger C, Rademacher A, Chappell D, Sadeghi-Azandaryani M, Heyn J. Plantar vein thrombosis due to busy night duty on intensive care unit. Clin Appl Thromb Hemost 2011; 17: 232–234

Siegal DS, Wu JS, Brennan DD, Challies T, Hochman MG. Plantar vein thrombosis: a rare cause of plantar foot pain. Skeletal Radiol 2008; 37: 267–269

Hallucis longus and Digitorum longus Intersection Syndrome

Buck FM, Gheno R, Nico MA, Haghighi P, Trudell DJ, Resnick D. Chiasma crurale: intersection of the tibialis posterior and flexor digitorum longus tendons above the ankle. Magnetic resonance imaging-anatomic correlation in cadavers. Skeletal Radiol 2010; 39: 565–573

Coughlin MJ, Mann R, Saltzman C. Surgery of the Foot and Ankle. Vol. I. 8thed. Philadelphia: Mosby / Elsevier; 2007

Lee RP, Hatem SF, Recht MP. Extended MRI findings of intersection syndrome. Skeletal Radiol 2009; 38: 157–163

Michelson J, Dunn L. Tenosynovitis of the flexor hallucis longus: a clinical study of the spectrum of presentation and treatment. Foot Ankle Int 2005; 26: 291–303

Sanhudo JA. Stenosing tenosynovitis of the flexor hallucis longus tendon at the sesamoid area. Foot Ankle Int 2002; 23: 801–803

Metatarsalgia

Coughlin MJ, Mann R, Saltzman C. Surgery of the Foot and Ankle. Vol. I. 8thed. Philadelphia: Mosby / Elsevier; 2007

Espinosa N, Maceira E, Myerson MS. Current concept review: metatarsalgia. Foot Ankle Int 2008; 29: 871–879

Plantar Warts

Coughlin MJ, Mann R, Saltzman C. Surgery of the Foot and Ankle. Vol. I. 8thed. Philadelphia: Mosby / Elsevier; 2007

Lichon V, Khachemoune A. Plantar warts: a focus on treatment modalities. Dermatol Nurs 2007; 19: 372–375

Wirth CJ, Zichner L. Orthopädie und orthopädische Chirurgie – Fuß. Stuttgart: Thieme; 2002: 382

Compartment Syndrome of the Interosseous Muscles

Fulkerson E, Razi A, Tejwani N. Review: acute compartment syndrome of the foot. Foot Ankle Int 2003; 24: 180–187

Myerson MS. Management of compartment syndromes of the foot. Clin Orthop Relat Res 1991: 239–248

Wirth CJ, Zichner L. Orthopädie und orthopädische Chirurgie – Fuß. Stuttgart: Thieme; 2002: 382

Chapter 7

Neurologic Diseases

7 Neurologic Diseases

M. Walther and U. Szeimies

7.1 Morton Neuroma

Definition

Morton neuroma is the benign swelling of a plantar intermetatarsal nerve. It occurs most commonly between the heads of the third and fourth metatarsals.

Symptoms

- Plantar pain on weight bearing
- Pain increased by walking on hard ground or wearing a tight-fitting shoe
- Pain radiates to the toes
- Dysesthesia in the interdigital space
- Positive Mulder click test
- Positive "doorbell" sign (point tenderness between the metatarsal heads in response to plantar pressure)

Predisposing Factors

- Thin plantar fat pad
- Peak age incidence between 40 and 60 years
- More common in women

Anatomy and Pathology

The plantar intermetatarsal nerve branch is compressed in the area of the deep intermetatarsal ligament. The normal diameter of the nerve is approximately 2 mm; enlargement to more than 5 mm is definitely abnormal. Histologic examination reveals fibrosis of the nerve and Schwann cells. The late stage is marked by perineural and epineural fibrosis with hypertrophy.

Imaging

Radiographs

Unrewarding.

Ultrasound

Longitudinal and transverse scans over the dorsal side of the metatarsal bones, usually the third or fourth, demonstrate an elliptical hypoechoic mass.

MRI

MRI is used to confirm the clinical impression and exclude other metatarsalgias (stress fracture, Köhler disease II, insufficiency of the plantar plate).

Interpretation Checklist

- Demonstrate the Morton neuroma
- Exclude a second Morton neuroma
- Evaluate other structures: metatarsophalangeal and interphalangeal joints (degenerative changes, activation processes); increased loads on bony structures, especially the metatarsal heads; plantar keratosis due to an antalgic gait

Examination technique

Contrast administration is not essential for demonstrating a Morton neuroma but is helpful in narrowing the differential diagnosis.

- *Standard protocol:* prone position, high-resolution multichannel coil
- *Sequences:*
  - Coronal and sagittal PD-weighted fat-sat
  - Coronal and axial T1-weighted (most important sequence)
  - Coronal and axial T1-weighted fat-sat after contrast administration

MRI Findings (▶ Fig. 7.1 and ▶ Fig. 7.2)

- Interdigital soft-tissue proliferation, usually located between the second and third or third and fourth metatarsophalangeal joints and extending toward the sole
- Most clearly depicted in the unenhanced coronal and axial T1-weighted sequences (the very cellular, hypointense tissue nodule with a bulbous or fusiform shape contrasts sharply with the intense fat signal from the plantar soft tissue)
- Enhancement after contrast administration is variable, depending on the degree of vascularity, and ranges from almost no enhancement to intense enhancement

Imaging Recommendation

Modality of choice: MRI.

Differential Diagnosis

- Metatarsal stress fracture
- Atrophy of the plantar fat pad
- Rupture of the plantar plate
- Osteonecrosis (Köhler disease II)
- Tarsal tunnel syndrome
- Neurofibroma
- Intermetatarsal bursitis

Treatment

Conservative

- Avoid high heels
- Wear shoes with a wide toebox
- Cushion the forefoot
- Local injections (corticosteroid, local anesthetic–alcohol mixture)

Operative

- Decompress the nerve by dividing the deep intermetatarsal ligament
- Excise the neuroma

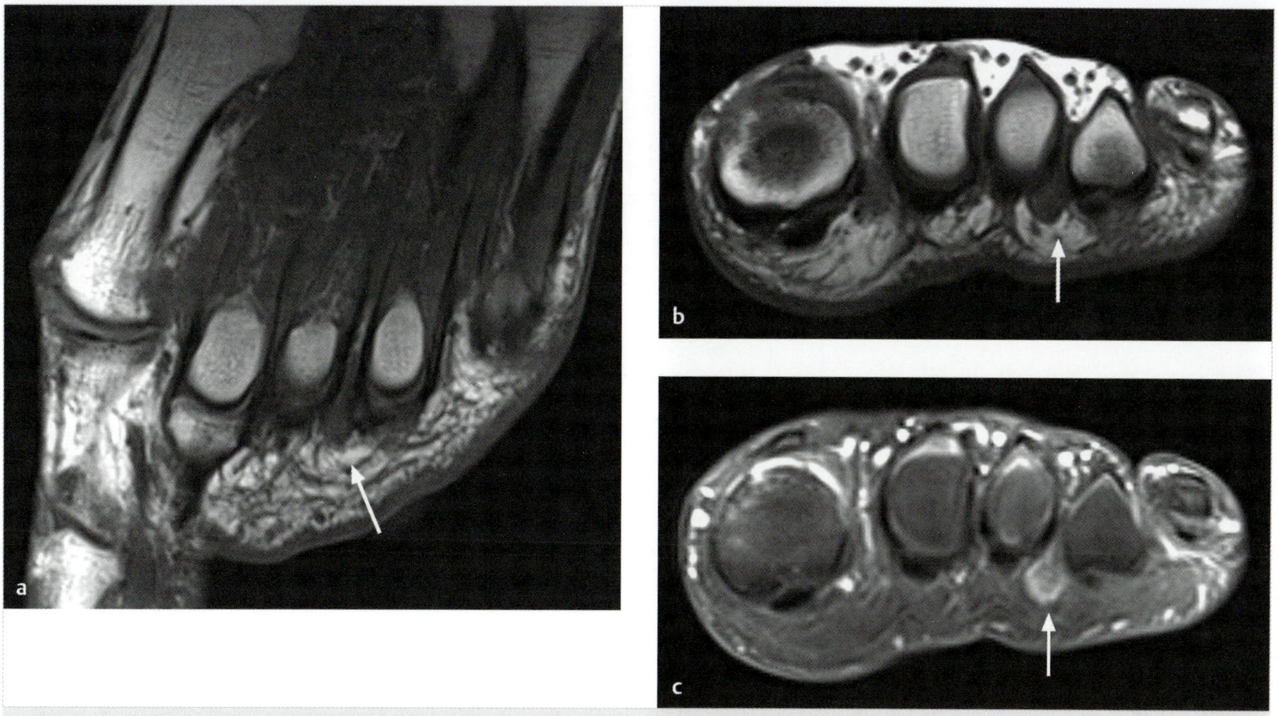

Fig. 7.1 a–c Typical MRI appearance of a Morton neuroma between the third and fourth metatarsals.
a Coronal T1-weighted sequence shows a small, hypointense, club-shaped soft-tissue mass (arrow) located between the third and fourth metatarsophalangeal joints.
b Axial T1-weighted sequence shows a hypointense structure extending toward the sole. The mass contrasts sharply with hyperintense plantar fat (arrow).
c Axial T1-weighted fat-sat sequence shows intense enhancement of the Morton neuroma after contrast administration (arrow).

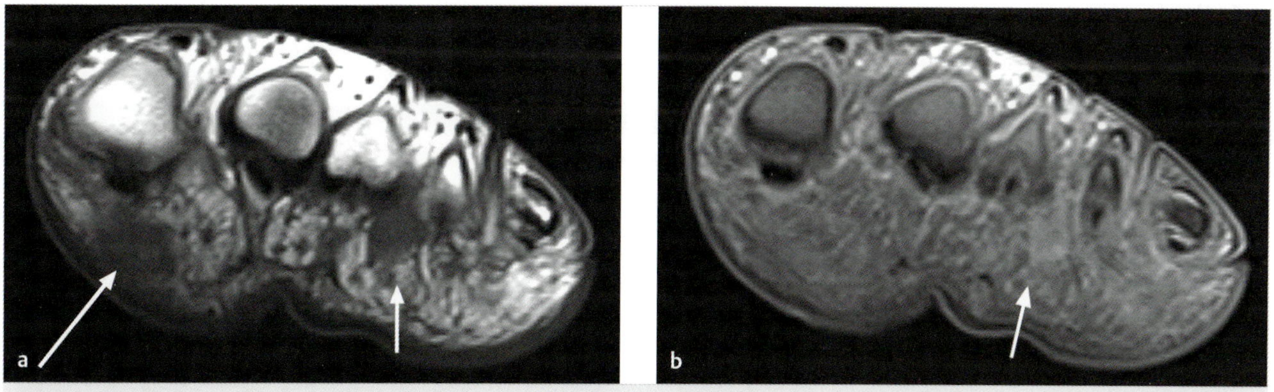

Fig. 7.2 a, b Chronic metatarsalgia in a 54-year-old woman with point pain and tenderness between the third and fourth metatarsal heads.
a Axial T1-weighted sequence shows a plantar interdigital soft-tissue mass located between the third and fourth metatarsal heads (short arrow). The image also demonstrates plantar keratosis below the first metatarsophalangeal joint due to the weight shift away from the lesion (long arrow).
b Axial T1-weighted fat-sat sequence after contrast administration shows only faint enhancement of a Morton neuroma with moderate vascularity (arrow).

Prognosis, Complications

Possible complications:

- Atrophy of the skin and plantar fat pad due to repeated corticosteroid injections
- Stump neuroma after the excision of a Morton neuroma
- Persistent, chronic pain

7.2 Other Nerve Compression Syndromes

Definition

▶ Table 7.1 lists the most common compression syndromes affecting the foot (mechanical injury to peripheral nerves from compression due to intrinsic or extrinsic causes).

Table 7.1 Nerve compression syndromes in the foot

Affected nerve	Site of compression	Causes	Symptoms	Comments
Tibial nerve	Tarsal tunnel	• Trauma (fractures, scarring) • Mass effect (ganglion, lipoma, varicosity, accessory muscles such as an accessory flexor digitorum longus) • Foot deformities (hindfoot valgus, pes planus, coalition) • Systemic diseases (diabetes mellitus, arterial occlusive disease)	Burning pain and paresthesias on the plantar side, extending to the toes, increased by weight bearing	Tarsal tunnel syndrome mainly causes sensory nerve damage; muscular deficits are rare
Baxter nerve (= inferior calcaneal nerve; first branch of the lateral plantar nerve)	Below the abductor hallucis fascia, causing nerve entrapment and compression at three sites of predilection: • At the fascia of a hypertrophic abductor hallucis (e.g., in long-distance runners) • The medial side of the quadratus plantae muscle • The medial calcaneus at the level of the fibro-osseous junction of the plantar aponeurosis	• Compression by adjacent enthesiophytes • Compression by fibrovascular reactive tissue due to plantar fasciitis • Occasional compression by a bony heel spur (▶ Fig. 6.4)	• Pain around the heel • Pain may radiate to the lateral side • Loss of sensation is rare	Baxter nerve innervates the abductor digiti minimi and portions of the quadratus plantae and digitorum brevis muscles
Medial plantar nerve	At the knot of Henry (intersection of flexor hallucis longus and flexor digitorum longus tendons in the region of the navicular tuberosity)	• Patients often have marked hindfoot valgus and pronation of the forefoot • Nerve is damaged at this site of predilection by repetitive trauma and overuse (jogging) • Compression of the nerve by shoe inserts for longitudinal arch support	• Pain in the heel and midfoot • Paresthesias on the medial side of the sole • Positive Hofmann–Tinel sign	Jogger's foot may increase the risk of premature osteoarthritis of the first metatarsophalangeal joint and damage to the medial plantar nerve
Calcaneal branch	At the tarsal tunnel or distal in the soft tissue	• Veins • Ganglia • Scars • External pressure from shoes	• Pain at the medial side of the calcaneus, proximal to the insertion of the plantar fascia • Hyposensitivity may be present at the medial calcaneus	Sensory branch of the tibial nerve; arises from the tibial nerve in the proximal tarsal tunnel and supplies sensory innervation to the medial calcaneus
Sural nerve	Anywhere in the course of the nerve	• Ganglia • Scarring after a sprain injury • Achilles tendon disease • Surgical scars in the course of the nerve	• Loss of sensation at the lateral foot • The area of hyposensitivity can be extremely variable in size	The sural nerve is often used as graft for the reconstruction of nerve injuries
Superficial peroneal nerve	At its site of emergence from the deep fascia in the lateral lower leg, one handwidth proximal to the ankle joint	• Muscle hernias • Direct nerve compression by the fascial border	• Pain, radiating to the dorsal aspect of the foot • Tenderness where the nerve penetrates the fascia ventrolateral at the calf, approximately 10 cm proximal to the ankle • Hoffmann–Tinel sign	• Can mimic degenerative arthritis of the midfoot • Damages to the lateral branches can be caused by ankle sprain

Table 7.1 continued

Affected nerve	Site of compression	Causes	Symptoms	Comments
Deep peroneal nerve	• Inferior retinaculum (anterior tarsal tunnel syndrome) • Intersection with the extensor hallucis longus tendon • Intersection with the extensor hallucis brevis tendon	• Chronic pressure • Tight shoe laces • Tendons	• Loss of sensation in the webspace between the 1st and 2nd toes	
Saphenous nerve	Anywhere in the course of the nerve	• Direct trauma • Surgical procedures	• Loss of sensation from the medial malleolus to the hallux	
Lateral plantar nerve	Between the deep fascia of the abductor hallucis and the medial border of the quadratus plantae	• Compression by a plantar heel spur or a thickened plantar fascia • Veins • Ganglia • Lipoma	• Reduced sensitivity at the lateral plantar surface of the foot • Atrophy of the muscles around the digiti minimi • Abducted position of the fifth toe due to the loss of function of the adductor digiti minimi	Pain radiates to the lateral side of the foot

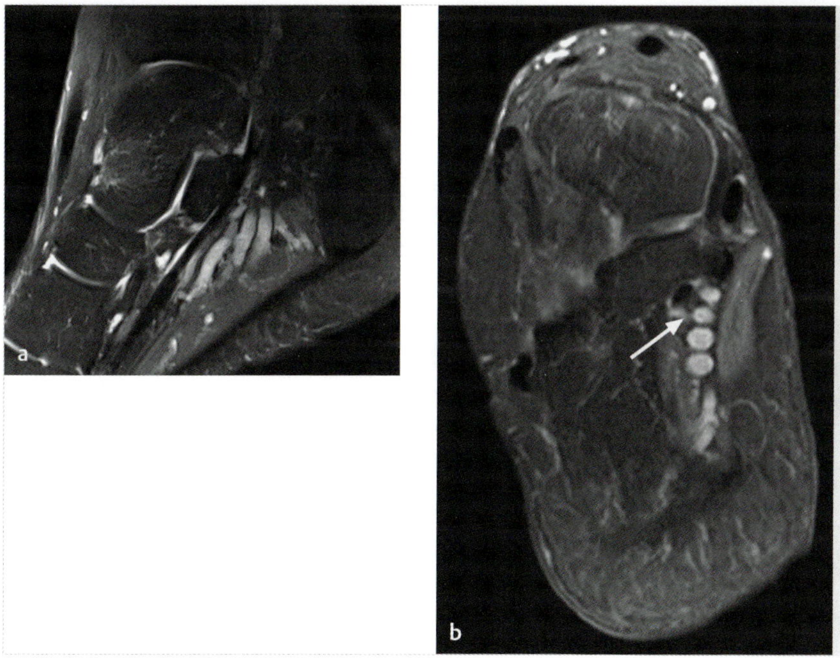

Fig. 7.3 a, b Tarsal tunnel syndrome.
a Sagittal PD-weighted fat-sat image shows marked varicosity with tibial nerve compression at the level of the tarsal tunnel.
b The dilated veins and flexor hallucis longus tendon have caused crowding of the tibial nerve (arrow).

Symptoms

- Pain radiating proximally and distally along the nerve pathway
- Hypoesthesia in the nerve distribution
- Atrophy of the innervated muscles
- Local tenderness at the site of nerve compression
- Positive Hofmann–Tinel sign
- Delayed nerve conduction velocity is not consistently detected

Predisposing Factors

- *Intrinsic compression:*
  - Anatomic variants
  - Osteophytes or other bony ridges
  - Ganglia
  - Scars
  - Hypertrophic tendons
  - Varicosity
  - Hyperpronation

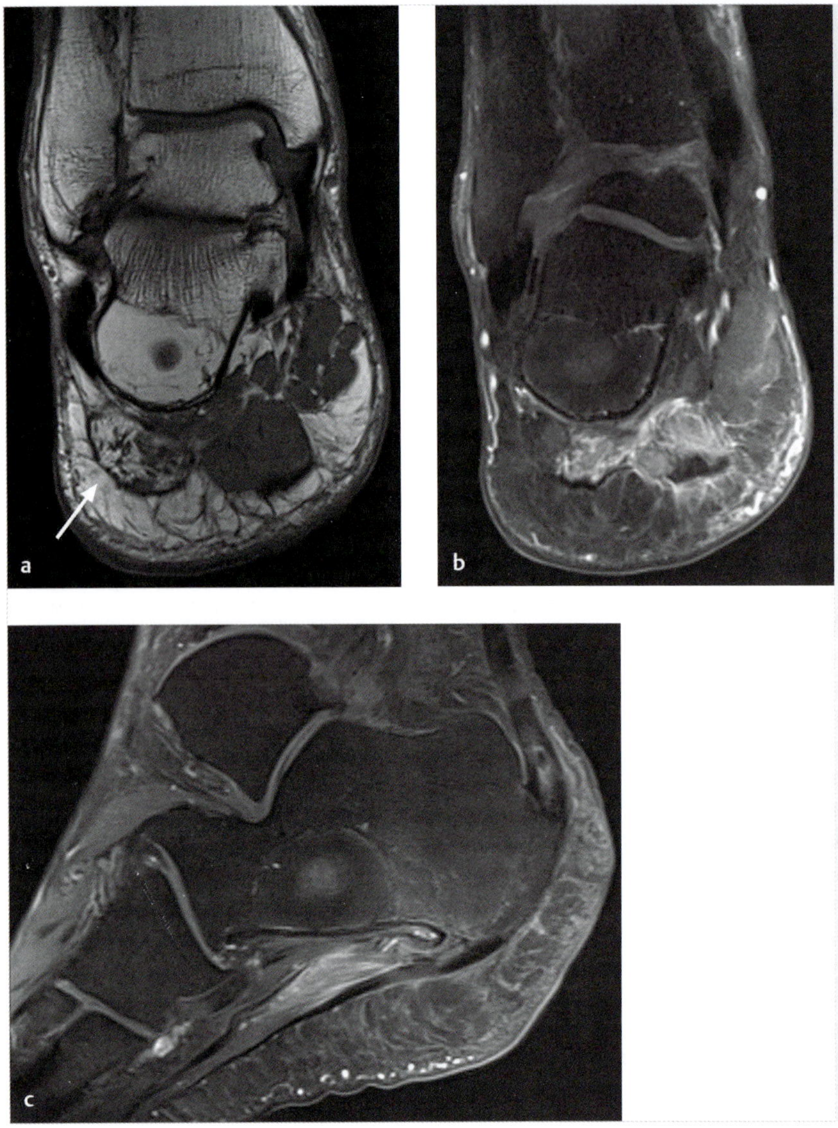

Fig. 7.4 a–c **Compression of the Baxter nerve.**
a Coronal T1-weighted image shows lipomatous involution of the abductor digiti minimi (arrow). Lipoma in the calcaneus with central regression is noted as an incidental finding.
b Coronal T1-weighted fat-sat image after contrast administration shows enhancement in portions of the abductor digiti minimi and quadratus plantae as evidence of denervation.
c Sagittal T1-weighted fat-sat image after contrast administration. An activated plantar heel spur with plantar fasciitis has caused the compression or irritation of the first branch of the lateral plantar nerve under the abductor hallucis fascia. The increased enhancement is consistent with acute denervation in the abductor digiti minimi.

- *Extrinsic compression:*
  - Tight shoe
  - Shoe laced too tightly
  - Shoe inserts

Anatomy and Pathology

The sensitivity of nerves to local pressure is highly variable in its degree. Hourglass narrowing of the affected nerve may be found at operation.

Imaging

Radiographs

Radiographs can exclude compression from a bony source (heel spur).

Ultrasound

Not indicated.

MRI

Interpretation Checklist

- Describe the location of the nerve damage
- Identify the cause (soft-tissue mass, crowding, anatomic variant, coalition, accessory muscle, adjacent inflammation, plantar fasciitis)
- Evaluate the innervated muscles (early damage, denervation edema, advanced stage, lipomatous involution)
- Exclude other possible diagnoses

Examination Technique

- *Standard protocol:* prone position, high-resolution multichannel coil
- *Sequences:*
  - Coronal and sagittal PD-weighted fat-sat
  - Coronal and axial T1-weighted
  - Sagittal and axial T1-weighted fat-sat after contrast administration

- The protocol should be adapted for the targeted investigation of a specific nerve, using high-resolution slices (2.0–2.5 mm) and a small field of view

MRI Findings

- *Tarsal tunnel syndrome* (▶ Fig. 7.3):
  - Accessory muscle within the tarsal tunnel (accessory flexor digitorum longus) or outside the tarsal tunnel (accessory soleus)
  - High-resolution scans (2.0–2.5 mm) can directly visualize the nerve and its pathology (edema, swelling, adjacent edema in perineural fat, possible contrast enhancement)
  - Denervation edema in the muscles is rare, as the sensory component is predominantly affected; watch for distal edema formation in the forefoot and midfoot muscles

- *Medial plantar nerve (jogger's foot):*
  - Abnormal enhancement of the tendon sheaths at the knot of Henry
  - Denervation edema with increased signal intensity in fat-suppressed water-sensitive sequences of the abductor hallucis and flexor digitorum brevis muscles
  - Lipomatous involution and fatty degeneration in T1- and T2-weighted sequences

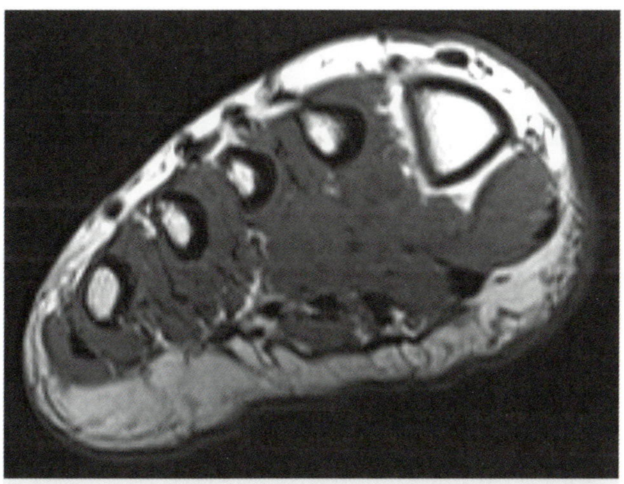

Fig. 7.5 Normal appearance of the foot muscles. Axial T1-weighted image shows normal, intact muscles at the level of the metatarsals.

- *Baxter neuropathy* (▶ Fig. 7.4):
  - Denervation edema, especially of the abductor digiti minimi
  - Subsequent lipomatous involution and atrophy
  - Visualization of florid plantar fasciitis

! Note

In patients with plantar fasciitis, particular care should be taken to describe the abductor digiti minimi in the T1-weighted sequence (edematous in the early stage). The clinical features of Baxter neuropathy are often nonspecific and difficult to classify. Even an electromyogram may be inconclusive.

Imaging Recommendation

Modality of choice: MRI. High-resolution imaging systems (3 T, high-resolution joint coils, thin slices) can directly visualize the nerve and any abnormalities (edema, increased enhancement) that may be present. MRI can localize and evaluate the causes of nerve compression and can provide early detection of late sequelae (denervation edema of the muscles).

! Note

Nerve entrapment and its effects are often missed in MRI of the foot. A peripheral nerve lesion caused by compression or entrapment should always be considered in the differential diagnosis of unexplained foot pain.

If a patient complains of unexplained pain and burning with or without limited motion while walking or at rest, and has previous negative radiographs and sectional images, the findings on clinical examination will often be equivocal. Nerve conduction velocity and electromyograms, if obtained, are not always abnormal in patients with a nerve entrapment syndrome. MRI may show no edema, no fluid collections, no masses, etc., and if contrast-enhanced images are obtained, they do not show abnormal enhancement, resulting in additional negative findings. Often, too little attention is given to the foot muscles in the plain T1-weighted sequence, and atrophy is simply overlooked. In dealing with unexplained complaints of this kind, therefore, the condition of the foot muscles should be closely scrutinized

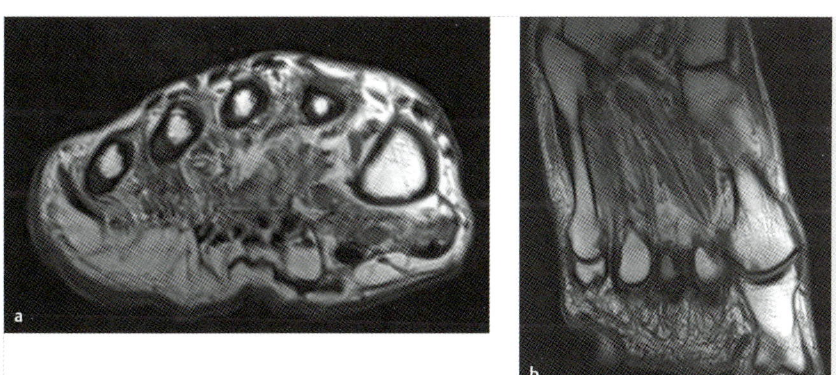

Fig. 7.6 a, b Muscular atrophy.
a Axial T1-weighted image shows atrophy and lipomatous infiltration of all muscles at the level of the metatarsals.
b Coronal T1-weighted image shows streaky lipomatous involution of the interosseous muscles.

(fatty degeneration or atrophy?) for possible signs of nerve entrapment (▶ Fig. 7.5 and ▶ Fig. 7.6).

Differential Diagnosis

- Nerve pathology at a more proximal level
- Other local pathologies in the painful areas

Treatment

- Eliminate external compression
- Corticosteroid injections
- If complaints persist and a mechanical cause has been identified: surgical nerve decompression

Prognosis, Complications

If the cause of the nerve compression can be eliminated, good results are reported in up to 80% of cases. Nerve regeneration will take 6 months or longer in 50% of patients, however.

7.3 Bibliography

Morton Neuroma

Adams WR. Morton's neuroma. Clin Podiatr Med Surg 2010; 27: 535–545

Beltran LS, Bencardino J, Ghazikhanian V, Beltran J. Entrapment neuropathies III: lower limb. Semin Musculoskelet Radiol 2010; 14: 501–511

Giannini S, Bacchini P, Ceccarelli F, Vannini F. Interdigital neuroma: clinical examination and histopathologic results in 63 cases treated with excision. Foot Ankle Int 2004; 25: 79–84

Hughes RJ, Ali K, Jones H, Kendall S, Connell DA. Treatment of Morton's neuroma with alcohol injection under sonographic guidance: follow-up of 101 cases. AJR Am J Roentgenol 2007; 188: 1535–1539

Lee KS. Musculoskeletal ultrasound: how to evaluate for Morton's neuroma. AJR Am J Roentgenol 2009; 193: W172

Markovic M, Crichton K, Read JW, Lam P, Slater HK. Effectiveness of ultrasound-guided corticosteroid injection in the treatment of Morton's neuroma. Foot Ankle Int 2008; 29: 483–487

Pace A, Scammell B, Dhar S. The outcome of Morton's neurectomy in the treatment of metatarsalgia. Int Orthop 2010; 34: 511–515

Sharp RJ, Wade CM, Hennessy MS, Saxby TS. The role of MRI and ultrasound imaging in Morton's neuroma and the effect of size of lesion on symptoms. J Bone Joint Surg Br 2003; 85: 999–1005

Stamatis ED, Karabalis C. Interdigital neuromas: current state of the art—surgical. Foot Ankle Clin 2004; 9: 287–296

Villas C, Florez B, Alfonso M. Neurectomy versus neurolysis for Morton's neuroma. Foot Ankle Int 2008; 29: 578–580

Womack JW, Richardson DR, Murphy GA, Richardson EG, Ishikawa SN. Long-term evaluation of interdigital neuroma treated by surgical excision. Foot Ankle Int 2008; 29: 574–577

Zanetti M, Saupe N, Espinosa N. Postoperative MR imaging of the foot and ankle: tendon repair, ligament repair, and Morton's neuroma resection. Semin Musculoskelet Radiol 2010; 14: 357–364

Zelent ME, Kane RM, Neese DJ, Lockner WB. Minimally invasive Morton's intermetatarsal neuroma decompression. Foot Ankle Int 2007; 28: 263–265

Other Nerve Compression Syndromes

Aktan Ikiz ZA, Uçerler H, Bilge O. The anatomic features of the sural nerve with an emphasis on its clinical importance. Foot Ankle Int 2005; 26: 560–567

Allen JM, Greer BJ, Sorge DG, Campbell SE. MR imaging of neuropathies of the leg, ankle, and foot. Magn Reson Imaging Clin N Am 2008; 16: 117–131, vii

Beltran LS, Bencardino J, Ghazikhanian V, Beltran J. Entrapment neuropathies III: lower limb. Semin Musculoskelet Radiol 2010; 14: 501–511

Chhabra A, Subhawong TK, Williams EH et al. High-resolution MR neurography: evaluation before repeat tarsal tunnel surgery. AJR Am J Roentgenol 2011; 197: 175–183

Daniels TR, Lau JT, Hearn TC. The effects of foot position and load on tibial nerve tension. Foot Ankle Int 1998; 19: 73–78

Dirim B, Resnick D, Ozenler NK. Bilateral Baxter's neuropathy secondary to plantar fasciitis. Med Sci Monit 2010;16(4): CS50–CS53

Donovan A, Rosenberg ZS, Cavalcanti CF. MR imaging of entrapment neuropathies of the lower extremity. Part 2. The knee, leg, ankle, and foot. Radiographics 2010; 30: 1001–1019

Gondring WH, Shields B, Wenger S. An outcomes analysis of surgical treatment of tarsal tunnel syndrome. Foot Ankle Int 2003; 24: 545–550

Peck E, Finnoff JT, Smith J. Neuropathies in runners. Clin Sports Med 2010; 29: 437–457

Takakura Y, Kumai T, Takaoka T, Tamai S. Tarsal tunnel syndrome caused by coalition associated with a ganglion. J Bone Joint Surg Br 1998; 80: 130–133

Watson TS, Anderson RB, Davis WH, Kiebzak GM. Distal tarsal tunnel release with partial plantar fasciotomy for chronic heel pain: an outcome analysis. Foot Ankle Int 2002; 23: 530–537

Chapter 8

Diseases Not Localized to a Specific Site

8

8 Diseases Not Localized to a Specific Site

U. Szeimies

8.1 Reflex Sympathetic Dystrophy, CRPS

Definition, Synonyms

Complex regional pain syndrome (CRPS), also called reflex sympathetic dystrophy or Sudeck atrophy, is a chronic pain condition involving bones, joints, and soft tissues.

Symptoms

The stages of CRPS are reviewed in ▶ Table 8.1.

! Note

The syndrome is characterized by a triad of sensory, sympathetic, and motor dysfunction.

Predisposing Factors

- Approximately 90% of cases are posttraumatic and are preceded by a soft-tissue injury, fracture, or contusion
- Some cases have a nontraumatic etiology—principally myocardial infarction or stroke
- No correlation exists between the severity of an injury and the subsequent development of reflex sympathetic dystrophy
- More common in females
- Peak age incidence is approximately the fifth decade of life, but CRPS may occur at any age
- Other predisposing factors: systemic bone diseases (osteoporosis, osteomalacia, hyperparathyroidism, osteogenesis imperfecta)
- Previous surgery
- Arthroscopy
- Infection
- Electrical injury
- Cold or heat injury
- Neurologic damage
- Vascular diseases
- Medications (tuberculostatics, thyrostatics, phenobarbital, cyclosporine)
- Metabolic disorders (diabetes mellitus, hyperlipidemia, gout)
- Alcohol abuse

Anatomy and Pathology

Dihlmann has described CRPS as a vasomotor dysregulation with associated dysfunction of the sympathetic nervous system. A nociceptive stimulus (triggered by a fracture, contusion, etc.)

Table 8.1 Stages of complex regional pain syndrome (CRPS) based on symptoms

Stage	Description	Symptoms
I	Hyperemic inflammatory stage	• Acute onset over several days • Burning pain • Skin changes (red or purple, moist and warm) • Swelling of soft tissues • Stiffness • Hypersensitivity of the skin • Pain at rest or with movement • Skin ulceration • Local warmth • Soft-tissue edema • Persistent pain recurring after at least 4 weeks • Cutaneous manifestations may be absent • No inflammatory markers • Patchy, predominantly subcortical bone marrow edema
II	Dystrophic stage	• Onset in weeks or months after trauma • Limitation of motion • Skin is cool, pale, and dry • Skin changes with trophic disturbances (hair, nails, fibrosis) • Contractures • Diminishing pain • Cold sensation • Cancellous bone appears blotchy, inhomogeneous, radiolucent
III	Atrophic stage	• Fibrosis • Contractures • Leathery skin • Atrophy of subcutaneous fat • Glossy skin • Muscular atrophy • Glassy appearance of bones on radiographs

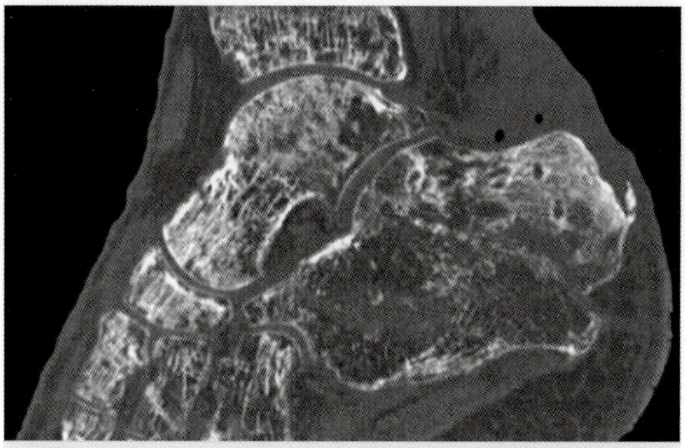

Fig. 8.1 Sagittal reformatted CT image of the hindfoot in severe, advanced reflex sympathetic dystrophy with pronounced decalcification.

activates the dorsal horn of the spinal cord via sensory fibers, which in turn activates the sympathetic trunk in the lateral horn of the spinal cord. The dysregulation spreads to the periphery via efferent sympathetic fibers on the spinal nerves and blood vessels, causing changes in blood flow and permeability that may produce a range of effects on bones and soft tissues (edema, skin thickening, atrophy, fibrosis, bone deficiency).

Imaging

Radiographs

X-rays appear normal in the early stage. After a period of weeks, radiographs show a loss of cancellous bone substance with increased lucency and patchy demineralization, accentuated bone contours, and eventual loss of the subchondral plate, cortical thinning, and subperiosteal resorption. The absence of joint-space narrowing distinguishes CRPS from arthritis. The changes are still reversible in stages I and II. Radiographs in stage III show "glassy" bones with occasional hypertrophic bone atrophy and thickened, rarefied trabeculae.

Ultrasound

Not indicated.

CT (▶ Fig. 8.1)

CT is negative in the early stage. Later scans show patchy demineralization and rarefied trabeculae, as seen on plain radiographs. The changes are difficult to distinguish from disuse osteopenia.

MRI

Interpretation Checklist

- Diagnosis
- Early detection in patients with equivocal pain symptoms
- Use MRI findings to narrow the differential diagnosis

Examination Technique

The MRI examination of reflex sympathetic dystrophy does not require IV contrast administration. The scan parameters depend on the location of the pain (hindfoot, midfoot, forefoot).

- *Standard protocol:* prone position, high-resolution multichannel coil.
- *Sequences:*
  - Changes are best displayed by STIR and PD-weighted fat-sat sequences
  - Hindfoot:
    - Sagittal STIR
    - Sagittal T1-weighted
    - Axial T2-weighted
    - Coronal PD-weighted fat-sat
  - Midfoot and forefoot:
    - Oblique coronal STIR
    - Oblique coronal T1-weighted
    - Axial T2-weighted
    - Sagittal PD-weighted fat-sat

MRI Findings (▶ Fig. 8.2)

Images typically show patchy diffuse bone marrow edema distributed throughout the skeleton. Subcortical edema, appearing as fine subchondral or subcortical lines or dots, is virtually pathognomonic in the early stage. There is associated soft-tissue edema, moderate effusion, and possible thickening and edema of the synovial membrane. Differentiation from disuse osteopenia may be difficult but is aided by the clinical presentation (less pain in disuse osteopenia, no skin changes), the absence of subcutaneous edema, and less-pronounced bone marrow edema. In transient bone marrow edema syndrome, the bone marrow edema is regional and confined to one bone, and it is considerably more intense and homogeneous. CRPS is distinguished from grade 0 Charcot arthropathy by noting that the edema in CRPS is more diffuse and is distributed throughout the tarsus; this differs from the monoarticular involvement and focal edema of Charcot arthropathy.

Imaging Recommendation

Modality of choice: MRI for early detection and differential diagnosis.

Differential Diagnosis

- Arthritis (inflammatory markers)
- Disuse osteopenia (distinguishing feature: less soft-tissue involvement)
- Diabetic Charcot foot in stage 0 (differentiated by pain)
- Transient bone marrow edema syndrome (changes are more focal)
- Osteomyelitis (loss of fatty marrow signal)

Treatment

Besides physical therapy and analgesics, bisphosphonates have become increasingly important in recent years. A variety of drugs are used, depending on the nature of the pain. They include nonsteroidal anti-inflammatory drugs (NSAIDs), gabapentin derivatives, selective serotonin-reuptake inhibitors, and opioids. Topical treatment with lidocaine and capsaicin has also been described. Treatment recommendations have changed several times in recent years, and many new agents are currently undergoing trials.

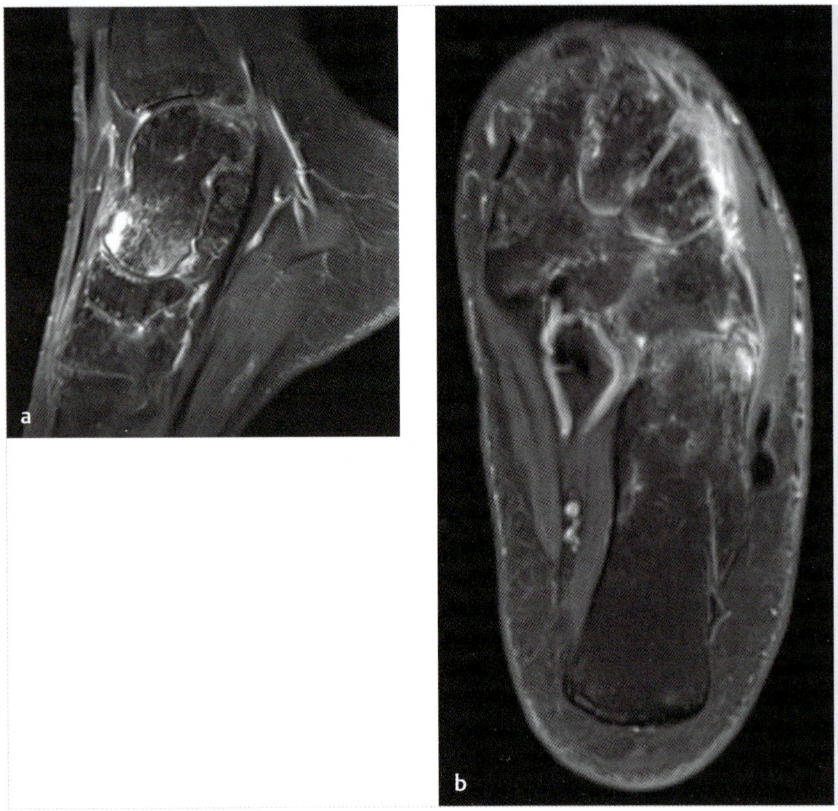

Fig. 8.2 a, b Reflex sympathetic dystrophy 2 months after an ankle sprain. Contrast administration is usually unnecessary in this condition, which can be adequately diagnosed with water-sensitive fat-suppressed MRI sequences.
a Sagittal T1-weighted fat-sat image after contrast administration shows a patchy bone marrow signal with typical spotty and linear hyperintensities and contrast enhancement in the subchondral region.
b Axial T1-weighted fat-sat image after contrast administration. Unlike transient bone marrow edema syndrome, reflex sympathetic dystrophy affects all bony areas and shows diffuse soft-tissue involvement.

Prognosis, Complications

The disease often runs a self-limiting course with reversible functional deficits. Irreversible changes may occur (joint contractures, secondary deformities, loss of function), and some may cause serious disability.

8.2 Bone Marrow Edema Syndrome

Definition

Transient bone marrow edema syndrome is a transitory osteoporosis, a painful juxta-articular bone disease associated with reversible bone marrow edema.

Symptoms

- Pain on weight bearing
- Pain at rest
- Tenderness to pressure

Predisposing Factors

- Usually occurs spontaneously without a precipitating cause
- Pregnancy (last trimester)
- Often preceded by minor trauma

Anatomy and Pathology

The etiology of bone marrow edema syndrome is not fully understood. Presumably it has a metabolic cause related to the group of reflex sympathetic dystrophies. Vasomotor dysfunction leads to the release of inflammatory mediators and to a disturbance of vascular permeability with painful bone marrow edema. The syndrome is manifested in weight-bearing joints, most commonly affecting the femoral head, knee, and foot. Associated findings are soft-tissue swelling and joint effusion.

Imaging

Radiographs

Negative findings in the early stage are followed within several weeks by signs of bone deficiency and increased radiolucency.

Ultrasound

Not indicated.

MRI

Interpretation Checklist

- Make a definitive diagnosis, identifying the cause of unexplained pain
- Evaluate extent
- Carefully evaluate the subchondral region and cortical layer (impending cortical collapse with small insufficiency fractures or early demarcation of necrotic areas)

Examination Technique

Contrast administration is unnecessary for the MRI evaluation of bone marrow edema syndrome. Scan parameters are tailored to the location of the pain (hindfoot, midfoot, forefoot).

- *Standard protocol:* prone position, high-resolution multichannel coil.

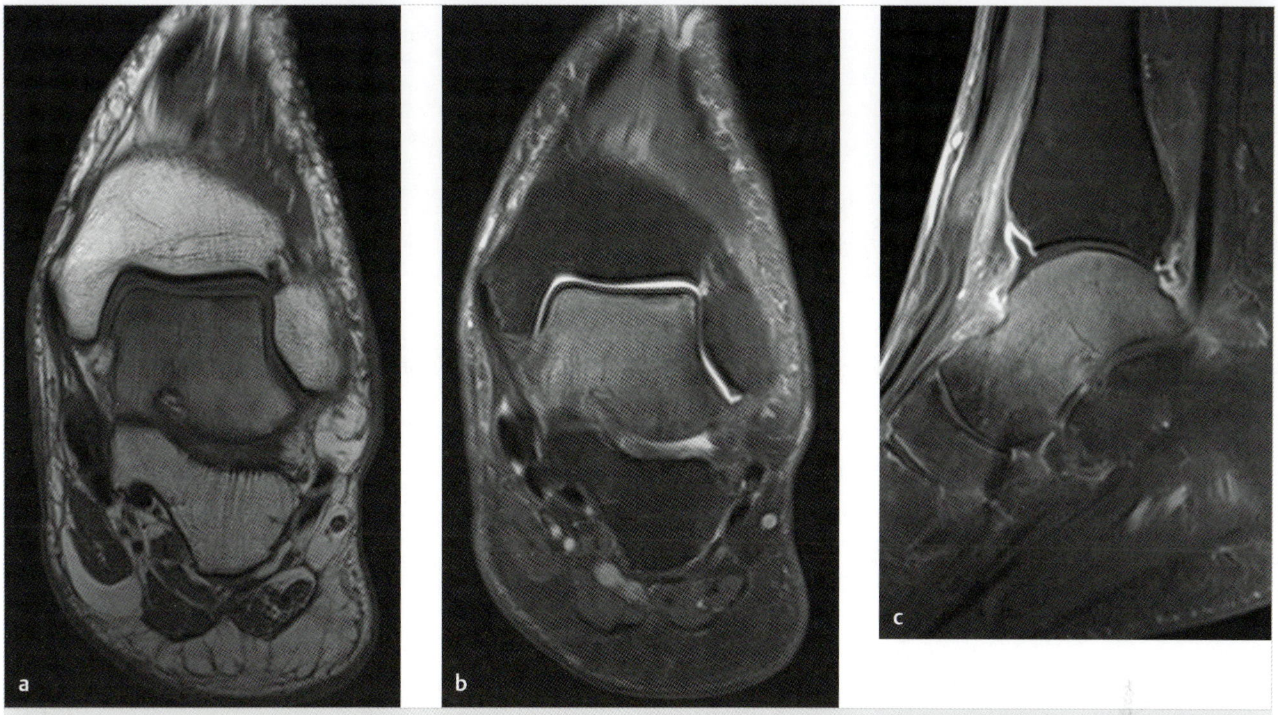

Fig. 8.3 a–c Pain at rest and during exercise in a 54-year-old woman with bone marrow edema syndrome of the talus.
a Coronal T1-weighted image shows diffuse low signal intensity in the talus with some preservation of the fatty marrow signal. This excludes osteonecrosis.
b Coronal PD-weighted fat-sat image shows typical homogeneous bone marrow edema in one bone area (here the talar dome) with normal signal intensity in adjacent bony structures. Slight signal irregularities are noted in the subchondral region on the lateral shoulder of the talus. There is no evidence of cortical collapse.
c Sagittal T1-weighted fat-sat image after contrast administration shows intense, homogeneous enhancement of the talar dome and neck sparing the talar head. Typical increased enhancement is also noted in the adjacent soft tissues.

- *Sequences:*
  - Changes are best displayed by STIR and PD-weighted fat-sat sequences
  - Hindfoot:
    - Sagittal STIR
    - Sagittal T1-weighted
    - Axial T2-weighted
    - Coronal PD-weighted fat-sat
  - Midfoot and forefoot:
    - Oblique coronal STIR
    - Oblique coronal T1-weighted
    - Axial T2-weighted
    - Sagittal PD-weighted fat-sat

MRI Findings (▶ Fig. 8.3 and ▶ Fig. 8.4)

- Areas of intense bone marrow edema uniformly occupying a bone or bone region, usually limited to one bone (e.g., the navicular or talar dome) with little or no edema in adjacent bones
- Associated soft-tissue edema
- Differentiating transient bone marrow edema syndrome from overuse edema:
  - Bone marrow edema syndrome has intense edema usually affecting the entire bone or the tarsals with adjacent soft-tissue edema and joint effusion
  - In a bone response to stress, the marrow edema is concentrated along the biomechanical stress line and is more localized
  - Fine hypointense lines indicating an incipient stress fracture are sometimes observed in transient bone marrow edema syndrome

Imaging Recommendation

Modality of choice: MRI.

Differential Diagnosis

- Monoarthritis
- Osteonecrosis
- Bone infarction
- Osteomyelitis
- Mechanical overload

Treatment

- Syndrome often resolves spontaneously in 3 to 6 months
- Resting the affected limb plus pain therapy (analgesics, NSAIDs or calcitonin, bisphosphonates, analogue of prostacyclin [e.g., iloprost])

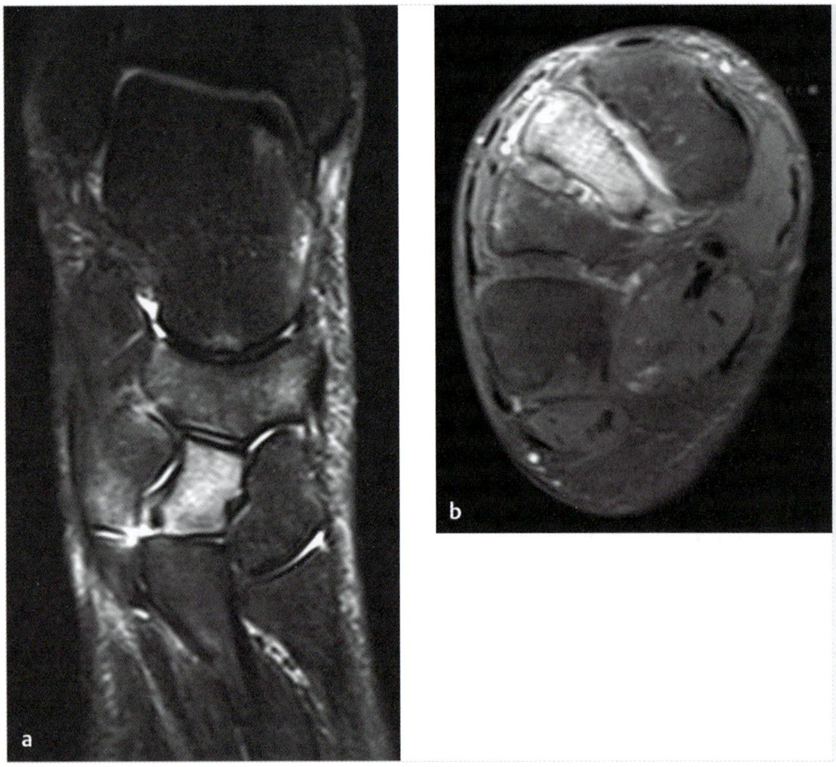

Fig. 8.4 a, b Classic findings in bone marrow edema syndrome affecting the intermediate cuneiform bone.
a Coronal STIR sequence shows intense edema in the intermediate cuneiform with only a slight increase of signal intensity in the navicular and lateral cuneiform.
b Axial T1-weighted fat-sat image after contrast administration shows homogeneous enhancement of the intermediate cuneiform with marked activation of adjacent soft tissues.

Prognosis, Complications

- Possible protracted course lasting 12 to 18 months
- Insufficiency fracture due to chronic edema
- Possible migration of the disease (saltatory or migratory edema) with involvement of other bone areas
- Recurrence is rare

8.3 Overuse Edema

Definition

Overuse edema is bone marrow edema that occurs in a setting of excessive or unphysiologic loads.

Symptoms

- Pain with movement
- Local tenderness
- Swelling

Predisposing Factors

- Unilateral repetitive loads without a recovery period
- Overweight
- Osteoporosis
- Posttraumatic after a long rest period
- Foot deformity

Anatomy and Pathology

Overuse edema develops in bone areas subjected to increased mechanical or point stresses. It may be the precursor of a stress fracture, often occurring as a compensatory response to altered biomechanics (e.g., in activated osteoarthritis of the first metatarsophalangeal joint, shifting weight to the lateral side of the foot while walking to avoid pain, and excessive loads on the head of the fifth metatarsal).

Imaging

Radiographs

Radiographs show no abnormalities.

Ultrasound

Not indicated.

MRI

Interpretation Checklist

- Determine precise anatomical localization
- Differentiate overuse edema from a stress fracture
- Narrow the differential diagnosis
- If possible, identify the cause of the bone overload (tendon pathology, ligament insufficiency)

Examination Technique

MRI evaluation of overuse edema does not require IV contrast administration. Scan parameters are tailored to the location of the pain (hindfoot, midfoot, forefoot).

- *Standard protocol:* prone position, high-resolution multichannel coil
- *Sequences:*
  - Changes are displayed best by STIR and PD-weighted fat-sat sequences
  - Hindfoot:
    - Sagittal STIR
    - Sagittal T1-weighted

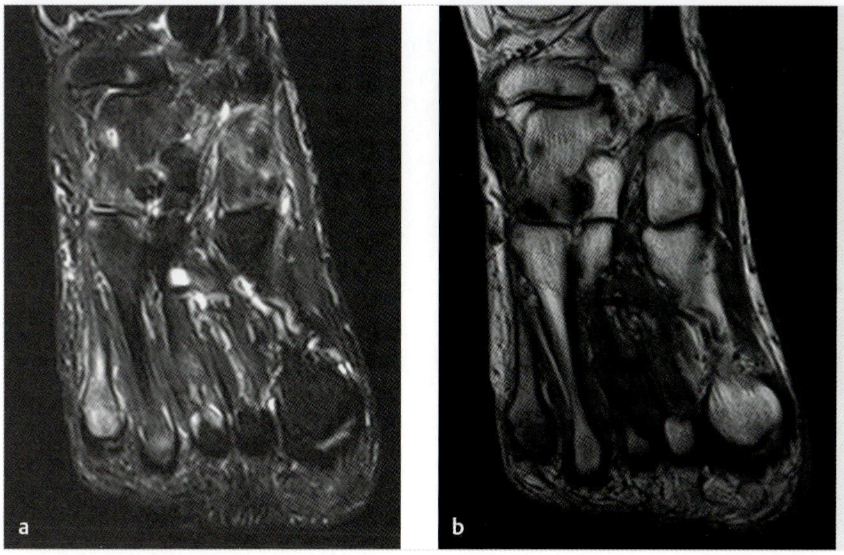

Fig. 8.5 a, b Overuse edema.
a Coronal STIR sequence shows bone marrow edema in the distal fifth metatarsal due to chronic unphysiologic loads (weight shifted to lateral side of foot during walking).
b Coronal T1-weighted sequence shows a decreased fatty marrow signal with no evidence of a fracture line.

  - Axial T2-weighted
  - Coronal PD-weighted fat-sat
- ○ Midfoot and forefoot:
  - Oblique coronal STIR
  - Oblique coronal T1-weighted
  - Oblique axial T2-weighted
  - Sagittal PD-weighted fat-sat

MRI Findings (▶ Fig. 8.5)

- Rather diffuse area of bone marrow edema with ill-defined margins, located in articulating bone ends or in one or more metatarsals
- Little or no edema of adjacent soft tissues
- Preservation of fatty marrow signal in the T1-weighted sequence
- Normal-appearing articular cartilage

Imaging Recommendation

Modality of choice: MRI.

Differential Diagnosis

- Stress fracture
- Bone marrow edema syndrome
- Osteonecrosis
- Osteomyelitis

Treatment

- Rest
- Immobilization
- Local pressure relief by custom-made insoles
- Modify walking stresses with a medial or lateral wedge
- Some deformities may require corrective surgery

Prognosis, Complications

The prognosis is good, and changes are completely reversible when causal stresses are relieved.

8.4 Stress Fractures, Microfractures

Definition

A stress fracture is a fracture that has been caused not by direct trauma but by abnormal loads. Two types are distinguished:

- *Stress or fatigue fracture:* abnormal stresses acting on normal bone
- *Insufficiency fracture:* normal stresses acting on abnormally unstable bone (e.g., due to osteoporosis, osteomalacia, Charcot arthropathy, rheumatoid arthritis)

Symptoms

- Pain worsened by weight-bearing activity
- Pain at rest
- Swelling
- Possible local warmth

Predisposing Factors

- Overuse ("march fracture", marathon runners, ballet dancers)
- Overweight
- Malalignment
- Unphysiologic loads

Anatomy and Pathology

Sites of predilection for stress fractures are the metatarsals (most commonly the second and third metatarsals in athletes and the fifth metatarsal in soccer and tennis players), the distal tibia, calcaneus, talar neck, sesamoids, and navicular. When soccer players make rapid accelerating and cutting maneuvers, different forces are exerted at the base and head of the metatarsals, giving rise to a bending stress along the metatarsal shaft that is strongest in the fifth metatarsal. A stress fracture of the second metatarsal has two sites of predilection: proximal near the base and distal in the shaft. The proximal fractures are more likely to take a chronic course with thickening of the cortex and are more aptly classified as insufficiency fractures. Common associated factors are low bone density, a shortened Achilles tendon, a length discrepancy between the first and second metatarsals, and multiple stress fractures. The more distal fractures of the second metatarsal are more likely to be "true" stress fractures caused by abnormal loads (increased training level).

Fractures are classified by their healing tendency as high-risk fractures (navicular, second metatarsal base, fifth metatarsal, sesamoids, medial malleolus) or low-risk fractures (calcaneus, distal metatarsals). High-risk fractures are at high risk for delayed union and refracturing.

Imaging

Radiographs

Radiographs are initially negative. Later they show a bone response with periosteal thickening, a sclerotic zone, a sclerotic fracture line, and soft-tissue swelling.

Ultrasound

A longitudinal scan over the affected bone (often the second metatarsal or talus) shows hypoechoic thickening over the echogenic, possibly disrupted bone line consistent with a periosteal hematoma or edema. Later examinations will show increasing echogenic callus formation. Ultrasound yields positive findings earlier than radiographs.

MRI

Interpretation Checklist

- Stage the stress fracture (early peripheral fracture or complete fracture)
- Determine the degree of activation and healing
- Exclude other differential diagnoses

! Note

There are a number of different classifications for stress fractures, and a generally valid system that takes into account clinical and MRI criteria has not yet been established. It is essential to differentiate between overuse edema and a fracture and to assess the degree of activation.

Examination Technique

Stress fractures can be imaged and evaluated by MRI without contrast administration. Scan parameters are tailored to the location of the pain (hindfoot, midfoot, forefoot).

- *Standard protocol:* prone position, high-resolution multichannel coil
- *Sequences:*
  - Changes are best displayed by STIR and T1-weighted sequences
  - Hindfoot:
    - Sagittal STIR
    - Sagittal T1-weighted
    - Axial T2-weighted
    - Coronal PD-weighted fat-sat
  - Midfoot and forefoot:
    - Oblique coronal STIR
    - Oblique coronal T1-weighted
    - Oblique axial T2-weighted
    - Sagittal PD-weighted fat-sat

MRI Findings (▶ Fig. 8.6)

Initial findings are intense bone marrow edema and associated edema of adjacent soft tissues. MRI is usually performed at a later stage, that is, not within days but after a period of 2 to 3 weeks or even later. Especially in the metatarsals, signs of bone stress (intense edema) coexist with periosteal thickening as evidence of repair. Edema typically shows an intense center with peripheral extensions that distinguish it from bone marrow edema syndrome (which affects the entire bone with fairly uniform intensity). The hallmark of a stress fracture is the presence of one or more hypointense, slightly wavy lines (e.g., located in the calcaneus) in the T1-weighted sequence. Fatty marrow signal is still visible within the T1-hypointense bone-marrow signal caused by edema, and this distinguishes the stress fracture from osteomyelitis and from a pathologic fracture resulting from a tumor.

Imaging Recommendation

Modalities of choice: radiography and ultrasonography, also MRI in suspicious cases owing to its sensitivity in the early stage. In addition, MRI can distinguish overuse edema from an actual stress fracture.

Differential Diagnosis

- Activated osteoarthritis
- Bone marrow edema syndrome
- Arthritis
- Osteomyelitis
- Pathologic fracture
- Fifth metatarsal: Jones fracture (fracture of the fifth metatarsal at the proximal metaphyseal–diaphyseal junction without involvement of the tarsometatarsal joint)

Treatment

- Rest, immobilization for 6 weeks, then gradual progression to full weight bearing
- Training below the pain threshold is usually possible (e.g., running athletes can perform endurance training on a bicycle ergometer or in water)
- If decreased bone density is found, diagnose osteoporosis
- High-risk stress fractures may be an indication for internal fixation
- Prophylaxis by training modification and, if necessary, the use of orthotic shoe inserts

Prognosis, Complications

With adequate immobilization, the fracture will usually heal with complete bony consolidation. Progression to an unstable fracture or nonunion is possible, especially if the causal stress is continued.

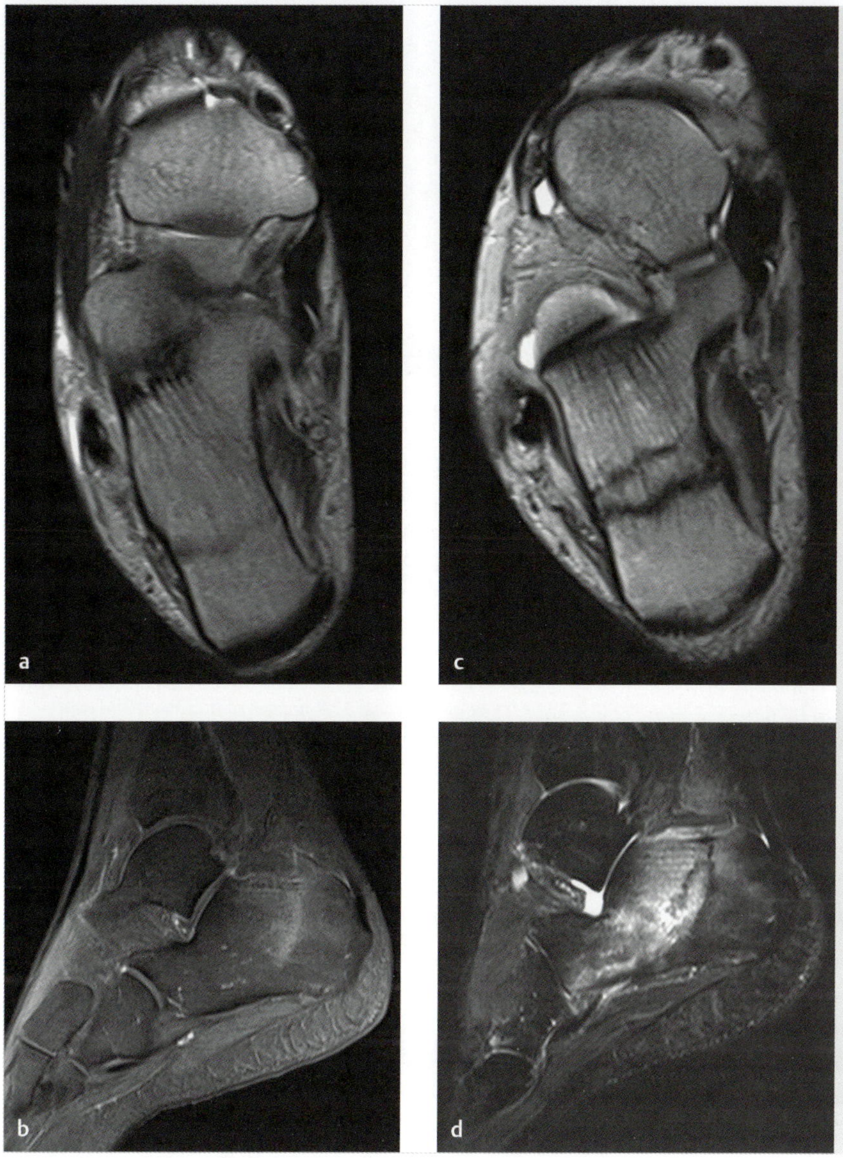

Fig. 8.6 a–d Stress fracture of the calcaneus followed over a 3-month period. This woman, a jogger, sustained a fatigue fracture of the calcaneus that was not adequately treated.
a Axial T2-weighted image shows a faint hypointense line through the calcaneus.
b Sagittal T1-weighted fat-sat image after contrast administration shows a moderately enhancing area in the overstressed bone that is most pronounced along the fracture line.
c Axial T2-weighted image at 3 months shows a complete fracture line and a more distal partial fatigue fracture through the calcaneus.
d Sagittal STIR image at 3 months shows conspicuous fracture edema in the calcaneus extending to the anterior process, accompanied by subtalar effusion and visible fracture lines.

8.5 Pediatric Bone Marrow Edema (Tiger-Stripe Pattern)

Pediatric bone marrow edema of the tarsal bones, called a “tiger-stripe” pattern due to its mottled imaging appearance, often poses a challenge to the clinician and radiologist: MRI is ordered for a young patient with unexplained spontaneous pain or persistent posttraumatic complaints of variable severity in the hindfoot and midfoot, which are usually worsened by physical activity. In children, it is normal to find a speckled bone marrow signal in the hindfoot and tarsals that shows high intensity in fat-suppressed sequences and is caused by persistent red bone marrow. The changes may be focal or patchy. Sometimes it is difficult to classify findings that are borderline between normal and pathologic. Even children may exhibit reflex dystrophic changes as well as migratory bone marrow edema. Studies vary considerably in their descriptions of symptomatology, severity, progression, correlations, and indications for treatment, and no standard recommendations have yet been established.

Definition

The “tiger-stripe” pattern describes a speckled, disseminated pattern of bone marrow edema that is found in children and predominantly affects the hindfoot and less commonly the tarsals.

Symptoms

- Diffuse pain of unknown cause
- Persistent pain after trauma
- Pattern may be detected incidentally in children without pain

Predisposing Factors

- Previous trauma
- Spontaneous

Anatomy and Pathology

Up until about the 15th year of life, it is normal to find hematopoietic bone marrow in the hindfoot (usually the calcaneus, occasionally the talus and navicular).

Imaging

Radiographs

Radiographs show no abnormalities.

Ultrasound

Not indicated.

MRI

Interpretation Checklist

- Try to classify the bone marrow edema
- Intensity
- Distribution pattern
- Predominantly subchondral
- Soft-tissue component

Examination Technique

MRI of the "tiger-stripe" pattern does not require contrast administration. Scan parameters are tailored to the location of the pain (hindfoot, midfoot, forefoot).

- *Standard protocol:* prone position, high-resolution multichannel coil
- *Sequences:*
  - Changes are best displayed by STIR and T1-weighted sequences
  - Hindfoot:
    - Sagittal STIR
    - Sagittal T1-weighted
    - Axial T2-weighted
    - Coronal PD-weighted fat-sat
  - Midfoot and forefoot:
    - Oblique coronal STIR
    - Oblique coronal T1-weighted
    - Oblique axial T2-weighted
    - Sagittal PD-weighted fat-sat

MRI Findings (▶ Fig. 8.7 and ▶ Fig. 8.8)

- Speckled pattern of bone marrow edema distributed diffusely in the talus and calcaneus (differentiate from hematopoietic bone marrow: the edematous foci show higher signal intensity in the STIR sequence and a broader distribution)
- Distinct foci of bone marrow edema in the navicular and subchondral regions: always suspicious
- Soft-tissue swelling
- Soft-tissue edema and effusion are rare

Imaging Recommendation

Modality of choice: MRI.

Differential Diagnosis

- Contusional edema
- Chronic recurring multifocal osteomyelitis

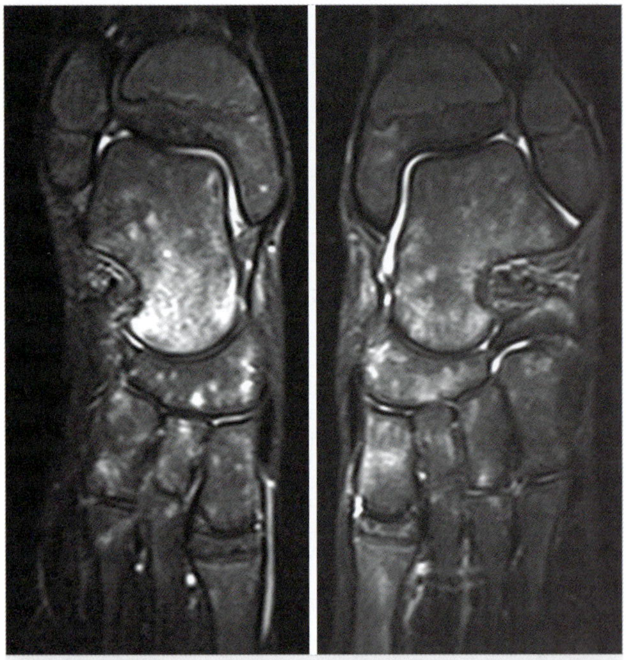

Fig. 8.7 Pediatric bone marrow edema with a "tiger-stripe" pattern in a 13-year-old girl. Coronal STIR images of both feet. The water-sensitive sequences show conspicuous speckled hyperintensities, with the most pronounced signal increase in the talar head. Since the patient was asymptomatic, the findings most likely represent growth processes that have no real pathologic significance.

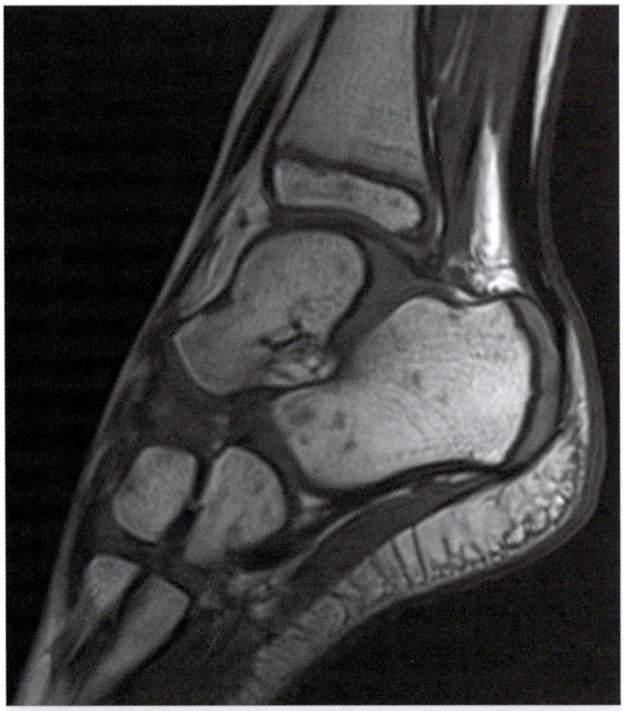

Fig. 8.8 Pediatric bone marrow edema ("tiger-stripe" pattern) in a 5-year-old girl with no clinical complaints (follow-up examination). Sagittal T1-weighted image shows scattered focal signal changes in the bone marrow that have no pathologic significance.

- Osteonecrosis
- Overuse edema
- Activated coalition

Treatment

- Immobilization (controversial)
- Symptomatic treatment for pain
- Physical therapy
- Temporary stress reduction

Prognosis, Complications

The prognosis varies according to etiology. Any outcome is possible, ranging from complete resolution to a chronic pain syndrome or a remitting and relapsing course.

8.6 Bibliography

Reflex Sympathetic Dystrophy, CRPS

Bohndorf K, Imhoff H, Fischer W. Radiologische Diagnostik der Knochen und Gelenke. 2nd ed. Stuttgart: Thieme; 2006: 26

Darbois H, Boyer B, Dubayle P, Lechevalier D, David H, Aït-Ameur A. MRI symptomology in reflex sympathetic dystrophy of the foot [Article in French] J Radiol 1999; 80: 849–854

Dihlmann W, Stäbler A. Gelenke des Fußes einschließlich des oberen Sprunggelenks. In: Dihlmann W, Stäbler A, eds. Gelenke – Wirbelverbindungen. 4th ed. Stuttgart: Thieme; 2010: 729

Mackey S, Feinberg S. Pharmacologic therapies for complex regional pain syndrome. Curr Pain Headache Rep 2007; 11: 38–43

Poll LW, Weber P, Böhm HJ, Ghassem-Zadeh N, Chantelau EA. Sudeck's disease stage 1, or diabetic Charcot's foot stage 0? Case report and assessment of the diagnostic value of MRI. Diabetol Metab Syndr 2010; 2: 60

Schmid MR, Hodler J, Vienne P, Binkert CA, Zanetti M. Bone marrow abnormalities of foot and ankle: STIR versus T1-weighted contrast-enhanced fat-suppressed spin-echo MR imaging. Radiology 2002; 224: 463–469

Schürmann M, Zaspel J, Löhr P et al. Imaging in early posttraumatic complex regional pain syndrome: a comparison of diagnostic methods. Clin J Pain 2007; 23: 449–457

Bone Marrow Edema Syndrome

Dihlmann W, Stäbler A. Gelenke des Fußes einschließlich des oberen Sprunggelenks. In: Dihlmann W, Stäbler A, eds. Gelenke – Wirbelverbindungen. 4th ed. Stuttgart: Thieme; 2010: 729

Fernandez-Canton G, Casado O, Capelastegui A, Astigarraga E, Larena JA, Merino A. Bone marrow edema syndrome of the foot: one year follow-up with MR imaging. Skeletal Radiol 2003; 32: 273–278

Hayes CW, Conway WF, Daniel WW. MR imaging of bone marrow edema pattern: transient osteoporosis, transient bone marrow edema syndrome, or osteonecrosis. Radiographics 1993; 13: 1001–1011, discussion 1012

Hofmann S, Engel A, Neuhold A, Leder K, Kramer J, Plenk H. Bone-marrow oedema syndrome and transient osteoporosis of the hip. An MRI-controlled study of treatment by core decompression. J Bone Joint Surg Br 1993; 75: 210–216

Judd DB, Kim DH, Hrutkay JM. Transient osteoporosis of the talus. Foot Ankle Int 2000; 21: 134–137

Kim YM, Oh HC, Kim HJ. The pattern of bone marrow oedema on MRI in osteonecrosis of the femoral head. J Bone Joint Surg Br 2000; 82: 837–841

Miltner O, Niedhart C, Piroth W, Weber M, Siebert CH. Transient osteoporosis of the navicular bone in a runner. Arch Orthop Trauma Surg 2003; 123: 505–508

Toms AP, Marshall TJ, Becker E, Donell ST, Lobo-Mueller EM, Barker T. Regional migratory osteoporosis: a review illustrated by five cases. Clin Radiol 2005; 60: 425–438

Wilson AJ, Murphy WA, Hardy DC, Totty WG. Transient osteoporosis: transient bone marrow edema? Radiology 1988; 167: 757–760

Overuse Edema

Elias I, Zoga AC, Raikin SM et al. Bone stress injury of the ankle in professional ballet dancers seen on MRI. BMC Musculoskelet Disord 2008; 9: 39

Niva MH, Sormaala MJ, Kiuru MJ, Haataja R, Ahovuo JA, Pihlajamaki HK. Bone stress injuries of the ankle and foot: an 86-month magnetic resonance imaging-based study of physically active young adults. Am J Sports Med 2007; 35: 643–649

Schweitzer ME, White LM. Does altered biomechanics cause marrow edema? Radiology 1996; 198: 851–853

Weishaupt D, Schweitzer ME. MR imaging of the foot and ankle: patterns of bone marrow signal abnormalities. Eur Radiol 2002; 12: 416–426

Zanetti M, Steiner CL, Seifert B, Hodler J. Clinical outcome of edema-like bone marrow abnormalities of the foot. Radiology 2002; 222: 184–188

Stress Fractures, Microfractures

Arni D, Lambert V, Delmi M, Bianchi S. Insufficiency fracture of the calcaneum: Sonographic findings. J Clin Ultrasound 2009; 37: 424–427

Banal F, Gandjbakhch F, Foltz V et al. Sensitivity and specificity of ultrasonography in early diagnosis of metatarsal bone stress fractures: a pilot study of 37 patients. J Rheumatol 2009; 36: 1715–1719

Boden BP, Osbahr DC. High-risk stress fractures: evaluation and treatment. J Am Acad Orthop Surg 2000; 8: 344–353

Brockwell J, Yeung Y, Griffith JF. Stress fractures of the foot and ankle. Sports Med Arthrosc 2009; 17: 149–159

Bui-Mansfield LT, Thomas WR. Magnetic resonance imaging of stress injury of the cuneiform bones in patients with plantar fasciitis. J Comput Assist Tomogr 2009; 33: 593–596

Chuckpaiwong B, Cook C, Pietrobon R, Nunley JA. Second metatarsal stress fracture in sport: comparative risk factors between proximal and non-proximal locations. Br J Sports Med 2007; 41: 510–514

Ekstrand J, Torstveit MK. Stress fractures in elite male football players. Scand J Med Sci Sports 2012; 22: 341–346

Gregg JM, Schneider T, Marks P. MR imaging and ultrasound of metatarsalgia—the lesser metatarsals. Radiol Clin North Am 2008; 46: 1061–1078, vi–vii

Hetsroni I, Nyska M, Ben-Sira D et al. Analysis of foot structure in athletes sustaining proximal fifth metatarsal stress fracture. Foot Ankle Int 2010; 31: 203–211

Mann JA, Pedowitz DI. Evaluation and treatment of navicular stress fractures, including nonunions, revision surgery, and persistent pain after treatment. Foot Ankle Clin 2009; 14: 187–204

Miller T, Kaeding CC, Flanigan D. The classification systems of stress fractures: a systematic review. Phys Sportsmed 2011; 39: 93–100

Muthukumar T, Butt SH, Cassar-Pullicino VN. Stress fractures and related disorders in foot and ankle: plain films, scintigraphy, CT, and MR Imaging. Semin Musculoskelet Radiol 2005; 9: 210–226

Orendurff MS, Rohr ES, Segal AD, Medley JW, Green JR, Kadel NJ. Biomechanical analysis of stresses to the fifth metatarsal bone during sports maneuvers: implications for fifth metatarsal fractures. Phys Sportsmed 2009; 37: 87–92

Rossi F, Dragoni S. Talar body fatigue stress fractures: three cases observed in elite female gymnasts. Skeletal Radiol 2005; 34: 389–394

Spitz DJ, Newberg AH. Imaging of stress fractures in the athlete. Radiol Clin North Am 2002; 40: 313–331

Yu JS, Solmen J. Stress fractures associated with plantar fascia disruption: two case reports involving the cuboid. J Comput Assist Tomogr 2001; 25: 971–974

Pediatric Bone Marrow Edema (Tiger-Stripe Pattern)

Kellenberger CJ, Epelman M, Miller SF, Babyn PS. Fast STIR whole-body MR imaging in children. Radiographics 2004; 24: 1317–1330

Kröger L, Arikoski P, Komulainen J, Seuri R, Kröger H. Transient bone marrow oedema in a child. Ann Rheum Dis 2004; 63: 1528–1529

Orr JD, Sabesan V, Major N, Nunley J. Painful bone marrow edema syndrome of the foot and ankle. Foot Ankle Int 2010; 31: 949–953

Shabshin N, Schweitzer ME, Morrison WB, Carrino JA, Keller MS, Grissom LE. High-signal T2 changes of the bone marrow of the foot and ankle in children: red marrow or traumatic changes? Pediatr Radiol 2006; 36: 670–676

Shabshin N, Schweitzer ME. Age dependent T2 changes of bone marrow in pediatric wrist MRI. Skeletal Radiol 2009; 38: 1163–1168

Zanetti M, Steiner CL, Seifert B, Hodler J. Clinical outcome of edema-like bone marrow abnormalities of the foot. Radiology 2002; 222: 184–188

Chapter 9

Systemic Diseases that Involve the Foot

9

9 Systemic Diseases that Involve the Foot

9.1 Inflammatory Joint Diseases

A. Roeser and A. Staebler

9.1.1 Rheumatoid Arthritis

Definition

Rheumatoid arthritis is a chronic inflammatory systemic disease in which the proliferation of inflammatory tissue leads to synovitis with joint effusions, tenosynovitis, and bursitis. The disease takes a progressive, episodic course characterized by the destruction of joints and tendons and the development of typical deformities. Extra-articular organ manifestations (in the eye, blood vessels, skin, nails, kidney, lung, heart, or nerves) may occur.

Symptoms

- ACR criteria (defined by the American College of Rheumatology)
- Joint swelling, effusion, angular deformity
- Tenosynovitis, tendon ruptures, development of secondary deformities
- Hindfoot: pes planovalgus, medioplantar callus below the talar head
- Forefoot: hallux valgus, varus fifth toe, bursitis of the distal first or fifth metatarsal, lateral deviation of the small toes, dorsal subluxation or dislocation of the small toes at the metatarsophalangeal joints, fixed hammer toe deformities, plantar calluses, ulcerations, loss of toe contact with the ground, pain on metatarsal compression (Gaenslen test)
- Differentiation from psoriatic arthritis: radial pattern of involvement

Predisposing Factors

- Affects 1 to 2% of the general population with a 3:1 female preponderance
- Positive family history
- Laboratory detection of anti-CCP antibodies (antibodies against cyclic citrullinated peptides) has a specificity of 96 to 98%

Anatomy and Pathology

Rheumatoid arthritis is the result of an autoimmune response whose precipitating factors are not yet fully understood.

Antigen presentation evokes the activation of T-helper cells (with a concomitant decrease in T-suppressor cell activity), and B-cells differentiate to immunoglobulin-producing plasma cells. This process culminates in the formation of autoantibodies that include rheumatoid factors.

Chronic synovitis (pannus tissue) incites a complement and cytokine activation (interleukin 1, lymphokines) which triggers the release of inflammatory mediators and collagenases. These in turn cause destructive changes in cartilage, tendons, tendon sheaths, ligaments, and joint capsules.

Imaging

Radiographs (▶ see Figs. 9.1–9.9)

- *Staging of radiographic joint destruction by the Larsen–Dale–Eek scale (1977):* LDE 0 through V, with reference tables for the forefoot, midfoot, and hindfoot
- *Weight-bearing radiographs of the foot in three planes:* to determine the extent of destruction and deformity
- *Weight-bearing radiographs of the ankle joint in two planes, Saltzman view:* to determine the extent of destruction and deformity

Ultrasound

What follows applies to all joints affected by arthritis: longitudinal and transverse ultrasound scans in exudative rheumatoid arthritis (as in activated osteoarthritis) will show a hypoechoic effusion and distended joint capsule early in the course of the disease. The synovial stripe below the echogenic fibrous capsule is thickened, may be hypoechoic to moderately echogenic, and shows a positive Doppler signal. Compression produces an "aquarium" effect due to the presence of floating villi and fibrotic elements. In chronic cases the fibrous joint capsule may appear increasingly echogenic while its contours become more irregular. In cases with a proliferative course, the synovium also becomes more echogenic, may show uneven thickening, and is poorly delineated from the joint capsule, especially when the process spreads to cartilage and bone. Bony changes consist of juxta-articular erosions, which may be associated with a positive power Doppler signal. Later in the course of the disease, echogenic osteophytes form due to secondary degenerative changes and the destruction of the echogenic articular surfaces.

The application and release of transducer pressure on a joint effusion yields information on its volume and viscosity and thus on its accessibility to needle aspiration. Differentiation from arthritis with an infectious cause cannot be reliably accomplished sonographically. Percutaneous joint injections and aspirations can be performed under ultrasound guidance, which may be very helpful in joints that are deeply situated or have undergone marked degenerative changes. Intra-articular injections can be monitored sonographically, helping to improve intraobserver reliability and patient compliance.

MRI

Interpretation Checklist

- Presence of synovitis
- Presence of solid, enhancing synovial proliferations
- Thinning of the articular cartilage
- Presence of bone defects or erosions
- Involvement pattern typical of rheumatoid arthritis

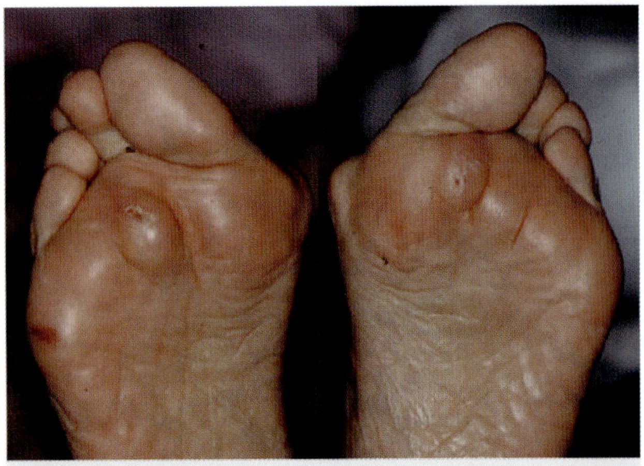

Fig. 9.1 Clinical appearance of forefoot deformity in rheumatoid arthritis.

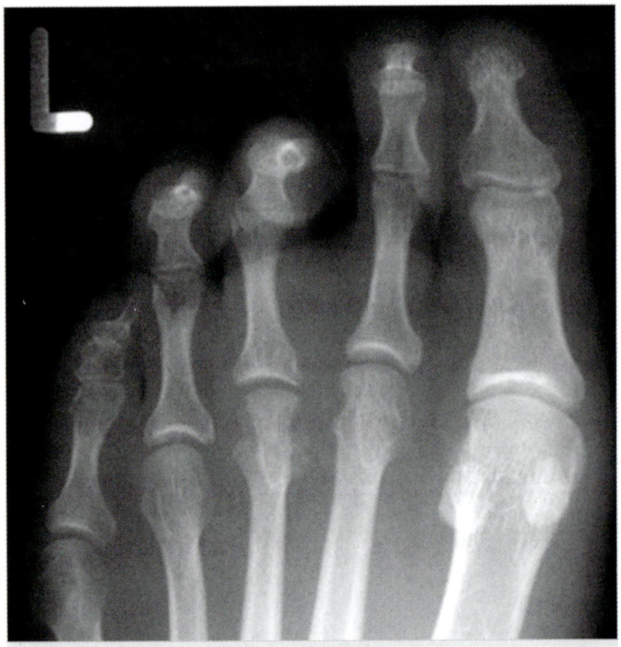

Fig. 9.2 Destruction of the second and third metatarsophalangeal joints in LDE stage II disease (Larsen–Dale–Eek scale). This is an indication for joint-preserving treatment: synovectomy with distal corrective osteotomies of the second and third metatarsals.

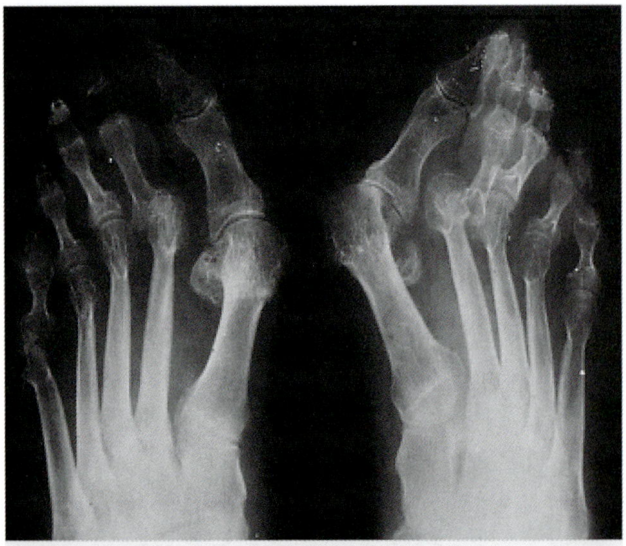

Fig. 9.3 Rheumatoid forefoot deformity with advanced destructive changes in LDE stage IV disease. This is an indication for resection arthroplasty of the first through fifth metatarsophalangeal joints.

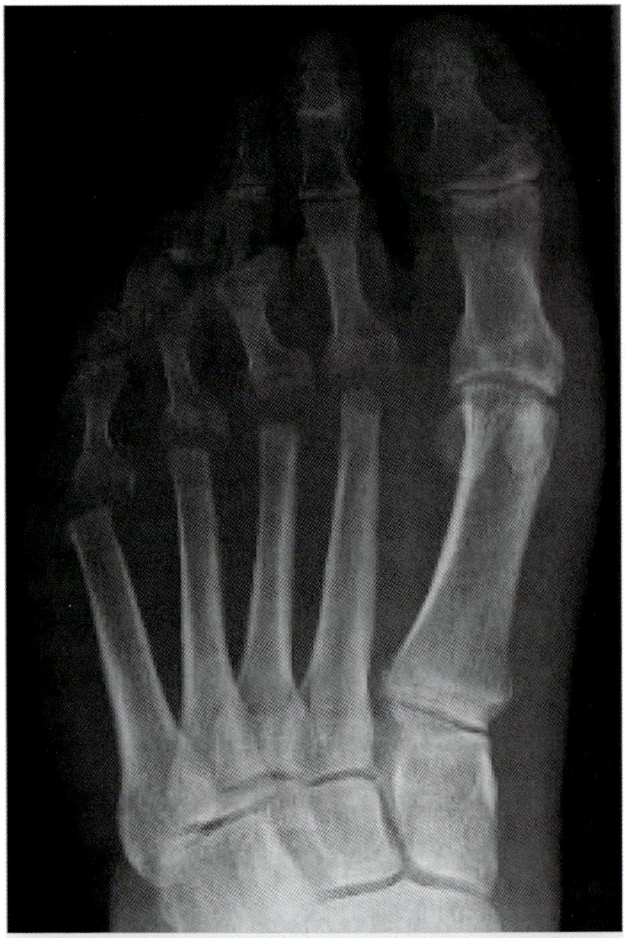

Fig. 9.4 Rheumatoid forefoot deformity. Appearance following resection arthroplasty of the first through fifth metatarsophalangeal joints.

Examination Technique

Sequences for evaluating the hindfoot, for example:

- Coronal T2-weighted and PD-weighted fat-sat
- Sagittal PD-weighted fat-sat
- Axial T2-weighted
- Sagittal and axial T1-weighted fat-sat after IV contrast administration

The axial postcontrast images should be angled perpendicular to the course of the tendon. Scanning the foot in the prone position tends to straighten out the hindfoot tendons. Synovial proliferation and pannus tissue are most clearly depicted in fat-suppressed sequences after contrast administration.

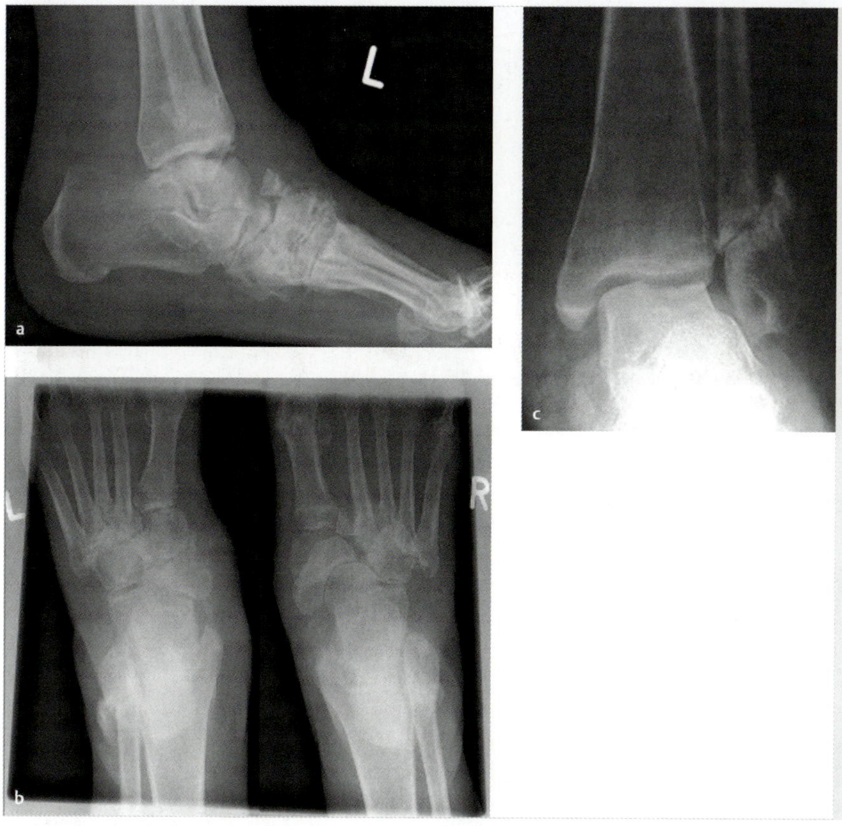

Fig. 9.5 a–c Destruction of the ankle joint, subtalar joint, and Lisfranc joint line in LDE stage IV disease. There is an associated pathologic fracture of the fibula. This is an indication for a reorienting hindfoot and Lisfranc arthrodesis.
a Lateral projection: instability in the Chopart joint.
b DP projection: medial dislocation of the navicular.
c DP view of the ankle joint: defect in the lateral talus and an insufficiency fracture of the fibula.

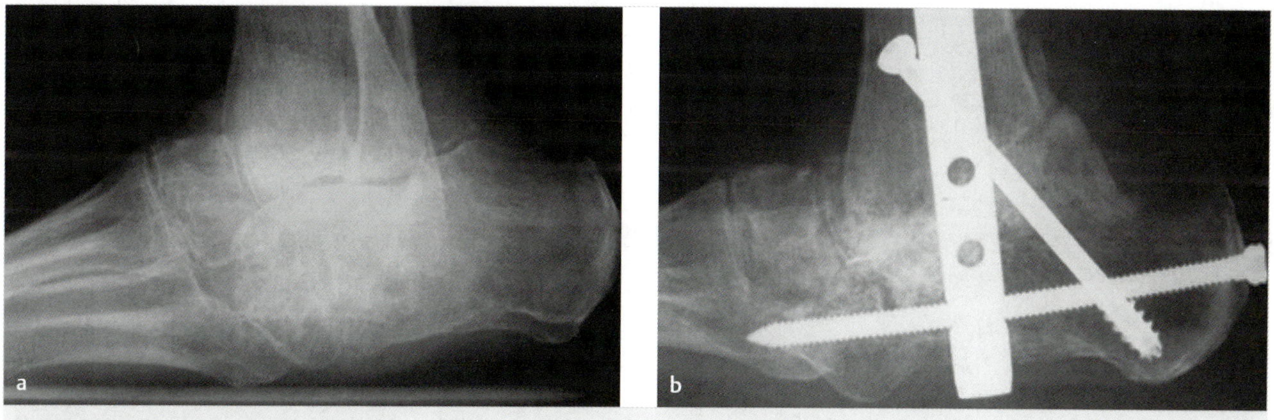

Fig. 9.6 a, b Rheumatoid hindfoot deformity.
a Subtalar dislocation.
b Plantar arthrodesis by retrograde nail insertion.

MRI Findings (▶ Fig. 9.10, ▶ Fig. 9.11, ▶ Fig. 9.12)

Rheumatoid synovitis leads to joint effusion and contrast enhancement in areas of synovial proliferation. The inflammatory pannus is hyperintense on water-sensitive sequences acquired in the acute inflammatory stage, but it appears less intense when fibrotic elements have formed in more protracted cases. If inflammatory pannus invades the bone, it displaces the hyperintense fatty marrow signal, and the erosions have low signal intensity in T1-weighted images. Articular cartilage undergoes a uniform, concentric thinning.

In the hindfoot, the talonavicular joint is particularly affected by rheumatoid arthritis (▶ Fig. 9.10). Joint space narrowing occurs without significant osteophytosis, and numerous signal cysts and erosions are found. With passage of time, secondary degenerative changes become superimposed upon the arthritic findings.

Synovitis in a tendon sheath leads to effusion in the sheath with peripheral enhancement. Solid proliferative foci show intense contrast uptake. T1-weighted fat-saturated images after contrast administration are also best for evaluating the tarsometatarsal (Lisfranc) and metatarsophalangeal joints based on the enhancement findings.

Imaging Recommendation

Modalities of choice: radiography and ultrasonography. Preoperative contrast-enhanced MRI can be used before synovectomy

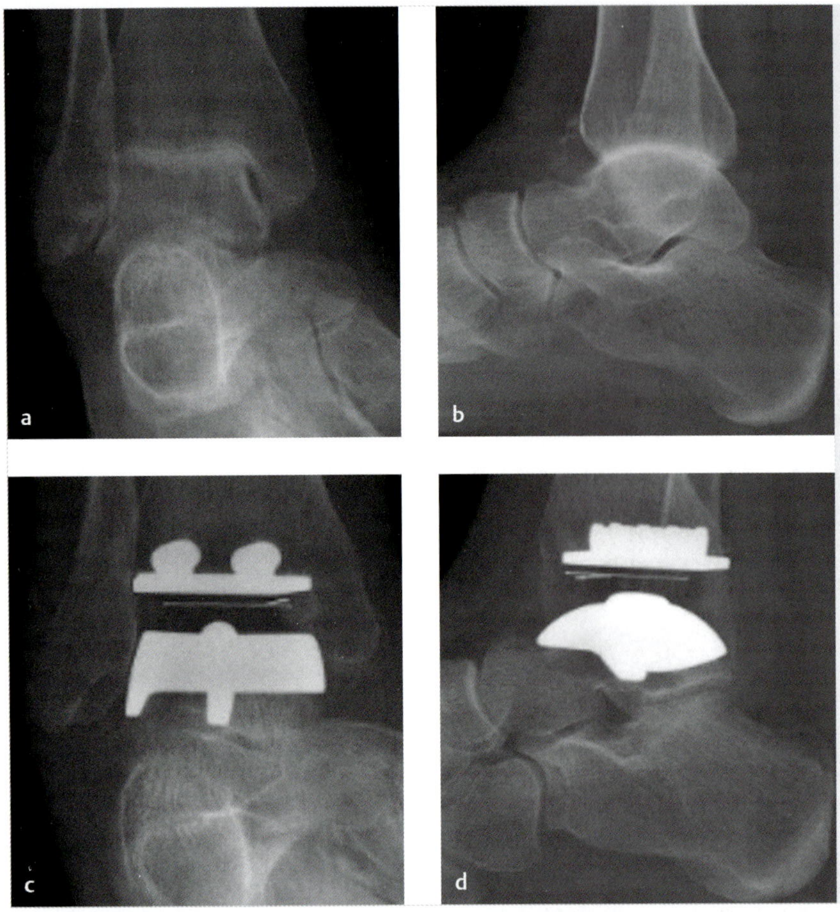

Fig. 9.7 a–d Postarthritic osteoarthritis of the ankle joint with LDE stage IV disease, treated by total ankle replacement.
a AP radiograph of the ankle joint: LDE stage IV with an obliterated joint space.
b Lateral radiograph of the ankle in **a**.
c AP radiograph after implantation of a STAR™ total ankle replacement.
d Lateral view of the ankle in **c**.

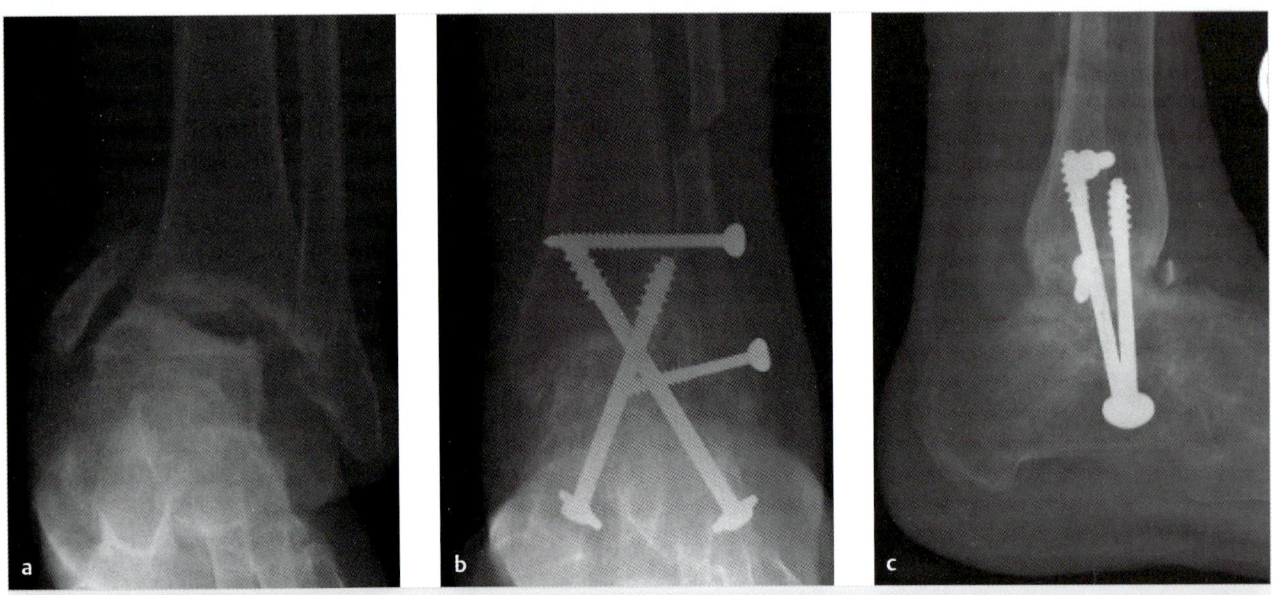

Fig. 9.8 a–c Postarthritic osteoarthritis of the ankle joint with LDE stage IV disease. Total ankle replacement is contraindicated in this case, which was managed by arthrodesis.
a AP radiograph of the ankle joint: postarthritic osteoarthritis (LDE stage IV).
b AP radiograph of the ankle joint after arthrodesis of the ankle and subtalar joints.
c Lateral radiograph of the ankle in **b**. The midtarsal joint is also obliterated.

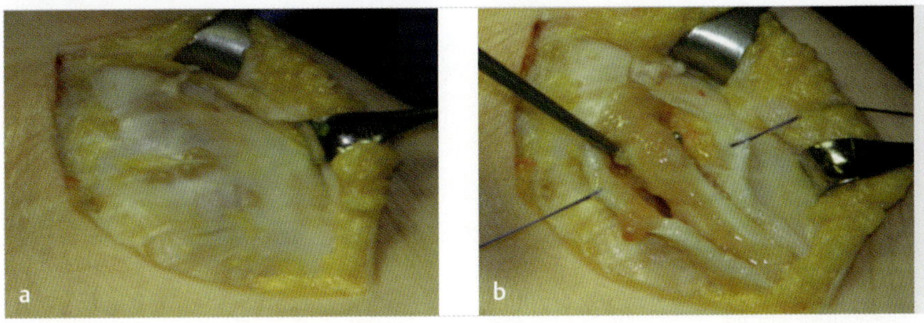

Fig. 9.9 a, b Intraoperative appearance of tenosynovitis of the posterior tibial and flexor digitorum longus tendons.
a The tendon sheath appears swollen due to extensive tenosynovitis.
b The tendon sheath is opened to expose the tenosynovitis surrounding the posterior tibial and flexor digitorum longus tendons.

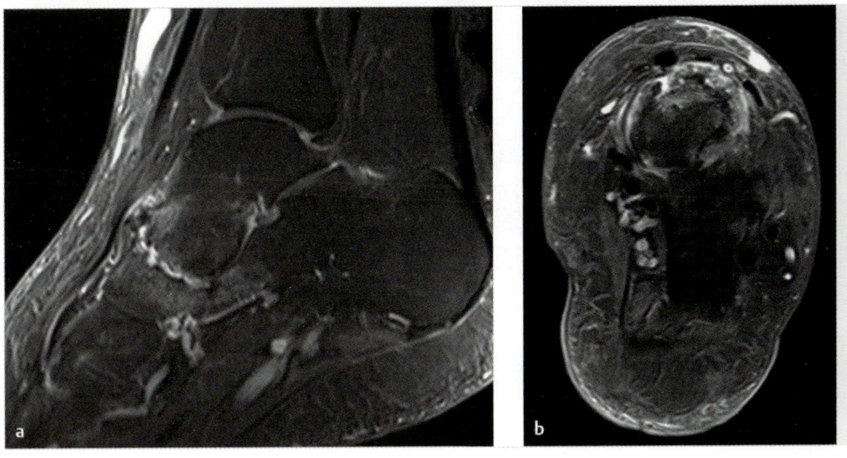

Fig. 9.10 a, b Typical imaging features of rheumatoid arthritis with talonavicular joint involvement in a 69-year-old woman.
a Sagittal T1-weighted fat-sat image after contrast administration shows advanced arthritic destruction of the talonavicular joint with slight concomitant involvement of the rest of the subtalar joint. Joint-space narrowing is present without significant osteophytosis. Numerous erosions are visible.
b Axial oblique T1-weighted fat-sat image after contrast administration shows rheumatoid synovitis with joint effusion and marked enhancement in areas of synovial proliferation.

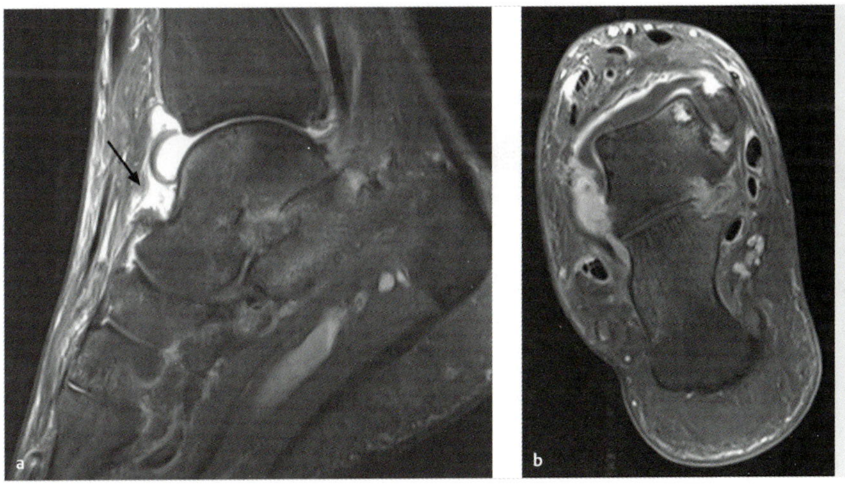

Fig. 9.11 a, b Rheumatoid synovitis in the ankle joint of a 65-year-old man with known rheumatoid arthritis.
a Sagittal T1-weighted fat-sat image after contrast administration shows severe thinning of the hyaline articular cartilage in the ankle joint. Postcontrast image shows intense enhancement of inflammatory pannus tissue (arrow). Also typical are the faint patches of bone marrow edema with associated areas of enhancement.
b Axial T1-weighted fat-sat image after contrast administration demonstrates effusion, peripheral sites of synovial proliferation, and the inflammatory pannus tissue, most pronounced on the lateral side.

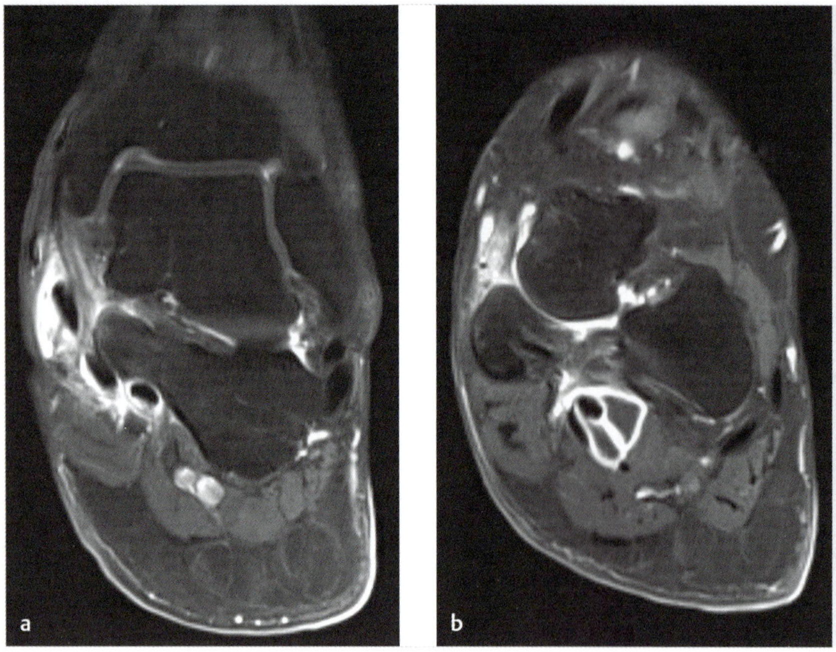

Fig. 9.12 a, b Rheumatoid arthritis with involvement of the tendon sheaths.
a Coronal T1-weighted fat-sat image after contrast administration shows synovitis in a tendon sheath with intensely enhancing solid proliferative foci.
b Coronal T1-weighted fat-sat image after contrast administration (more distal level) shows synovitic enhancement at the periphery of the flexor hallucis longus and flexor digitorum longus tendon sheaths. As a general rule, effusion in the flexor hallucis longus tendon sheath is not pathologic, whereas peripheral contrast enhancement is an abnormal finding.

for the accurate assessment and localization of synovial proliferation.

Differential Diagnosis

Activated osteoarthritis, reactive forms of arthritis, gouty and infectious arthritis:

- Detection of antinuclear antibodies: connective tissue diseases
- Human leukocyte antigen (HLA)-B27: ankylosing spondylitis
- Reactive arthritis (*Chlamydia*, *Yersinia*, *Shigella*, or *Borrelia* species), Reiter disease
- Crystal arthropathies (calcium pyrophosphate)
- Uric arthritis (gout)
- Hemochromatosis, ochronosis
- Activated osteoarthritis, polyarthrosis
- Suppurative arthritis (determination of microbial etiology, generally confined to one joint)

Treatment

Rheumatoid arthritis is managed by a combination of systemic medications, orthopedic therapies, and preventive measures (therapeutic exercises, orthopedic footwear, ergotherapy).

Conservative

- Insoles
- Custom-made shoes
- Therapeutic exercises

Operative

With involvement and deformity of multiple joints in the lower limb, the problems are addressed in a proximal-to-distal fashion. Treatment measures are classified as preventive or reconstructive.

Preventive

Disease-modifying antirheumatic drugs (DMARDs) are used to moderate the course of the disease and slow the progression of degenerative changes. Often, however, radiologic joint erosions are still observed in the early stages of the disease (< 2 years after initial diagnosis). Poor pharmacologic reduction of inflammatory activity with persistent synovitis or tenosynovitis for 3 to 6 months after the start of DMARD therapy or the presence of LDE stage 0–II or III radiologic changes is an indication for early synovectomy or early tenosynovectomy (open or arthroscopic). Radiosynoviorthesis is recommended for 6 to 8 weeks postoperatively. A late synovectomy can be performed by open or arthroscopic technique, again followed by radiosynoviorthesis for 6 to 8 weeks.

Reconstructive

- *Goal:* stable, plantigrade ground contact of the foot during gait
- *Treatments recommended for specific affected joints:*
  - Resection arthroplasty: first through fifth metatarsophalangeal joints (Hoffmann/Tillmann or Lelievre technique)
  - Arthrodesis: ankle and subtalar joints, tarsus, proximal and distal interphalangeal joints, first metatarsophalangeal joint
  - Arthroplasty: first metatarsophalangeal joint, ankle joint
- *Treatments recommended for specific LDE stages:*
  - Ankle joint:
    - LDE 0–II/III: synovectomy
    - LDE III–V: arthrodesis or arthroplasty (third generation, cementless)
  - Subtalar joint:
    - LDE 0–II: prescription footwear
    - LDE III–V: reorienting arthrodesis appropriate for the involvement and deformity (isolated talonavicular or subtalar, double talonavicular and subtalar, triple talonavicular, subtalar and calcaneocuboid)

- Tarsometatarsal (Lisfranc) joint line:
  - LDE III–V: arthrodesis
  - LDE 0–II: prescription footwear
- Metatarsophalangeal joints, LDE 0–III:
  - First through fifth metatarsophalangeal joints: synovectomy
  - First metatarsal: joint-preserving hallux valgus correction (distal, diaphyseal, proximal osteotomy; for instability in the first tarsometatarsal joint: Lapidus procedure)
  - Second through fifth metatarsals: distal corrective osteotomy for subluxation or metatarsalgia
  - Fifth metatarsal: correction of varus fifth toe deformity by distal, diaphyseal or proximal osteotomy
- Metatarsophalangeal joints, LDE IV and V:
  - Second through fifth or first through fifth metatarsals: resection arthroplasty
  - First metatarsophalangeal joint: arthrodesis or arthroplasty (silicone stent)
- Proximal and distal interphalangeal joints:
  - LDE III–V: resection arthroplasty or arthrodesis
  - LDE 0–II: prescription footwear, synovectomy

- *Treatments recommended for different grades of pes planovalgus:*
  - Grade IV pes planovalgus with destruction of the ankle and subtalar joints: plantar arthrodesis (nail)
  - Grade III pes planovalgus with destruction of the subtalar joint: double arthrodesis
  - Grade II pes planovalgus: joint-preserving hindfoot correction by a calcaneal sliding osteotomy, combined if necessary with a lateral lengthening osteotomy and flexor digitorum longus transfer
  - Grade I pes planovalgus: tenosynovectomy of the posterior tibial tendon, combined if necessary with a medial slide calcaneal osteotomy
- *Forefoot:* combination of tendon lengthening or transposition, temporary K-wire soft-tissue splinting or transfixation

Prognosis, Complications

DMARDs should be withheld perioperatively to avoid wound-healing problems and infection. Other risks are nonunion, secondary dislocation due to osteoporosis from prolonged corticosteroid use, and immobility. Prescription footwear is usually essential after surgery.

Rheumatoid arthritis cannot be cured. The goals are to make an early diagnosis and achieve a partial remission (ACR-20, ACR-50, ACR-70 response criteria). Partial remission means at least a 20% improvement in designated parameters such as the number of swollen or painful joints and the reduction of acute phase parameters (e.g., C-reactive protein). A partial remission can be achieved only through complex management of the systemic disease, preferably at a specialized rheumatoid center or unit.

9.1.2 Seronegative Spondylarthropathies

Definition

A seronegative spondylarthropathy is a chronic inflammatory joint disease with a negative serologic status.

Approximately 20% of chronic inflammatory joint diseases have seronegative laboratory findings, that is, rheumatoid factors are absent, the histocompatibility antigen HLA-B27 is often positive, and a genetic disposition is found. Seronegative spondylarthropathies usually take a more benign course than seropositive arthritis. The group of seronegative spondylarthropathies includes the following disorders:

- Ankylosing spondylitis with peripheral joint involvement
- Psoriatic arthritis with or without cutaneous manifestations
- Reactive arthritides (special form is Reiter disease characterized by enteritis, urethritis, conjunctivitis, and arthritis)
- Enteropathic arthritides (in Crohn disease and ulcerative colitis)
- Juvenile oligoarthritis type 2
- Undifferentiated spondylarthropathies

Symptoms

- *Ankylosing spondylitis:* chronic heel pain consistent with an enthesopathy. In adolescents, monoarthritis of the ankle joint may signal the arthritic precursor of ankylosing spondylitis.
- *Psoriasis:*
  - Skin changes in the form of psoriasis vulgaris:
    - Dry, red skin lesions with well-defined margins, most common on the extensor surfaces of the elbow and knee
    - Scalp
  - Nail changes:
    - White stippling
    - Transverse ridges
    - Thickening
  - Joints:
    - Radial pattern of involvement; involvement is not symmetrical as in rheumatoid arthritis
    - Sausage toe: involvement of the distal and proximal interphalangeal joints and metatarsophalangeal joint with soft-tissue swelling and redness
    - Transverse involvement of all distal interphalangeal joints with no changes in the proximal interphalangeal and metatarsophalangeal joints
    - Firm swelling of the joint capsule (vs. soft, doughy swelling in rheumatoid arthritis)
    - Insertional tendinopathy on the calcaneus

Predisposing Factors

- *Ankylosing spondylitis:*
  - Male predominance
  - Positive family history
  - HLA-B27 association
- *Psoriasis:*
  - 6 to 39% of all patients have psoriasis vulgaris
  - 20% of all seronegative polyarthritides
  - Detection of HLA-B13 or HLA-B17

Anatomy and Pathology

- *Ankylosing spondylitis:* Changes mainly affect the sacroiliac joints and spinal column; destructive peripheral joint involvement at the end stage of the disease most commonly affects the hip and knee, with possible involvement of the ankle joint. Fibro-osseous junction involvement (enthesitis) is typically present.

- *Psoriasis:* chronic inflammatory joint disease, generally coexisting with psoriasis vulgaris. Bony excrescences and proliferative tissue formation are often present in addition to destructive joint changes. There may be preexisting seronegative polyarthritis; involvement of the sacroiliac joints and spinal column is also possible. A cytokine, TNF-α (tumor necrosis factor), and activated T-cells have a special role in the pathogenesis of psoriasis, which is marked by a mixed pattern of destructive joint changes (erosions) and proliferative changes (protuberances). Possible forms:
  - Predominant involvement of the interphalangeal joints and nails
  - Severe joint destruction with ankylosis or mutilating changes
  - Symmetrical polyarthritis resembling rheumatoid arthritis; benign course
  - Mono- or oligoarthritis
  - Involvement of the spinal column (psoriatic spondyloarthritis)
- Psoriasis in the foot most commonly affects the hindfoot, especially the Achilles bursa, the Achilles tendon attachments, plantar fascia, and the Achilles tendon itself. The great majority of asymptomatic psoriasis patients show involvement of the hindfoot on MRI.

Imaging (▶ see Figs. 9.13–9.21)

Radiographs

A hallmark of the seronegative spondylarthropathies is new bone formation with associated sclerosis. Calcifications and ossifications are found close to tendon insertions on the calcaneus. But there are also characteristic erosions extending, for example, from the Achilles bursa into the upper part of the calcaneal tuberosity. While ankylosing spondylitis is typically manifested in the distal part of the Achilles tendon, psoriatic

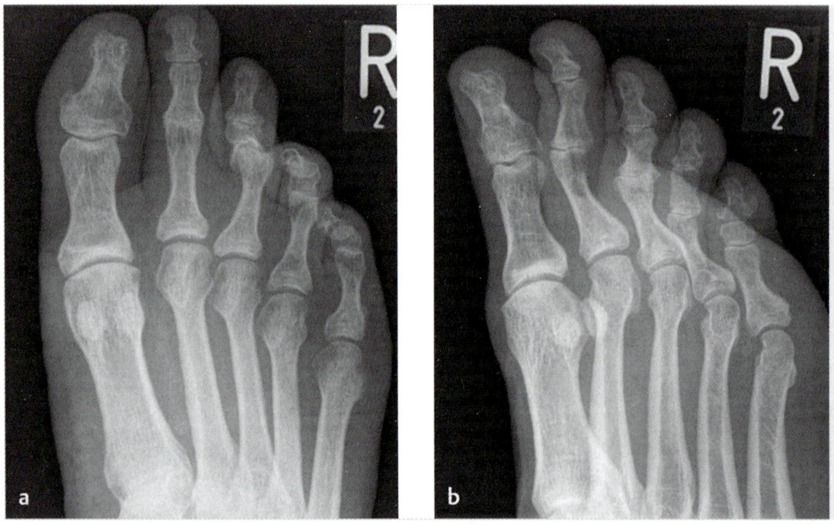

Fig. 9.13 a, b Boutonniere deformity of the third phalanx and postarthritic osteoarthritis of the second proximal interphalangeal joint. Films show an abnormal soft-tissue shadow and protuberances on the distal phalanges of the fourth and fifth toes.
a DP projection.
b Oblique projection.

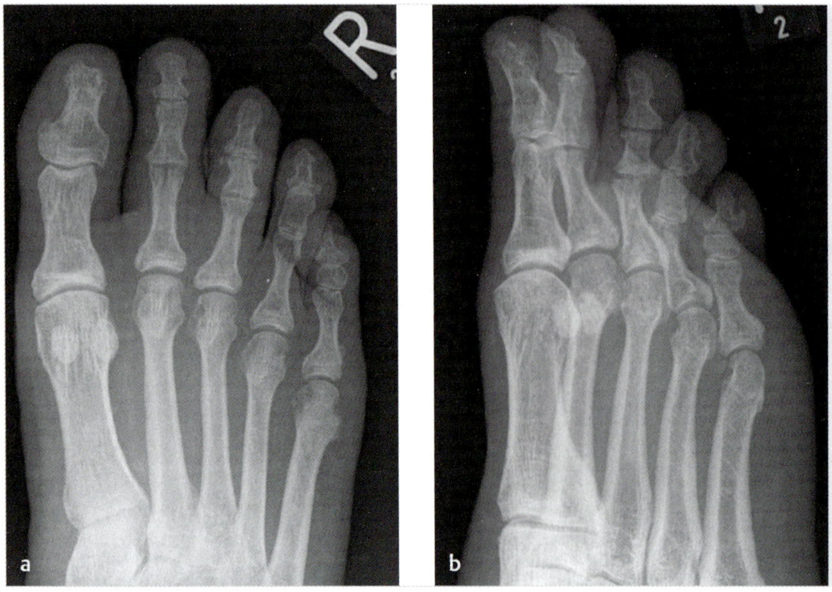

Fig. 9.14 a, b Same case as in Fig. 9.13, following treatment by resection arthroplasty of the second and third proximal interphalangeal joints and the third distal interphalangeal joint.
a DP projection.
b Oblique projection.

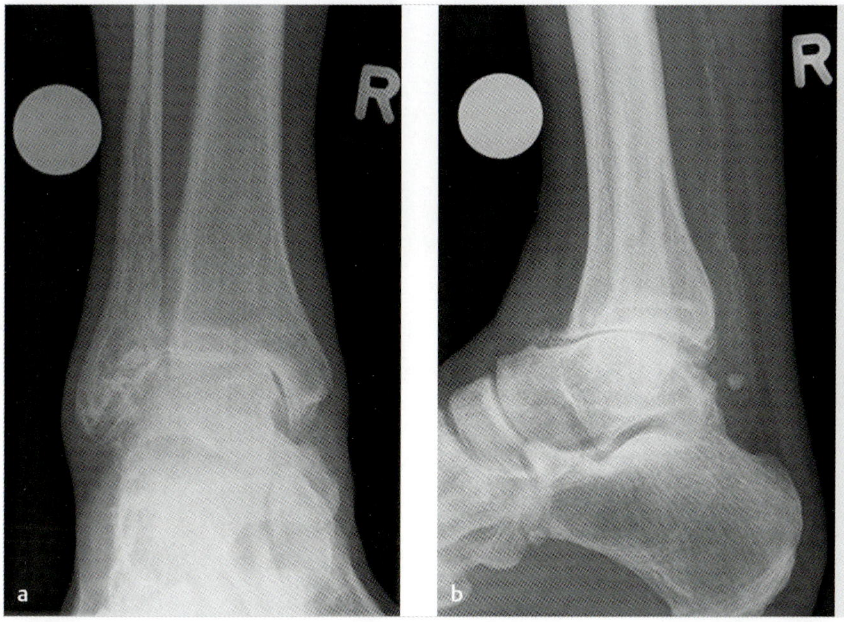

Fig. 9.15 a, b Postarthritic psoriatic arthropathy of the ankle joint.
a AP projection.
b Lateral projection.

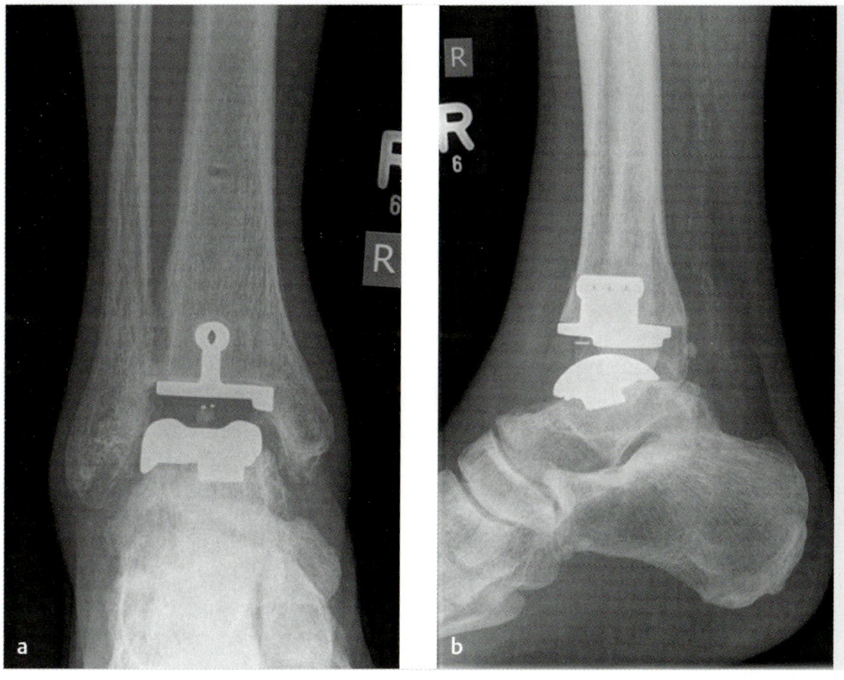

Fig. 9.16 a, b Postarthritic psoriatic arthropathy of the ankle joint, managed by total ankle replacement.
a AP projection.
b Lateral projection.

arthritis more commonly affects the metatarsophalangeal and interphalangeal joints.

Psoriasis has the following radiographic features:

- Forefoot: radial or transverse pattern of involvement
- Coexistence of erosions and protuberances
- Pencil-in-cup deformity
- Rarely, juxta-articular osteoporosis

Ultrasound

Sites of predilection are the small joints of the fingers and toes, but the sternoclavicular and knee joints may also be involved. Ultrasound scanning displays a mixed pattern of proliferative and destructive changes.

MRI

Interpretation Checklist

- Presence of arthritic bone edema
- Intact articular cartilage and articular pillar
- Presence of a soft-tissue reaction with thickening and edema

Examination Technique

Water-sensitive sequences are important for demonstrating soft-tissue changes. Contrast administration is helpful for detecting synovitis, bursitis, and possible enthesitis.

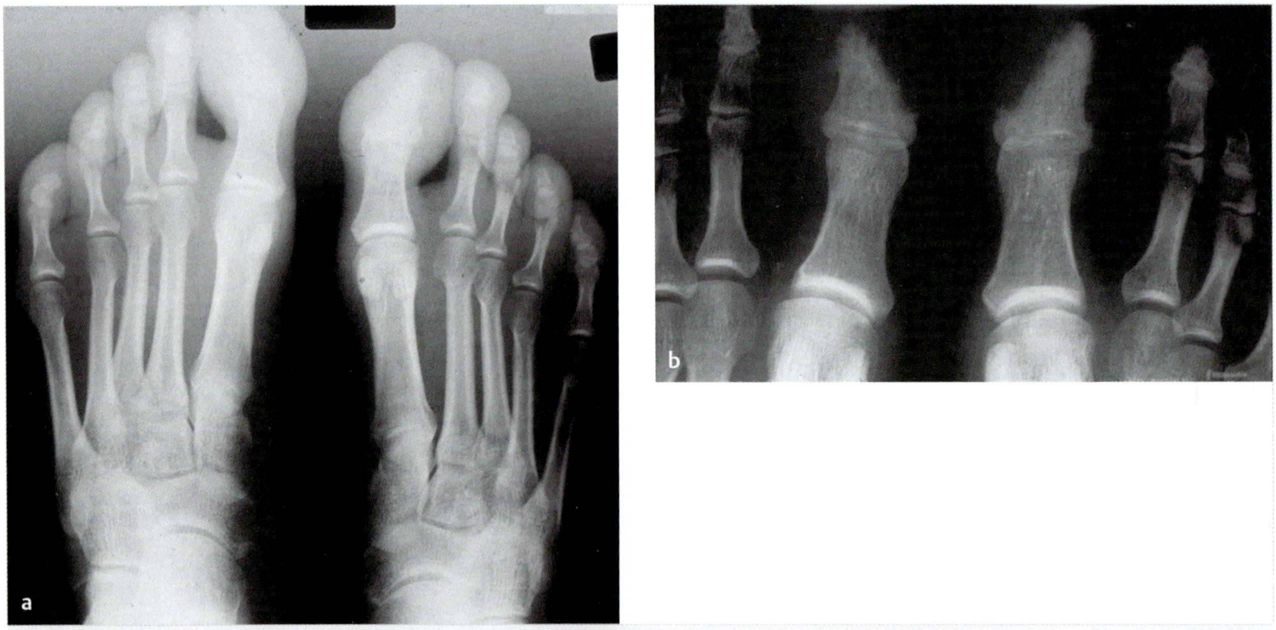

Fig. 9.17 a, b Psoriatic arthropathy with involvement of the big toes.
a DP radiographs of the both forefeet show conspicuous soft-tissue swelling of both big toes, which is typical of psoriatic arthropathy (sausage toes).
b Bony erosions are visible in the medial surface of the distal phalanges of the big toes.

MRI Findings

While bone edema is rarely found in rheumatoid arthritis, it is a characteristic feature of psoriatic arthritis. Moreover, as in the fingers, soft-tissue swelling along the ray creates a "sausage toe" appearance. Seronegative spondylarthropathies are typically manifested by Achilles tendon enthesopathy with Achilles bursitis and possible erosive or proliferative bone changes.

Imaging Recommendation

Modalities of choice: radiography, ultrasonography, scintigraphy, MRI.

Differential Diagnosis

- Heel pain: dorsal heel spur, chronic Achilles tendinopathy, plantar fasciitis, plantar heel spur
- Seropositive rheumatoid arthritis

Any disease from the group of seronegative spondylarthropathies may present similar radiographic features.

Treatment

- *Ankylosing spondylitis:*
  - DMARDs
  - Physical therapy and exercises to preserve motion
  - Rare cases may require synovectomy of joints in the foot and ankle
- *Psoriasis:*
  - DMARDs
  - Distal and proximal interphalangeal joints: arthrodesis or resection arthroplasty combined with synovectomy
  - Tarsometatarsal joints or subtalar joint: arthrodesis
  - Ankle joint: arthrodesis or arthroplasty
  - Conservative: prescription footwear, insoles
  - Concomitant treatment of skin and nail changes

Prognosis, Complications

- *Ankylosing spondylitis:* limitation of spinal motion and impaired respiratory function are limiting factors in ankylosing spondylitis, hence the goals are early diagnosis and partial remission.
- *Psoriasis:* usually takes a slowly progressive course, as opposed to the relapsing and remitting course of rheumatoid arthritis. The goal is early diagnosis and treatment to prevent advanced destructive joint changes. A partial remission is evaluated on the basis of psoriatic arthritis response criteria. DMARDs should be withheld perioperatively to avoid wound-healing problems, infection, nonunion, secondary dislocation due to osteoporosis from long-term corticosteroid use, and immobility.

9.2 Gouty Arthropathy

A. Staebler

Definition

Gouty arthropathy is marked by the deposition of uric acid crystals causing joint inflammation that may progress to cartilage destruction and osteoarthritis.

Gout is a disease of purine metabolism characterized by elevated uric acid levels in the blood (hyperuricemia), which are increased to >6.5 mg/dL. Deposition of uric acid crystals occurs in bradytrophic tissues, most notably the capsules and ligaments, cartilage, bursae, and tendons. The term "gouty

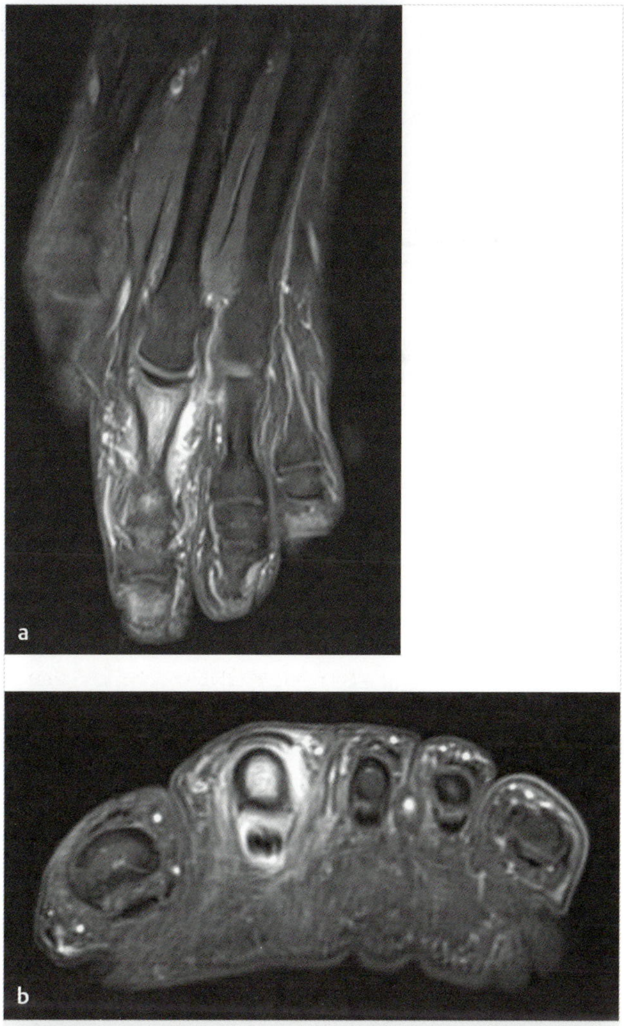

Fig. 9.18 **a, b Soft-tissue involvement of the second toe in psoriatic arthropathy.**
a Coronal T1-weighted fat-sat image after contrast administration shows enhancing soft tissue with bone marrow edema, which is typical of psoriasis. Most enhancement is concentrated in the proximal phalanx of the second toe.
b Axial T1-weighted fat-sat image after contrast administration shows synovitis with involvement of the flexor tendon sheath.

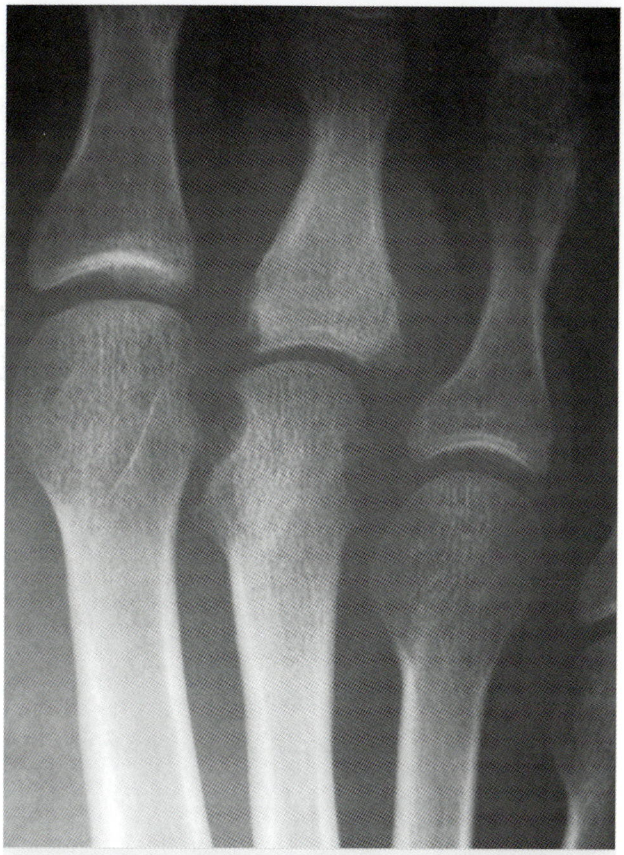

Fig. 9.19 **DP radiograph of the forefoot in psoriatic arthropathy demonstrates typical marginal bone erosions in the metatarsal head.** Patchy areas of increased sclerosis are indicative of chronic bone marrow edema.

arthritis" or "uric arthritis" reflects the articular involvement by the disease. Gout is classified among the crystal arthropathies along with hydroxyapatite and calcium pyrophosphate dihydrate crystal deposition disease.

Symptoms

An elevated uric acid level does not necessarily lead to symptoms (asymptomatic phase). Gout generally becomes symptomatic in the form of an acute attack, most commonly affecting the first metatarsophalangeal joint (podagra). Other joints in the foot, including the ankle joint, may also be involved. The joint is reddened, swollen, and extremely painful and tender. Besides an elevated uric acid level, laboratory tests show an elevated white blood count and erythrocyte sedimentation rate. The patient may remain asymptomatic for years following a gout attack. Chronic gout that goes untreated may eventually lead to renal damage and the formation of gouty tophi, which form just beneath the skin and may erupt, discharging a chalky mass of uric acid crystals.

Predisposing Factors

- Males predominate by 20:1
- Affects 1 to 2% of men 40 to 60 years of age in affluent regions
- Consumption of large amounts of alcohol, meats, and purine-rich foods

Anatomy and Pathology

Gout is classified as primary or secondary, with primary congenital gout accounting for < 1% of cases. Diagnosis is based on laboratory findings; a single uric acid level within normal limits does not exclude gout. It is diagnosed from radiographic findings and, if necessary, by the direct detection of urate crystals in joint aspirate.

Imaging

Radiographs (▶ Fig. 9.22)

Radiographs in an acute gout attack are normal. With chronic gout, the calcium urate crystal deposits lead to the formation of gouty tophi, which appear as soft-tissue opacities. The joint

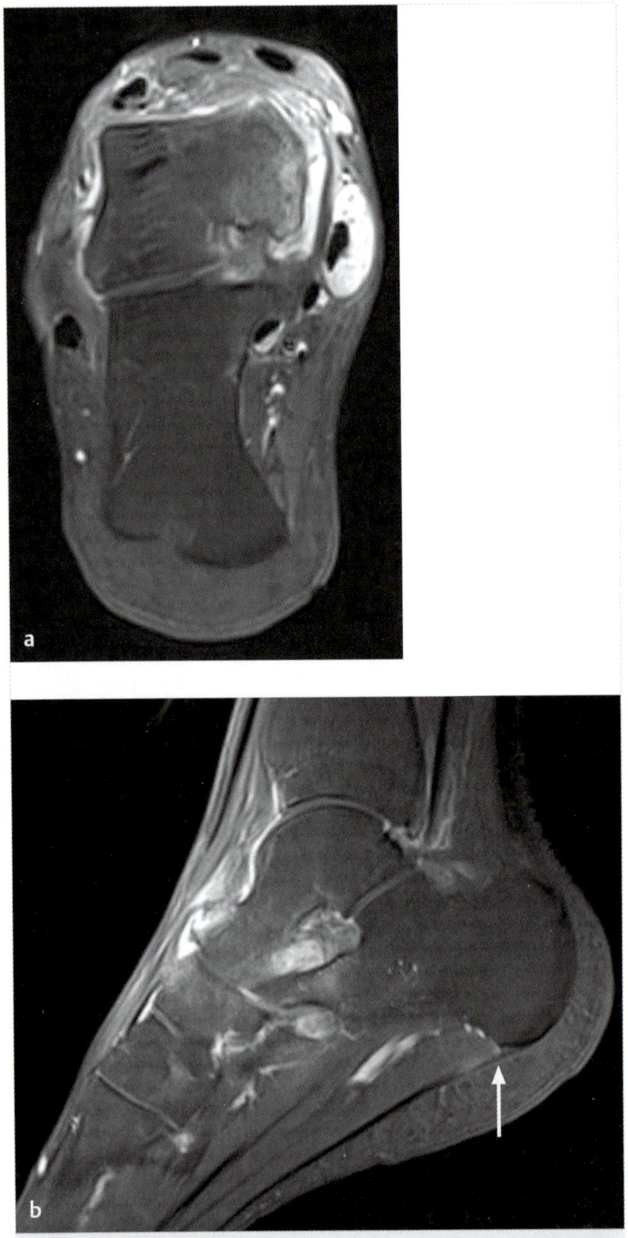

Fig. 9.20 a, b Seronegative spondylarthropathy with tendon involvement in a 40-year-old woman.
a Axial oblique T1-weighted fat-sat image after contrast administration shows pronounced synovitic enhancement
b Sagittal T1-weighted fat-sat image shows features of talonavicular arthritis with loss of articular cartilage, inflammatory pannus formation, and typical faint bone marrow edema in the talar head, navicular, and anterior calcaneal process. Mild enthesopathy of the plantar aponeurosis (arrow) is also seen. Enthesopathies affecting the Achilles tendon or plantar fascia, for example, are typical of seronegative spondylarthropathies and help to distinguish them from rheumatoid arthritis.

space in gout remains relatively normal for some time, with principal changes consisting of submarginal erosions and osteolytic foci. Osteolysis may incite local bone proliferation leading to a sharp spicule. Typical findings are tophaceous spicules, overhanging bone margins, mutilating joint changes, and punched-out defects.

Ultrasound

With involvement of the ankle joint, first metatarsophalangeal joint, or knee joint, which are the most commonly affected sites, a longitudinal scan over the anterior side of the joint will show a hypoechoic mass with bulging of the joint capsule and a possible hypoechoic synovial rim that has a positive power Doppler signal.

CT

CT can demonstrate osteolytic lesions and calcium urate deposits (tophi). The deposits have a mean attenuation value of approximately 160 HU (Hounsfield units). Threshold-based 3D renderings of CT data can provide detailed views of the deposits.

MRI

Interpretation Checklist

- Presence of gout
- Synovitis only, or presence of tophus-related tissue
- Bone erosion or destruction
- Joint still intact?

Examination Technique

With involvement of the first metatarsophalangeal joint, for example, the forefoot is imaged with a high-resolution multichannel coil using the following sequences:

- Coronal T1-weighted and PD-weighted fat-sat
- Sagittal PD-weighted fat-sat
- Axial T1-weighted
- Axial and coronal T1-weighted fat-sat after IV contrast administration
- If necessary, coronal susceptibility-sensitive gradient echo sequence

MRI Findings (▶ Fig. 9.23)

Acute gout has nonspecific findings with an inflammatory soft-tissue response showing increased signal intensity in water-sensitive sequences and increased enhancement in the periarticular soft tissues and associated synovitis. Tophaceous gout with urate crystal deposits in the tissue (gouty tophus) is isointense to soft tissue in T1-weighted sequences. Signal intensity on water-sensitive sequences is variable and ranges from hypointensity with heavy calcium deposits to hyperintensity. Postcontrast images show inhomogeneous, circumscribed, markedly increased signal intensity, with calcified areas showing low signal intensity.

Imaging Recommendation

Modalities of choice (diagnostic cascade): radiography, ultrasound, CT, MRI.

Differential Diagnosis

- Calcium pyrophosphate dihydrate deposition (pseudogout, tumorous calcinosis)
- Infectious arthritis
- Rheumatoid arthritis and other rheumatic forms of arthritis
- Seronegative spondylarthropathy
- Cellulitis

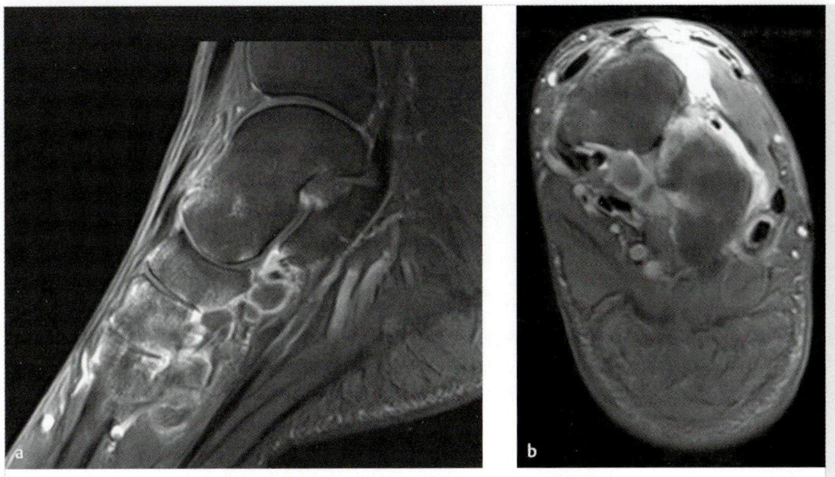

Fig. 9.21 a, b **A 70-year-old woman with chronic foot pain unresponsive to osteoarthritis therapy.** Several months passed before a seronegative spondylarthropathy was diagnosed.
a Sagittal T1-weighted fat-sat image after contrast administration shows massive irritation in the midfoot with patchy bone marrow edema in the tarsals and effusion in the intertarsal, tarsometatarsal, and subtalar joints. Intense synovitic enhancement is noted throughout the midfoot, especially on the plantar side, with visualization of inflammatory pannus tissue. The areas of bone marrow edema are a typical differentiating feature from rheumatoid arthritis.
b Axial oblique T1-weighted fat-sat image after contrast administration shows intense synovitic enhancement and pannus tissue in the talonavicular joint.

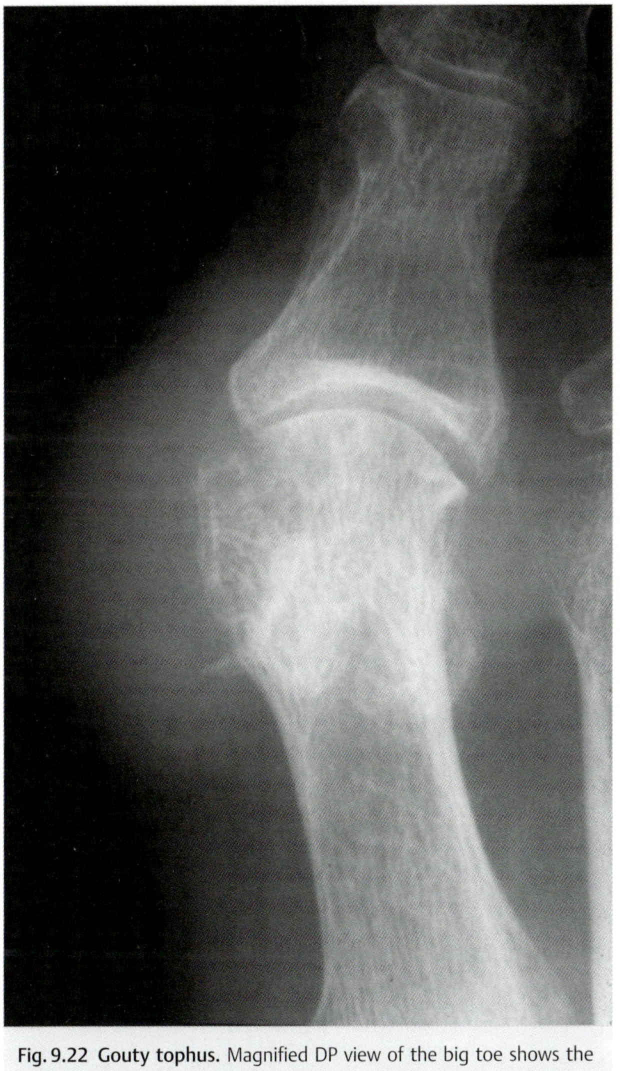

Fig. 9.22 **Gouty tophus.** Magnified DP view of the big toe shows the typical radiographic appearance of gouty arthropathy of the first metatarsophalangeal joint with soft-tissue opacity caused by deposition of calcium urate crystals. Submarginal erosions and osteolysis are visible on the medial side, and a tophaceous spicule has formed on the proximal joint margin. Relatively good joint-space preservation despite marked arthritic changes is typical of gouty arthropathy.

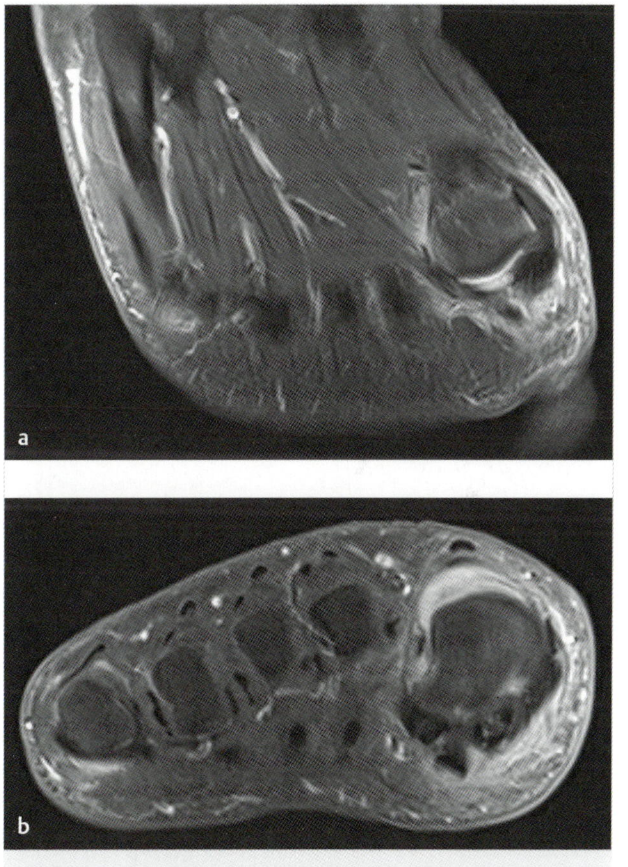

Fig. 9.23 a, b **A 57-year-old man presented with an acute gout attack and severe pain in the first metatarsophalangeal joint.**
a Coronal T1-weighted fat-sat image after contrast administration shows soft-tissue edema and increased periarticular enhancement about the first metatarsophalangeal joint and along the capsule and ligaments.
b Axial T1-weighted fat-sat image after contrast administration displays marked circumferential synovitis in acute gout.

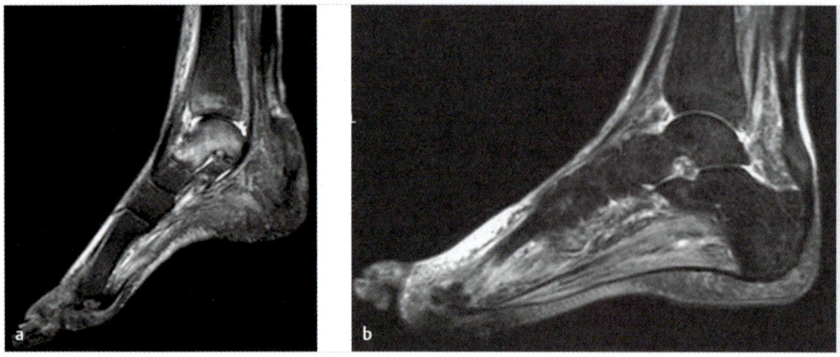

Fig. 9.24 a, b Early stages of diabetic osteoarthropathy.
a MRI demonstrates edema throughout the talus.
b Image 7 months later documents complete resolution of the edema.

Treatment

- *Acute gout attack:*
  - Nonsteroidal anti-inflammatory drugs
  - Corticosteroids
  - Colchicine
- *Chronic gout:*
  - Dietary modification
  - Weight reduction
  - Alcohol restriction
  - Uricosuric agents
  - Uricostatic agents

Prognosis, Complications

The prognosis is good with pharmacologic therapy and dietary modification.

9.3 Diabetic Osteoarthropathy, Charcot Arthropathy

S. Kessler and A. Staebler

Definition

The Charcot foot is characterized in advanced cases by significant, often painful deformity resulting from fractures of bones in the foot or distal tibia. The deformities may lead to ulceration and severe infection. Early forms present with edema of bones and soft tissues and with atypical bone fractures. Less experienced examiners will often misinterpret the findings as osteomyelitis.

Synonyms for this condition are Charcot foot, osteoarthropathy, neuropathic osteoarthropathy (NOAP), and diabetic neuropathic osteoarthropathy (DNOAP).

Symptoms

A Charcot foot is diagnosed clinically in patients with neuropathy, usually secondary to diabetes mellitus, who present with spontaneous swelling or a painless deformity. However, all other conditions which affect the peripheral nerve system can cause a NOAP (e.g., alcohol, drugs, bacterial, or viral infection). To avoid complications, the disease must be detected in its early stage. The differential diagnosis includes malignancies and inflammatory disorders, especially osteomyelitis, but these entities are rarely considered. Despite the typical symptomatology, most Charcot patients are misdiagnosed and treated as osteomyelitis patients.

Primary (hematogenous) osteomyelitis presents entirely different features. Aside from the fact that it is very rare, osteomyelitis is an acute, painful, rapidly progressive disease with high levels of inflammatory markers. It is responsive to antibiotic therapy in its early stage. Purulent liquefaction with spontaneous perforation soon develops in cases that have not been treated by surgical drainage.

In approximately 98% of cases, a patient with neuropathy who develops painful swelling and deformity without significant antecedent trauma has a Charcot foot—even if the neuropathy was not previously diagnosed. Alternative diagnoses, especially osteomyelitis in the absence of prior soft-tissue damage, are very rare.

Predisposing Factors

The etiology is unknown. A significant factor is neuropathy, which is present in all Charcot feet and usually results from diabetes mellitus. Many Charcot patients have serious co-morbid conditions:

- Diabetes mellitus
- Peripheral arterial occlusive disease
- Renal failure
- Coronary heart disease
- Chronic obstructive pulmonary disease, etc.

Anatomy and Pathology

Primary Changes

- *Edema phase:* The initial stage is marked by edema in one or more bones and surrounding soft tissues. The edema may involve only part of the bone (▶ Fig. 9.24).
- *Osteopenic phase:* If weight bearing is continued, substantial bone loss may occur due to demineralization and osteoclast activation (▶ Fig. 9.25 and ▶ Fig. 9.26).
- Repair phase: Edema and osteopenia will regress completely in cases where bone or cartilage defects have not yet occurred. This requires a sufficiently long period of non-weight bearing on the affected foot.

Secondary Changes

Secondary changes occur when weight bearing is continued during the osteopenic phase, resulting in bone fractures that

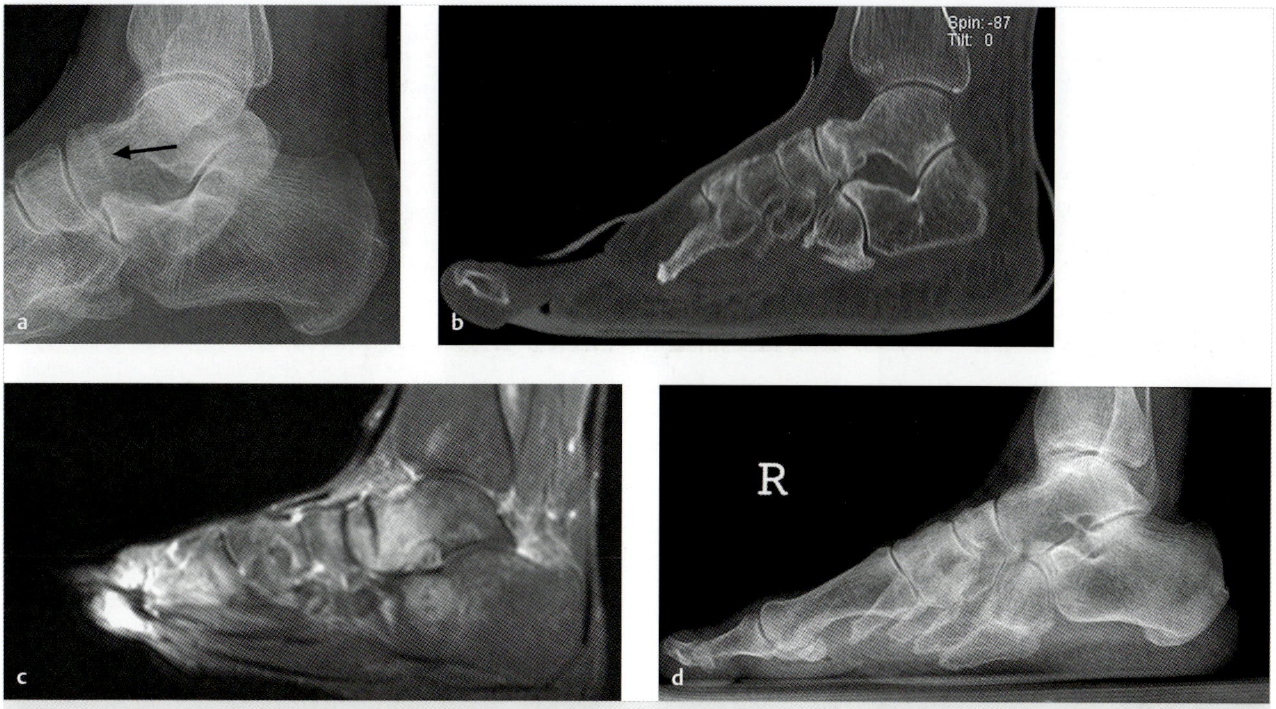

Fig. 9.25 a–d Early stages of diabetic osteoarthropathy.
a Lateral radiograph. A sclerotic line (arrow) is visible on the dorsal aspect of the talar head.
b CT shows a fissure passing completely through the talar head with no visible bone resorption.
c MRI shows perifocal edema bordering the fissure.
d By 3 months the fissure is no longer visible on a conventional radiograph.

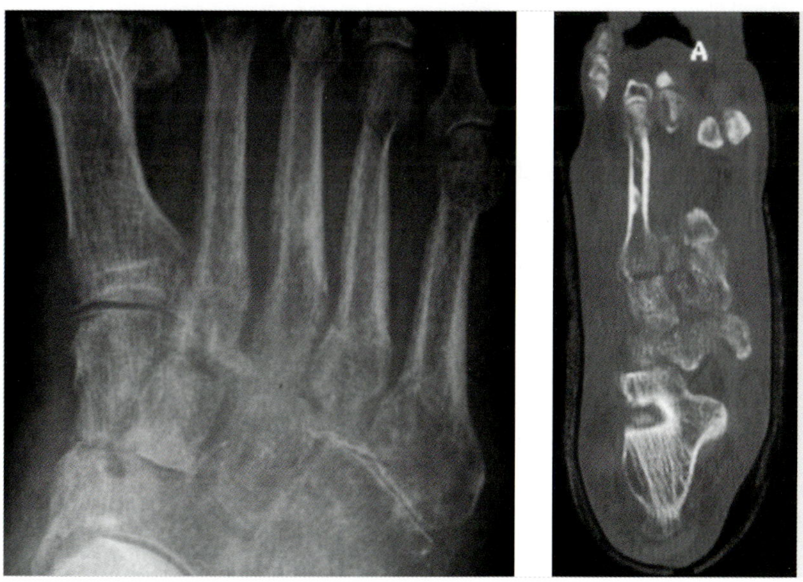

Fig. 9.26 a, b Early stages of diabetic osteoarthropathy: demineralization.
a Conventional radiograph shows significant demineralization, which is most advanced in the cuboid, lateral cuneiform, and lateral portion of the navicular. A number of joint spaces have been narrowed or obliterated, showing that the process in this region has already gone beyond pure demineralization. Mineral content appears unchanged in the small imaged portion of the talar head.
b CT displays demineralization in the navicular and the lateral and intermediate cuneiforms, plus the narrowing of multiple joint spaces with an essentially normal calcium content in the calcaneus.

trigger a cascade of complications. Most of the fractures are compression fractures, which initially cause instabilities and eventually result in fixed deformities (pes planus, varus or valgus) (▶ see Figs. 9.27–9.34). The deformities give rise to abnormal bony prominences, which cause pressure injury to local soft tissues. Avulsion fractures may occur rarely (▶ Fig. 9.32 b), in which case the fragments are displaced by muscle traction from the triceps surae or tibialis posterior, for example, or by passive traction from the plantar joint capsules. The bone fragment to which the capsule or tendon is attached may be so small that it goes undetected on radiographs; this is particularly common in the midfoot due to superimposed structures. Due to the neuropathy and loss of pain sensation, patients continue to bear weight on the foot despite the bony prominences, initially leading to callus formation and later to ulcerations and eventual infection (▶ Fig. 9.35). In the absence of infection, the fracture may go on to bony union either spontaneously or in response to conservative therapy, although any bone loss or deformity will

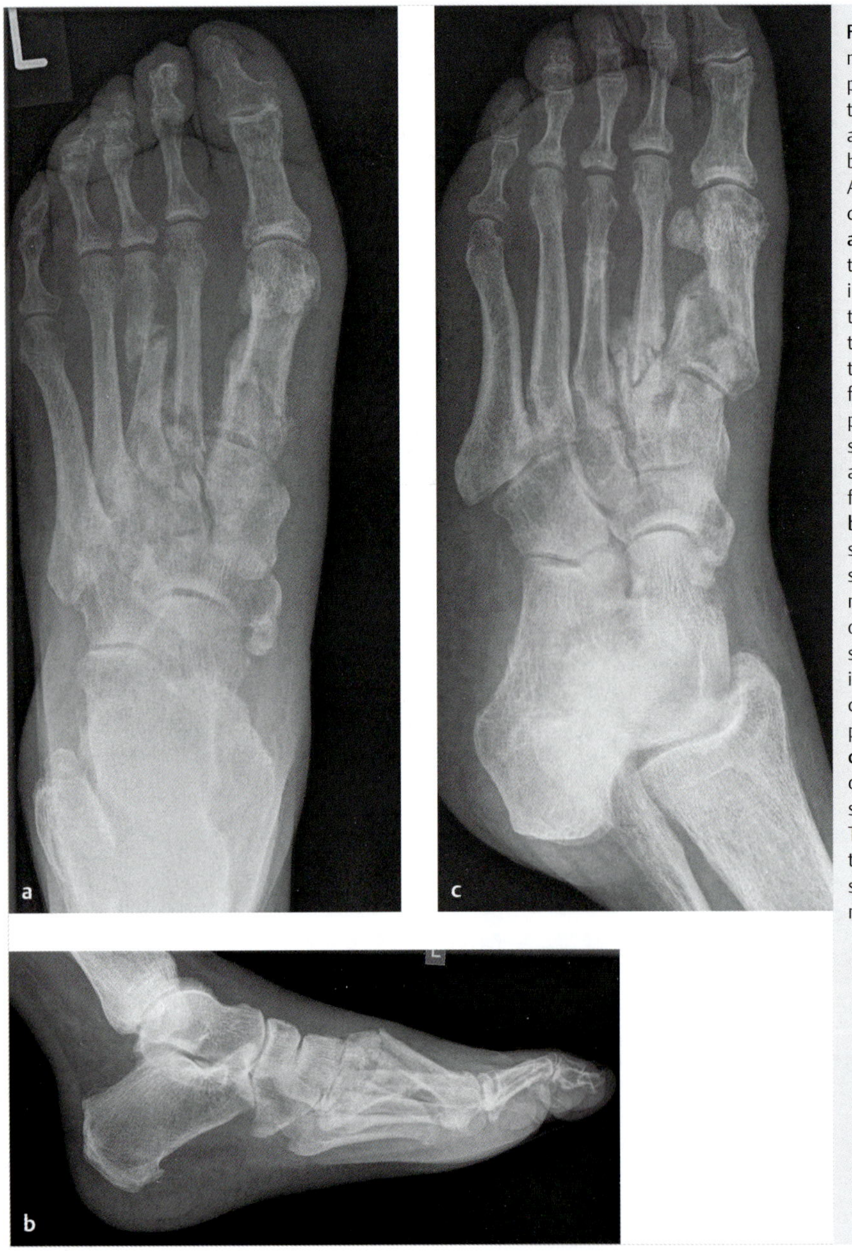

Fig. 9.27 a–c Metatarsal fractures. For several months the patient, a 63-year-old woman, had painless swelling of the left forefoot with no soft-tissue changes, normal inflammatory markers, and no antecedent trauma. Osteomyelitis had been diagnosed (inaccurately) from MRI findings. Antibiotics were initiated but did not result in clinical improvement.
a DP radiograph reveals fractures of the first through third metatarsals. The oblique fracture in the proximal third of the first metatarsal extends into the articular surface. The fracture in the proximal epimetaphysis of the second metatarsal extends close to the joint. The midshaft fracture of the third metatarsal has been displaced by the width of the shaft. All the fractures show copious new bone formation that suggests advanced consolidation. This degree of new bone formation excludes osteomyelitis.
b Oblique radiograph. The advanced bony consolidation is even more apparent in the first and second metatarsals. The fourth and fifth tarsometatarsal joint spaces are narrowed. The head of the first metatarsal bears several cystlike lesions consistent with typical osteoclast activation in a Charcot foot. When such lesions enlarge and coalesce, pathologic fracture may occur in response to ordinary loads.
c Lateral radiograph shows a dorsiflexed position of the first metatarsal fracture. This has not significantly altered the load-bearing pattern. Treatment began with weight bearing in a custom-molded shoe. Follow-up at 3 months showed further progression of consolidation with no change in bone position.

persist. Calluses and ulcerations will not heal as long as local peak pressure persists, due to bony deformities.

Mild instabilities and deformities can be left alone when suitable footwear is prescribed. Higher grades require qualified conservative treatment or surgical intervention (▶ Fig. 9.29, ▶ Fig. 9.32, ▶ Fig. 9.33). Dislocations in the subtalar joint may damage the artery of the tarsal canal, disrupting blood flow to the talus and causing osteonecrosis of that bone (▶ Fig. 9.32 e). Infections that are initially confined to the area around an ulcer will spread to tendon sheaths, joint spaces, bones, etc. and may eventually threaten the foot or lead to sepsis.

Sites of Occurrence

Charcot fractures may occur in the toes, metatarsals, large and small tarsal bones, ankle joint, or tibia. Clinical manifestations depend on the fracture location and associated deformity, the magnitude of the loads placed on the foot, and on co-morbid conditions such as peripheral arterial occlusive disease, heart failure, obesity, etc. Charcot fractures are located principally in the small tarsal bones, becoming less frequent at more proximal and more distal sites.

- *Toes, metatarsals:* Rare fractures in the toes and metatarsals may affect one or more metatarsal bones with variable degrees of fragment displacement. Generally there is no associated soft-tissue damage (▶ Fig. 9.27).
- *Distal tarsus:* The distal tarsus (= the small tarsal bones = the navicular, cuneiforms, and cuboid plus adjacent portions of the talus and calcaneus and the metatarsal bases) may show flattening of the plantar arch leading to a flatfoot (▶ Fig. 9.28) or in extreme cases to a rocker-bottom-foot deformity (▶ Fig. 9.29). With collapse of the distal tarsal bones, traction from the triceps surae tends to increase the equinus position of the hindfoot while traction from the dorsiflexors causes

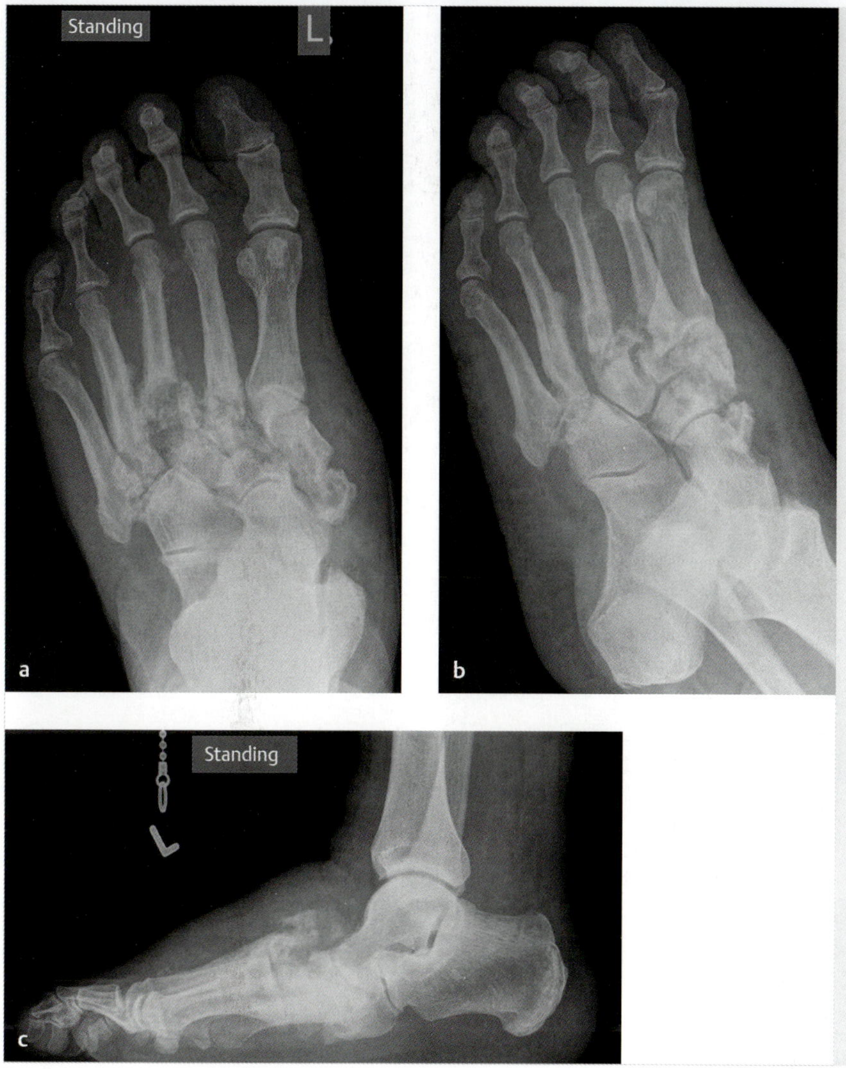

Fig. 9.28 a–c Grade 1 midfoot collapse in a 68-year-old man with painless swelling of the left midfoot with no calluses or instability. The foot was examined incidentally when the patient was hospitalized for a different disease.
a, b DP radiograph (**a**) and oblique radiograph (**b**) show destructive changes and dislocations of the navicular, the lateral and intermediate cuneiforms, and the base of the third metatarsal. Dissociations are most pronounced in the third tarsometatarsal joint, and superficial destructive changes are noted in the fourth and fifth tarsometatarsal joints. Sites of periosteal new bone formation indicate that the collapse has been present for several weeks.
c The lateral radiograph demonstrates the collapse at the level of the small tarsal bones, with the hindfoot showing inevitable displacement into an equinus position—in this case by half the shaft width. There is no abnormal bone contact with the plantar surface of the foot. Incidental finding: motor neuropathy and flatfoot have caused hammer toe deformity in all the toes, posing a risk of ulceration. The soft tissues are not at risk by radiographic or clinical findings. Bony bridging of the fracture zone is not visible on conventional radiographs but cannot be excluded. This case should be managed conservatively with orthopedic footwear.

extension of the forefoot, perpetuating the pes planus deformity. Charcot arthropathy in this region is manifested clinically by instability or deformity plus callosity or ulceration of the plantar, medial or lateral midfoot (▶ Fig. 9.35). The greater the degree of arch collapse, the greater the risk of ulceration and infection. Schon developed a system for classifying the severity of collapse in the sagittal plane: Type A is a mild deformity that does not collapse to the level of the plantar surface (▶ Fig. 9.28). Type B signifies moderate midfoot collapse, and type C represents collapse below the level of the plantar surface, creating a rocker-bottom foot (▶ Fig. 9.29). As long as the collapse is still flexible and reducible, it can be treated conservatively with a supportive insole that corrects for the pes planus deformity. The efficacy of this treatment can be assessed by pressure measurement and by lateral weight-bearing radiographs of the foot with and without a shoe. If surgery is needed, it is important to determine the extent of osteolytic changes and bone loss when planning the placement of implants (▶ Fig. 9.30).

- *Subtalar joint:* Charcot fractures in the subtalar joint, which are located in the lower talus or upper calcaneus, usually lead to valgus or rarely varus angulation of the calcaneus (▶ Fig. 9.31). This deviation of the calcaneus may be missed on radiographs; apparent absence of the subtalar joint in the lateral view is an important clue. Significant deformity with angulation of the calcaneus is best appreciated on an AP radiograph of the ankle joint or the Saltzman view. CT can provide detailed visualization.
- *Talus:* Charcot fractures of the talus are relatively common (▶ Fig. 9.32). The fractures are rarely limited to the medial or lateral border of the talus. Often they destroy large portions of the talar body while sparing the talar head (▶ Fig. 9.32 a). In some cases the entire talus, including the tail and even portions of the calcaneus, is lysed or destroyed (▶ Fig. 9.32 b, c). Loss of the talus means a loss of stability at the tibiotalar joint; this allows the foot to tilt out of alignment and may even cause the patient to walk on the malleolus (▶ Fig. 9.32 d). Charcot collapse may also compromise blood flow to the body of the talus, causing osteonecrosis (▶ Fig. 9.32 e). The necrotic bone creates an ideal culture medium for bacteria as it protects them from host defenses and systemic antibiotics.
- *Ankle joint:* Fractures of the ankle joint in Charcot arthropathy pose special challenges for operative treatment and rehabilitation and require differentiation from traumatic fractures. The absence of adequate trauma with minimal ankle pain would be consistent with a Charcot fracture. Radiographs

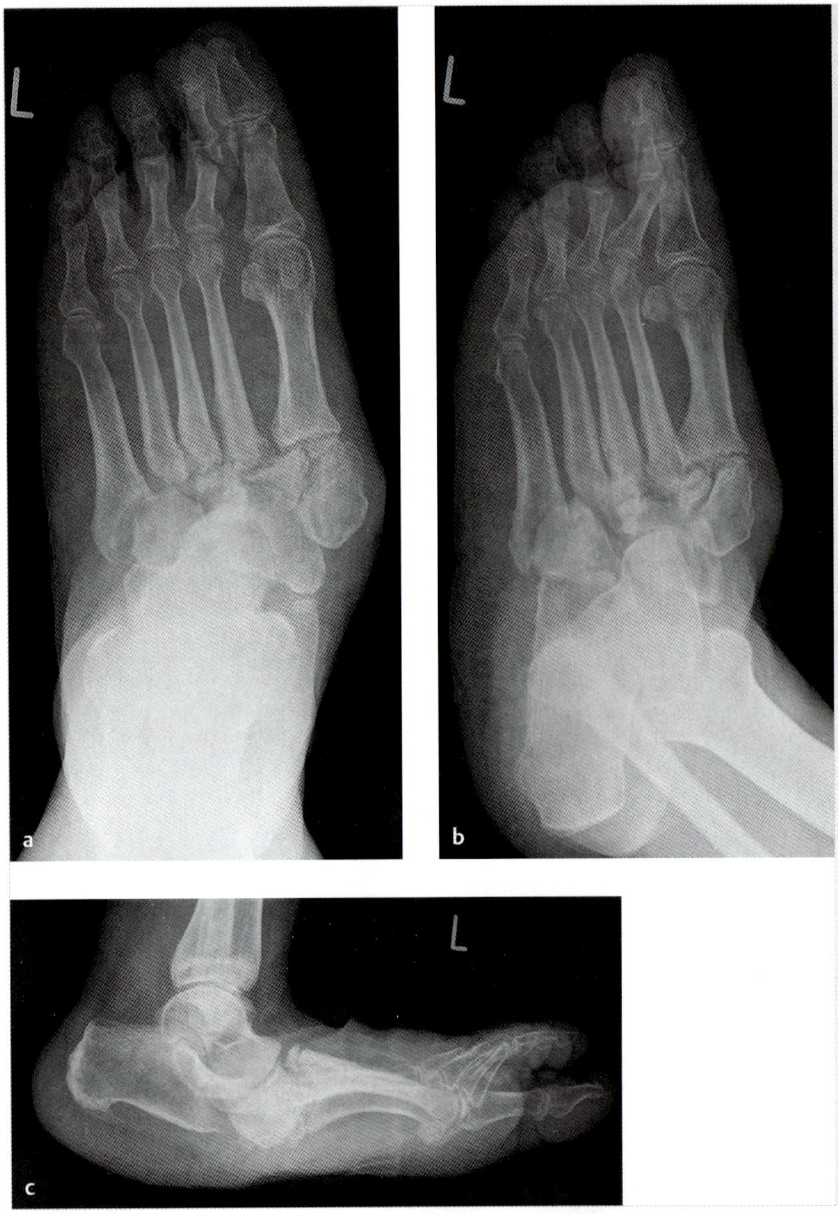

Fig. 9.29 a–c Grade 3 collapse of the midfoot with an ulcer. The foot ulcer in this 70-year-old man had been present for 1 year.
a DP weight-bearing radiograph shows abduction of the forefoot with a first tarsometatarsal angle of 30° plus fractures and substantial loss of the intermediate and lateral cuneiforms. The talonavicular joint appears narrowed due to a projection error. The joint between the cuboid and fourth and fifth metatarsals is subluxated. The articulating bone ends along the Lisfranc joint line show varying degrees of damage.
b The oblique radiograph does not add significant information in this case.
c The lateral first tarsometatarsal angle is 25°, and there is associated flattening of the calcaneus. The cuneiforms are displaced downward at the tarsometatarsal joints and are pressing on the plantar surface of the foot. The underlying soft-tissue defect can be seen.

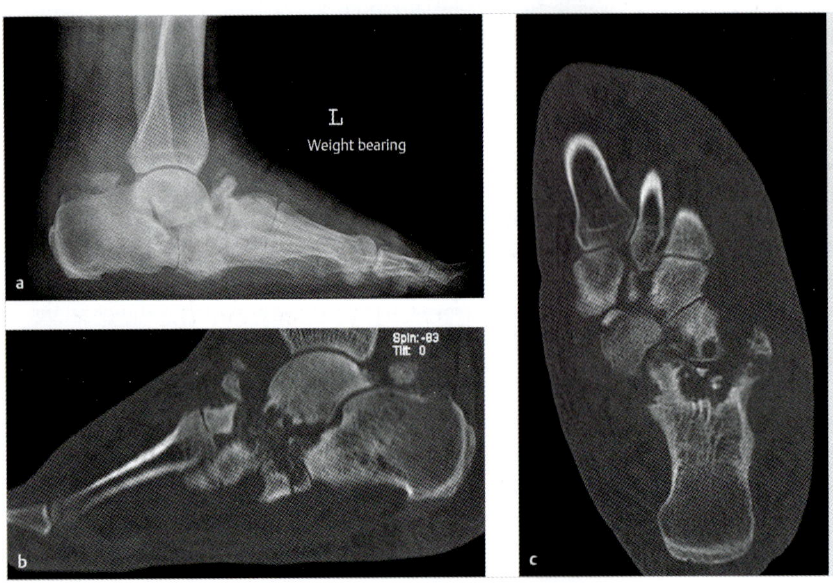

Fig. 9.30 a–c Charcot osteolysis.
a Lateral radiograph shows longitudinal arch collapse secondary to bone loss in the talar head and navicular. It is uncertain how much bone is still available for anchoring the implants for a fusion operation.
b Sagittal reformatted CT image defines the extent of osteolysis in the talar head and navicular.
c Axial reformatted image documents bone loss in the anterior calcaneus and cuboid.

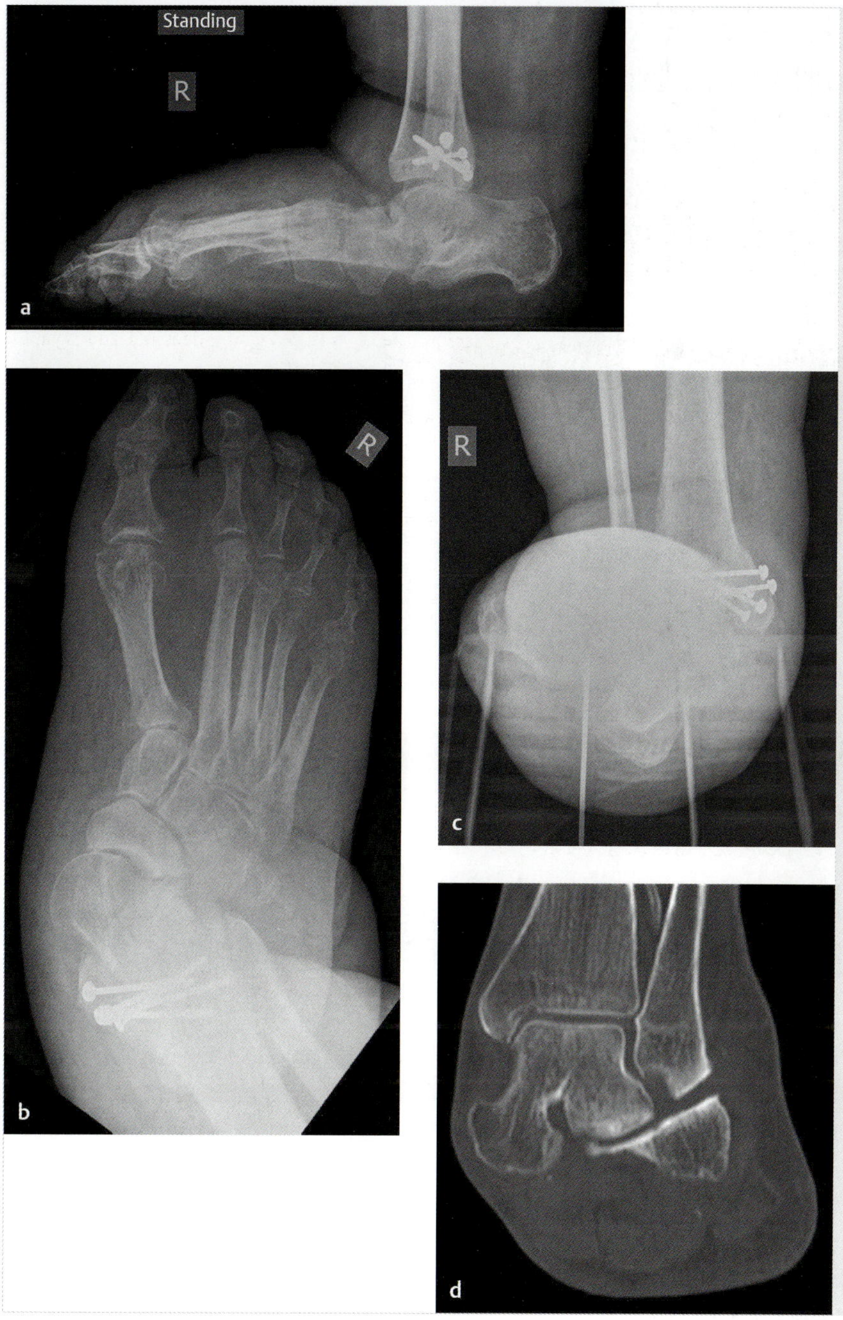

Fig. 9.31 a–d Dislocation of the subtalar joint.
a Lateral radiograph shows bone collapse with flattening of the plantar arch, with collapse occurring principally in the naviculocuneiform joint. The first tarsometatarsal angle is 45°. The pes planus deformity has caused flexion of the toes, with the result that the first metatarsal head is no longer in contact with the ground and the lesser toes are contracted in a hammer-toe position. The talocalcaneal joint (subtalar joint) is not visualized due to significant angulation of the hindfoot, which is seen more clearly in the other projections.
b DP radiograph shows almost complete dislocation of the talonavicular joint. The degree of forefoot abduction is not accurately represented by the first tarsometatarsal angle due to opposing adduction at the first tarsometatarsal joint. Forefoot abduction relative to the second metatarsal equals 55°.
c Saltzman view shows 45° valgus angulation of the calcaneus.
d CT image from a different patient shows advanced lateral angulation and translation of the calcaneus.

show fracture patterns that do not occur with trauma (▶ Fig. 9.33 a). Atypical fracture patterns also occur in the distal tibial metaphysis (tibial pilon) with collapse occurring on the medial, lateral, or posterior side (▶ Fig. 9.33 b–d). The reliable detection of bony consolidation after surgical stabilization is important to ensure that weight bearing is not resumed prematurely, jeopardizing the result of treatment. While there are a few patients who can tolerate a rigid nonunion, this is not true of most patients, especially where the ankle joint is concerned. External callus formation can mimic fracture union on plain radiographs. In doubtful cases, therefore, CT scans should be ordered for the reliable assessment of bony consolidation (▶ Fig. 9.33 e).

- *Tibia, calcaneus:* The tibia and calcaneus are rare sites of occurrence for Charcot fractures. If the fracture is not identified as Charcot-related, it is likely that healing complications will develop, especially in the tibia.

Therapeutically relevant findings and classification

Older classifications of Charcot arthropathy do not have therapeutic implications. It is essential to describe the findings of the clinical evaluation (edema, instability, callosity, ulceration and infection, abscess formation, cellulitis, empyema) and imaging studies (edema, osteopenia, resorption, fracture, deformity: unstable or fixed, dislocations, type and degree of bone pressure on soft tissues). The following points should be addressed:

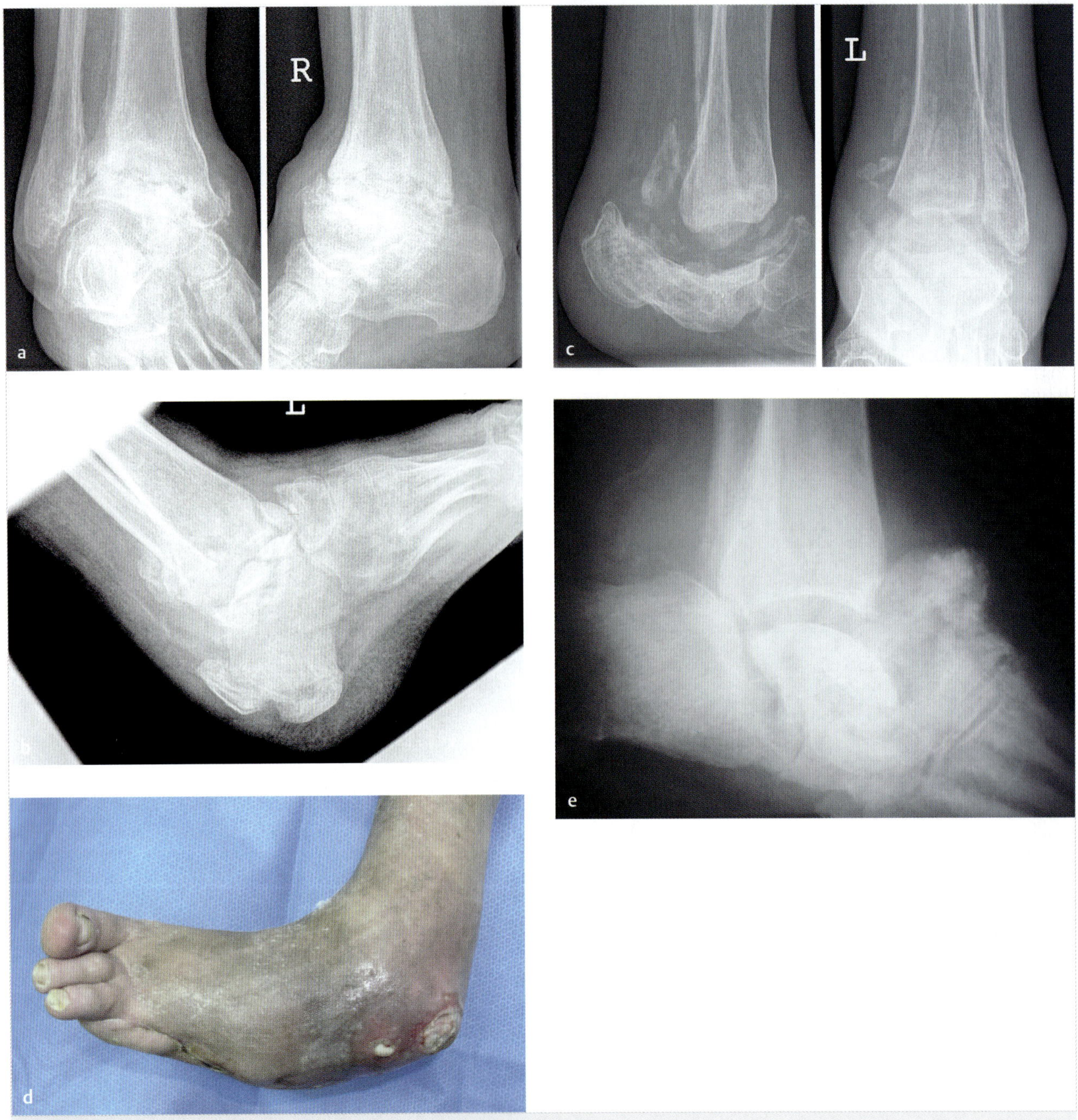

Fig. 9.32 a–e Fractures of the talus in various patients.
a A large portion of the talar body has collapsed in this patient, with associated destruction of the ankle joint. The talar head and talonavicular joint are intact.
b The talus in this patient has been mostly destroyed by a compression fracture, leaving just a few small bone remnants. There is also an avulsion fracture at the Achilles tendon attachment on the posterosuperior calcaneus. It appears that bony bridging has already occurred in this position.
c This patient cannot bear weight on her foot due to severe instability. Conventional radiograph shows that the entire talus and large portions of the calcaneus have been lost. General nephrogenic osteoporosis is noted as an incidental finding.
d Extreme varus deformity has caused this patient to walk on the lateral edge of his foot and lateral malleolus, resulting in ulcerations with exposed tendons and sites of infected tendon necrosis.
e Clinically, this patient had an acquired flatfoot deformity with swelling and a purulent draining sinus tract. Besides collapse in the Charcot region with loss of the talar head, navicular, and portions of the cuneiforms, the radiograph shows reactive new bone formation along with anterior and plantar dislocation of the talus. This dislocation ruptured the artery of the tarsal canal, causing loss of blood flow to the talus. Osteonecrosis of the talus accounts for the increased radiopacity of the bone.

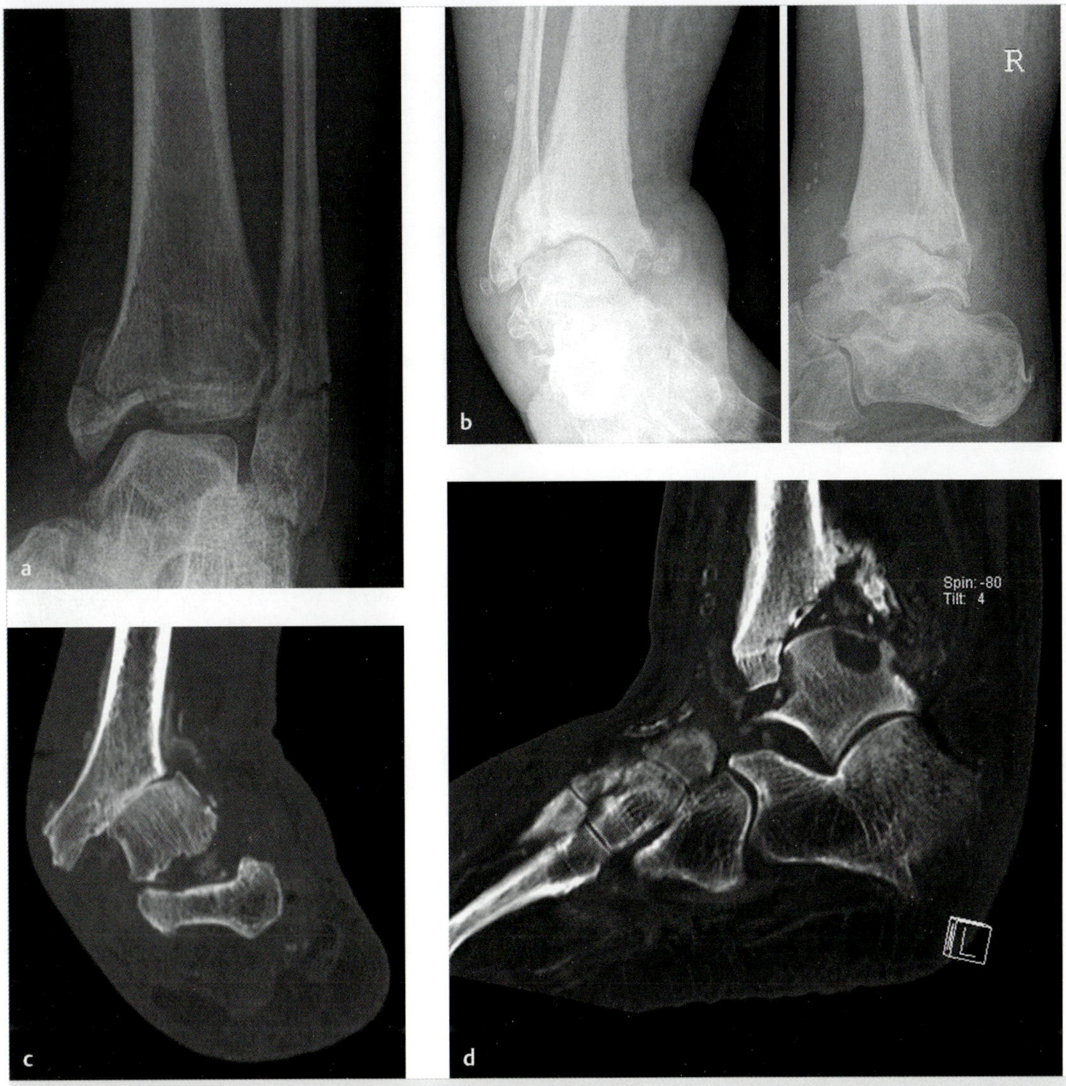

Fig. 9.33 a–f Fractures of the ankle joint and pilon in various patients.
a The bimalleolar fracture in this patient has a medial malleolar fragment that includes part of the tibial articular surface and distal metaphysis and has caused an articular step-off at the medial joint space. The lateral malleolar fracture runs perpendicular to the long axis of the fibula. These patterns are not found in traumatic ankle fractures and should raise immediate suspicion of a Charcot fracture.
b Medial pilon in a different patient. PA and lateral radiographs show collapse of the medial tibial articular surface with consequent varus angulation of the talus and foot. The joint space is narrowed. Reactive bone formation shows that the fracture has been present for some time.
c Lateral pilon. Osteolysis of the lateral tibial plateau in this patient has resulted in significant valgus deformity of the ankle joint.
d Extensive osteolysis of the posterior pilon. Sagittal reformatted CT image shows loss of the posterior portions of the tibial pilon. The talus is dislocated backward and upward. Osteolysis is also present in the body of the talus. Slight new bone formation is noted in the posterior part of the ankle joint but is insufficient to stabilize the joint for weight bearing.

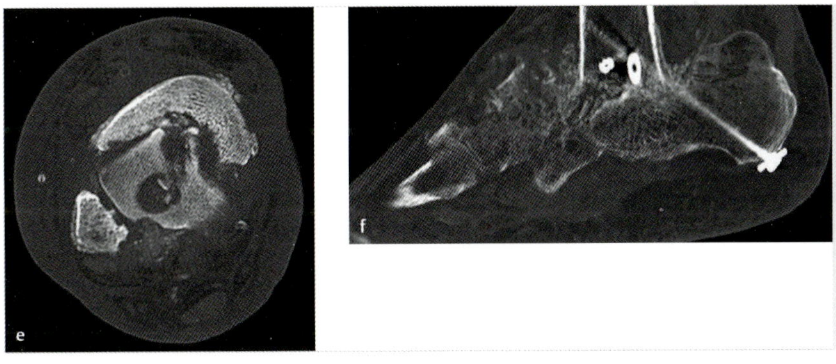

e Axial CT scan of the patient in **d** shows both central and lateral osteolysis. Nevertheless, most of the bone in the talus is still intact—a fact that is important in planning surgical treatment.
f CT in a different patient documents bony consolidation 8 weeks after surgical fusion of the tibia, calcaneus, navicular, and cuboid. Bony bridging between the posterior portions of the tibia and calcaneus and between the calcaneus and cuboid is well advanced, while union is still incomplete between the tibia and calcaneus anteriorly and between the tibia and navicular.

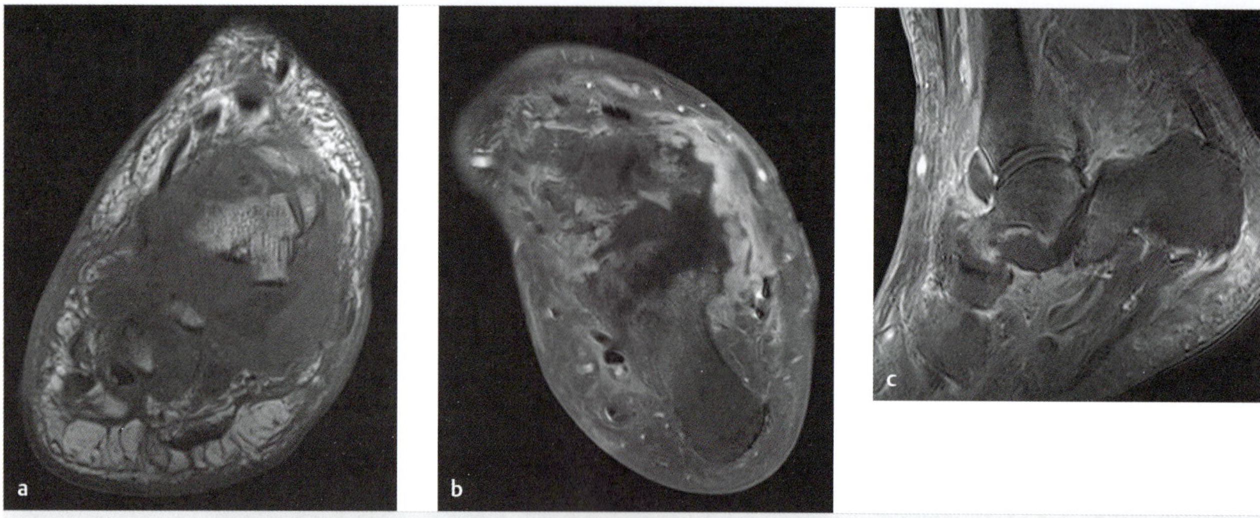

Fig. 9.34 a–c Advanced diabetic osteoarthropathy (Charcot arthropathy).
a Coronal T1-weighted image shows anatomical disruption with destruction of the right tarsus in the Chopart joint line.
b Axial T1-weighted fat-sat image after contrast administration shows distinct fluid inclusions in the joint spaces and intense granulation tissue. Signs of mechanical instability are typically present in Charcot arthropathy. There is no evidence of osteomyelitis or bone necrosis.
c Sagittal T1-weighted fat-sat image after contrast administration shows destruction of the ankle joint with depression of the anterior calcaneus and destruction of the articulation between the talus, navicular, calcaneus, and cuboid. There is conspicuous plantar keratosis and plantar fasciitis.

- Which bones are fractured?
- What fracture patterns are present? Is there any bone loss?
- What are the resulting deformities?
- Which bone is exerting pressure on soft tissues?
- What is the soft-tissue damage?
- Has an infection developed?

Imaging

Radiographs

Radiographs are the primary tool for imaging evaluation. In contrast to sectional imaging studies, radiographs can image the weight-bearing foot to detect any instability and identify sites of abnormal bone pressure. Radiographs can display the foot in its entirety. Deformities such as flatfoot and abduction or adduction are easily recognized on X-ray films and can be quantified by angle measurements. The first tarsometatarsal angle is determined in the lateral and DP projections to assess the degree of flatfoot and lateral deviation.

Radiographs show no abnormalities in the initial edematous phase of Charcot arthropathy. Advanced osteopenia can be identified, while initial stages of osteopenia or fractures will elude radiographic detection and require CT. Early fractures and destructive joint changes as well as displacements and dislocations are demonstrable by CT or MRI, while MRI is used to detect osteomyelitic destruction, early osteomyelitis without bone destruction, and to investigate a possible active process. Weight-bearing radiographs are excellent for the diagnosis of instabilities. Abnormal bone pressure on the skin can be detected along with the spontaneous or postoperative fusion of bones. CT is more reliable for detecting the initial bony bridging of fracture sites.

Ultrasound

Echo-free or hypoechoic joint effusions are occasionally found in a setting of activated, secondary osteoarthritis. Ultrasound in patients with chronic degenerative changes will show associated changes in echogenic bony subchondral structures, soft-tissue edema in a Charcot foot, and possible abscess formation in incipient osteomyelitis.

CT

Charcot arthropathy is relatively easy to evaluate by CT. Demineralization and intraosseous and superficial osteolysis are detectable even in their early stage. CT provides a nonsuperimposed view of displacements, dislocations, and deformities in the Lisfranc or Charcot joints as well as fractures and bone disintegration. CT can also detect subtle new bone formation and bony bridging of fracture sites. For reliable information on whether bony consolidation has occurred after a spontaneous fusion or arthrodesis, for example, CT is required. CT is limited in its ability to depict soft-tissue changes, however.

MRI (▸ Fig. 9.34)

MRI provides detailed visualization of intra- and extraosseous soft-tissue changes even in their early stage. It displays inflammatory changes, especially fistulous tracts, abscesses in soft tissues and joint lines, and osteomyelitis. It is also used to detect osteonecrosis and assess bone vitality. Another application of MRI is for the detection or exclusion of other possible diagnoses, especially osteomyelitis and malignancies. The visualization of changes in mineralized tissues—bone resorption, fractures, new bone formation, bony bridging—is less impressive than with CT, and MRI cannot evaluate bony consolidation. It can,

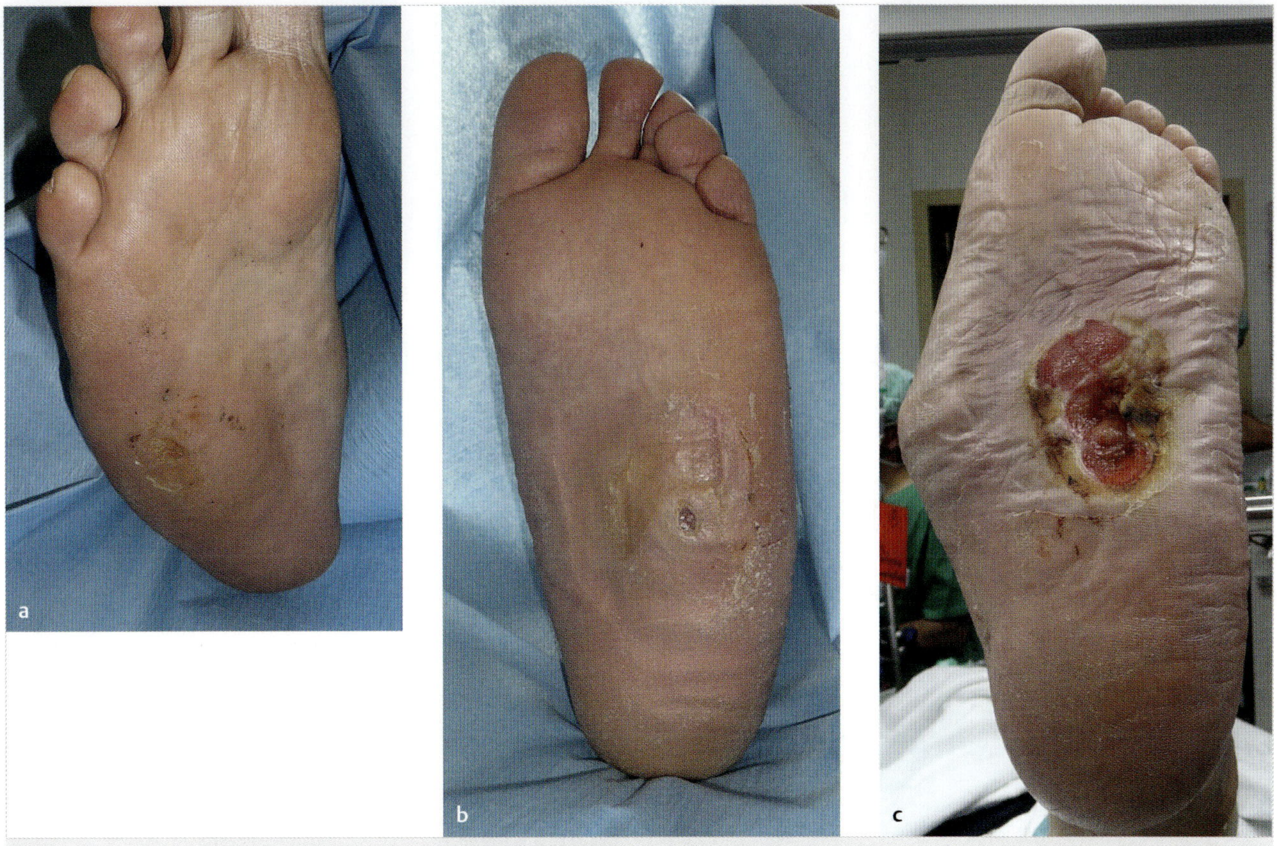

Fig. 9.35 a–c Soft-tissue changes on the sole of the foot after midfoot collapse.
a Callus.
b Small ulcer.
c Large ulcer.

however, demonstrate malalignments, dislocations, and displacements as well as cartilage lesions.

Imaging Recommendation

Modality of choice: weight-bearing radiographs in three planes should always be the initial imaging study.

- *MRI:*
  - Early signs of Charcot arthropathy
  - Signs of abscess formation (ultrasound, MRI)
  - Bone vitality
- *CT:*
  - Degree of osteoclastic activity
  - Details of bone displacement and destruction
  - Bony consolidation after surgical fusion

Differential Diagnosis

- Osteoclastic metastasis
- Osteomyelitis

Treatment

The treatment is multidisciplinary and includes bone and joint surgeons as well as orthopedic technicians, podiatrists, vascular surgeons, and multiple disciplines dealing with diabetes-related problems.

The aim of the treatment is a stable, plantigrade hindfoot which can be supplied with a custom orthopedic shoe and allows ambulation of the patient.

Conservative

In early stages of the disease with no pre-existent deformity, adequate external stability with a walker or orthopedic shoes can be sufficient. The Charcot fracture can be reduced in a custom-molded shoe.

If calluses or ulcers are present, local pressure reduction is mandatory to prevent ulcers or allow pre-existent ulcers to heal. External devices like walkers or total contact casts have proven to be effective. In addition, a surgical removal of bony lumps can be considered.

Operative

In cases with instability, extended fusion with external fixator or hybrid techniques can be used to realign the foot.

If infection of an ulcer has already caused septic metabolic conditions, if severe vascular disease cannot be improved or if the bony destruction does not allow any reconstruction, primary amputation has to be considered. Often amputations can be limited to achieve a resilient stump (e.g., Pirogoff amputation).

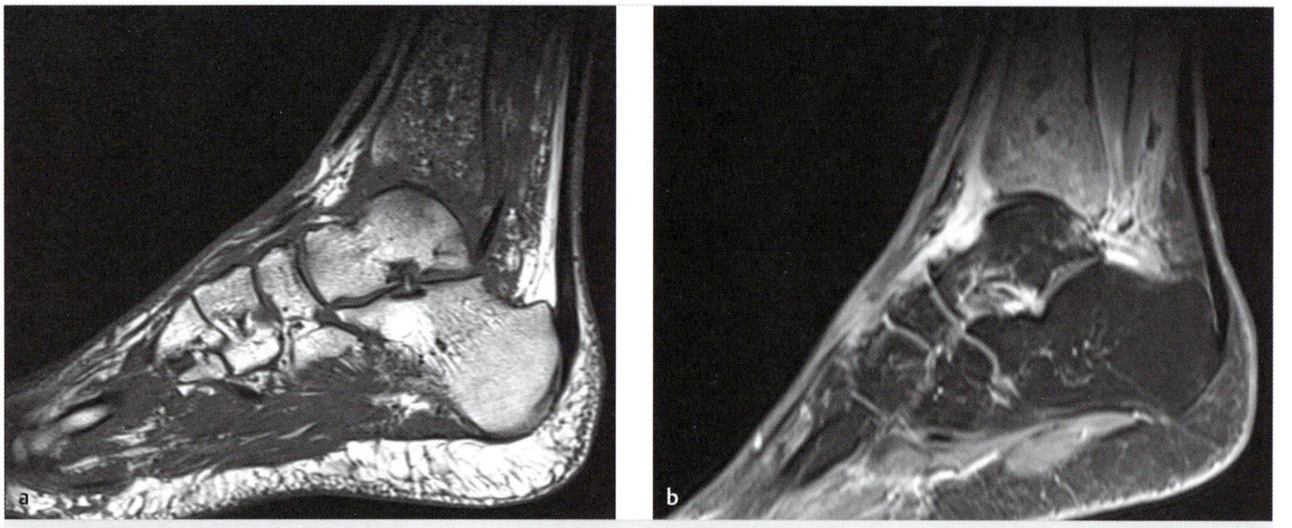

Fig. 9.36 a, b Acute osteomyelitis.
a Sagittal T1-weighted image documents hyperintense fat globules in the distal tibia. These foci of fat necrosis are pathognomonic for acute osteomyelitis.
b Sagittal T1-weighted image after contrast administration shows intense enhancement of the tibia and adjacent soft tissues with a granular image pattern of the tibial medullary cavity and isolated larger areas of hypointense fat necrosis.

9.4 Osteitis, Osteomyelitis

A. Staebler

Definition

Osteomyelitis is an inflammation of the bone marrow caused by infectious organisms. A better term for bone inflammation is osteitis, since all portions of the bone including the cortex, periosteum, and articular pillar may be involved in addition to the medullary cavity.

Symptoms

Osteomyelitis can be classified as acute, subacute, or chronic depending on the time course and duration of the disease:

- *Acute osteomyelitis:* Acute osteomyelitis is characterized by swelling, redness, local warmth, pain, and inflammatory markers with elevated C-reactive protein and an elevated white blood count.
- *Subacute osteomyelitis:* A partially encapsulated inflammatory process, such as a Brody abscess in children and adolescents or vertebral body osteomyelitis, often takes a subacute course. Inflammatory markers are not necessarily elevated.
- *Chronic osteomyelitis:* Chronic osteomyelitis may run an insidious course for years or decades with exacerbations and with sequestration, fistulation and abscess formation in the medullary cavity or adjacent soft tissues.

Predisposing Factors

- Focus of bacterial infection, such as sinusitis, endocarditis, urinary tract infection, soft-tissue or organ abscess
- Open fracture, surgical operation
- Host defenses compromised due to diabetes mellitus, immunosuppression, malnutrition, alcoholism, etc.

Anatomy and Pathology

Hematogenous osteomyelitis, in which the causative organisms spread to the bone via the bloodstream, is distinguished from exogenous osteomyelitis, which results from direct contamination of a traumatic or surgical wound with infectious organisms or contiguous spread from a local soft-tissue abscess or infection.

The main causative organisms of osteomyelitis are *Staphylococcus aureus* (75–80% of cases) and β-hemolytic streptococci. Enterobacteria such as *Escherichia coli*, *Serratia marcescens*, *Pseudomonas aeruginosa*, or Klebsiella species may be causative in adults. Osteomyelitis in Eastern and African countries may be caused by *Mycobacterium tuberculosis* and atypical mycobacteria, brucellosis, and actinomycetes. *Haemophilus influenzae* may also be causative in children, and enteric salmonella may cause osteomyelitis in young patients with sickle cell anemia.

Imaging (▶ Fig. 9.36, ▶ Fig. 9.37, ▶ Fig. 9.38)

Radiographs

Radiographs in acute osteomyelitis show no abnormalities initially. As decalcification progresses, destructive changes may appear as moth-eaten or permeative lesions in the medullary cavity and cortex and/or circumscribed foci of bone destruction.

! Note

Cortical bone destruction is considered the most important radiographic criterion, especially in the foot.

Over time, osteitis, or osteomyelitis will eventually produce sclerotic changes. As bone areas become devitalized and form sequestra, the affected bone can no longer participate in bone metabolism, especially osteoclastic bone resorption, and so the

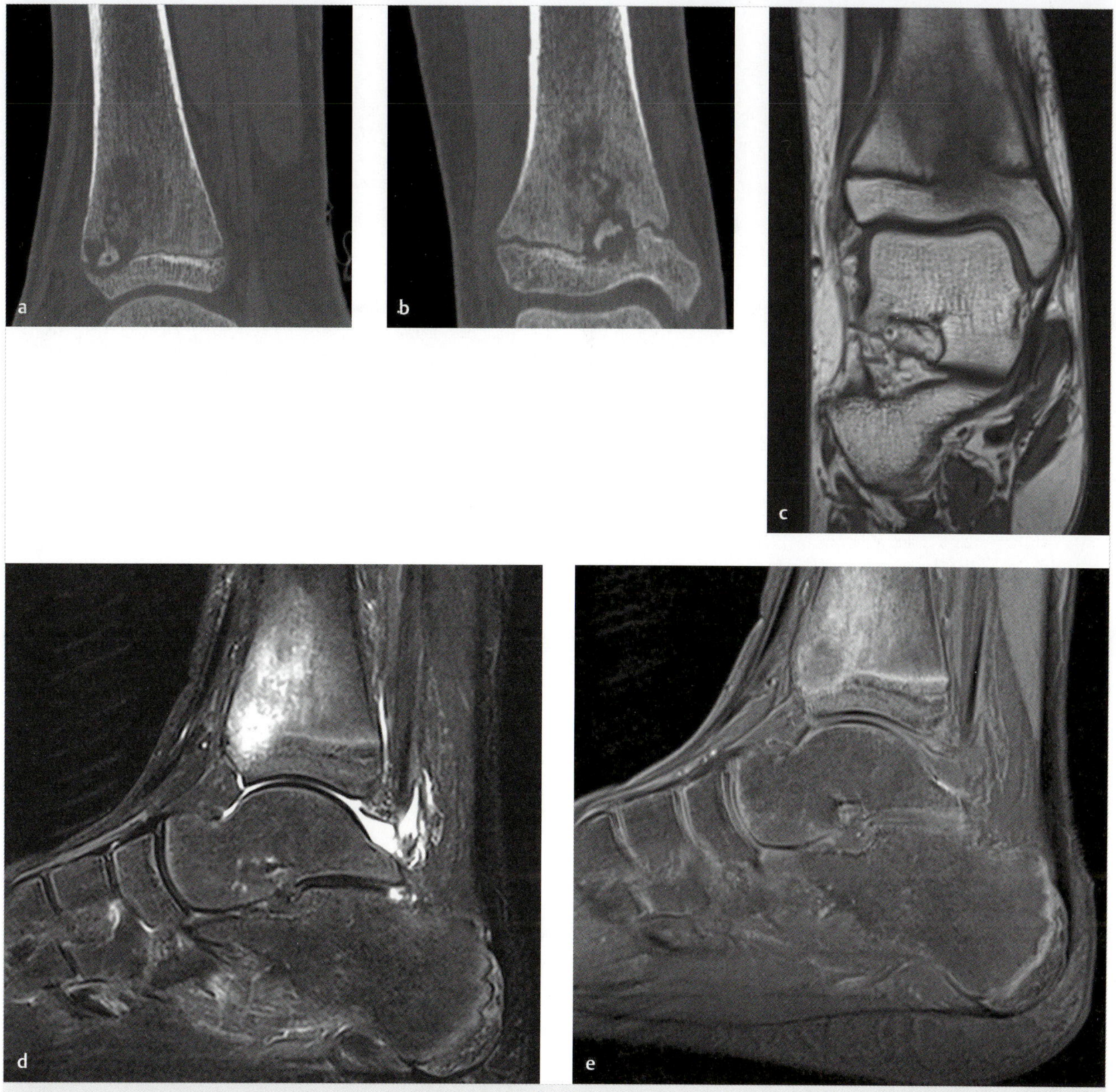

Fig. 9.37 a–e Acute osteomyelitis with sequestrum formation in a 14-year-old boy.
a, b CT images. Sagittal reformatted CT image (**a**) shows acute osteomyelitis with metaphyseal and epiphyseal bone destruction. The process extends through the anterior epiphyseal plate in the distal right tibia with bone sequestration. Coronal reformatted CT image (**b**) shows the presence of multiple bone sequestra, the largest of which features an osteolytic rim and increased sclerosis.
c–e MR images 2 months after CT and after sequestrectomy, still demonstrating florid osteomyelitis. **c** Coronal T1-weighted image. The most important sequence for diagnosing osteomyelitis is the T1-weighted sequence, which shows segments in which the hyperintense fatty marrow signal is almost completely lost, in this case obliterating the contours of the epiphyseal plate. **d** Sagittal STIR sequence shows intense edema formation in the area affected by osteomyelitis. **e** Sagittal T1-weighted fat-sat image after contrast administration shows enhancement of the osteomyelitic focus. The STIR and T1-weighted sequences in themselves are often sufficient for evaluating an inflammatory process in the medullary cavity (especially in cases where contrast medium cannot be used). Contrast administration is recommended to exclude articular and soft-tissue involvement.

bone density increases. Other possible causes of increased sclerosis are chronic reactive hyperemia and reactive new bone formation in response to destructive changes.

Vascular calcifications in the small arteries of the foot due to medial sclerosis are a sign of diabetes mellitus and are a common finding in osteomyelitis involving the hindfoot.

Ultrasound

With acute osteomyelitis in the ankle region, longitudinal and transverse scans over the affected bone may show hypoechoic areas of periosteal elevation. The underlying echogenic bone surface may have a stippled consistency or may show lamellar

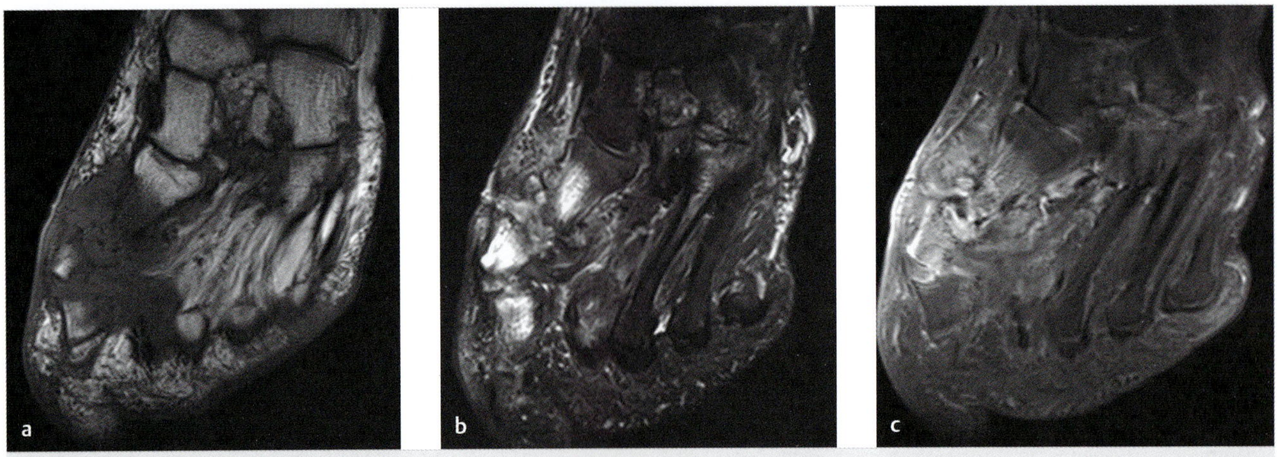

Fig. 9.38 a–c Infection with acute osteomyelitis after hallux valgus surgery in a 58-year-old man.
a Coronal T1-weighted image shows osteomyelitis in the proximal fragment of a metatarsal osteotomy with loss of fatty marrow signal, which also shows some initial distal spread.
b Coronal STIR image shows intense bone marrow edema in the dislocated metatarsal segments and remnant of the proximal phalanx.
c Coronal T1-weighted fat-sat image after contrast administration shows distinct cellulitic enhancement in the adjacent soft tissues.

densities and calcifications that hamper ultrasound visualization. The power Doppler signal is positive.

Sites of cortical destruction may be found but are not consistently detectable, which is why ultrasonography is not routinely ordered. The medullary cavity cannot be satisfactorily evaluated with ultrasound.

MRI

Interpretation Checklist

- Presence of osteomyelitis or a different cause of bone edema such as reactive edema in response to mechanical stress or overuse, reflex sympathetic dystrophy, or in a setting of tumorlike lesions such as osteoid osteoma
- Precise extent of the change in the medullary cavity
- Signs of abscess formation in the bone or soft tissues
- Early appearance of signal voids in the hypointense cortex in unenhanced T1-weighted images
- Sequestration or necrosis

Examination Technique

- *Standard protocol:* high-resolution multichannel coil in the supine position, or high-resolution multichannel coil in the prone position
- *Sequences:*
  - Oblique coronal T1-weighted and STIR
  - Sagittal and axial oblique PD-weighted fat-sat
  - Oblique coronal and axial T1-weighted fat-sat after IV contrast administration
  - Most important sequence: T1-weighted image without contrast administration

MRI Findings

- Absence of fatty marrow signal in the T1-weighted sequence, intense bone marrow edema
- Location: often borders on concentrated stress zones (malleolar region, metatarsal heads) or in continuity with soft-tissue defects
- Most important criterion: cortical signal void on unenhanced T1-weighted images and cortical destruction
- Abscesses, fistulation, peripheral enhancement in adjacent soft tissues
- Acute or peracute osteomyelitis may cause fat necrosis manifested by the appearance of small fat globules with very high signal intensity in the unenhanced T1-weighted image. This pattern is pathognomonic for highly acute bacterial osteomyelitis (see ▶ Fig. 9.36).

CT

High-resolution multislice CT with volume acquisition, overlapping reconstructions, and MPRs can provide detailed, nonsuperimposed views of bony and cortical destruction with high sensitivity. CT is also advantageous in the detection of bone sequestra. Sequestra are sclerotic bone fragments that are no longer in continuity with the parent bone (▶ Fig. 9.37 a, b).

Scintigraphy

Scintigraphic studies including Tc-99 m methylene diphosphonate scintigraphy, leukocyte scintigraphy, and sequential 18F-FDG PET/CT have only a minor role in the investigation of suspected osteomyelitis in the foot.

Imaging Recommendation

Modalities of choice: radiography and MRI.

Differential Diagnosis

- Neurogenic or Charcot arthropathy
- Osteoid osteoma
- Stress- or overuse-related reactive bone edema, stress and fatigue fractures
- Ewing sarcoma, osteosarcoma
- Differentiation between neuropathy and osteomyelitis is the most difficult. Neuropathy has the following characteristics:
- Joint malalignments

- Slight displacement and subluxation initially, followed later by severe dislocation
- Valgus deformity of the hindfoot
- Disruption of the Charcot or Lisfranc joint line
- Subchondral erosions and cysts
- Bone fragments
- Intra-articular loose bodies
- Involvement of multiple joints
- Areas of reactive bone marrow edema with some preservation of fat marrow signal in the T1-weighted sequence
- Even a Charcot joint sometimes shows almost a complete loss of fat marrow signal due to reactive sclerosis

Treatment

- Surgical treatment usually consists of amputation at the level of the toes or forefoot
- Surgical removal of all affected bone marrow, generally combined with antibiotic therapy (gentamicin beads)
- Immobilization, if necessary with an external fixation device

Prognosis, Complications

The amputation of toes, the midfoot, or the entire foot may be necessary. Septic complications may also arise. While acute and subacute osteomyelitis will resolve completely in most patients, chronic osteomyelitis may last a lifetime.

9.5 Bibliography

Rheumatoid Arthritis

Egerer K, Feist E, Burmester GR. The serological diagnosis of rheumatoid arthritis: antibodies to citrullinated antigens. Dtsch Arztebl Int 2009; 106: 159–163

Larsen A, Dale K, Eek M. Radiographic evaluation of rheumatoid arthritis and related conditions by standard reference films. Acta Radiol Diagn (Stockh) 1977; 18: 481–491

Seronegative Spondylarthropathies

Erdem CZ, Tekin NS, Sarikaya S, Erdem LO, Gulec S. MR imaging features of foot involvement in patients with psoriasis. Eur J Radiol 2008; 67: 521–525

Ghanem N, Uhl M, Pache G, Bley T, Walker UA, Langer M. MRI in psoriatic arthritis with hand and foot involvement. Rheumatol Int 2007; 27: 387–393

Hettenkofer HJ. Rheumatologie: Diagnostik–Klinik–Therapie. 5th ed. Stuttgart: Thieme; 2003

McQueen F, Lassere M, Østergaard M. Magnetic resonance imaging in psoriatic arthritis: a review of the literature. Arthritis Res Ther 2006; 8: 207

Müller-Ladner U. Evidenzbasierte Therapie in der Rheumatologie. 2nd ed. Bremen: UNI-MED; 2007

Tan AL, McGonagle D. Psoriatic arthritis: correlation between imaging and pathology. Joint Bone Spine 2010; 77: 206–211

Weiner SM, Jurenz S, Uhl M et al. Ultrasonography in the assessment of peripheral joint involvement in psoriatic arthritis : a comparison with radiography, MRI and scintigraphy. Clin Rheumatol 2008; 27: 983–989

Gouty Arthropathy

Carter JD, Kedar RP, Anderson SR et al. An analysis of MRI and ultrasound imaging in patients with gout who have normal plain radiographs. Rheumatology (Oxford) 2009; 48: 1442–1446

Dalbeth N, Doyle A, Boyer L et al. Development of a computed tomography method of scoring bone erosion in patients with gout: validation and clinical implications. Rheumatology (Oxford) 2011; 50: 410–416

Gerster JC, Landry M, Dufresne L, Meuwly JY. Imaging of tophaceous gout: computed tomography provides specific images compared with magnetic resonance imaging and ultrasonography. Ann Rheum Dis 2002; 61: 52–54

Lagoutaris ED, Adams HB, DiDomenico LA, Rothenberg RJ. Longitudinal tears of both peroneal tendons associated with tophaceous gouty infiltration. A case report. J Foot Ankle Surg 2005; 44: 222–224

Morrison WB, Ledermann HP, Schweitzer ME. MR imaging of inflammatory conditions of the ankle and foot. Magn Reson Imaging Clin N Am 2001; 9: 615–637, xi–xii

Yu JS, Chung C, Recht M, Dailiana T, Jurdi R. MR imaging of tophaceous gout. AJR Am J Roentgenol 1997; 168: 523–527

Diabetic Osteoarthropathy, Charcot Arthropathy

Donovan A, Schweitzer ME. Use of MR imaging in diagnosing diabetes-related pedal osteomyelitis. Radiographics 2010; 30: 723–736

Höpfner S, Krolak C, Kessler S et al. Preoperative imaging of Charcot neuroarthropathy in diabetic patients: comparison of ring PET, hybrid PET, and magnetic resonance imaging. Foot Ankle Int 2004; 25: 890–895

Ledermann HP, Morrison WB. Differential diagnosis of pedal osteomyelitis and diabetic neuroarthropathy: MR Imaging. Semin Musculoskelet Radiol 2005; 9: 272–283

Ranachowska C, Lass P, Korzon-Burakowska A, Dobosz M. Diagnostic imaging of the diabetic foot. Nucl Med Rev Cent East Eur 2010; 13: 18–22

Rozzanigo U, Tagliani A, Vittorini E, Pacchioni R, Brivio LR, Caudana R. Role of magnetic resonance imaging in the evaluation of diabetic foot with suspected osteomyelitis. Radiol Med (Torino) 2009; 114: 121–132

Schon LC, Easley ME, Weinfeld SB. Charcot neuroarthropathy of the foot and ankle. Clin Orthop Relat Res 1998: 116–31

Zampa V, Bargellini I, Rizzo L et al. Role of dynamic MRI in the follow-up of acute Charcot foot in patients with diabetes mellitus. Skeletal Radiol 2011; 40: 991–999

Osteitis, Osteomyelitis

Ahmadi ME, Morrison WB, Carrino JA, Schweitzer ME, Raikin SM, Ledermann HP. Neuropathic arthropathy of the foot with and without superimposed osteomyelitis: MR imaging characteristics. Radiology 2006; 238: 622–631

Collins MS, Schaar MM, Wenger DE, Mandrekar JN. T1-weighted MRI characteristics of pedal osteomyelitis. AJR Am J Roentgenol 2005; 185: 386–393

Donovan A, Schweitzer ME. Use of MR imaging in diagnosing diabetes-related pedal osteomyelitis. Radiographics 2010; 30: 723–736

Johnson PW, Collins MS, Wenger DE. Diagnostic utility of T1-weighted MRI characteristics in evaluation of osteomyelitis of the foot. AJR Am J Roentgenol 2009; 192: 96–100

Ledermann HP, Morrison WB, Schweitzer ME. MR image analysis of pedal osteomyelitis: distribution, patterns of spread, and frequency of associated ulceration and septic arthritis. Radiology 2002; 223: 747–755

Toledano TR, Fatone EA, Weis A, Cotten A, Beltran J. MRI evaluation of bone marrow changes in the diabetic foot: a practical approach. Semin Musculoskelet Radiol 2011; 15: 257–268

Chapter 10

Tumorlike Lesions

10 Tumorlike Lesions

A. Staebler

10.1 Osteoid Osteoma

Definition

Osteoid osteoma consists of a soft or partially calcified, reddish nidus surrounded by a zone of reactive sclerosis. It is a benign bone-forming tumor characterized by its small size, limited growth potential, and relatively severe pain.

Symptoms

- Pain disproportionate to the size of the tumor
- Pain worse at night
- Pain relieved by salicylates

Predisposing Factors

- Peak age incidence in adolescents and young adults
- 50% of cases in the second decade of life, 20% each in the first and third decades (90% of all osteoid osteomas occur before age 40), with the remaining 10% occurring between the ages of 40–49 years
- Males predominate by 2:1

Anatomy and Pathology

Between 10 and 12% of all benign bone tumors are osteoid osteomas, which account for 2 to 3% of all primary bone tumors. Osteoid osteoma is less than 1.5 cm in diameter. The actual tumor, or nidus, consists of osteoid tissue with a variable degree of calcification and ossification. Osteoid osteomas are most commonly located in the cortex but may also arise in periosteum or cancellous bone. Osteoid osteomas can also be classified as intra-articular or extra-articular. Intra-articular lesions lead to reactive or concomitant synovitis and monoarthritis, and there may be associated growth stimulation and joint deformities (as in the hip). Approximately 13% of osteoid osteomas are intra-articular.

Approximately 31% of osteoid osteomas are located in the femur (femoral neck and trochanter), 25% in the tibia, 11% in the foot, 10% in the hand, 6% in the humerus, and 5% in the vertebral column. Typical sites of occurrence in the foot are the neck of the talus (periosteal location) and the talar trochlea. They may also arise in other tarsal bones such as the calcaneus or cuboid and in the phalanges.

Imaging (▶ Fig. 10.1 and ▶ Fig. 10.2)

Radiographs

Radiographs show a frequently eccentric zone of reactive sclerosis or hyperostosis in a long bone with thickening of the diaphyseal or metaphyseal cortex and no demonstrable nidus. The soft nidus may undergo variable ossification and appear as a rounded osteolytic zone with relatively well-defined margins. It resembles a bone sequestrum in chronic osteomyelitis, except that the osteoid osteoma nidus is small and surrounded by considerable new bone formation and sclerosis.

Ultrasound

Not indicated. Sonography may detect a joint effusion associated with juxta-articular lesions.

CT

High-resolution thin-slice CT with multiplanar reformatting (MPR) is the best method for detection and localization of the nidus. The degree of nidus calcification is visible on CT scans. CT should be used whenever MRI shows an unexplained focus of intense bone edema, and osteoid osteoma is suspected on clinical grounds, even though MRI has not shown a definite nidus. The nidus may be purely osteolytic or may show variable degrees of calcification or ossification. A periosteal nidus is often heavily ossified and outlined by a faint lucent rim.

Bone Scintigraphy

Radionuclide bone scans are no longer used for this indication. They could theoretically be used to exclude osteoid osteoma, since the nidus shows strong tracer uptake.

MRI

Interpretation Checklist

- Osteoid osteoma with a detectable nidus
- Precise location of the nidus and its accessibility to a radiofrequency probe
- Synovitis in an adjacent joint
- Secondary changes such as growth disturbance or secondary osteoarthritis

Examination Technique

- *Standard protocol:* prone position, high-resolution multichannel coil
- *Sequences:*
  - Water-sensitive sequences for detection of reactive bone edema
  - Contrast administration with frequency-selective fat suppression to localize the nidus and display reactive tissue changes such as enhancing bone edema and synovitis
  - Sagittal and coronal PD-weighted fat-sat
  - Coronal T1-weighted
  - Axial T2-weighted (angled to plane of ankle joint)
  - Axial and sagittal T1-weighted fat-sat after contrast administration

MRI Findings

The hallmark of osteoid osteoma is an intense, rounded or hemispherical focus of bone edema. The nidus is located at the virtual center of the bone edema. It has variable signal intensity in water-sensitive sequences, ranging from hypointense to hyperintense depending on the degree of vascularity and ossification. A characteristic feature is intense bone edema that does not have an obvious cause. The bone edema is relatively well demarcated from nonedematous bone marrow. Usually the

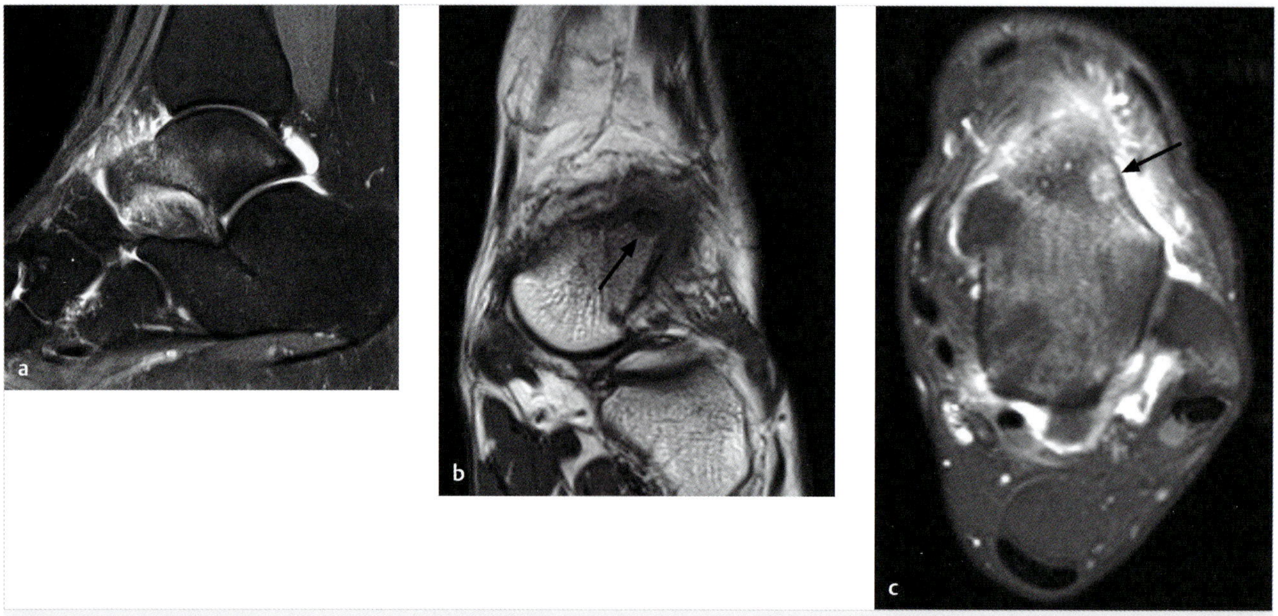

Fig. 10.1 a–c Typical imaging appearance of osteoid osteoma in a 26-year-old woman with a 6-year history of ankle swelling and pain that was worse at night and relieved by aspirin.
a Sagittal PD-weighted fat-sat image shows bone marrow edema in the talar neck with conspicuous edema. Fluid accumulation is noted in adjacent soft tissues.
b Coronal T1-weighted image demonstrates a hypointense lentiform lesion approximately 6 mm in diameter (arrow) on the subperiosteal bone surface of the anterolateral talar neck.
c Axial T1-weighted fat-sat image after contrast administration shows enhancement of the lentiform lesion (arrow), pronounced synovitis throughout the ankle joint, and diffuse enhancement in the local soft tissues on the anterolateral aspect of the ankle joint.

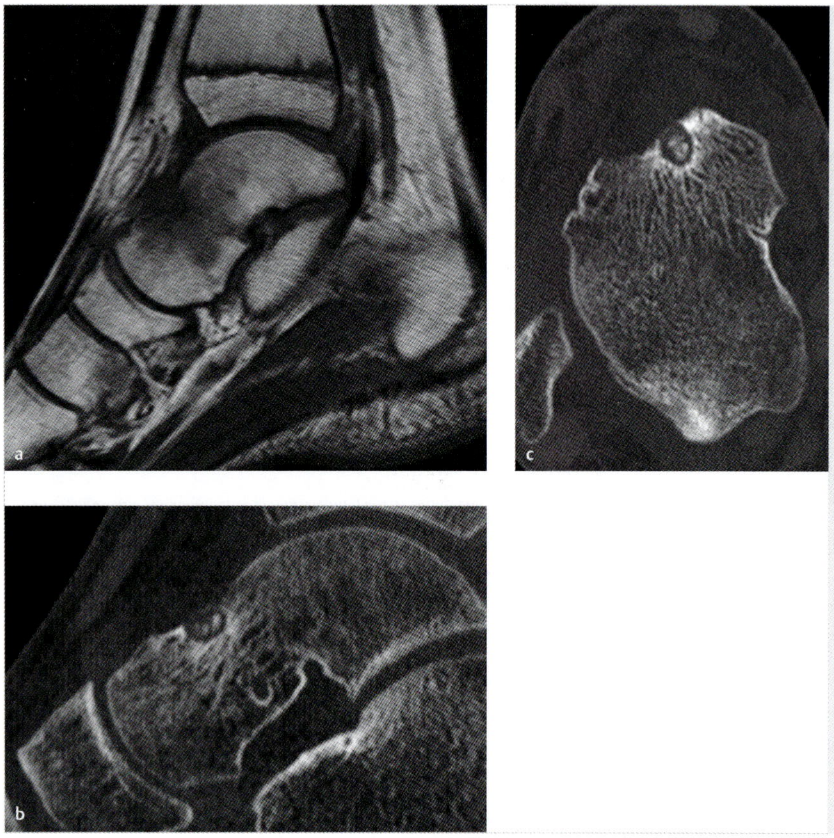

Fig. 10.2 a–c Osteoid osteoma in a 12-year-old boy.
a Sagittal T1-weighted MRI shows an edematous zone at the junction of the neck and body of the talus.
b Sagittal reformatted CT of the edematous zone demonstrates an osteoid osteoma on the dorsal aspect of the talar neck with an elliptical osteolytic lucency in the cortex, a sclerotic rim, and a central sclerotic nidus.
c Axial reformatted CT shows the subperiosteal location of the sclerotic nidus.

fatty marrow signal is not completely lost on T1-weighted images. Intra-articular and periosteal lesions are often associated with synovitis, and reactive hyperemia may lead to increased bone growth (e.g., coxa magna) in patients who have not reached skeletal maturity.

Imaging Recommendation

Modality of choice: MRI is the recommended initial study for investigating unexplained pain in younger patients. If osteoid osteoma is suspected in a patient with intense, localized bone edema but no clearly detectable nidus, CT should be performed to identify the nidus.

Differential Diagnosis

- Subacute or chronic osteomyelitis
- (Periosteal) osteosarcoma
- Ewing sarcoma
- Fatigue or stress fracture
- Cortical hemangioma (extremely rare)

Treatment

- Radiofrequency ablation or laser ablation
- Surgical removal (by drilling or excision)

Prognosis, Complications

The overresection of an osteoid osteoma may lead to pathologic fracture or instability. Excessive heat generation during radiofrequency or laser ablation in the spinal column may result in neurogenic injury or spinal cord damage.

10.2 Lipoma

Definition

The World Health Organization (WHO) defines lipoma as a benign neoplasm composed of adipocytes, which develops in the medullary cavity, cortex, or surface of a bone or within soft tissue.

Symptoms

Lipomas are generally asymptomatic. Intraosseous lipomas are usually detected incidentally. Soft-tissue lipomas can be detected by their local mass effect; pressure from the lesions may lead to bone resorption and occasionally to clinical complaints. Soft-tissue lipomas may become symptomatic through their mass effect on blood vessels and nerves, for example. Calcaneal lipomas have been described that mimic plantar fasciitis.

Predisposing Factors

None are known.

Anatomy and Pathology

Soft-tissue lipomas are the most common tumors in the human body. They are composed of lobulated fatty tissue that may contain zones of increased density, ossifications, and internal septa. Intraosseous lesions often display regressive changes with necrotic areas, possible calcifications, and occasional zones of pseudocystic liquefaction. Differential diagnosis is difficult in lesions that show regressive changes with cyst formation. There are reports of lesions classified radiographically as calcaneal lipomas that were identified histologically as bone cysts. Many lesions are not true neoplasms but are regressive changes in an anatomical area that contains copious fat.

Intraosseous lipomas in the foot occur predominantly in the calcaneus between the principal trabecular stress lines.

Imaging

Radiographs

Radiographs show a well-circumscribed elliptical osteolytic area, often outlined by a sclerotic rim and with typical central calcification or ossification in a setting of fat necrosis. Cyst formation and fat necrosis are associated with peripheral calcifications in the cyst. The calcaneus is a typical site of occurrence for intraosseous lipoma.

Ultrasound

Ultrasonography demonstrates a circumscribed, usually subcutaneous mass with an organized internal echo pattern. The mass is well demarcated in dynamic scans and is hyperechoic to subcutaneous fat.

CT (▶ Fig. 10.3)

CT shows an osteolytic lesion of fat attenuation. It is usually well encapsulated with a distinct sclerotic rim. Calcifications, ossifications, and cystic components may be visible at the center of the mass. The soft-tissue portion of the mass has fat attenuation and may contain septations.

MRI

Interpretation Checklist

- Fatty tumor
- Calcifications or ossifications
- Regressive cystic changes
- Solid enhancing soft-tissue structures inside the fat-containing mass or at its periphery
- Size of osteolytic area
- Risk for spontaneous or surgical fracture

Examination Technique

T1-weighted and frequency-selective fat-suppressed sequences are mandatory. If unenhanced images show evidence of intralesional solid tissue not corresponding to fat, contrast-enhanced images should be acquired, preferably with frequency-selective fat suppression, in order to detect any enhancing solid tumor components.

- *Standard protocol:* prone position, high-resolution multichannel coil
- *Sequences:*
  - Sagittal and coronal PD-weighted fat-sat
  - Coronal T1-weighted
  - Axial T2-weighted (angled to plane of ankle joint)
  - Axial and sagittal T1-weighted fat-sat after contrast administration

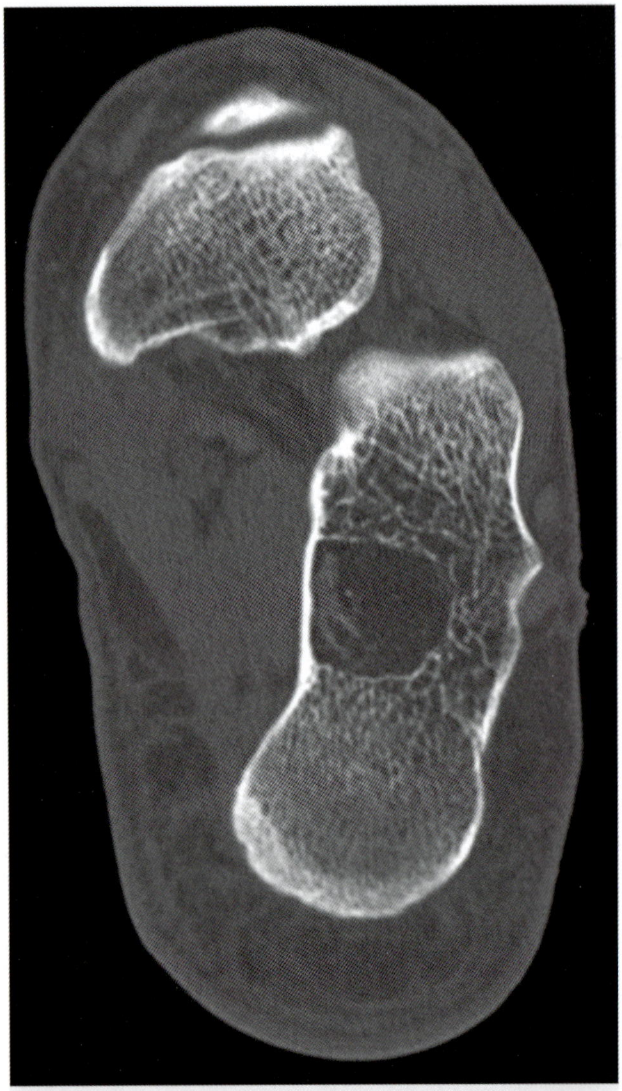

Fig. 10.3 **Intraosseous lipoma detected incidentally in the left calcaneus of an asymptomatic 46-year-old man.** Axial CT scan (0.5-mm slice thickness) shows an intraosseous lipoma extending to the medial cortex with no evidence of cortical thinning. Fine, faint calcifications are visible within the lipoma near its medial border.

MRI Findings (▶ Fig. 10.4 and ▶ Fig. 10.5)

Lipomas have a very characteristic signal pattern based on their signal intensity in T1-weighted sequences. They have the high signal intensity of subcutaneous fat in fast T2-weighted spin-echo sequences, while they appear as signal voids in frequency-selective fat-suppressed sequences. They do not enhance after IV contrast administration. Some lesions contain fine fibrous septa and have capsulelike margins. If regressive cystic changes develop in intraosseous lipomas, possibly associated with calcifications and ossifications, the necrotic or cystic components will have water-equivalent signal intensities while calcifications and ossifications appear as signal voids.

Imaging Recommendation

Modalities of choice: sonography for soft-tissue lipomas. If ultrasound shows a growth tendency or equivocal findings, MRI should be employed to detect or exclude a liposarcoma. Preoperative MRI is useful for tumor localization and defining its relationship to blood vessels and nerves. CT can help narrow the differential diagnosis in difficult cases.

Differential Diagnosis

Differentiation from simple bone cysts is difficult in lesions with regressive cystic changes. Lesions with coarse calcifications and little fat may be difficult to distinguish from chondrosarcoma. The differential diagnosis should also include chondroma, chondromyxoid fibroma, and fibrous dysplasia.

Treatment

Lipomas that are not causing complaints do not require treatment. This particularly applies to lipomas of the calcaneus. Treatment by excision and cancellous bone grafting is reserved for lesions that pose a fracture risk or show signs of activation on MRI.

Prognosis, Complications

Since most intraosseous lipomas are detected incidentally, it is unlikely that complications will arise. There have been scattered reports of soft-tissue lipomas undergoing malignant transformation. Large calcaneal lipomas may cause a pathologic fracture.

10.3 Aneurysmal Bone Cyst

Definition

As defined by the WHO, an aneurysmal bone cyst is a benign cystic lesion composed of blood-filled spaces with connective tissue septa and giant cells. Aneurysmal bone cysts may occur as primary lesions or may develop secondarily in a pre-existing benign or malignant bone tumor or after trauma.

Symptoms

- Pain, usually mild
- Palpable swelling in some cases
- Occasionally manifested by a pathologic fracture

Predisposing Factors

Over 50% of cases occur in the second decade of life. Approximately 82% of patients are less than 22 years of age. Both sexes are affected equally. Approximately 8% of aneurysmal bone cysts are located in the foot and ankle region.

Anatomy and Pathology

Aneurysmal bone cysts are rare, comprising only about 1.0 to 3.4% of all bone tumors. The blood-filled channels that make up the tumor communicate with one another. The cyst contains fine internal septa, typically with a connective tissue that includes fibroblasts, giant cells, and osteoid. Irregular bony trabeculae may also be present.

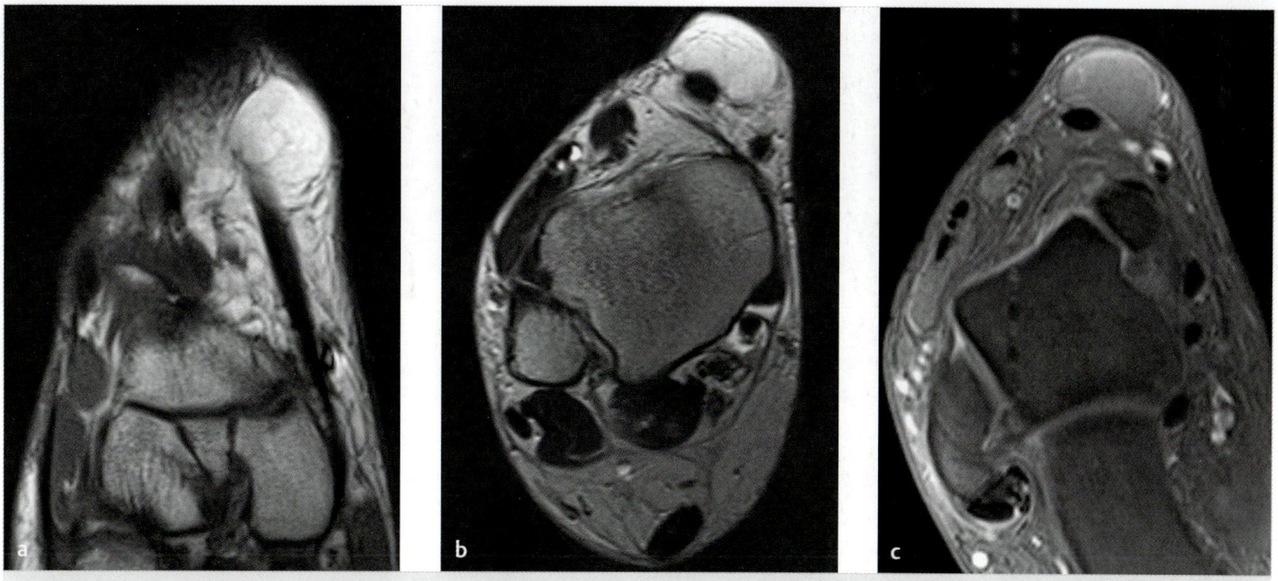

Fig. 10.4 a–c MRI examination of a 64-year-old woman with a circumscribed mass in the anteromedial ankle joint. MRI was ordered for further differentiation of the mass.
a Coronal T1-weighted image shows a spherical mass with internal fat intensity bordering on the anterior tibial tendon and located in subcutaneous fat at the level of the right ankle joint.
b Axial T2-weighted image shows the lipoma abutting on the anterior tibial tendon. The fatty tissue within the lipoma is permeated by fine septa.
c Axial T1-weighted fat-sat image after contrast administration. Since fat signals are suppressed in the fat-sat sequence, no enhancing soft tissue is visible within the lipoma.

Imaging

Radiographs

Radiographs show a cystic osteolytic area that may be rimmed by sclerosis. A thin periosteal shell is often present. The lesions display an eccentric metaphyseal or central diaphyseal location. Cysts also may be numerous and contain septa and trabeculae. The cortex may show sites of resorbing osteolysis.

Ultrasound

Not indicated.

MRI

Interpretation Checklist

- Aneurysmal bone cyst
- Fracture risk?
- Exact location in the bone
- Relationship to nearby joints (e.g., does the lesion involve the articular surface of the talar dome?)

Examination Technique

The most important sequences are T2-weighted and PD-weighted fat-sat images to detect fluid levels, which should be clearly visualized. Imaging planes that are parallel to the fluid levels (e.g., coronal slices of the ankle joint in the supine patient) will not detect them. Also, T2-weighted sequences are better than T1-weighted sequences for revealing sedimentation effects in the blood-filled spaces. Imaging in all three planes is helpful for joint evaluation. Intravenous contrast should be administered to identify enhancing solid tumor elements and provide differentiation from, say, a giant cell tumor. Internal fibrous septa will enhance after contrast administration. The contrast-enhanced images should be acquired with frequency-selective fat suppression.

- *Standard protocol:* prone position, high-resolution multichannel coil
- *Sequences:*
  - Sagittal, axial and coronal PD-weighted fat-sat
  - Coronal T1-weighted
  - Axial T2-weighted (angled to plane of ankle joint)
  - Axial and sagittal T1-weighted fat-sat after contrast administration

MRI Findings (▶ Fig. 10.6)

The relationship of the lesion to subchondral bone and articular cartilage is particularly important because a joint in close proximity to an aneurysmal bone cyst is at risk for deformity, softening, and articular surface collapse. Bone cysts on MRI invariably show cystic cavities, enhancing cyst wall, internal septa, a relatively hypointense margin, and are clearly demarcated from the bone and surrounding soft tissues. Less common features are scalloped margins and cortical expansion. Diverticula like outpouchings of the cyst walls may be found. Edema in adjacent soft tissues is rarely present.

Imaging Recommendation

Modality of choice: multiplanar MRI with T2-weighted sequences and IV contrast administration. Thin-slice CT may be helpful for assessing the fracture risk and the deformity of the subchondral plate.

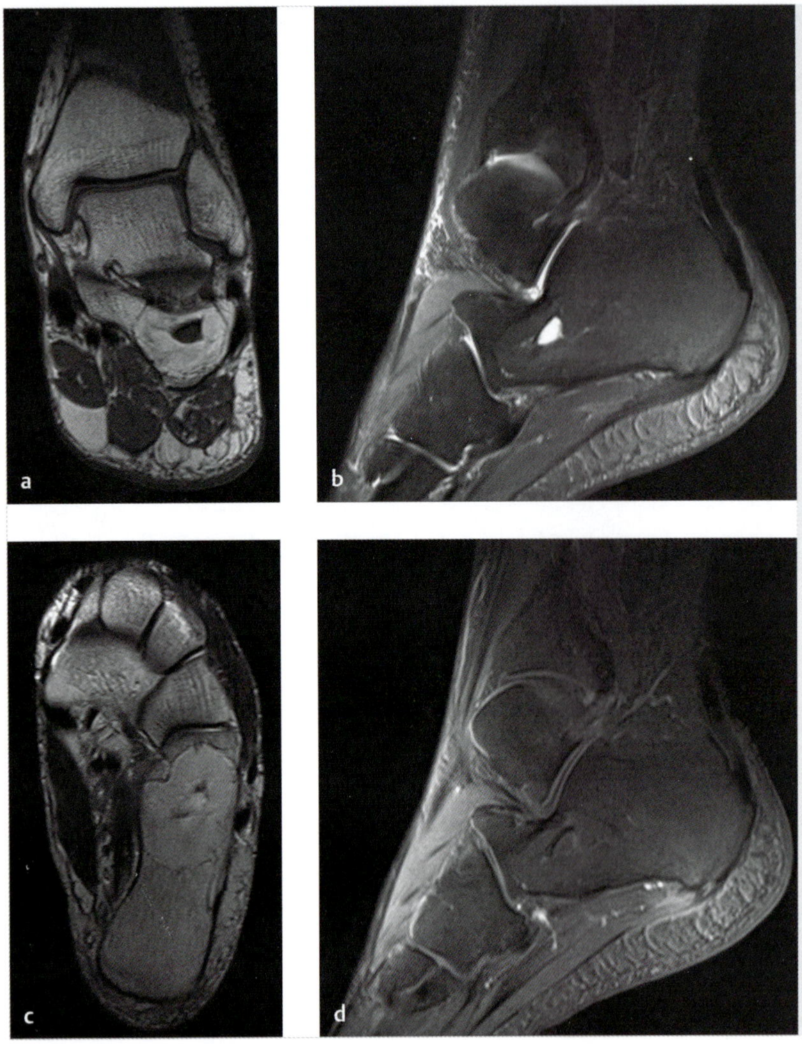

Fig. 10.5 a–d MRI of an intraosseous lipoma in the calcaneus, detected incidentally in a 66-year-old man with plantar fasciitis.
a Coronal T1-weighted image shows fat signal intensity within the calcaneus with central cystic or regressive change.
b Sagittal PD-weighted fat-sat image shows central cystic fat necrosis with homogeneous suppression of other internal signals from the lipoma.
c Axial T2-weighted image displays the lipoma in the calcaneus, which has an intact cortex.
d Sagittal T1-weighted fat-sat image after contrast administration shows no abnormal enhancement of the lipoma. Florid plantar fasciitis is noted as an incidental finding.

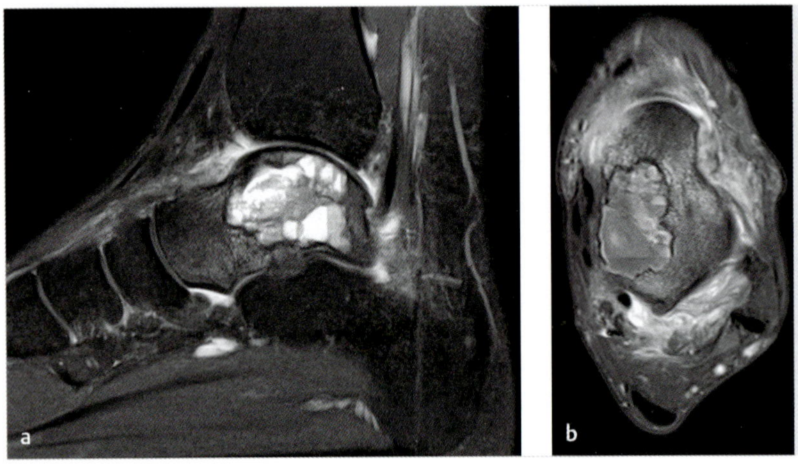

Fig. 10.6 a, b Aneurysmal bone cyst in a 24-year-old man with a 2-month history of ankle pain.
a Sagittal PD-weighted fat-sat image shows subtotal permeation of the talar dome by a cystic, multiloculated mass with blood–fluid levels, typical of an aneurysmal bone cyst.
b Axial T1-weighted fat-sat image after contrast administration shows an enhancing cyst wall with no increased enhancement of solid tissue components.

Differential Diagnosis

- *Giant cell tumor:* Patients with aneurysmal bone cyst are younger (first or second decade of life, versus third and fourth decades for giant cell tumors). Giant cell tumors may contain fluid levels and typically have solid enhancing components that are not present in an aneurysmal bone cyst.
- *Reparative giant cell granuloma:* This entity is very rare, and there are few published cases involving the foot. It is also referred to as a solid aneurysmal bone cyst. Reparative giant cell granuloma is histologically indistinguishable from a solid aneurysmal bone cyst, nor can it be positively distinguished from a brown tumor.

- *Brown tumor:* Brown tumors in a setting of secondary hyperparathyroidism are a very rare occurrence. In the foot, they have been described in the metatarsals and calcaneus.
- *Telangiectatic osteosarcoma:* This tumor may contain fluid levels. It is extremely rare in the foot.

Treatment

Formerly, aneurysmal bone cysts were treated by surgical resection or curettage followed by cancellous bone grafting of the defect. But given the relatively high recurrence rate of 20 to 70%, there have been recent attempts to find alternatives to extirpation: radionuclide therapy, arterial embolization therapy, and the instillation of sclerosing agents. Pharmacologic therapies also appear promising, and aneurysmal bone cysts have been successfully treated by radiotherapy.

Prognosis, Complications

High recurrence rates have been reported after surgical excision.

10.4 Hemangioma

Definition

The WHO describes a hemangioma as a vessel-forming neoplasm or a developmental disturbance of endothelial cells. The benign lesions are composed of capillaries or cavernous blood vessels. Hemangiomas occur in bones and soft tissues.

Symptoms

There have been no published reports of intraosseous hemangiomas in the bones of the foot. Soft-tissue hemangiomas may be located superficially in the skin or subcutaneous tissue or may infiltrate the muscle. There may be an associated local mass effect that causes complaints.

Predisposing Factors

None.

Anatomy and Pathology

The lesions consist of endothelial-lined cavities with no cellular atypias, no proliferative foci, and a fibrous wall. The cavities are usually filled with blood. Diffuse infiltration and permeation of muscles may occur in the soft tissues. Phleboliths may form at sites of venous ectasia.

Imaging

Radiographs

Hemangiomas do not occur in the bones of the foot. Soft-tissue hemangiomas may be detectable indirectly on radiographs by the presence of phleboliths and a soft-tissue opacity.

Ultrasound

A Doppler study may be performed for the differentiation of hemangioma, lymphangioma, and vascular malformation.

MRI

Interpretation Checklist

- Extent of the soft-tissue mass
- Involvement or infiltration of muscles
- Involvement of vessels and/or nerves

Examination Technique

Unenhanced T1-weighted images can help furnish a specific diagnosis by the detection of fat and blood constituents. T2-weighted images, fat-suppressed images, and fat-suppressed T1-weighted images after contrast administration will aid in delineation and classification of the lesion.

- *Standard protocol:* prone position, high-resolution multichannel coil
- *Sequences:*
  - Sagittal and coronal PD-weighted fat-sat
  - Coronal T1-weighted
  - Axial T2-weighted (angled to plane of ankle joint)
  - Axial and sagittal T1-weighted fat-sat after contrast administration

MRI Findings (▶ Fig. 10.7 and ▶ Fig. 10.8)

- Circumscribed or diffusely permeating soft-tissue mass with low T1-weighted signal intensity
- Typical areas of high signal intensity representing fatty components or blood constituents
- Typical very high signal intensity is found in water-sensitive and T2-weighted sequences
- Possible signal voids from phleboliths

Imaging Recommendation

Modality of choice: contrast-enhanced MRI to demonstrate extent, infiltration or permeation of muscle, and neurovascular involvement prior to possible surgery.

Differential Diagnosis

- *Lymphangioma:* A cystlike, frequently lobulated mass of water signal intensity is seen in all pulse sequences; does not enhance after IV contrast administration.
- *Ganglion cysts:* These are sometimes more lobulated, have water signal intensity in all sequences, and show slight peripheral rim enhancement with no solid tissue components. Ganglion cysts arise from the mucoid degeneration of a capsuloligamentous structure and expand into soft tissue or into bone, establishing contact with the bone surface at the site of a ligament attachment.
- *Paget disease:* Like hemangioma, Paget disease exhibits a honeycomb structure with thickened trabeculae.

Treatment

Hemangioma may be left untreated, but troublesome symptomatic lesions may be excised or treated locally by sclerotherapy, alcohol injection, or interstitial laser therapy. Radiotherapy may be used if needed.

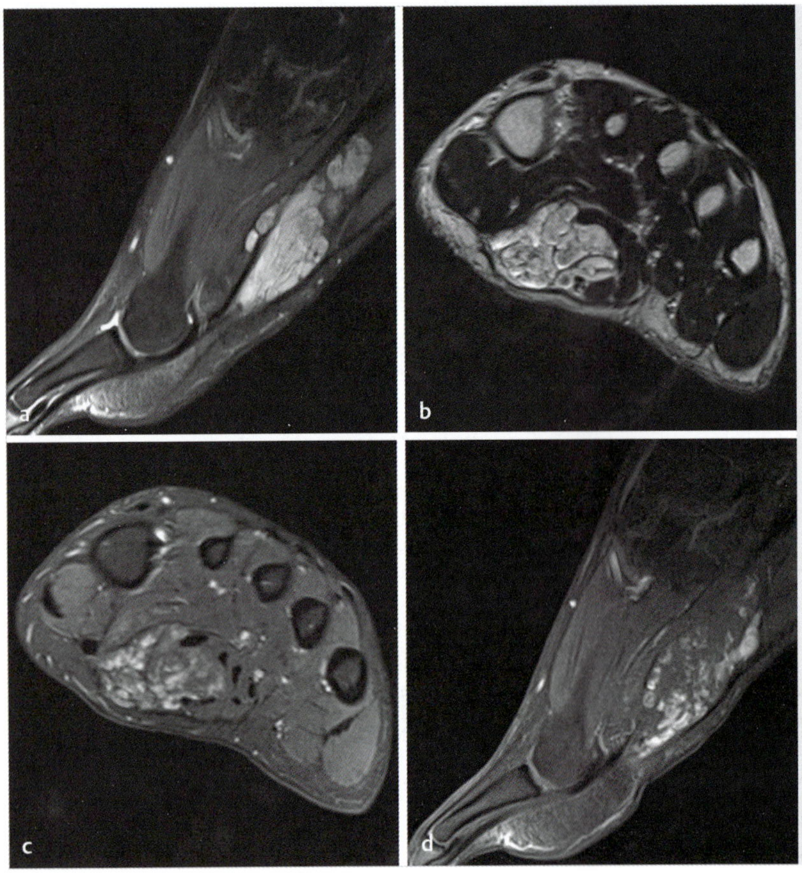

Fig. 10.7 a–d Typical MRI features of a soft-tissue hemangioma in a 20-year-old man referred with an indeterminate mass in the plantar soft tissues.
a Sagittal PD-weighted fat-sat image shows a diffuse, hyperintense mass in the left plantar soft tissues along the first through third metatarsals, displacing the tendons and muscles and showing intermuscular extension into the plantar arch.
b Axial T2-weighted image shows typical high signal intensity from fat components and blood constituents.
c Axial T1-weighted fat-sat image after contrast administration shows a spongy, hyperperfused soft-tissue mass producing a local mass effect.
d Sagittal T1-weighted fat-sat image after contrast administration. Fat suppression in this sequence displays the relatively large lipomatous component of the hemangioma.

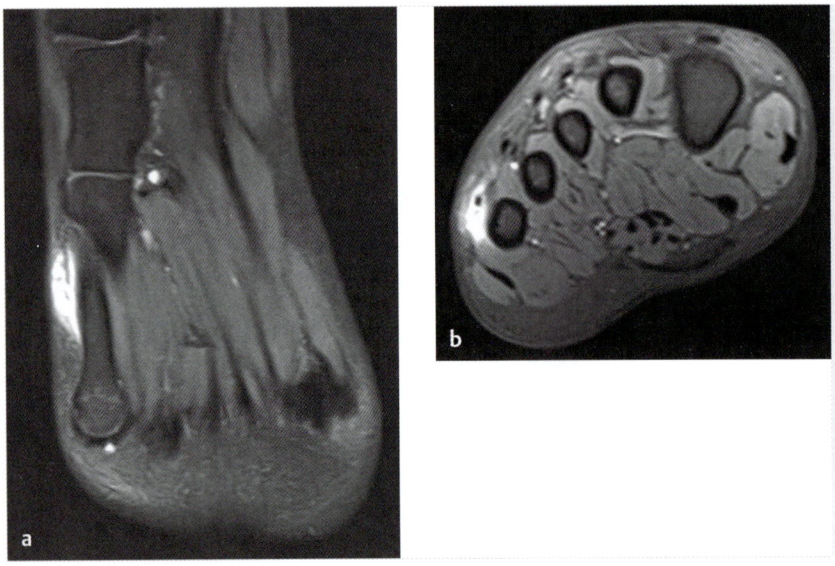

Fig. 10.8 a, b Example of a somewhat atypical soft-tissue hemangioma without a fatty component.
a Coronal PD-weighted fat-sat image shows a dorsolateral hemangioma of high signal intensity partially involving the extensor tendon along the fifth metatarsal.
b Axial T1-weighted fat-sat image after contrast administration shows intense enhancement of the mass.

Prognosis, Complications

- Hemangiomas are often not fully responsive to local treatments.
- Hemangiomas do not undergo secondary malignant transformation.
- Complications may result from tissue damage caused by local therapy.

10.5 Ganglion

Definition

Ganglia, also called ganglion cysts, occur within bones and soft tissues. They arise from the mucoid degeneration of fibrous ligamentous tissue and are bounded by a fibrous wall. Unlike degenerative subchondral cysts, they do not communicate with the joint cavity, and the overlying articular cartilage is intact.

Symptoms

Intraosseous ganglion cysts may be painful, especially if MRI shows adjacent enhancing bone edema.

Predisposing Factors

- More common in males than females
- Mechanical loads predispose to the development of ganglion cysts

Anatomy and Pathology

Ganglion cysts, whether intraosseous or in soft tissue, result from excessive loads on fibrous ligamentous structures leading to mucoid degeneration. Through the vascularization of a ligament at its attachment to bone, fluid deposition occurs and causes initial bone resorption, presumably due to intraligamentous pressure. Once an intraosseous lesion has formed, the ganglion cyst can develop further on its own. Intraosseous ganglion cysts are self-limiting and do not transcend the boundaries of the affected bone. All cases must have a demonstrable connection between the ganglion cyst and bone surface. The connection extends into the attachment of a capsuloligamentous structure but does not damage the hyaline articular cartilage. Intraosseous ganglion cysts of the tarsus occur mostly in the talus. Sites of predilection in soft tissues are the sinus tarsi, tarsal tunnel, and plantar tarsus at the level of the tarsometatarsal joint line.

Imaging

Radiographs

An intraosseous ganglion appears as a lytic lesion with a sclerotic rim. Often the connection with the ligament attachment is visible in the radiograph.

Ultrasound

The ultrasound scan shows a localized, rounded, echo-free mass arising from a joint or tendon sheath. It has echo-free contents and shows posterior acoustic enhancement. Often it is poorly compressible with the probe but can be aspirated with a percutaneous needle, if necessary under sonographic guidance.

MRI

Interpretation Checklist

- Accurately describe the ganglion cyst and its extent, identifying its site of origin whenever possible (this may be difficult if a long stalk is present) as an aid to preoperative planning
- Check presence of intraosseous ganglion cysts
- Look out for effects of pressure from the cysts on adjacent structures (especially nerves [tarsal tunnel syndrome])
- Determine degree of capsuloligamentous pathology and degree of vascularity
- Exclude a different mass

Examination Technique

The fluid-filled cysts have high signal intensity in T2-weighted and PD-weighted fat-sat sequences. Imaging should employ thin slices and an expanded matrix for improved resolution to define the connection of the intraosseous ganglion cyst to the ligament attachment. Contrast-enhanced sequences should employ frequency-selective fat suppression for the sensitive detection of mild-to-moderate degrees of peripheral enhancement. High-resolution cartilage images are necessary for differentiation from subchondral cysts.

- *Standard protocol:* prone position, high-resolution multichannel coil
- *Sequences:*
  - Sagittal and coronal PD-weighted fat-sat
  - Coronal T1-weighted
  - Axial T2-weighted (angled to plane of ankle joint)
  - Axial and sagittal T1-weighted fat-sat after contrast administration

MRI Findings (▶ Fig. 10.9 and ▶ Fig. 10.10)

Ganglion cysts located in bone or soft tissue have water signal intensity in all pulse sequences and show only peripheral, generally faint contrast enhancement. The chronic pressure from the ganglion causes osteonecrosis at the cyst margins. With symptomatic ganglion cysts, enhancing bone edema may be observed in adjacent bone marrow. Circumscribed vascularization is often noted at the fibro-osseous junction with the attaching ligament structure, creating a starting point for development of the intraosseous ganglion cyst.

Imaging Recommendation

Modalities of choice: Ultrasound is useful for the detection of soft-tissue ganglia. Intraosseous ganglion cysts are best demonstrated by high-resolution MRI. Contrast administration is occasionally helpful for distinguishing between symptomatic and asymptomatic ganglion cysts and can narrow the differential diagnosis in equivocal cases.

Differential Diagnosis

- Juvenile bone cyst
- Aneurysmal bone cyst
- Hemangioma
- Lymphangioma

Treatment

- Excision of the cyst into its site of origin
- Cancellous bone grafting of intraosseous ganglion cysts

Prognosis, Complications

Soft-tissue ganglia may cause nerve compression.

10.6 Pigmented Villonodular Synovitis

Definition

Pigmented villonodular synovitis (PVNS) is a diffuse type of giant cell tumor that is associated with a destructive proliferation of synoviumlike cells and often infiltrates the bone. The tumor may occur in synovial membrane, bursae, joints, and

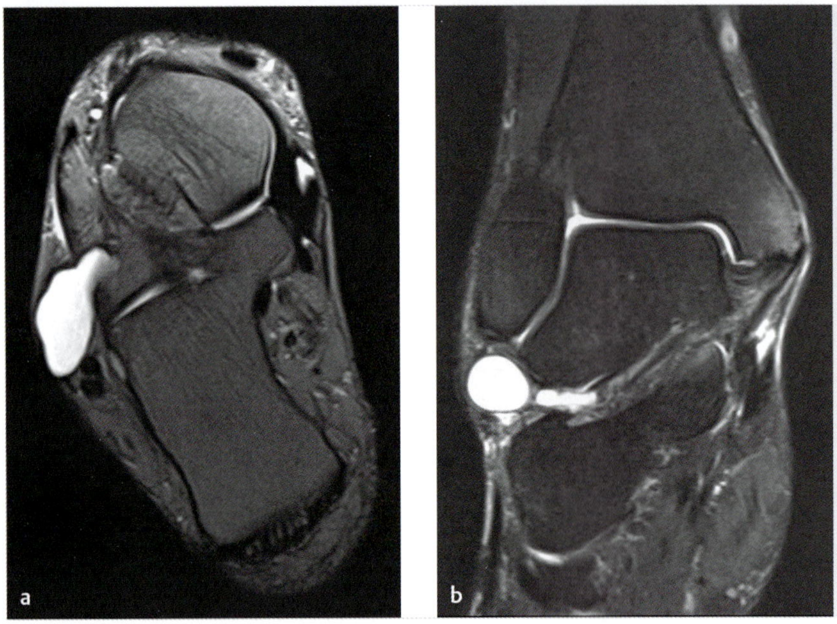

Fig. 10.9 a, b Ganglion in a 52-year-old woman with recurrent swelling and pain of the ankle joint.
a Axial T2-weighted image shows a cystic mass extending far into the soft tissues over the lateral malleolus anterior to the peroneal tendons.
b Coronal PD-weighted fat-sat image shows a ganglion on the subtalar joint arising from the sinus tarsi and talocalcaneal ligament (cervical ligament). The image displays the origin of the ganglion with smaller cysts radiating into portions of the ligament.

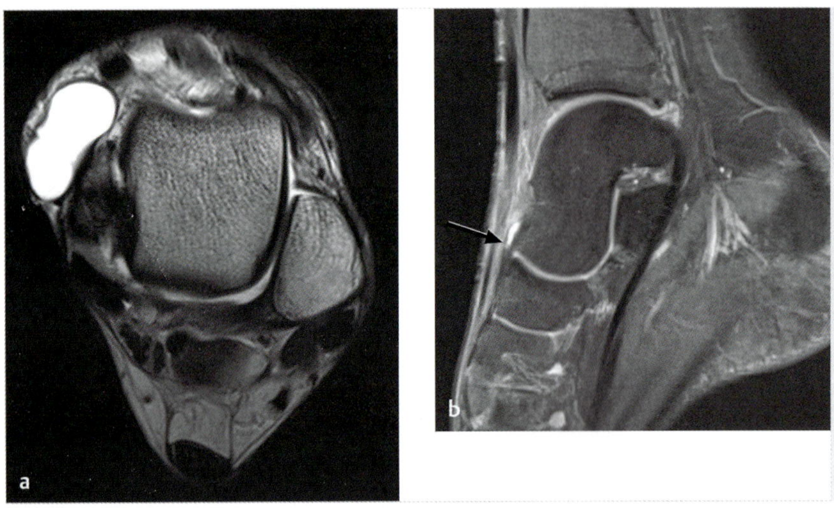

Fig. 10.10 a, b Investigation of unexplained swelling over the lateral malleolus in a 34-year-old woman with a known ganglion cyst.
a Axial T2-weighted image reveals a large cystic mass with a fine pseudocapsule.
b Sagittal PD-weighted fat-sat image demonstrates the origin of the ganglion (arrow) with a small, oblong cystic protrusion in the talonavicular joint capsule.

tendon sheaths and belongs to the class of fibrohistiocytic soft-tissue tumors.

Symptoms

Many patients have long-standing, nonspecific joint complaints with associated swelling or effusion.

Predisposing Factors

- More common in young adults, with both sexes affected equally
- 2 to 10% of PVNS cases involve the joints of the foot or ankle
- Possible association with athletic activity and sports-related trauma

Anatomy and Pathology

PVNS is characterized by a diffuse, focal, or nodular involvement of one joint (monoarticular) with reddish-brown staining of the tissue due to previous hemorrhage and iron deposition.

Imaging

Radiographs

Radiographs in the diffuse form of PVNS show soft-tissue opacities that resemble the hemorrhages found in hemophilia and gout. Bony involvement leads to cystlike osteolytic areas with sclerotic margins that are caused by pressure and often involve both of the articulating bone ends. The joint space remains unaffected for some time.

Ultrasound

Ultrasound scanning can demonstrate effusion and synovial proliferation in the joint cavity.

MRI

Interpretation Checklist

- Decreased signal intensity due to spin dephasing from blood breakdown products
- Blood flow to areas of synovial proliferation

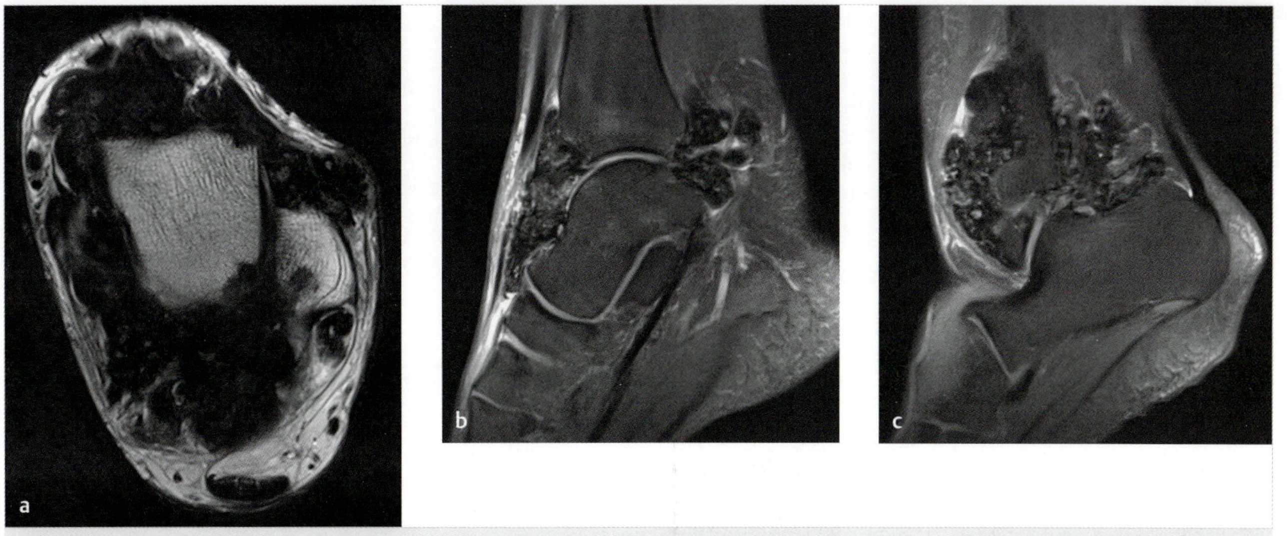

Fig. 10.11 a–c Typical MRI appearance of pigmented villonodular synovitis (PVNS) with extensive involvement of the ankle joint in a 32-year-old man with a long history of ankle pain and swelling.
a Axial T2-weighted image shows plaquelike tissue thickening all around the ankle joint with conspicuous, hypointense areas of synovial proliferation.
b Sagittal T1-weighted fat-sat image after contrast administration reveals a combination of diffuse and nodular, tumorlike proliferates showing moderate enhancement.
c Sagittal T1-weighted fat-sat image after contrast administration. PVNS shows markedly low signal intensity in all pulse sequences due to hemosiderin deposits.

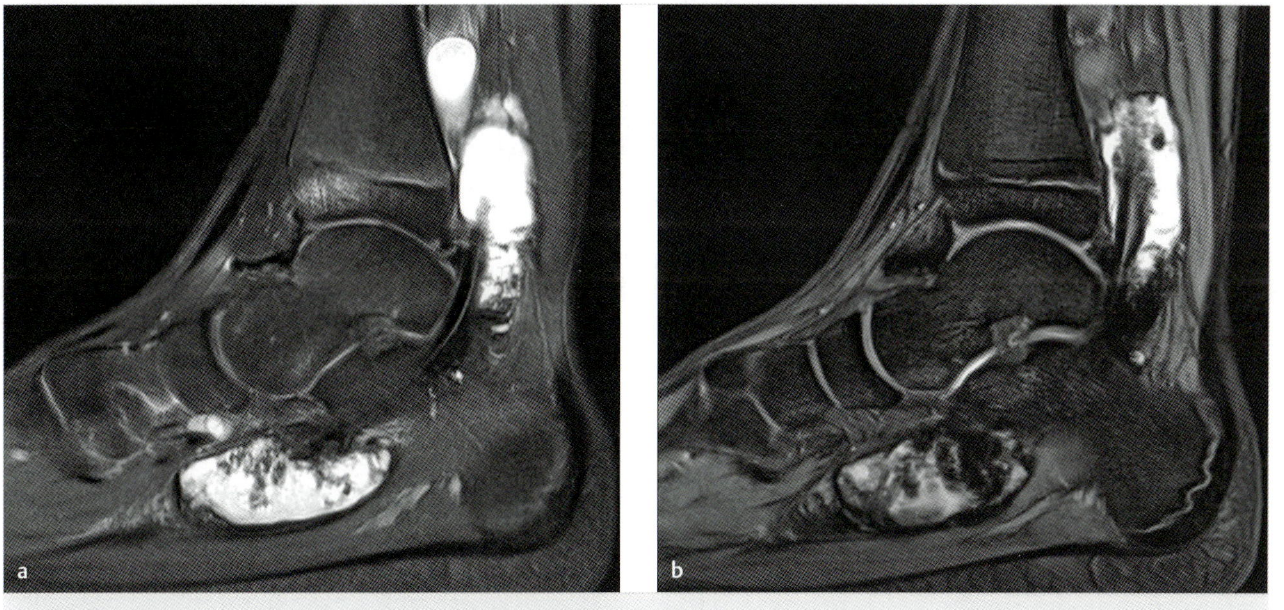

Fig. 10.12 a, b Pigmented villonodular synovitis (PVNS) in a 14-year-old boy.
a Sagittal PD-weighted fat-sat image shows polypous, villuslike sites of synovial proliferation along the flexor tendon sheaths.
b Sagittal T2-weighted gradient echo sequence. Complete signal voids are a common finding in susceptibility-sensitive gradient echo sequences and are typical of PVNS.

- Articular cartilage lesions
- Infiltration of the bone

Examination Technique

A standard protocol with unenhanced T1-weighted and PD-weighted fat-sat sequences will detect effusion, synovial proliferation, and sites of bone destruction that are in contact with the joint. Synovial proliferation has markedly low signal intensity in the susceptibility-sensitive gradient echo sequence due to the presence of iron and hemosiderin deposits. IV contrast administration is helpful because sites of synovial proliferation in PVNS are perfused with blood and appear hyperintense on frequency-selective fat-sat images, even in remote joint areas.

- *Standard protocol:* prone position, high-resolution multichannel coil
- *Sequences:*
    - Sagittal and coronal PD-weighted fat-sat
    - Coronal T1-weighted
    - Axial T2-weighted (angled to plane of ankle joint)
    - Axial and sagittal T1-weighted fat-sat after contrast administration

MRI findings (▶ Fig. 10.11 and ▶ Fig. 10.12)

Areas of synovial proliferation may be focal, tumorlike (nodular), diffusely distributed in the joint with plaquelike tissue thickening, or may appear as polypous, villuslike proliferative foci. Markedly low signal intensity in all pulse sequences is particularly evident on susceptibility-sensitive gradient echo sequences, and complete signal voids are often found. With intraosseous involvement, images will almost always show the bone lesion communicating with the bone surface and with the joint.

Imaging Recommendation

Modality of choice: high-resolution multiplanar MRI using gradient echo sequences and IV contrast administration.

Differential Diagnosis

- Proliferative synovitis
- Chondromatosis with associated synovitis
- Synovial hemangioma (hyperintense on T2-weighted images, unlike PVNS)
- Intracapsular osteoid osteoma with reactive synovitis
- Amyloidosis with intraosseous lesions

Treatment

Treatment consists of surgical removal. This can sometimes be done endoscopically for ankle and subtalar joint lesions. There have been attempts to lower the recurrence rate by combining surgery with radiosynoviorthesis.

Prognosis, Complications

Often the tumor cannot be removed completely, which accounts for the relatively high recurrence rate. The process may eventually lead to joint destruction.

10.7 Bibliography

Osteoid Osteoma

Allen SD, Saifuddin A. Imaging of intra-articular osteoid osteoma. Clin Radiol 2003; 58: 845–852

Dahin DC. Bone Tumors. Springfield: CC Thomas; 1989

Freyschmidt J, Ostertag H, Jundt G. Knochentumoren. 3rded. Berlin: Springer; 2010: 113

Rhee JH, Lewis RB, Murphey MD. Primary osseous tumors of the foot and ankle. Magn Reson Imaging Clin N Am 2008; 16: 71–91, vi

Schajowicz F. Tumors and Tumorlike Lesions of Bone and Joints. Berlin: Springer; 1994

Van Dyck P, Vanhoenacker FM, Gielen JL, De Schepper AM, Parizel PM. Imaging of tumours of the foot and ankle. JBR-BTR 2004; 87: 252–257

Woertler K. Soft tissue masses in the foot and ankle: characteristics on MR Imaging. Semin Musculoskelet Radiol 2005; 9: 227–242

Lipoma

Diard F, Hauger O, Moinard M, Brunot S, Marcet B. Pseudo-cysts, lipomas, infarcts and simple cysts of the calcaneus: are there different or related lesions? JBR-BTR 2007; 90: 315–324

Freyschmidt J, Ostertag H, Jundt G. Knochentumoren. 3rded. Berlin: Springer; 2010: 555

Greenspan A, Raiszadeh K, Riley GM, Matthews D. Intraosseous lipoma of the calcaneus. Foot Ankle Int 1997; 18: 53–56

Huch K, Werner M, Puhl W, Delling G. Calcaneal cyst: a classical simple bone cyst? [Article in German] Z Orthop Ihre Grenzgeb 2004; 142: 625–630

Karthik K, Aarthi S. Intraosseous lipoma of the calcaneus mimicking plantar fascitis. Foot Ankle Surg 2011; 17: 25–27. doi:10.1016/j.fas.2010.10.004

Aneurysmal Bone Cyst

Bush CH, Adler Z, Drane WE, Tamurian R, Scarborough MT, Gibbs CP. Percutaneous radionuclide ablation of axial aneurysmal bone cysts. AJR Am J Roentgenol 2010; 194: W84-W90

Cebesoy O, Karakok M, Arpacioglu O, Baltaci ET. Brown tumor with atypical localization in a normocalcemic patient. Arch Orthop Trauma Surg 2007; 127: 577–580

Chowdhry M, Chandrasekar CR, Mohammed R, Grimer RJ. Curettage of aneurysmal bone cysts of the feet. Foot Ankle Int 2010; 31: 131–135

Cottalorda J, Bourelle S. Modern concepts of primary aneurysmal bone cyst. Arch Orthop Trauma Surg 2007; 127: 105–114

Dahlin DC, McLeod RA. Aneurysmal bone cyst and other nonneoplastic conditions. Skeletal Radiol 1982; 8: 243–250

Davies AM, Evans N, Mangham DC, Grimer RJ. MR imaging of brown tumour with fluid-fluid levels: a report of three cases. Eur Radiol 2001; 11: 1445–1449

Doğan A, Algün E, Kisli E, Harman M, Kösem M, Tosun N. Calcaneal brown tumor with primary hyperparathyroidism caused by parathyroid carcinoma: an atypical localization. J Foot Ankle Surg 2004; 43: 248–251

Freyschmidt J, Ostertag H, Jundt G. Knochentumoren. 3rd ed. Berlin: Springer; 2010

Ilaslan H, Sundaram M, Unni KK. Solid variant of aneurysmal bone cysts in long tubular bones: giant cell reparative granuloma. AJR Am J Roentgenol 2003; 180: 1681–1687

Keenan S, Bui-Mansfield LT. Musculoskeletal lesions with fluid-fluid level: a pictorial essay. J Comput Assist Tomogr 2006; 30: 517–524

Lingg G, Roessner A, Fiedler V et al. Das reparative Riesenzellgranulom der Extremitäten. Fortschr Röntgenstr 1985; 142: 185–188

Mankin HJ, Hornicek FJ, Ortiz-Cruz E, Villafuerte J, Gebhardt MC. Aneurysmal bone cyst: a review of 150 patients. J Clin Oncol 2005; 23: 6756–6762

Park YK, Joo M. Multicentric telangiectatic osteosarcoma. Pathol Int 2001; 51: 200–203

Schajowicz F. Tumors and Tumorlike Lesions of Bone and Joints. Berlin: Springer; 1994

Sundaram M, Totty WG, Kyriakos M, et al. Imaging findings in pseudocystic osteosarcoma. AJR Am J Roentgenol 2001;176:783–788

Van Dyck P, Vanhoenacker FM, Vogel J et al. Prevalence, extension and characteristics of fluid-fluid levels in bone and soft tissue tumors. Eur Radiol 2006; 16: 2644–2651

Varshney MK, Rastogi S, Khan SA, Trikha V. Is sclerotherapy better than intralesional excision for treating aneurysmal bone cysts? Clin Orthop Relat Res 2010; 468: 1649–1659

Wörtler K, Blasius S, Hillmann A et al. MR-Morphologie der primären aneurysmatischen Knochenzyste: Retrospektive Analyse von 38 Fällen. Fortschr Röntgenstr 2000; 172: 591–596

Hemangioma

Baek HJ, Lee SJ, Cho KH et al. Subungual tumors: clinicopathologic correlation with US and MR imaging findings. Radiographics 2010; 30: 1621–1636

Bakotic BW, Robinson M, Williams M, Van Woy T, Nutter J, Borkowski P. Aggressive epithelioid hemangioendothelioma of the lower extremity: a case report and review of the literature. J Foot Ankle Surg 1999; 38: 352–358

Bousson V, Hamzé B, Wybier M et al. Soft tissue tumors and pseudotumors of the foot and ankle [Article in French] J Radiol 2008; 89: 21–34

Chang JJ, Lui TH. Intramuscular haemangioma of flexor digitorum brevis.Musculus: flexor:digitorum brevis Foot Ankle Surg 2010; 16: e8–e11

Kransdorf MJ. Benign soft-tissue tumors in a large referral population: distribution of specific diagnoses by age, sex, and location. AJR Am J Roentgenol 1995; 164: 395–402

Llauger J, Palmer J, Monill JM, Franquet T, Bagué S, Rosón N. MR imaging of benign soft-tissue masses of the foot and ankle. Radiographics 1998; 18: 1481–1498

Mitsionis GI, Pakos EE, Kosta P, Batistatou A, Beris A. Intramuscular hemangioma of the foot: A case report and review of the literature. Foot Ankle Surg 2010; 16: e27–e29

Requena L, Luis Díaz J, Manzarbeitia F, Carrillo R, Fernández-Herrera J, Kutzner H. Cutaneous composite hemangioendothelioma with satellitosis and lymph node metastases. J Cutan Pathol 2008; 35: 225–230

Sartoris DJ, Resnick D. Magnetic resonance imaging of pediatric foot and ankle disorders. J Foot Surg 1990; 29: 489–494

Van Dyck P, Vanhoenacker FM, Gielen JL, De Schepper AM, Parizel PM. Imaging of tumours of the foot and ankle. JBR-BTR 2004; 87: 252–257

Waldt S, Rechl H, Rummeny EJ, Woertler K. Imaging of benign and malignant soft tissue masses of the foot. Eur Radiol 2003; 13: 1125–1136

Woertler K. Soft tissue masses in the foot and ankle: characteristics on MR Imaging. Semin Musculoskelet Radiol 2005; 9: 227–242

Yarmel D, Dormans JP, Pawel BR, Chang B. Recurrent pedal hobnail (Dabska-retiform) hemangioendothelioma with forefoot reconstructive surgery using a digital fillet flap. J Foot Ankle Surg 2008; 47: 487–493

Ganglion

Blitz NM, Amrami KK, Spinner RJ. Magnetic resonance imaging of a deep peroneal intraneural ganglion cyst originating from the second metatarsophalangeal joint: a pattern of propagation supporting the unified articular (synovial) theory for the formation of intraneural ganglia. J Foot Ankle Surg 2009; 48: 80–84

Delfaut EM, Demondion X, Bieganski A, Thiron MC, Mestdagh H, Cotten A. Imaging of foot and ankle nerve entrapment syndromes: from well-demonstrated to unfamiliar sites. Radiographics 2003; 23: 613–623

Fujita I, Matsumoto K, Minami T, Kizaki T, Akisue T, Yamamoto T. Tarsal tunnel syndrome caused by epineural ganglion of the posterior tibial nerve: report of 2 cases and review of the literature. J Foot Ankle Surg 2004; 43: 185–190

Schrank C, Meirer R, Stäbler A, Nerlich A, Reiser M, Putz R. Morphology and topography of intraosseous ganglion cysts in the carpus: an anatomic, histopathologic, and magnetic resonance imaging correlation study. J Hand Surg Am 2003; 28: 52–61

Woertler K. Soft tissue masses in the foot and ankle: characteristics on MR Imaging. Semin Musculoskelet Radiol 2005; 9: 227–242

Pigmented Villonodular Synovitis

Hughes TH, Sartoris DJ, Schweitzer ME, Resnick DL. Pigmented villonodular synovitis: MRI characteristics. Skeletal Radiol 1995; 24: 7–12

Kottal RA, Vogler JB, Matamoros A, Alexander AH, Cookson JL. Pigmented villonodular synovitis: a report of MR imaging in two cases. Radiology 1987; 163: 551–553

Masih S, Antebi A. Imaging of pigmented villonodular synovitis. Semin Musculoskelet Radiol 2003; 7: 205–216

Ottaviani S, Ayral X, Dougados M, Gossec L. Pigmented villonodular synovitis: a retrospective single-center study of 122 cases and review of the literature. Semin Arthritis Rheum 2011; 40: 539–546

Saxena A, Perez H. Pigmented villonodular synovitis about the ankle: a review of the literature and presentation in 10 athletic patients. Foot Ankle Int 2004; 25: 819–826

Schnirring-Judge M, Lin B. Pigmented villonodular synovitis of the ankle-radiation therapy as a primary treatment to reduce recurrence: a case report with 8-year follow-up. J Foot Ankle Surg 2011; 50: 108–116

Sharma H, Jane MJ, Reid R. Pigmented villonodular synovitis of the foot and ankle: Forty years of experience from the Scottish bone tumor registry. J Foot Ankle Surg 2006; 45: 329–336

Sierens P, Shahabpour M, Gombault V, Machiels F, Kichouh M, De Maeseneer M. Pigmented villonodular synovitis of the midfoot. JBR-BTR 2010; 93: 207–209

Chapter 11

Normal Variants

11 Normal Variants

U. Szeimies

11.1 Accessory Muscles, Low-Lying Muscle Belly

11.1.1 Peroneus quartus

The peroneus quartus muscle is a normal variant with a reported prevalence of 10% among the normal population. However, it can cause clinical symptoms as swelling over the lateral malleolus. The muscle and its tendon run medial and posterior to the peroneal tendons, arising from the posterior intermuscular septum and from the peroneus brevis muscle. The peroneus quartus has variable insertions, most commonly inserting into a bony prominence (peroneal tubercle) on the lateral side of the calcaneus, on the long or short peroneal tendon, and on the cuboid. This normal variant may be a rare cause of lateral ankle complaints. It has been suggested that involvement by tendinosis and partial tears of the peroneus brevis tendon may have causal significance.

11.1.2 Flexor Digitorum Accessorius Longus

This muscle is reportedly present in up to 15% of the general population. It has two bellies, arises from the flexor retinaculum and calcaneus, and fuses to a single tendon that inserts distally into the flexor digitorum longus and flexor hallucis longus tendons. The presence of this normal variant may be associated with a nerve compression syndrome (tarsal tunnel syndrome).

11.1.3 Accessory Soleus (▶ Fig. 11.1)

This is the most common variant. The accessory soleus has a separate muscle belly and a separate tendon in the hindfoot. It occurs when the soleus splits during embryonic development to form a separate muscular rudiment that arises anterior to the soleus and inserts into the calcaneus anteromedial to the Achilles tendon. The accessory soleus may aggravate a clubfoot deformity and prevent its correction.

This normal variant may be an incidental asymptomatic finding or may become clinically symptomatic during the increased physical activity of adolescence. In this case it may become hypertrophic and cause an unexplained hindfoot mass medial to the Achilles tendon with associated tenderness and exercise-dependent pain in young runners. An awareness of this normal variant is important in making a differential diagnosis.

11.1.4 Extensor Hallucis Capsularis

This normal variant is located medial to the extensor hallucis longus tendon and arises from either the extensor hallucis longus tendon or the muscle itself. It inserts on the first metatarsophalangeal joint capsule. It can provide donor material for a possible tendon transfer.

11.1.5 Peroneocalcaneus Internus

The peroneocalcaneus internus muscle, also called the "false flexor hallucis longus," is rare. An awareness of this variant is important for preoperative planning, however. The flexor hallucis longus is an important landmark for hindfoot arthroscopy as it forms the medial boundary of the neurovascular bundle. Consequently, the presence of a "false" flexor hallucis longus could pose a risk of neurovascular injury.

11.1.6 Abnormal Musculotendinous Junction

Muscle–tendon junctions are subject to considerable variations whose clinical importance is debated in the literature. An example is the low-lying peroneus brevis muscle belly, which may predispose to tendon tears. A low-lying muscle belly may rarely cause nerve compression syndromes or impingement syndromes, and their imaging may be important in preoperative planning (e.g., soleus insertion point in the Achilles tendon for an Achilles tendon reconstruction).

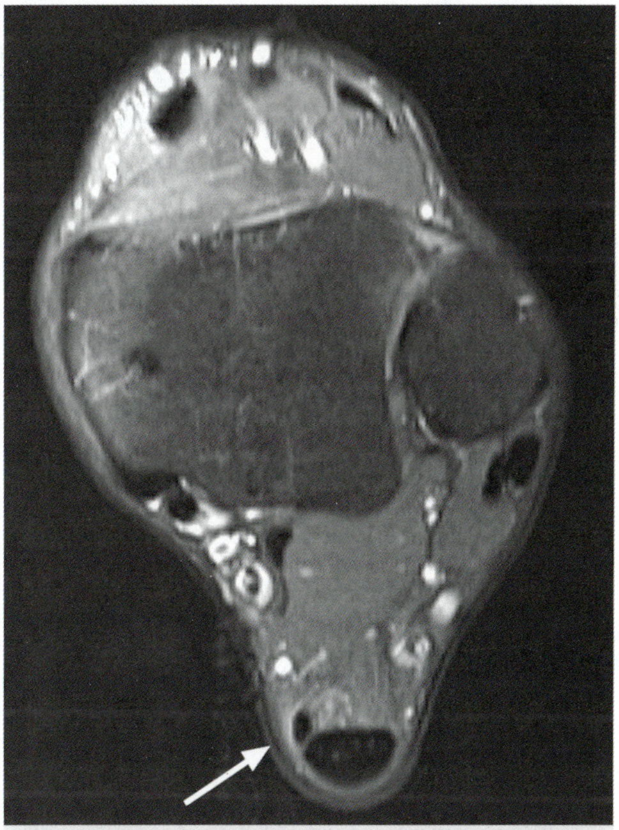

Fig. 11.1 Axial T1-weighted fat-sat image after contrast administration in an athletically active adolescent male with medial Achilles tendon pain. MRI shows tissue irritation with increased enhancement in the peritenon of the accessory soleus tendon (arrow).

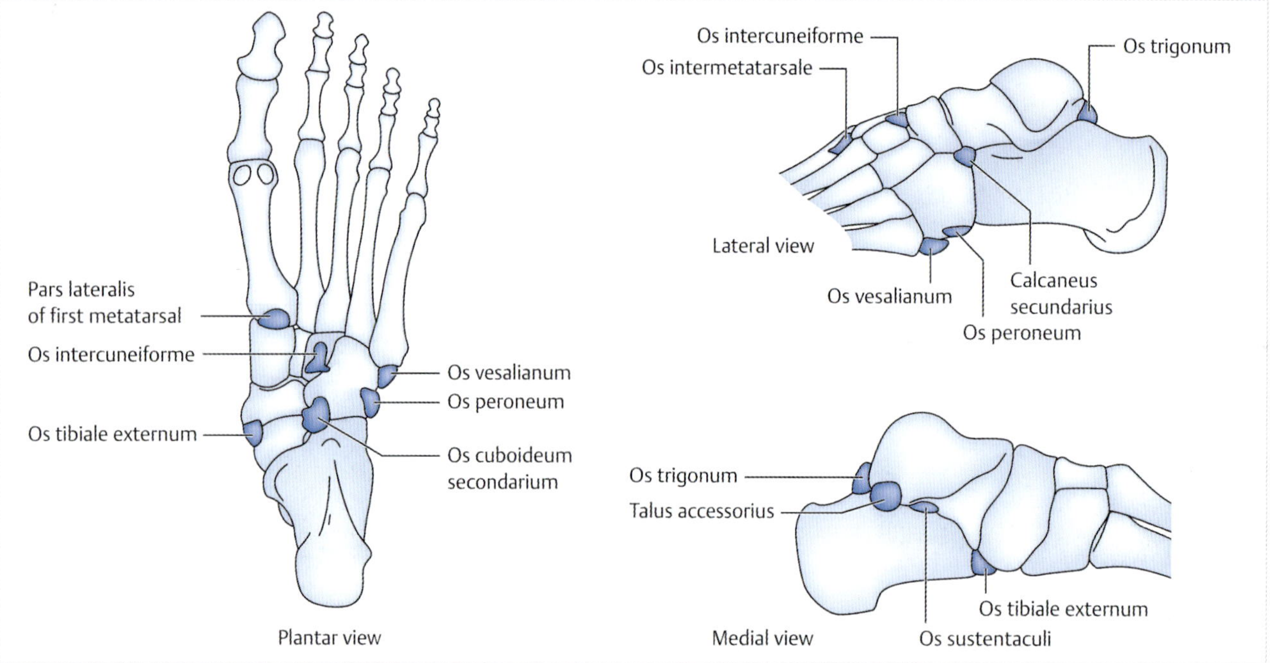

Fig. 11.2 Important accessory ossicles in the foot (source: Dihlmann and Stäbler 2010, Fig. 16.62).

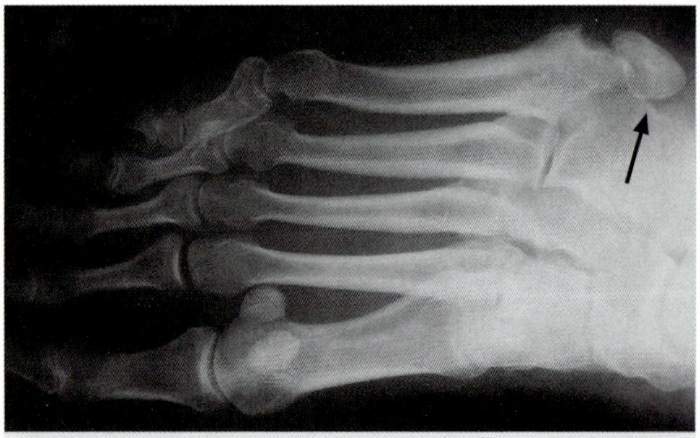

Fig. 11.3 Os vesalianum. Oblique radiograph of the midfoot. The os vesalianum results from failure of the apophysis to fuse with the base of the fifth metatarsal. Awareness of this accessory ossicle (arrow) is important in distinguishing it from a fracture.

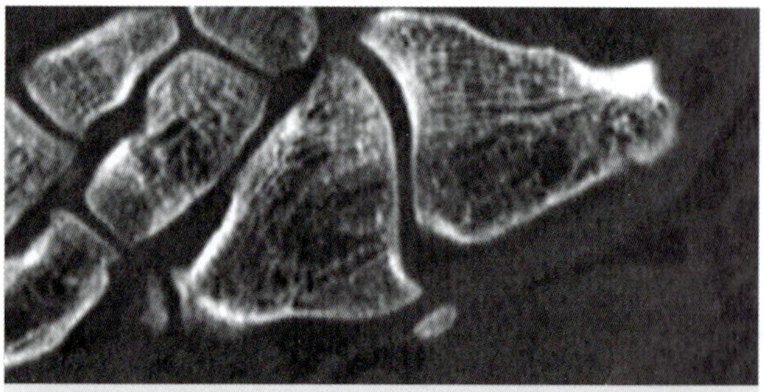

Fig. 11.4 Os peroneum. Oblique sagittal reformatted CT demonstrates the sesamoid bone in the peroneus longus tendon (os peroneum), located lateral and plantar to the cuboid bone.

11.2 Accessory Ossicles

The most common accessory ossicles in the foot are listed below and are discussed elsewhere in this book under separate headings based on their anatomic locations (▸ Fig. 11.2):

- *Accessory navicular:* see Accessory Navicular (p. 115) in Chapter 3 (Ankle and Hindfoot). Synonyms: os tibiale externum, os naviculare externum, os naviculare secundarium, accessory tarsal navicular
- *Cornuate navicular:* fusion of the ossification center of the tuberosity with the actual navicular, causing a hornlike protrusion, local tenderness, and a painful callus (see ▸ Fig. 11.5)
- *Os trigonum:* see the section on Os Trigonum Syndrome (p. 72) in Chapter 3 (Ankle and Hindfoot)
- *Os peroneum:* see ▸ Fig. 11.4
- *Os vesalianum:* very rare (prevalence 0.1–1%), proximal to the base of the fifth metatarsal within the peroneus brevis tendon. Caused by failure of fusion of the fifth metatarsal apophysis, usually asymptomatic. Awareness is important in differentiating a fracture of the fifth metatarsal base from an ossified apophysis of the metatarsal base or Iselin disease (apophysitis of the fifth metatarsal base). Rarely, the os vesalianum may cause a painful callus

Symptoms

- Local pain
- Persistent posttraumatic complaints
- Impingement symptoms
- Pain radiating along the tendon

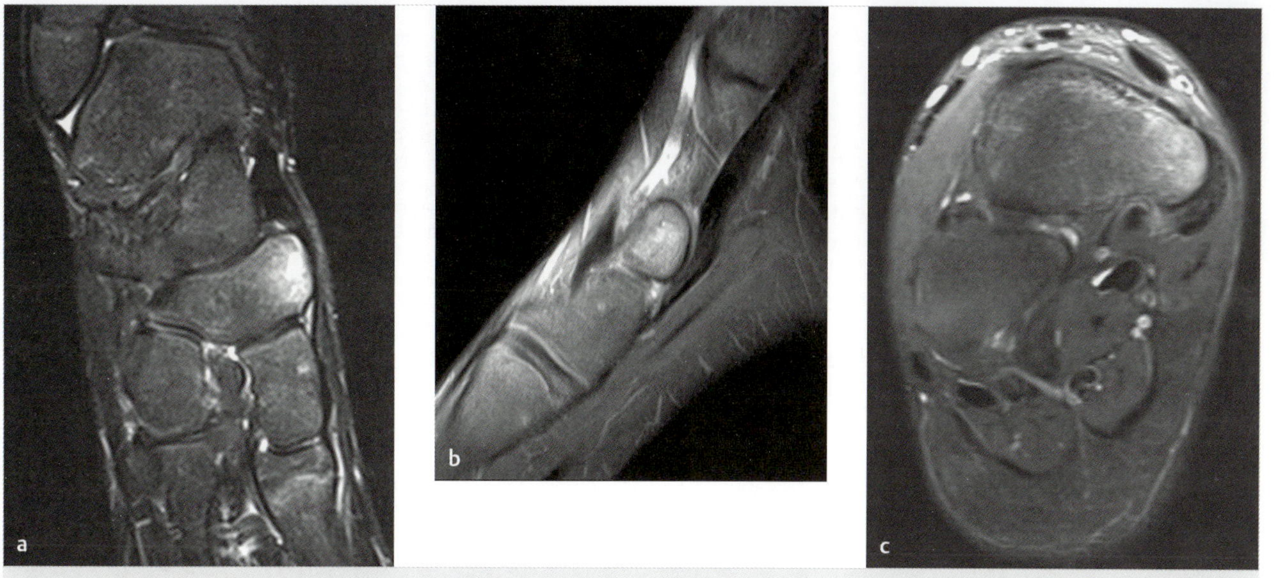

Fig. 11.5 a–c Cornuate navicular. The cornuate navicular results from fusion of the ossification center of the os tibiale externum with the navicular bone, resulting in a painful bony protuberance (a "horned" navicular).
a Coronal STIR image shows an activated, hornlike protrusion of the navicular with local tenderness.
b Sagittal PD-weighted fat-sat image shows displacement of the posterior tibial tendon by the bony protuberance.
c Axial PD-weighted fat-sat image. Because of the protuberance and its bony activation, the patient could wear only special footwear.

Predisposing Factors

In cases with fibrous attachment of the ossicle to the parent bone, the attachment may be loosened ("activated") as a result of trauma.

Anatomy and Pathology

Sesamoid bones and accessory ossification centers may develop into ossicles that have a synchondrotic attachment to the parent bone. Accessory ossicles are present in 20% of patients. An accessory navicular is the most common type, accounting for one-half of cases.

Imaging

Radiographs (▶ Fig. 11.3)

Accessory ossicles are generally well depicted on plain radiographs.

Ultrasound

Accessory ossicles are usually located in the course of tendons as well as ligaments. Longitudinal and transverse scans show a short, frequently convex, echogenic bony surface contour with acoustic shadowing. A complete survey of the affected connective-tissue structure will yield information on mobility, impingement, etc.

CT (▶ Fig. 11.4)

CT is sometimes used for detailed imaging (slice thickness 0.5 mm with multiplanar reformatting) to distinguish an accessory ossicle (e.g., sesamoid) from a fracture.

MRI

Interpretation Checklist

- Shape and consistency of the bone
- Bony or fibrous attachment
- Activation (bone marrow edema in the accessory ossicle and adjacent bone, soft tissues, tendon sheath, peritendinitis, tendinosis)

Examination Technique

- *Standard protocol:* prone position, high-resolution multichannel coil
- *Sequences:*
  - Sagittal and coronal PD-weighted fat-sat
  - Coronal T1-weighted
  - Axial T2-weighted (angled to joint plane)
  - Axial oblique (angled to tendon plane) and sagittal T1-weighted fat-sat after contrast administration

MRI Findings (▶ Fig. 11.5)

- Bone marrow edema and contrast enhancement in and around the accessory ossicle
- Local soft-tissue irritation with synovitis
- Increased enhancement along the tendon sheath and into the fibro-osseous junction
- Ossicular fracture or necrosis in rare cases

Imaging Recommendation

Modalities of choice: radiography for initial evaluation, MRI to assess activation.

Differential Diagnosis

- Osteochondral avulsion
- Intra-articular loose bodies
- Posttraumatic calcification

It may be difficult to distinguish a bony avulsion from an accessory ossicle in acute trauma cases. Sectional imaging (rounded bone edges, fracture edema, soft-tissue edema) will facilitate the diagnosis. Differentiation from an old bony avulsion and nonunion is accomplished by noting enhancement characteristics on MRI. With the de-novo appearance of a bony structure, the differential diagnosis should include heterotopic ossification and the inflammatory or posttraumatic ossification of a cartilaginous anlage.

Treatment

- Insoles to relieve mechanical stresses on the activated region
- If complaints persist: surgical removal of the ossicle
- In rare cases: rigid internal fixation to the parent bone

Prognosis, Complications

If conservative treatment is unsuccessful, surgical fusion or removal of the accessory ossicle can relieve complaints in more than 80% of patients.

11.3 Bibliography

Accessory Muscles, Low-Lying Muscle Belly

Boyd N, Brock H, Meier A, Miller R, Mlady G, Firoozbakhsh K. Extensor hallucis capsularis: frequency and identification on MRI. Foot Ankle Int 2006; 27: 181–184

Burks JB, DeHeer PA. Tarsal tunnel syndrome secondary to an accessory muscle: a case report. J Foot Ankle Surg 2001; 40: 401–403

Buschmann WR, Cheung Y, Jahss MH. Magnetic resonance imaging of anomalous leg muscles: accessory soleus, peroneus quartus and the flexor digitorum longus accessorius. Foot Ankle 1991; 12: 109–116

Chepuri NB, Jacobson JA, Fessell DP, Hayes CW. Sonographic appearance of the peroneus quartus muscle: correlation with MR imaging appearance in seven patients. Radiology 2001; 218: 415–419

Cheung YY, Rosenberg ZS, Ramsinghani R, Beltran J, Jahss MH. Peroneus quartus muscle: MR imaging features. Radiology 1997; 202: 745–750

Christodoulou A, Terzidis I, Natsis K, Gigis I, Pournaras J. Soleus accessorius, an anomalous muscle in a young athlete: case report and analysis of the literature. Br J Sports Med 2004; 38: e38

Hill RV, Gerges L. Unusual accessory tendon connecting the hallucal extensors. Anat Sci Int 2008; 83: 298–300

Holzmann M, Almudallal N, Rohlck K, Singh R, Lee S, Fredieu J. Identification of a flexor digitorum accessorius longus muscle with unique distal attachments. Foot (Edinb) 2009; 19: 224–226

Karapinar L, Kaya A, Altay T, Ozturk H, Surenkok F. Congenital clubfoot associated with an accessory soleus muscle. J Am Podiatr Med Assoc 2008; 98: 408–413

Kendi TK, Erakar A, Oktay O, Yildiz HY, Saglik Y. Accessory soleus muscle. J Am Podiatr Med Assoc 2004; 94: 587–589

Phisitkul P, Amendola A. False FHL: a normal variant posing risks in posterior hindfoot endoscopy. Arthroscopy 2010; 26: 714–718

Pichler W, Tesch NP, Grechenig W, Leithgoeb O, Windisch G. Anatomic variations of the musculotendinous junction of the soleus muscle and its clinical implications. Clin Anat 2007; 20: 444–447

Saupe N, Mengiardi B, Pfirrmann CW, Vienne P, Seifert B, Zanetti M. Anatomic variants associated with peroneal tendon disorders: MR imaging findings in volunteers with asymptomatic ankles. Radiology 2007; 242: 509–517

Trono M, Tueche S, Quintart C, Libotte M, Baillon J. Peroneus quartus muscle: a case report and review of the literature. Foot Ankle Int 1999; 20: 659–662

Unlu MC, Bilgili M, Akgun I, Kaynak G, Ogut T, Uzun I. Abnormal proximal musculotendinous junction of the peroneus brevis muscle as a cause of peroneus brevis tendon tears: a cadaveric study. J Foot Ankle Surg 2010; 49: 537–540

Wachter S, Beekman S. Peroneus quartus. A case report. J Am Podiatry Assoc 1983; 73: 523–524

Wittmayer BC, Freed L. Diagnosis and surgical management of flexor digitorum accessorius longus-induced tarsal tunnel syndrome. J Foot Ankle Surg 2007; 46: 484–487

Zammit J, Singh D. The peroneus quartus muscle. Anatomy and clinical relevance. J Bone Joint Surg Br 2003; 85: 1134–1137

Accessory Ossicles

Abramowitz Y, Wollstein R, Barzilay Y et al. Outcome of resection of a symptomatic os trigonum. J Bone Joint Surg Am 2003; 85-A: 1051–1057

Bashir WA, Lewis S, Cullen N, Connell DA. Os peroneum friction syndrome complicated by sesamoid fatigue fracture: a new radiological diagnosis? Case report and literature review. Skeletal Radiol 2009; 38: 181–186

Boya H, Ozcan O, Tandoğan R, Günal I, Araç S. Os vesalianum pedis. J Am Podiatr Med Assoc 2005; 95: 583–585

Dihlmann W, Stäbler A. Gelenke des Fußes einschließlich des oberen Sprunggelenks. In: Dihlmann W, Stäbler A, eds. Gelenke – Wirbelverbindungen. 4th ed. Stuttgart: Thieme; 2010: 731

Dorrestijn O, Brouwer RW. Bilateral symptomatic os vesalianum pedis: a case report. J Foot Ankle Surg 2011; 50: 473–475

Jeppesen JB, Jensen FK, Falborg B, Madsen JL. Bone scintigraphy in painful os peroneum syndrome. Clin Nucl Med 2011; 36: 209–211

Leonard ZC, Fortin PT. Adolescent accessory navicular. Foot Ankle Clin 2010; 15: 337–347

Mendez-Castillo A, Burd TA, Kenter K, et al. Radiologic case study. Os trigonum syndrome. Orthopedics 1999;22(12):120–1202, 1208

Mouhsine E, Crevoisier X, Leyvraz PF, Akiki A, Dutoit M, Garofalo R. Post-traumatic overload or acute syndrome of the os trigonum: a possible cause of posterior ankle impingement. Knee Surg Sports Traumatol Arthrosc 2004; 12: 250–253

Perdikakis E, Grigoraki E, Karantanas A. Os naviculare: the multi-ossicle configuration of a normal variant. Skeletal Radiol 2011; 40: 85–88

Schratt E, Bosch U, Thermann H. Os trigonum-Syndrom Zeichen. J Unfallchirurg 1999; 102: 320–323

Scott AT, Sabesan VJ, Saluta JR, Wilson MA, Easley ME. Fusion versus excision of the symptomatic Type II accessory navicular: a prospective study. Foot Ankle Int 2009; 30: 10–15

Sobel M, Pavlov H, Geppert MJ, Thompson FM, DiCarlo EF, Davis WH. Painful os peroneum syndrome: a spectrum of conditions responsible for plantar lateral foot pain. Foot Ankle Int 1994; 15: 112–124

Index

P

Q

R

S